Cosmeceuticals and Cosmetic Ingredients

Cosmeceuticals and Cosmetic Ingredients

FIRST EDITION

Leslie Baumann, MD
CEO, Baumann Cosmetic and Research Institute
Miami, FL

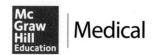

New York   Chicago   San Francisco   Athens   London   Madrid   Mexico City
Milan   New Delhi   Singapore   Sydney   Toronto

COSMECEUTICALS AND COSMETIC INGREDIENTS, FIRST EDITION

2 3 4 5 6 7 8 9 0   CTP/CTP 19 18 17 16 15

ISBN 978-0-07-179398-8
MHID 0-07-179398-4

This book was set in Stempel Schneidler Std by MPS Limited.
The editors were Anne Sydor and Regina Y. Brown.
The production supervisor was Richard Ruzycka.
Project management was provided by Asheesh Ratra of MPS Limited.
The cover designer was Anthony Landi.
Image Credit: © Jutta Klee/ableimages/Corbis
China Translation & Printing Services, Ltd. was the printer and binder.

This book is printed on acid-free paper.

Library of Congress Cataloging-in-Publication Data
Baumann, Leslie, author.
  Cosmeceuticals and cosmetic ingredients / Leslie Baumann.
      p. ; cm.
  Includes index.
  ISBN 978-0-07-179398-8 (hardcover : alk. paper)—ISBN 0-07-179398-4
  I. Title.
  [DNLM: 1.   Dermatologic Agents—pharmacology. 2.   Cosmetics—pharmacology.
  3.   Plant Preparations—pharmacology. 4.   Skin—drug effects. 5.   Skin Care.   QV 60]
  RL801
  616.5'061—dc23
                                                                                    2014028271

McGraw-Hill Education books are available at special quantity discounts to use as premiums and sales promotions or for use in corporate training programs. To contact a representative, please visit the Contact Us pages at www.mhprofessional.com.

This book is dedicated to Edmund Weisberg, my Managing Editor for over a decade and a half.

Contents

Preface

This book was inspired by a passion for skin care, science, the history of the cosmeceutical industry, and almost two decades of treating patients with cosmeceutical products. Its goal is to help the reader understand the history of cosmeceutical ingredients, the science behind them, as well as the challenges of using them in a skin care regimen, and learn how to choose what type of ingredients are appropriate for various Baumann Skin Types®. This book is meant to dispel myths and misperceptions about what certain ingredients can and cannot do. It provides an unbiased, brand-agnostic approach to the subject. (I work for almost all of the companies and I do not have my own skin care line.) It will explain the various studies on the ingredients and provide detailed references so that the reader can go back and read the original study if they have doubts. It is divided into sections to help the reader classify ingredients in a simple manner; however, some ingredients work for more than one purpose. For this reason, we have provided two "Table of Contents": One is by type of ingredient such as cleanser, moisturizer, or antiaging agent, and the second is in alphabetical order by ingredient. As I am a dermatologist and not a formulator, this book does not attempt to teach you how to formulate skin care products, but instead helps you know what ingredients should work for various types of skin and why. In other words, we provide the ingredients, but we do not provide the recipe. In order to understand how this book came about and the passion that went into writing it, one must understand the history of my career as a cosmetic dermatologist.

In 1997, when I was asked by William Eaglstein, MD, Chairman of the prestigious Department of Dermatology at the University of Miami, to become the Director of the country's first Division of Cosmetic Dermatology, I was skeptical at first. At that time, Botox and hyaluronic acid dermal fillers like Restylane and Juvéderm had not yet been approved by the FDA and there was not much scientific research supporting skin care products (with the notable exception of the individual work by Drs. Albert Kligman, Jim Leyden, Sheldon Pinnell, and Eugene Van Scott). Dr. Eaglstein and my other mentor, Dr. Francisco Kerdel, knew of my passion for skin care science and my love of the history of the cosmetic skin care industry. I collected vintage cosmetic advertisements, face powders, soaps, and even an old tin of Burt's Bees furniture polish. I cherished books written by industry pioneers such as Helena Rubenstein, Elizabeth Arden, Mary Kay, Estée Lauder, and Charles Revson. I was 30 years old, with lots of energy, and was willing to accept the challenge. Drs. Eaglstein and Kerdel explained that they had heard about a new product called "Botox" and thought "it might cause changes in the dermatology industry, and increase interest in in-office cosmetic procedures and skin care."

To put it into perspective, "skin care lectures" at that time consisted of subjective opinions and little data. Companies just were not spending money and effort on researching their products for efficacy, and few dermatologists sold skin care products. Rodan and Fields had recently launched Proactiv and changed the way people thought about acne treatments and proved that there was money to be made in the acne skin care business. I decided to join those rising to the challenge of raising the bar of cosmetic science and founded the Division of Cosmetic Dermatology. Soon thereafter, our department became the leading center for cosmetic dermatology research, performing the research trials that led to FDA approval of Botox, Dysport, Hylaform, Juvéderm, Sculptra, Voluma, Tri-Luma, and many other products and procedures. I began studying cosmetic skin care products for over 50 companies such as Elizabeth Arden, Unilever (Ponds and Dove), Johnson and Johnson (Neutrogena, Aveeno, Roc), and L'Oréal and served on numerous advisory boards and committees. My vintage compact collection grew as did my experience and knowledge.

In 2001, I began writing a monthly column called "Cosmeceutical Critique" on cosmetic ingredients for *Skin and Allergy News*, a journal for dermatologists. I still write this column and it can be found online. In 2002, I published the first textbook devoted to cosmetic dermatology, *Cosmetic Dermatology: Principles and Practice* (McGraw-Hill), which has been translated into several languages and is the bestselling cosmetic dermatology book in the world. In 2004–2005, I developed a skin typing system used to divide patients into 16 unique "Baumann Skin Types®" that are used to properly match ingredients and products to skin type. This system resulted in a *New York Times* bestselling book *The Skin Type Solution* (Bantam, 2005) and a PBS Special of the same name in 2010. During this time, I ran a busy cosmetic dermatology clinic and saw 6,000 to 7,000 Botox and filler patients a year – all of whom were put on customized skin care regimens using the skin typing system. Doctors around the world began using the Baumann Skin Typing System in their practices and giving us data and feedback. The skin typing system is described in Chapter 1 of this book and in several leading textbooks and multiple publications in the fields of dermatology, plastic surgery, and facial plastic surgery.

In 2009, my team developed www.virtualtrialfacility.com, a website that allows people to register to try various skin care products and provide an unbiased opinion. This online survey system, my live clinical research trials, and my busy clinical practice, allowed me to test different ingredients on the various Baumann Skin Types and identify which ingredients worked best in each setting. I was able to test and "type" tens of thousands of skin care products around the world. The "SkinIQ" quiz that was developed in 2003–2005 was tested on hundreds of thousands of people online and in dermatologic practices around the world. In 2009–2010, we found that when the Baumann Skin Typing System was used in dermatology practices to prescribe skin care products, product return rates were significantly lowered and patient outcomes were improved.

By 2012, my Yahoo blog at www.skinguru.com had over 3 million readers – many of whose comments revealed that there was still much misinformation about skin care science and people just did not know who or what to believe. It seemed that all of the "experts" had something to sell, and even dermatologists were getting confused. I realized that dermatologists did not have the time in their busy schedules to adequately educate their patients on the multiple important details of skin care. That year, we launched STS Franchise System, LLC, a turn-key skin care retail solution for medical practices that identifies and tests products from around the world and matches them to the 16 Baumann Skin Types.

All of these activities and experiences led to the knowledge that there is no unbiased encyclopedic reference of cosmeceutical ingredients that helps aestheticians, skin care specialists, and doctors properly match cosmeceutical ingredients to skin type.

After 14 years of writing my monthly column on cosmeceutical ingredients for dermatologists and researching skin care products for the STS Franchise system, I decided to put all of my ingredient knowledge together in one place. Thanks to my managing editor Edmund Weisberg, we were able to rewrite and update the "Cosmeceutical Critique" columns, add new chapters, and organize them into a manageable structure. This project has been a labor of love and the book is much longer than originally planned because I just could not stop adding ingredients. I had to choose my favorite ingredients because of space constraints, so not all ingredients are included. I hope that whether you are a doctor, aesthetician, nurse, cosmetic scientist, skin care retailer, or a lover of skin care technology and science that this book will help you understand the fascinating science of cosmeceuticals. We have set up a YouTube channel at youtube.com/ingredientbook and will post videos to supplement some of the information in this book and keep you up to date.

My goal with this book is to empower you to understand cosmeceutical science so that you can decipher marketing claims and make better skin care decisions for your patients, your clients, your family, and yourself.

Acknowledgments

I met Edmund in the late 1990s when he was an editor for my monthly column at the dermatology magazine *Skin and Aging*. We developed a great rapport and enjoyed working together. One day he suggested that I write a textbook on cosmetic dermatology. I had no idea how to do a book proposal and he generously offered to help me. We decided to send the proposal to McGraw-Hill because they were the publisher of all of the great medical books, such as *Harrison's Principles of Internal Medicine* and *Fitzpatrick's Dermatology in General Medicine*. We were thrilled to get a book deal with them and wrote and published the first edition of *Cosmetic Dermatology* in 2002. It rapidly became a bestseller. Somewhere during that time, I was asked to write a column in *Skin and Allergy News* and I asked Edmund to become my editor. We have worked together for over 15 years now on various projects including the "Cosmeceutical Critique" column that led to this book. We are currently working on the 3rd edition of *Cosmetic Dermatology* – which remains the bestselling cosmetic dermatology textbook in the world. We share a love of literature, food, and chocolate and have become good friends. Although Edmund's title is Managing Editor, his role was far more. He functioned as a research assistant, cowriter, and psychologist throughout the process. Although this book is finished, I anticipate continuing working with Edmund for years to come.

Thank you Edmund – you are one of the easiest people to work with that I have ever met. You are reliable, organized, funny, and if you get stressed out – I never see it. It is so funny when you make fun of my misspellings and typos and turn them into jokes. Your limericks keep me laughing and your enthusiasm keeps me writing. We are a great team and I look forward to many more years of working together.

Leslie Baumann

Cosmeceuticals and Cosmetic Ingredients

CHAPTER 1

The Importance of Skin Type: The Baumann Skin Type System

The Baumann Skin Type System (BSTS) is a skin-type classification system comprised of 16 distinct skin phenotypes. This approach to categorizing skin type was developed in 2004 by dermatologist Leslie Baumann, M.D., to subdivide research participants into specific distinct phenotypes in order to facilitate data collection and analysis as well as subject recruitment. The 16 Baumann Skin Types have been used in genetic research aimed at identifying the genes that contribute to skin characteristics such as dryness, oiliness, aging, pigmentation, and sensitivity. The BSTS optimizes communication between researchers, dermatologists, cosmetic scientists, aestheticians, advertisers, consumers, and educators. The classification system has been adopted by aestheticians, dermatologists, consumers, and retailers worldwide to match cosmeceutical ingredients and skin care product recommendations to specific skin types. It is applicable to all ethnicities, ages, and genders.

The Baumann Skin Type (BST) is determined by a scientifically validated questionnaire, known as the Baumann Skin Type Indicator (BSTI). In the United States, the 16 Baumann Skin Types have been the subject of the *New York Times* bestselling book *The Skin Type Solution* (Bantam 2005, 2010) and a public television special *Skin Type Solutions with Dr. Leslie Baumann* (2010, 2011). *The Skin Type Solution* has also been published in other countries including Australia, the United Kingdom, Brazil, Turkey, China, Vietnam, and South Korea.

BST can change with the use of a new skin care regimen, advancing age, travel or a move to a different geographic location, or a change in hormone status. It is recommended that patients retake the BSTI when one of these changes has occurred or when one's current skin care regimen does not seem to be working.

THE PARAMETERS

The BSTS is based on the identification and combination of four main skin characteristics or parameters that apply to facial skin:

1. Dry versus Oily
2. Sensitive versus Resistant
3. Pigmented (uneven skin toned) versus Non-pigmented (even toned)
4. Wrinkle prone versus Tight (non-wrinkle prone).

One option from each of these parameters is assigned to the BST; therefore, 16 possible skin types emerge from the four skin-type parameters (Figure 1-1). For example, one BST is DSPW or dry, sensitive, pigmented, and wrinkled while another is ORNT or oily, resistant, non-pigmented, and tight. The 16 skin phenotypes are much more than just different combinations of basic skin characteristics. The individual parameters interact and express themselves in 16 unique skin "syndromes" that predispose certain skin types to specific dermatological issues

OSPW	OSPT	OSNW	OSNT
ORPW	ORPT	ORNW	ORNT
DSPW	DSPT	DSNW	DSNT
DRPW	DRPT	DRNW	DRNT

▲ **FIGURE 1-1** The 16 Baumann skin types.

and challenges, and dictate the courses of prevention and treatment. It is crucial to take all four of the factors into consideration when evaluating facial skin.

Color Dot System

In order to simplify the BSTS, a color dot system was developed that assigns a color and number to each skin type. Consumers, cosmetic companies, and retailers can use this color dot system to effectively communicate using mobile applications, web sites, product labels, shelf displays, or other visual aids (Figure 1-2).

Weight and Severity of the Parameters

Each of these four parameters is weighted to indicate the severity of each of the relevant skin issues. The calculations used to determine these scores and the resulting skin type are proprietary and were developed after years of research, and are also beyond the scope of this chapter. Suffice it to say that the BSTI questionnaire that determines skin type is preferentially tallied by a computer program that takes several factors into account. A complicated mathematical formula is used in the process to analyze the BSTI scores and to determine the BST designations.

SKIN HYDRATION: DRY (D) VERSUS OILY (O)

In the BSTS, the D or O designation is designed for simplicity of use. However, the designation of D versus O is actually much more complex than it seems at first glance.

Score Numbering of the Dry and Oily Skin Types

A dry skin type is assigned a 1-4 numerical value depending on the way the questions are answered in the questionnaire. A higher number indicates severe dryness and a lower number indicates slight dryness. A D_3, for example, is much dryer than a D_2. Similarly, an oily skin type is also assigned a 1-4 numerical

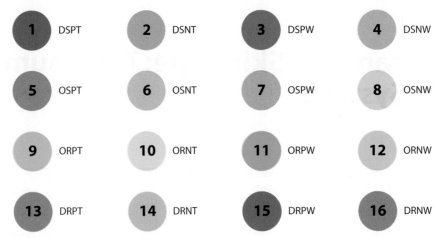

▲ **FIGURE 1-2** Each Baumann skin type is assigned a color and a number.

value. Accordingly, a higher number indicates severe oiliness and a lower number indicates slight oiliness. An O_3, for example, is much oilier than an O_2.

Dry Skin

Dry skin is characterized by the lack of moisture in the stratum corneum (SC). Water is the major plasticizer of the skin, and when levels are low, cracks and fissures occur.[1] The increase in transepidermal water loss (TEWL) that leads to dry skin results when a defect in the permeability barrier allows excessive water to be evaporated off of the skin and lost to the atmosphere. Dry skin is a result of decreased water content in the SC, which leads to abnormal desquamation of corneocytes and, eventually, to skin roughness.[2] For the skin to appear and feel normal, the water content of the SC must be greater than 10 percent.[3] When the water level in skin is less than 10 percent, study subjects experience symptoms that we specifically ask about in the BSTI. Questions about these symptoms were developed and shown to correlate with TEWL in skin.[4]

Many factors play a role in skin hydration. Sebum production is an important one, but certainly not the determining factor of dry skin. Sebum creates a lipid-based occlusive film on the skin, which has an effect on skin hydration by preventing water evaporation from the skin.[5] However, those with decreased sebum production will not be designated as a "D" (dry) skin type if TEWL and skin water content are within normal limits.

Oily Skin

Diet, stress, and hormones play a role in sebum production, but there is a significant genetic link,[6] and twin studies have shown that identical twins have similar sebum secretion rates. In humid climates, the sebum is more fluid and subjects perceive sebum secretion to be greater even if it is not. Studies have also shown that subjects are unable to correctly estimate the amount of sebum secretion on their skin in many cases.[7] To validate the BSTI, studies were performed to evaluate questions answered by subjects about their perception of skin oiliness in order to identify which questions correlated with actual measured sebum secretions using a Sebumeter®. It was found that certain combinations of questions could correctly determine whether a subject was a low, medium, or high producer of facial sebum.[8] Greatly increased sebum production causes an oily skin phenotype that is designated as an "O" for "oily" in the BSTS.

Combination Skin

There are two main types of combination skin: 1) skin that is dry for parts of the year and oily during other parts of the year; and 2) skin that is oily in the T-zone and dry on the sides of the face.

SEASONAL SKIN Skin that is dry for one part of the year and oily during another part of the year likely has a defect in TEWL that worsens in low-humidity conditions such as winter. Such skin requires heavier moisturizer use in winter or in a dry climate. This skin type is the most impacted by geographic and weather changes and will likely require two skin regimens, one for humid climates, and one for dry climates and during winter. Individuals with such skin will test differently on the BSTI depending on the climate in which they are when taking the questionnaire. They may be O types in the summer and D types in the winter. For this reason, when the questions are answered on the BSTI, they should be answered according to how the skin is behaving at the time the BSTI is taken.

T-ZONE SKIN Skin that is oily in the T-zone and dry on the sides has decreased TEWL that is offset in the T-zone by increased sebum production. Individuals with such skin need cleansers that will strip excess oil from the T-zone combined with moisturizers that will improve the skin barrier without being occlusive. This type of combination skin type usually remains the same until middle age, when hormone activity changes.

Combination skin types will be designated as O or D depending on which deficiencies are found by the BSTI questionnaire. In some cases, the T-zone type of combination skin would benefit by applying moisturizers only to the dry parts of the skin, avoiding the T-zone.

Normal Skin

Normal skin types are designated as O_1 in the BSTS. Normal skin displays a normal baseline level of sebum secretion and an intact skin barrier with normal TEWL. Therefore, it does not receive the dry designation, but instead receives the designation of "O_1" to illustrate the normal function of the sebum glands. Conversely, skin with below normal sebum secretion, an intact skin barrier, and normal TEWL receives a designation of "D_1." Individuals with such skin may believe they have normal skin but in reality external moisturizing agents would be beneficial to them to compensate for the lack of sebum production, so they are designated as a dry type.

SKIN SENSITIVITY: SENSITIVE (S) VERSUS RESISTANT (R)

Resistant Skin

Resistant skin has a strong SC that confers protection to skin cells, keeping allergens and other irritating substances out. It rarely develops erythema unless sunburned, and rarely develops acne. Those with resistant facial skin can usually use any skin care product without developing a rash, acne, or a stinging sensation. However, resistant skin may also be impervious to penetration of active ingredients so that it is more difficult to see beneficial effects from less concentrated products.

SCORE NUMBERING OF RESISTANT SKIN Resistant skin is not weighted like sensitive skin. That is, a person either has resistant skin or not. In the BSTS, resistant skin is defined as skin that does not show signs of inflammation. Resistant skin that also exhibits D_2 or D_3 characteristics would be suspected to have an impaired skin barrier, but because inflammation is absent, the skin type is considered resistant. Either the skin's dryness is not caused by an impaired barrier, but by a defect in natural moisturizing factor, aquaporin, or a yet to be discovered ailment, or the skin has some sort of mechanism(s) protecting it from inflammation. Regardless of the reason, the skin would be considered resistant to inflammation. On the other hand, if the skin exhibits O_2 or O_3 characteristics and is resistant, then the person has protective mechanisms against acne. For some reason, this person either has less *Propionibacterium acnes* in the presence of copious sebum, or has an internal protective mechanism against acne in the presence of bacteria and sebum. Absence of acne, rosacea, stinging sensations, and dermatitis in combination with other characteristics gives important clues about underlying mechanisms that determine skin type.

Sensitive Skin

In the early 1990s, more than 40 percent of patients were claiming to have sensitive skin,[9] with healthy, premenopausal women presenting with this complaint more often than other demographic groups. However, the number of people presenting with such complaints has steadily increased, particularly among men,[10] in the last two decades. In addition, a majority of women in the United States, Europe, and Japan are thought to believe that they have sensitive skin.[11] In fact, a 2009 study with 1,039 subjects revealed a 68.4 percent prevalence of self-reported sensitive skin, with no gender differences observed.[10] Finding the best skin care product for a particular manifestation of sensitive skin is complicated by the fact that there are five very different subtypes of sensitive skin:

1. acne subtype
2. rosacea subtype
3. stinging subtype
4. allergic subtype
5. seborrheic dermatitis.

It is important to note that inflammation is the common denominator among all sensitive skin subtypes. Sunburn susceptibility is not considered a factor in the sensitive skin designation in this skin-typing system.

SCORE NUMBERING OF THE SENSITIVE SKIN TYPES The S score is calculated differently than the other parameters. Each subtype of sensitive skin contributes a number to the score. For example, an individual with acne would be designated as S_1 while an individual with stinging would be S_3. Combinations are possible, so, for example, an individual with acne, rosacea, and stinging would be $S_1S_2S_3$. These numbers do not indicate severity; however, a subject with more than one subtype would suffer from more skin problems than a subject with only one subtype.

COMBINING THE D/O AND S/R PARAMETERS

Eczema

Patients with an impaired skin barrier, manifested by dry skin, are more likely to suffer from eczema, which is now known to be a genetic defect of filaggrin. Those with eczema often test out as having a DS_4 or DS_3S_4 skin type. Subjects that do not have eczema but experience allergic reactions to allergens placed on the skin often also have dry skin because they have an impaired barrier.[12] These skin types are designated as DS_4.

Acne

People with OR types may have a pimple here and there, but do not suffer frequently from acne. For this reason, we know that oil alone is not enough to cause acne. Other factors such as genetic predisposition, high volume of *P. acnes*, and abnormal keratinization must be present. Although most S_1 types are also classified as oily (OS_1), there are some acne sufferers that have dry skin (DS_1). Individuals with DS_1 skin have very different skin care needs than acne sufferers with oily skin (OS_1). This is one of many reasons that all four of the BSTS parameters must be identified before a skin care regimen is prescribed.

Rosacea

S_3 types experience stinging of the skin. Those with rosacea (S_2), and dry skin (D) often experience stinging. Therefore, DS_2S_3 is a common skin type for those with rosacea.

SKIN PIGMENTATION: PIGMENTED (P) VERSUS NON-PIGMENTED (N)

This parameter measures the proclivity to develop unwanted solar-induced dark patches on the face, known as melasma or solar lentigos. These can be prevented and treated with skin care products and procedures. While intrinsic or genetic factors contribute to uneven pigmentation, extrinsic factors such as ultraviolet light and heat play an important role.

Score Numbering of the Pigmented Skin Types

A pigmented skin type may be assigned a 1-4 numerical value depending on how likely the skin is to develop skin pigmentation issues such as postinflammatory hyperpigmentation or melasma. This score can be used to screen candidates for dermatologic procedures in order to predetermine their risk for dyspigmentation after a procedure. The higher number indicates a higher risk for dyschromia and the lower number indicates less risk. An individual designated P_4, for example, would not be a good candidate for laser resurfacing procedures. The designation P for pigmented is often used without a number when used for the purpose of recommending skin care. Individuals with P skin types will benefit from skin-lightening ingredients.

SKIN ELASTICITY: WRINKLED (W) VERSUS TIGHT (T)

This parameter is affected by age and ethnicity in addition to lifestyle habits; however, this is the only BSTS parameter over which an individual has significant control. That is, while a person cannot alter the genetic component of skin aging, an individual can certainly change her/his behavior to reduce the risk of incurring exposure to and manifesting the signs of extrinsic aging, which is due to external factors such as smoking, excessive use of alcohol, poor nutrition, and, most importantly, sun exposure. In fact, 80 percent of facial aging is ascribed to sun exposure.[13]

COMBINING THE P/N AND W/T PARAMETERS

Photoaging

The pigmented lesions caused by sun exposure are typically associated with other signs of skin aging such as wrinkles, so a person with a P skin type and a significant history of sun exposure often falls into the W category. Photoaged skin would likely be designated as a PW type.

COMBINING THE PARAMETERS TO DESIGNATE BAUMANN SKIN TYPE

BST is calculated by a software program that assigns one letter from each parameter and, if applicable, a sensitive subtype, as described above. One example of the former designation is DRPW (dry, resistant, pigmented, and wrinkle prone), while DS_2S_3NW is an example of the latter (dry, non-pigmented type

prone to rosacea, stinging, and wrinkles). The letters are an extremely accurate way to categorize skin types in order to properly prescribe treatments and follow results.

DETERMINING THE BAUMANN SKIN TYPE

The BSTI questionnaire is the only validated method to determine BST. It is constantly updated as new data are considered and the software increases in sophistication. The most recent version of the BSTI is available at www.skintypesolutions.com.

REFERENCES

1. Takahashi J, Kawasaki K, Tanaka M, et al. The mechanism of stratum corneum plasticization with water. In: Marks R, Payne PA, eds. *Bioengineering and the Skin*. Lancaster: Cardiff MTP Press Limited; 1980:67–73.
2. Wildnauer RH, Bothwell JW, Douglass AB. Stratum corneum biomechanical properties. I. Influence of relative humidity on normal and extracted human stratum corneum. *J Invest Dermatol*. 1971;56:72.
3. Draelos ZD. Therapeutic moisturizers. *Dermatol Clin*. 2000;18:597.
4. Data on file Baumann Cosmetic and Research Institute (a).
5. Orton DI, Wilkinson, JD. Cosmetic allergy: Incidence, diagnosis, and management. *Am J Clin Dermatol*. 2004;5:327.
6. Mehta SS, Reddy BS. Cosmetic dermatitis – Current perspectives. *Int J Dermatol*. 2003;42:533.
7. Youn SW, Kim SJ, Hwang IA, et al. Evaluation of facial skin type by sebum secretion: discrepancies between subjective descriptions and sebum secretion. *Skin Res Technol*. 2002;8:168.
8. Data on file Baumann Cosmetic and Research Institute (b).
9. Jackson EM. The science of cosmetics. *Am J Contact Dermat*. 1993;4:108.
10. Farage MA. How do perceptions of sensitive skin differ at different anatomical sites? An epidemiological study. *Clin Exp Dermatol*. 2009;34(8):e521.
11. Kligman A. Human models for characterizing "Sensitive Skin." *Cosm Derm*. 2001;14:15.
12. Jovanovic M, Poljacki M, Duran V, et al. Contact allergy to Compositae plants in patients with atopic dermatitis. *Med Pregl*. 2004;57:209.
13. Uitto J. Understanding premature skin aging. *N Engl J Med*. 1997;337:1463.

CHAPTER 2

Basic Cosmetic Chemistry

There are entire books, courses, and academic societies dedicated to cosmetic chemistry. This chapter is intended to cover the basics only. Understanding these few basic chemistry items is crucial in order to decipher the language used in reference to personal care products.

■ COSMETIC INGREDIENT NOMENCLATURE

The cosmetic industry uses nomenclature that differs from that established by the International Union of Pure and Applied Chemistry (IUPAC), which is taught in organic chemistry. The Cosmetic Toiletry and Fragrance Association, which changed its name to the Personal Care Products Council in 2007, compiled a standardized list of ingredients and published it in 1973.[1] This system is now known as the International Nomenclature of Cosmetic Ingredients (INCI). A comprehensive description of this system appears in Chapter 4 of *Beginning Cosmetic Chemistry*.[2] Understanding the stem terms facilitates reading product labels. For the most up-to-date information on INCI nomenclature, visit the website for the Personal Care Products Council (http://www.personalcarecouncil.org/). In some cases, the nomenclature varies between the United States (US) and the European Union (EU). Botanical ingredients (those derived from plants), in particular, are labeled differently in the US and the EU. In the EU, the Latin binomial (genus and species names) is used, while in the US the name includes the Latin binominal, the common name of the plant, the plant part, and the type of preparation. Oatmeal extract is a good example to illustrate the divergent approaches to classification. In the EU, the INCI name for oatmeal extract is Avena Sativa. In the US, the INCI name is Avena Sativa (Oat) Kernel Extract. The biggest differences between names in the US and EU seem to be found in the names of botanicals, colorants, denatured alcohols, fragrances, and flavors.[3]

■ SIGNIFICANCE OF THE pH

Measurements of pH are used both in formulating and testing product stability. The pH of skin or hair is also a necessary consideration in cosmetic chemistry. pH is the measure of the activity of the hydrogen atom.

Measure of the activity of the hydrogen atom:

$$pH = -\log_{10}(a_{H+}) = \log_{10}\left(\frac{1}{a_{H+}}\right)$$

The higher the pH, the more basic or alkaline is the solution; the lower the pH, the more acidic the solution. The irritation or stinging induced by a product is often directly related to how low the pH is.

Obviously, pH is an important consideration when formulating personal care products. It affects shelf stability, bacterial growth, how well ingredients combine, and how the product interacts with skin or hair. Measurements of pH can be used to reflect the stability of a product. For example, if components in

the product hydrolyze, free acid would be released, which would lower the pH of the formulation and provide evidence that ingredient degradation has occurred. Changes in pH during shelf life can promote bacterial and fungal growth in the formulation. The pH of exfoliating skin care products such as hydroxy acids affects their efficacy. Acid products with a lower pH are more likely to cause exfoliation than a neutral pH preparation. (Water, for example, has a pH of 7.) The pH of a formulation can also play a role in the penetration of cosmetic ingredients into the stratum corneum. It is well known that ascorbic acid penetrates best at a pH of 2.0.[4]

■ ACID DISSOCIATION CONSTANT, K_a AND PK_a-

The pK_a of a substance is a quantitative measure of the strength of an acid in solution and it measures the capacity of that substance to donate protons. If HA is an acid, it can dissociate into its conjugate base (A−) and a hydrogen ion (H+). H+ is essentially a proton.

The generic acid HA dissociates into A− and H+.

$$HA \rightleftharpoons A^- + H^+$$

The larger the value of the pK_a, the less dissociation occurs; therefore, a weak acid has a high pK_a. A strong acid has a p$K_a \leq$ to −2.

The equations used to calculate the K_a and the more commonly used pK_a:

The dissociation constant called the K_a is written in mol/L:

$$K_a = \frac{[A-][H+]}{[HA]}$$

It is more common to use a logarithmic measure of the acid dissolution constant called the pK_a:

$$pK_a = -\log_{10} K_a$$

Another way to think about the acid dissociation constant is that the pK_a is the pH at which the level of free acid is the same as the level of the salt form of the acid. When the pH is less than the pK_a, the free acid form predominates; when the pH is greater than the pK_a, the salt form predominates.

The concept of pK_a is important in formulating cosmetic products. It is particularly pertinent when talking about products with exfoliating or peeling capabilities such as α-hydroxy acid (AHA) or β-hydroxy acid (BHA). In order to use AHAs and BHA properly, one must understand the pK_a and how the pH of a peel affects its efficacy. In the case of peeling agents, the acid form of the cosmetic ingredient is the "active form" in the peel because it provokes exfoliation. The proper balance of the salt and acid forms is necessary in order to yield an efficacious peel with minimal irritation. The pK_a for salicylic acid is 2.97 while 3.83 is the pK_a for the array of AHAs.[5,6] Because the pK_a of BHA differs from that of the AHA family, it is difficult to formulate an AHA and BHA combination product that can achieve an optimal pH.

For example, in a combination AHA–BHA product with a pH of 3.5, the AHA *acid* form would predominate but the BHA *salt* form would predominate. The effects of BHA would be rendered suboptimal.

MAILLARD REACTION OR GLYCATION

The Maillard reaction is a chemical reaction between an amino acid and a sugar that is also known as glycation. It usually requires heat. Louis-Camille Maillard first described this reaction in 1912 when he observed that amino acids can react with sugar to create brown or golden brown compounds. The Maillard reaction is a well-known phenomenon in cooking because it changes the flavors in food. Caramelizing sugar or onions, browning a turkey, and baking cookies all involve this process. In the personal care product world, the Maillard reaction is demonstrated in the darkening of skin that occurs with sunless tanning products that contain dihydroxyacetone (DHA). Scientists did not recognize the importance of glycation in health until the 1980s. Currently, many antiaging products are designed to prevent this response because the Maillard reaction can lead to protein crosslinks thought to contribute to aging and cancer in the skin and other organs.

Chemistry of the Maillard Reaction

In the Maillard reaction, heat and other circumstances cause a molecule of sugar to open its structure and glue itself (glycate) to a protein molecule. This sugar + protein molecule is called a Schiff base (Figure 2-1). The Schiff base is unstable and rapidly degrades to a more stable structure called an Amadori product. Amadori products can cause proteins to crosslink each other, which is the source of the problem. These crosslinked proteins are called advanced glycation endproducts or AGEs (Figure 2-2). Free radicals enhance this process resulting in an increased amount of dangerous AGEs. Many have touted the use of antioxidants as a method of preventing AGEs. Although antioxidants are beneficial for many reasons, they do not seem helpful in preventing the glycation process primarily because once the Schiff base is formed, it is highly unstable. Using antioxidants may result in blocking one pathway, but the Schiff base is free to move down another pathway still amassing harmful AGEs.

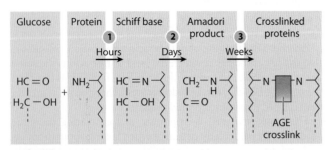

▲ **FIGURE 2-1** The Schiff base is the intermediate product formed when the Maillard Reaction occurs.

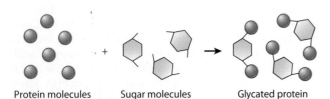

Protein molecules   Sugar molecules   Glycated protein

▲ **FIGURE 2-2** Advanced glycation endproducts (AGEs).

Glycation and Disease

Most of the research on glycation has been conducted to determine how diabetes affects the body. Diabetics have increased sugar in their blood, which leads to damaging protein crosslinks that manifest as coronary artery disease, poor circulation, and vision problems. This is the reason that the focus of diabetes treatment is to lower blood sugar levels using insulin and other medications. When doctors check how well a patient is keeping their blood sugar down, they order a test called hemoglobin A1c or HbA1c. This test measures the levels of glycated hemoglobin, which is an Amadori byproduct of sugar binding the hemoglobin in blood.

AGE crosslinks bind vital proteins such as elastin, which is needed to give skin and organs elasticity and the ability to bounce back. When the AGE crosslinks damage elastin, the arteries lose elasticity, which is one cause of high blood pressure. The ability of the heart to pump blood is also impaired. AGEs can damage the nerves, kidneys, and many other organs. They also hinder many types of proteins including collagen. It is important to know that sugars are not the only etiologic elements in glycation. Fats such as triglycerides also lead to AGEs. For this reason, healthy diets should be relatively low in saturated fat and carbohydrates (sugars).

Glycation and Skin Aging

Two main proteins, collagen and elastin, which are found in the dermal layer of the skin, play a major role in skin appearance. Collagen imparts strength to the skin, and elastin, flexibility. Glycosylated collagen and elastin are believed to play a role in the appearance of aged skin because glycation causes crosslinks in these fibers that alter their function (Figure 2-3). [7] The importance of these components is discussed at length in Chapter 5, Epidermis and Dermis.

REACTIVE OXYGEN SPECIES AND FREE RADICALS

Reactive oxygen species, also called free radicals, are chemically reactive molecules containing oxygen. Stable oxygen has an even number of electrons. When something consumes or removes one of the electrons from oxygen (such as ultraviolet exposure), oxygen is left with an unpaired electron that renders it reactive. "Free radicals" are another name for oxygen that has an uneven number of electrons; thus, they are inherently unstable. Free radicals steal electrons from other cellular components to regain an even number of electrons. It is the instability of the odd number of electrons that makes free radicals harmful. Free radicals can take electrons from DNA, lipids in cell membranes (such as low-density lipoproteins, also

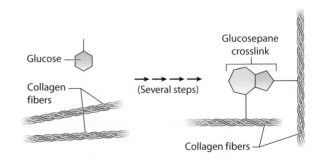

▲ **FIGURE 2-3** Glycation produces crosslinks in collagen fibers.

known as LDL or "bad cholesterol"), proteins, and other vital structures, leaving them impaired. Free radicals can be caused by ultraviolet exposure, cigarette smoking, normal cellular processes such as oxidative phosphorylation, as well as sunscreens and other chemicals upon decomposition. Antioxidants supply free radicals with the electrons they crave, thereby neutralizing them or rendering them harmless (see Chapter 46, Antioxidants).

CONCLUSION

Knowing this basic chemistry will enhance your understanding of the discussions throughout this book. While some sections may refer to the traditional uses of barely processed ingredients, the ultimate focus here will be on topical formulations used or potentially useful in the modern dermatologic armamentarium.

SUGGESTED READING

Schueller R, Romanowski P. *Beginning Cosmetic Chemistry.* 2nd ed. Allured Publishing, 2003.
Barel AO, Paye M, Maibach HI, eds. *Handbook of Cosmetic Science and Technology.* 3rd ed. INFRMA-HC; 2009.
Moore RJ, Wilkinson JB. *Harry's Cosmeticology*, 7th ed. Chemical Publishing Company; 1982.

WEBSITES

Society of Cosmetic Chemists: http://www.scconline.org/website/index.shtml
Personal Care Products Council: http://www.personalcarecouncil.org/

REFERENCES

1. Personal Care Products Council: A Centennial History of the Personal Care Products Council. http://www.personalcarecouncil.org/about-us/history?page=2. Washington, DC 2012. Accessed July 29, 2012.
2. Schueller R, Romanowski P. Cosmetic ingredient nomenclature. In: *Beginning Cosmetic Chemistry: An Overview for Chemists, Formulators, Suppliers and Others Interested in the Cosmetic Industry.* 2nd ed. Carol Stream, IL: Allured Publishing; 2003:21–27.
3. Schueller R, Romanowski P. INCI names: Differences between the US and the EU. In: *Beginning Cosmetic Chemistry: An Overview for Chemists, Formulators, Suppliers and Others Interested in the Cosmetic Industry.* 2nd ed. Carol Stream, IL, Allured Publishing; 2003:29–34.
4. Pinnell SR, Yang H, Omar M, et al. Topical L-ascorbic acid: Percutaneous absorption studies. *Dermatol Surg.* 2001;27:137.
5. Davies M, Marks R. Studies on the effect of salicylic acid on normal skin. *Br J Dermatol.* 1976;95:187.
6. Kligman A. A comparative evaluation of a novel low-strength salicylic acid cream and glycolic acid products on human skin. *Cosmet Dermatol Suppl.* 1997;10:11.
7. Pageon H, Bakala H, Monnier VM, et al. Collagen glycation triggers the formation of aged skin in vitro. *Eur J Dermatol.* 2007;17:12.

CHAPTER 3

Organic Ingredient Labeling

As pressure grows on cosmetics companies to use more environmentally-friendly ingredients and packaging, we are seeing a profound increase in organic/natural claims on "green" beauty products. Terms such as "active naturals," "botanical," "natural," "green," and "organic" are bandied about regularly; however, these terms are meaningless without standard consensus definitions. Of these categories, only the term "organic" has a set of requirements associated with its labeling. Unfortunately, standards and definitions in the United States (US) and other countries vary.

"ORGANIC" ORIGIN

The term "organic" was coined in 1940 by J.I. Rodale, who founded the Rodale book and magazine publishing empire with the publication *Organic Farming and Gardening*. In 1992, the US Department of Agriculture (USDA) created the National Organic Program (NOP) and approved the Organic Label within its accompanying standards; however, this "organic seal" is applied mainly to agricultural foods and practices. It is often used on personal care products, although it primarily takes into account the practices of growing the ingredients for food, so it is not always suitable for personal care products that contain modified agricultural materials and multicomponent packaging. For example, the seal does not mean that the packaging of the skin care product is recyclable.

ORGANIC REGULATION

There was no recognized "organic" label for personal skin care products until May 2002. The USDA made it clear then in a policy statement about the NOP that manufacturers of nonfood products (such as personal care products) containing agricultural ingredients were eligible to seek certification under the NOP. This allowed producers of nonfood items to display the iconic round, green "USDA Organic" seal to attest to "authentic" organic claims on their labels. However, in April 2004, the USDA issued a surprising "Guidance Statement" reversing this position, indicating that producers of personal care products would not be eligible to seek certification and had to cease use of their green symbol. There was vacillation on this decision for many months until August 2005 when the Organic Consumers Association (OCA), representing more than 500,000 members, won a major victory in a lawsuit against the USDA again allowing nonfood products to be certified with the organic seal. This NOP Standard offers three different kinds of organic certification: If a product contains 100 percent organic ingredients, it can be labeled as 100 percent organic and use the seal on the front of the package; if a product contains 95 percent organic ingredients, it can be labeled as "organic" and use the seal on the front of the package; if a product contains between 70 and 94 percent organic ingredients, it can be labeled as "made with (name of) organic ingredient" and the seal may not be used on the package. The nonorganic ingredients in the remaining 5 to 30 percent must also be screened to ensure that they conform to organic food standards.

THE RULES OF ORGANIC PRODUCTION

In organic farming, of food crops or those intended for topical products, farmers avoid the use of synthetic pesticides, hormones, genetically modified crops, and chemical products. Organic farming also follows traditional agricultural practices that enrich the soil, use resources in an environmentally sound manner, and treat livestock humanely. Specifically, a grower of organic ingredients must meet these baseline criteria in order for the products to be certified as organic:

1. Abstain from the application of prohibited materials (including synthetic fertilizers, pesticides, and sewage sludge) for three years prior to certification and then continually throughout their organic license.

2. Prohibit the use of genetically modified organisms, irradiation, and petrochemical solvents.

3. Employ positive soil building, conservation, manure management, and crop rotation practices.

4. Avoid contamination during the processing of organic products.

5. Keep records of all operations (courtesy of OCA).

REGULATORY BODIES FOR PERSONAL CARE PRODUCTS

For personal care products, the USDA seal is the one we see most commonly in the US, but because it applies to food products, many new standards have been created. However, no one standard has been agreed upon at a national level in the US. Standards and regulations also vary from country to country. In addition, some regulatory bodies are for-profit businesses that will certify products for a fee. Obviously, this presents an inherent bias.

In Europe, one organization that offers certification is the European Cosmetics Standards Working Group's Cosmetics Organic Standard (COSMOS). This group formed nearly 10 years ago, officially launched COSMOS in 2008, and released their certification standards in February 2011. COSMOS is an amalgamation of several other European associations, including BIOFORUM from Belgium, Cosmebio and Ecocert from France, Bundesverband der Industrie- und Handelsunternehmen (BDIH) from Germany, Associazione Italiana Agricoltura Biologica (AIAB) and Istituto per la Certificazione Etica e Ambientale (ICEA) from Italy, and the Soil Association from the United Kingdom. These seven organizations represent manufacturer associations, standards and certifying bodies, and consumer groups working in the field of organic and natural cosmetic products that have united to form COSMOS. For more information, visit http://www.cosmos-standard.org/.

Another popular certifying organization for natural and organic cosmetics is Na True from Belgium (www.natrue.org). Na True and COSMOS seem to be the most popular certifying bodies in the US currently. Not surprisingly, this is a competitive field right now and all organizations with an interest in labeling skin care products want to be recognized as the one defining the standards for natural and organic cosmetics. Other certifying bodies in the US include the National Sanitation Foundation (NSF International), which developed the American National Standards Institute (ANSI) 305 criteria (similar to Na True criteria) and OASIS, which was created by a coalition of beauty product manufacturers. Each certifying body has its own standards for what constitutes "organic." There is a discrepancy among them about such guidelines. For example, each standard differs in allowed preservatives, calculations for extracts, processing aids, etc.

ORGANIC TOPICAL PRODUCTS

While there are no long-term studies documenting the effects of using topical organic products or ingredients, consumers of organic products are typically as interested in what products *do not contain* as in what they *do* contain. The organic label intends to assure that the key cleansing and conditioning ingredients are derived from organically grown plant products, rather than conventionally grown plants, synthetic chemicals, or petroleum byproducts. In addition, topical organic products exclude or minimize any ingredients that could be considered potentially harmful to people, animals, waterways, or the environment. The rules about which ingredients can and cannot be included vary from regulatory body to regulatory body.

"NATURAL" INGREDIENTS

Natural Standard for Personal Care Products

It is important to note that a product that is touted as "natural" is not necessarily organic. There is much confusion about what the term "natural" means. The Natural Products Association (NPA), a nonprofit organization founded in 1936 as the American Health Foods Association that has since undergone several name changes, represents the interests of manufacturers and consumers in marketing and certifying products that are at least 95 percent natural. The NPA's "Natural Seal" can be displayed on products that meet this 95 percent science-based standard (95 percent natural ingredients or ingredients from natural sources, not counting water) as certified by independent third-party auditors. Although the NPA issues guidelines on whether or not a product can be deemed "natural," there is no governmental requirement to have this certification in order to use the term "natural" on the product label. The NPA seal should be thought of as a guideline to help conscientious consumers choose products that meet certain standards. The NPA seal certifies that a company has met standards pertaining to natural ingredients, safety, sustainability, and responsibility. The Natural Standard for Personal Care Products requires that companies be transparent, fully disclosing their ingredients accurately and truthfully. They should strive to maximize their use of recyclable and postconsumer recycled content in packaging. No animal testing in the development of the product is allowed. For more information and a list of ingredients that can be included in products, visit http://www.npainfo.org.

Active Naturals

"Active naturals" is a term popularized by the skin care product manufacturer Aveeno to describe ingredients that are found in nature but that have been enhanced in the laboratory. A good example is feverfew, which naturally contains the sesquiterpene lactone parthenolide. Topical applications of formulations containing parthenolide can lead to skin irritation; blisters in the mouth can develop when parthenolide is taken orally. Aveeno products contain feverfew that has had the parthenolide component removed. The "active soy" preparations found in Neutrogena and Aveeno products were developed in a similar manner. They contain soy that has had the estrogenic components removed. These products, while containing a form of natural ingredients, would not be eligible for the NPA certification because the constituents were adulterated in the laboratory to increase efficacy.

PITFALLS OF ORGANIC AND NATURAL PRODUCTS

Although natural and organic products are thought to be safer for the environment, they come with their own share of problems. For instance, many natural and organic brands contain certain fragrances and essential oils that can cause dermatitis. Oil of bergamot, and balsam of Peru are both highly allergenic, so even an organic product containing them could irritate sensitive individuals. Organic products containing strong essential oils like peppermint or rosemary can also irritate or inflame sensitive skin. Chamomile, generally considered a gentle and soothing herb, can induce allergies in some people (who may also tend to be allergic to ragweed). Some natural products contain a "perfume mix" to mask their odor. Components of the perfume mix are rarely listed on the product label since each company uses its own proprietary blend. Even a product listed as 95 percent organic could contain a perfume mix that might induce allergic reactions in some people. Organic products follow the International Fragrance Association (IFRA) restrictions that limit the kinds of fragrances used, so they are no more likely to cause fragrance allergy than synthetic products.

Manufacturers of organic and natural products have a tough challenge to face. These products are very appealing to bacteria and fungi and the kinds of preservatives that can be used in a product labeled as natural or organic are limited. For example, parabens are a very effective preservative ingredient shunned in the natural/organic product world and certainly omitted from the list of approved ingredients by the NPA. The more earth-friendly types of preservatives can, in fact, cause a skin allergy in the user. Companies struggle to find environmentally-friendly preservatives. At this time, phenoxyethanol is the most commonly used preservative in organic and natural products.

THE PRECAUTIONARY PRINCIPLE

Sometimes certain ingredients are excluded from products based on research. In other cases, exclusions are based on the "precautionary principle," which holds that until the cumulative impacts and exposures to a broad range of ingredients can be fully assessed, it is best to err on the side of *caution* and limit use. For example, though many chemical ingredients used in cosmetics are widely considered safe for use, some safety factors have not been fully studied. It is virtually impossible to assess the *cumulative effects* of repeated exposures from multiple sources. This is important because consumers, especially women, use several skin, hair, and beauty products per day. The ingredients in these products could potentially interact, or lead to a higher combined rate of exposure to certain ingredients than is usually evaluated by studying the safety of a single ingredient in the laboratory. Further, to accurately establish the baseline of the chemical exposures people can safely tolerate, it would be necessary to account for *all* chemical exposures from food, urban smog, industrial waste, and other sources.

Many consumers who choose organic foods and topical products prefer to limit chemical exposures as a precaution. Use of natural products is recommended for pregnant or breast-feeding women, young children, and others concerned about the impact that the creation and disposal of personal care products can have on the environment.

THE FUTURE OF ORGANICS

Very few product lines can meet the standards of these regulatory organizations (or, more accurately, self-regulatory organizations, as they are not governmental bodies with enforcement authority) because it is expensive and time consuming to achieve and maintain this standard. Luckily, there are successful brands that are forging the path for advances in this area, and raising the standards of natural products. Burt's Bees, for example, is a company that certifies to the NPA Natural Personal Care standard and has the top selling lip balm stock-keeping unit (SKU) across all categories (not just the natural categories). Other companies that make natural products include Jurlique, Dr. Hauschka, Suki, Sophyto, Toms, Organix, Alba, Jason, Avalon, Kiss My Face, Weleda, Pangea Organics, and Natural Gate.

It is important to remember that the terms "organic," "natural," or "sustainable" do not imply efficacy. None of the organic or natural certifications require efficacy data, so many of these products have not undergone the strict scrutiny of scientific investigation to evaluate efficacy. It is understandable that these companies are slower to perform clinical trials because the research process is expensive and they have already incurred such costs to meet the organic/natural standards. However, it is my hope that as sales increase, so will the scientific data.

CHAPTER 4

Cosmeceutical Marketing Claims

More than a quarter of a century since Albert Kligman, M.D., Ph.D., introduced the term "cosmeceutical," the existence of this group of compounds has never been officially or legally recognized, leaving this category of products largely unregulated.[1] The United States Food and Drug Administration (USFDA) classifies personal care products as a drug, cosmetic, or both [e.g., antidandruff shampoos or moisturizers with sun protection factor (SPF)]. Cosmeceutical products, which are personal care products that may actually yield a biologic impact, fall between the cracks of these incomplete designations.

Most manufacturers of cosmeceutical formulations have established the clinical merit of their products despite the lack of official oversight, but some doubt is inevitable given the regulatory loophole, particularly when companies make extraordinary claims. Manufacturers typically test main ingredients and finished products in small *in vivo* trials, but rarely if ever publish results in the peer-reviewed literature.

Even though cosmeceuticals are not regulated by the FDA, there are standards and guidelines for good practices in many cases. Manufacturers that try to skirt this self-policing system risk a greater likelihood that their product(s) will not succeed. It is important for practitioners and consumers alike to be familiar with these standards. That is, claims made on cosmeceutical products routinely use the same terms or expressions none of which are made patently clear but are somewhat consistently used across manufacturers. Given the absence of regulatory oversight of these products, this chapter will read between the lines and explain the language used in cosmeceutical marketing claims. These terms and expressions are defined below, and further described according to the typical data used to support their marketing.

ADVERTISING OMISSIONS

Allergen-free

No standard definition has been established for "allergen-free" either, and no testing is required of companies. More often than not, "allergen-free" indicates that the product includes no fragrances on the European Union's "List of Substances Which Cosmetic Products Must Not Contain Except Subject to Restrictions and Conditions Laid Down" or other compounds typically identified as allergens. Some manufacturers use human repeated insult patch testing (HRIPT) for allergy testing.

Hypoallergenic

Each manufacturer defines this term in its own way, often using it liberally, as no standard definition of hypoallergenicity has been established. HRIPT of about 100 to 200 subjects and cumulative irritation testing (smaller panel) are the common methods of evaluation. Occasionally, photoreactivity testing is conducted, depending on the product type.

Unscented/Fragrance-free

When a product lacks common fragrance ingredients, particularly those most often linked to allergic sensitivity, or a traditional fragrance intended to impart scent to a product, its manufacturer can label the formulation as fragrance-free. However, the appearance of the expression "fragrance-free" on a product does not necessarily mean that a fragrance is not included. Companies sometimes include fragrance subcomponents or botanicals to render a cosmetic or preservative effect that, concomitantly, delivers a scent or pleasant aroma to a formulation. If the primary reason for including the "fragrance" is not related to scent, such as acting as a preservative, then the manufacturer is not required to label the ingredient as a fragrance but can label the product as fragrance-free.

It is also worth noting that some ingredients, including preservatives like phenoxyethanol (the most often used one in organic and natural products), background wax odors from long chain/paraffins, or unfragranced sunscreens, are not considered fragrances, but do impart an odor and can provoke reactions in individuals sensitive or allergic to fragrance.

Formulations labeled as "unscented" typically have no detectable odor, but the product may have a "masking" fragrance included to disguise background odor. Therefore, "unscented" does not necessarily translate to no added fragrance. In an age in which companies have been compelled into advertising the absence of the preservative parabens, consumers have come to expect that if an ingredient is excluded from a product, it really is excluded. That said, this lack of clarity in advertising is likely not problematic for any but the most sensitive individuals. It is nonetheless important to understand how the process works.

ORGANIC OR NATURAL

In the last two decades, interest has increased greatly regarding the use of what consumers perceive to be the healthiest quality ingredients in skin care products, not to mention food and clothing. Manufacturers have responded to the call by using terms and expressions such as "organic," "natural," "naturally derived," and "botanical" on their product label claims. Consumers are left to puzzle as to exactly what these descriptions mean (see Chapter 3, Organic Ingredient Labeling, for a more detailed explanation).

Organic

In 2005, the US Department of Agriculture (USDA) issued new organic standards for skin care products. According to these guidelines, a product labeled as "organic" must contain at least 95 percent organic ingredients; one said to be "made with organic ingredients" must be composed of at least 75 and up to 94 percent organic ingredients. These standards are based on organic food standards, and prohibit the use of synthetic preservatives and most chemical processing of ingredients. Consequently, organic skin care products are derived from organically grown plant products, not conventionally grown plants, synthetic chemicals, or petroleum byproducts. To meet these standards, producers also exclude or minimize ingredients considered potentially deleterious to people, animals, waterways, or the environment.

Natural, Naturally Derived, Botanical

Products labeled as "natural" may or may not be organic. Such products contain ingredients derived from plants but can also contain chemicals added to act as preservatives or to improve its texture. In the next step further removed from what consumers might envision is natural are the so-called "naturally derived" ingredients, which find their origins in plants but are enhanced in the laboratory. None of these terms have any legal meaning. "Botanical" refers to products that were made from or contain some plant constituents. This in no way means that the product is exclusively made from plant components. Consumers can easily be misled in this regard or by the fact that while there are several effective botanical products on the market, generic versions with similar ingredients and packaging may not be as effective. The order of ingredients, pH, and temperature when ingredients were added are all patented trade secrets that influence the effectiveness of a product.

TESTING AND APPROVAL

Clinically Tested

Typically, these products have indeed been investigated through some form of clinical testing, but the test could be a simple 48-hour patch test for irritancy. There are no rules about how many subjects or the type of trial required for a formulation to be considered "clinically tested," and it is not always clear whether the finished formulation was tested or only components. When a product is described as "clinically tested," each word is carefully chosen (e.g., clinically tested "technology" or clinically tested "formula") to offer clarity to the attentive reader.

Clinical testing is distinct from more ordinary "consumer" testing, which could include focus groups and simple patient use questionnaires. Clinical tests are typically run with scientific/medical experts, using an approved protocol, specified statistical analysis, and enough subjects to provide statistical significance, based on the study design. The new sunscreen monograph allows for as few as 10 subjects per panel for SPF. Other types of assessments (moisturization, antiacne, etc.) would typically use more subjects, perhaps from 30 to 100.

Clinically Proven

"Proven," according to the National Advertising Division of the Council of Better Business Bureaus (NAD), requires two similar well-controlled clinical studies to make this claim. This is the standard for the major television networks with regard to broadcast advertising of a product. The Office of Broadcast Standards and Practices reviews ads and the data to support any claims before accepting them for broadcast. If there has been just one study, the wording might be limited to clinically "shown" or "tested." Sometimes, one study on the "technology" and another study on the final formulation will satisfy the network's requirements for "clinically proven."

Despite attempts at rigor, the "clinically proven" claim can be unclear for consumers, as they are unable to determine if it was only the ingredient or the actual final formulation that is clinically "proven." Furthermore, the advertising regulation does not apply to package labeling. If only the ingredient rather than the final formulation was tested, the wording usually is carefully crafted (e.g., "with an ingredient that has been clinically proven to X").

Dermatologist Tested

This claim conjures images of a dermatologist applying a lotion to the face, assessing it as cosmetically acceptable, and subsequently approving the formulation. While "dermatologist tested" generally means much more than this, the claim is highly variable. Often if a formulation is "dermatologist tested," a dermatologist has reviewed the clinical study and signed off on it, but s/he may have simply reviewed the formula or a study report. The doctor may or may not be involved in the conduct of the study and/or analysis of results.

Nonetheless, this claim is usually based on a specific clinical trial with a protocol, and the final formula sold in stores has been tested. Panel size depends on the company, but the general rule is a minimum of 30 subjects for claims of efficacy. In this case, a certified dermatologist signs off and oversees the testing. However, this is not required to make the claim "dermatologist tested."

Dermatologist Approved

This claim only requires one dermatologist to approve the product in some fashion, perhaps based on an assessment of safety, efficacy, or just a brief review of ingredients. Typically, a small company doing infomercials may just use one dermatologist, who may also be its consultant or a stockholder in the company. Larger companies typically sample four or five independent dermatologists with data to be reviewed, depending on the claim and the size of the company. This wording is not as common as "dermatologist recommended," which is typically based on a questionnaire that is sent to many dermatologists.

The Role of Monographs

A monograph is a statement detailing the kind and amount of active ingredients that, when used at the concentration range stipulated, can be included in product claims. Claim language preapproved by the FDA is allowed on a product monograph without supplying additional data. Generally, manufacturers are required to follow the wording used in the monograph for its claims. However, companies can provide additional claims (e.g., "moisturizes," "cleans," "brightens") for products not sold over the counter. To better illustrate this point, consider acne products. Companies must have an approved monograph listing active ingredients, such as benzoyl peroxide, salicylic acid, or sulfur, within the approved range. Companies are not required to test this formulation for effectiveness in treating acne as long as they meet the range requirement. However, they are not permitted to combine acne actives or other monograph actives. In other words, a formulation may not contain benzoyl peroxide and ultraviolet screens and then claim that it treats acne and imparts an SPF factor without undergoing FDA review and approval.[2]

PROBLEMS WITH PROPRIETARY DATA

Even though companies may perform extensive research on their cosmeceutical products, their findings most often remain unpublished. Consequently, dermatologists cannot easily access this scientific evidence to evaluate the efficacy of the myriad marketed products. Bereft of such evidence, physicians, who are taught to practice evidence-based medicine, have scant reason to believe that any of these products are actually effective. Therefore, the medical establishment dismisses such products as useless even though some of these formulations may potentially offer benefits to patients. Essentially, internal company research that is kept under proprietary wraps thwarts the peer-review process. Peer review has long been considered necessary to validate the research findings of scientists. Without the peer review of research findings, the scientific community as well as the public-at-large is left with no reasons to have confidence in study results.

APPEARANCE CLAIMS

Each company has its own research standards and some companies do not do any research at all to support its claims because research trials are not required by the FDA or FTC. Some cosmetic companies try the study product on five of its employees, all who know the identity of the cream and are obligated to their employers. This of course is not the ideal study design but is frequently used. Many companies perform "research trials" in-house, do not share the design and results of the trials, and do not attempt to publish the results. Other companies use an independent dermatologist to assess subjects in an open-label trial (the subject and the investigator know the identity of the study product). It is much preferred that the trial be a double-blinded vehicle-controlled trial.

Although some trusted manufacturers exist in the cosmeceutical realm and a number of formulations have proven their clinical merit, the lack of official oversight, the proprietary nature of the formulations, and the disincentive for research data leaves room for doubt about the efficacy claims of personal care products. Some reputable formulators test both the main ingredients and finished products through *in vivo* (in living human skin) trials, but most rely on the ingredient manufacturers *in vitro* (in test tubes or cell cultures) investigations of the individual ingredient and not the final formulation. It is almost impossible for consumers to know the specifics of the research study design by reading a product label but a few clues may reside in the language used. The following terms and expressions do not have regulated or legal definitions but are thought to convey the common connotations below:

Antiaging

Claims that a product confers an antiaging benefit are often based on an ingredient claim. Often included in this claim is a grading by consumers or experts. SPF is known to gauge the ability of a product to prevent photodamage and premature photoaging, and new label revisions allow SPF products to make this claim. However, manufacturers of antiaging products often tout the "antiaging" effects of their formulations based on ingredients other than UV screens. For example, AHAs and vitamin A derivatives are popular ingredients in "antiaging" products.

"…Appearance of Wrinkles"

For cosmetic products, this claim is typically supported by a dermatologist's *in vivo* or photographic assessment of subjects at the end of the trial compared to baseline. In some cases, bioinstruments (e.g., fringe projection, image analysis) are used or a consumer study with questionnaire is used to support this claim. Normally, only a drug product, like tretinoin, for exam-

ple, can make scientific claims of "increasing collagen production" or stimulating fibroblasts to produce collagen. To avoid that issue, companies will instead say "improves the appearance of wrinkles" and avoid the biological explanation of why the improvement occurred.

Brightening

The meaning of brightening is unclear but it seems to pertain to light reflection off of the skin's surface. This is also referred to as radiance or clarity. Decreasing melanin levels in the skin lead to "brightening" because melanin absorbs light. When there is less melanin, the skin reflects more light, making it appear brighter or more radiant. Often visual elements are placed in the formulations to reflect light and cause brightening. For this reason, brightening can be noticed instantly upon application of the product. There are multiple approaches for assessing "brightening" effects. This is typically performed via clinical evaluation, with dermatologists grading brightness on a scale (e.g., from very dull/not bright to very bright/no dullness) over the course of treatment. Results may also be obtained through measurement of luminosity image analysis such as photographs.

Deep Cleaning

This claim is made, but with no accompanying standard definition. That said, several approaches have been suggested. A standard compound can be applied to the skin and allowed to equilibrate, followed by a standardized washing procedure. Typically, a new cleansing product (or device) is compared to either one or all of the following: a competitor, water alone, bar soap, or an older formulation (device). The amount of residual material can be quantified using laboratory instruments. For instance, tape stripping is used to measure depth, and a sebumeter is used to demonstrate sebum reduction. Determining "cleanliness" may also be performed by consumers or expert graders.

Firming

Expert assessment and/or subject self-assessments are the foundation used to buttress a firming claim. Although some instrumental measurements have been applied (currently limited to ballistometry), few publications are available on this method and its validity is questionable. Occasionally, a firming claim is based on the inclusion of an ingredient with no actual testing performed.

Lifting

Three main methods are used to exhibit "lifting": bioinstruments (change in volume based on imaging software), expert graders, or consumer questionnaires. Live grading can be conducted split-face, if subjects are symmetrical, or three-dimensional imaging can be used for grading of lifting. Sometimes calculations can be performed on the images to measure in millimeters the appearance of visible lifting.

Lightening

Lightening means a decrease in the amount of melanin or brown in the skin. Lightening can be assessed with any combination or single method of evaluation, including bioinstrumentation, clinical expert assessment, or consumer questionnaire. Clinical studies typically include dermatologist assessments of overall skin fairness, overall evenness, and instrumental measurements such as L*a*b* values from chromameters. Image analysis for pigmented spots can be done on high-resolution images, and dark marks can be followed for size and intensity compared to nearby skin. Photographic assessment is commonly used.

Noncomedogenic

There is no standard definition associated with this claim. However, industry practice suggests the use of comedogenicity patch testing on the upper back in 10 to 20 subjects, based on the modified Kligman method in which cyanoacrylate follicular biopsies are then reviewed under a microscope.

Plumping

Lip cosmetics often make this claim. Companies may use dermatologist assessments (from one to three physicians) of lip volume, plumpness, color, or shape. Subject self-assessment may also be used by companies, as subjects sometimes say they can "feel" the plumpness. This claim is also based on the use of digital imaging and grading by experts; advanced three-dimensional imaging techniques can even allow quantification of volume changes. Plumping may simply be a claim based on the incorporation of ingredients that engender an increase in blood flow, thus temporarily expanding the size of the lips.

Pore Reducing

The observation of a pore size reduction may be made by dermatologist reviewers/graders in person or through before/after photograph comparisons. Images can also be evaluated with bioinstrumentation (e.g., the software in the Visia system by Canfield) that measures pore size changes. More often, though, effects on pore size are self-assessed by subjects and graded on a questionnaire.

Smoothing

Smoothing can be measured in many ways. It may be as simple as a claim based on feedback from consumers or subjects. A dermatologist may assess texture tactilely; improvements in tactile roughness would support a smoothing claim. Rarely, three-dimensional imaging or replicas are used to support this claim.

Volumizing

This is a common claim associated with eye cosmetics because any coating on the eyelash will expand the volume based on the volume equation $\pi r^2 h$. Thus, a doubling of the hair shaft radius will quadruple the volume (i.e., a 400 percent increase in the volume of the lash). Typically, photo assessments are completed, but there are no regulations on the number of subjects needed to claim that a product confers a plumping effect.

FTC GUIDELINES ON PRODUCT ENDORSEMENTS AND TESTIMONIALS

In 2009, the Federal Trade Commission (FTC) updated its "Guides Concerning the Use of Endorsements and Testimonials in Advertising," which covers endorsements by consumers, experts, organizations, and celebrities, as well as the disclosure of important connections between advertisers and endorsers. The previous version of the guidelines was published in 1980.[3] Advertisers can no longer issue a "results not typical" disclaimer;

instead, they are required to clearly state the results that consumers should usually expect.[3,4]

In addition, the revised guides added new examples to show that payments or free products exchanged between advertisers and endorsers must be divulged (e.g., bloggers paid to write a review or celebrity endorsements on a talk show). Similarly, if a company refers in an advertisement to the findings of a research organization that conducted research sponsored by the company, the advertisement must reveal the connection between the advertiser and the research organization.

The FTC guidelines are nonbinding administrative interpretations of the law intended to help advertisers comply with the FTC Act.

CAVEAT EMPTOR: BUYER BEWARE

Cosmetic company insiders have noted, somewhat cynically, that the most reliable claim on a package is the product size, since this can be objectively measured. All other claims can be exaggerated based on limited or non-product-specific data or even, rarely, nothing at all. Even when a company tests a product, the study may be conducted under unrealistic conditions or with such tight controls that a consumer's actual use pattern will not likely yield similar results. For example, a manufacturer may claim that its product improves wrinkles after 51 percent of consumers report a self-assessed benefit, which, of course, translates to roughly a 50/50 chance of a given consumer deriving a benefit.

Nevertheless, well-formulated products can elicit benefits. "Clinically proven" claims, supported by research studies with independent dermatologists, are reliable indicators of potential product efficacy. Another strong indicator of likely benefits from products are television ads on the three major networks. A television ad on one of the traditional major networks that refers to a product as "clinically proven" is also a good indication of product effectiveness. Such claims are most likely to be brandished by brand name products with strong research and development divisions. Consumers should be wary of generic store brands that urge comparisons to other products. Manufacturers of these products are trying to piggyback off of the reputation of the "innovator" and are unlikely to have conducted any studies. Generic products may contain the same ingredients as another brand, but are unlikely to be identical to the original products. The generic version can only be thought to deliver the same efficacy if its final formulation has been clinically proven.

It may take extra work, but for reliability, consumers should be advised to consider the history and reputation of the company selling the product and note the efficacy claimed as well as any new reports on the product or manufacturer. Larger companies generally will conduct clinical research and testing aimed at verifying claims, since their competitors are likely to challenge any false advertising. Smaller companies are less likely to be scrutinized; therefore, they can more easily operate under the radar and perhaps get away with making more unfounded or less scrupulous claims.

CONCLUSION

It is prudent for consumers to always remember that companies are in business to make profits for their shareholders. This is more likely if a quality product is proffered, but that is not always the case. With lax or a lack of regulations regarding various product claims, there are many opportunities for cosmeceutical manufacturers to make misleading or false claims while also making money. Claims are not often clearly defined or objectively determined. An objective, standardized approach to product assessment would best serve patients and dermatologists alike. This murky information void is especially important to consider when discussing in-office physician dispensing of products. Such doctors should certainly understand the science of formulations and their claims and be very clear with their patients, keeping the best interest of patients at the forefront of the process. Preserving patient trust and the sanctity of the physician–patient relationship should be placed on the same level as patient welfare as the highest priorities.

REFERENCES

1. Kligman A. Cosmeceuticals: do we need a new category? In: Elsner P, Maibach H, eds. *Cosmeceuticals*. New York: Marcel Dekker Inc.;2000:1.
2. Kessler DA. Rules and regulations, acne. *Fed Reg.* 1991; 56(159):41020.
3. FTC Publishes Final Guides Governing Endorsements, Testimonials. http://www.ftc.gov/opa/2009/10/endortest.shtm.
4. Federal Trade Commission 16 CFR Part 255. Guides Concerning the Use of Endorsements and Testimonials in Advertising. October 15, 2009;74:198.

CHAPTER 5

Epidermis And Dermis

The appearance of the skin is affected by both the outer layer of the skin, the epidermis, and the middle layer of the skin, the dermis. The deepest layer is composed of a subcutaneous fat layer. The thickness and contour of the fat layer can also affect the appearance of the skin. The fat layer and muscle layer below it are too deep to be influenced by topical skin care agents so they will not be discussed in this book. Instead, the epidermis and dermis will be explored. (For a more in-depth review of basic skin science, see *Cosmetic Dermatology: Principles and Practice*, 2nd edition, Chapters 1–8.) The epidermis and dermis contain many types of cells. Only the ones known to play an important role in skin care will be discussed here (Figure 5-1).

KERATINOCYTES

Keratinocytes constitute the outer layer of skin called the epidermis. The epidermis is very important in skin appearance because it provides protection, keeping skin hydrated while preventing the penetration of caustic agents, and significantly contributes to skin radiance, evenness of color, and smoothness.

The epidermis is made up of layers of keratinocyte cells that resemble a brick wall. The youngest cells are found at the base and are called the basal layer. The stem cells also reside in the basal layer. The next layer contains spiny attachments that tightly hold the keratinocyte cells together to give skin strength. This layer is called the spinous layer. The next layer of cells is very productive, synthesizing fats, proteins, and sugars as well as other cellular components in "factories" inside the cells. When viewed through a microscope these factories (cellular organelles) appear as multicolored granules. For this reason, this important layer is called the granular layer. After the granular layer, the cells begin to lose activity, the granules disappear, and the cells flatten out. This layer of flattened inactive cells is the most outer layer and is termed the stratum corneum (SC).

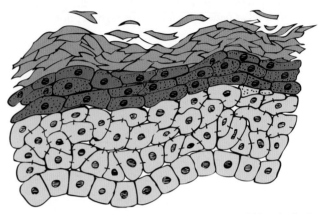

▲ **FIGURE 5-2** Normal epidermis showing the cuboidal basal cells, the spinous layer, granular layer, and stratum corneum. The top layer of the SC is exhibiting the process of desquamation.

The outermost cells are known as *squamous cells* from the Latin *squama* meaning "scale." They are "dead" or *apoptotic* and flake off into the environment. At some point in the SC the attachments that hold these squamous cells together loosen, allowing the cells to fall from the surface in an action known as desquamation, from the Latin *desquamare* meaning "to scrape the scales off" (Figure 5-2).

Aged skin is thinner and more fragile than young skin because the middle dermal layer thins with age. In contrast, the top layer, the epidermis, is often thickened in aged skin. The thickened epidermis is caused by an excess of keratinocyte cells in the SC. This occurs because the keratinocytes normally migrate toward the skin's surface, and as the keratinocytes die, they accumulate at the surface of the skin. Normally, naturally occurring enzymes degrade the connections between the SC cells, releasing them from the cells below and allowing them to desquamate. Older, aged skin or dehydrated skin lacks these enzymes. The result is a buildup of dead squamous skin cells on the surface of the skin (Figure 5-3). This amassing of dead cells prevents the skin from reflecting light. People often complain that the skin looks "dull and tired." People with darker skin types often describe their dry or aged skin as "ashy" in appearance (Figure 5-4). Cosmetic products can be used to make the skin look smoother and more radiant (see Video 1 for a more detailed explanation).

Keratinocytes can lose the ability to undergo apoptosis (programmed cell death) and become cancerous. They begin to replicate and produce multiple copies of themselves. When superficial keratinocyte cells become cancerous, it is known as squamous cell carcinoma (SCC). When the deeper, or basal, keratinocytes become cancerous, this is known as basal cell carcinoma (BCC). SCCs and BCCs are more common in people with a history of significant sun exposure. SCCs and BCCs are usually treated surgically, which can lead to scarring. There is some evidence that antioxidants and retinoids may play a role in the prevention of SCCs and BCCs.[1,2]

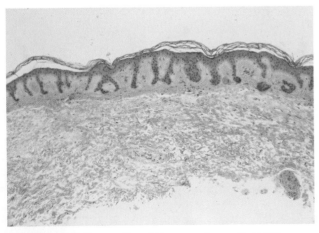

▲ **FIGURE 5-1** Cross-section of skin as seen from a microscope.

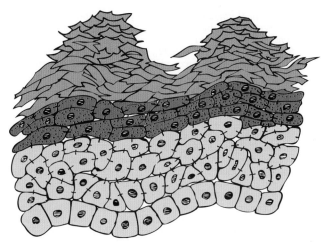

▲ **FIGURE 5-3** The upper layer of keratinocytes cling together creating heaps and valleys that form scales and make skin look dull and ashy.

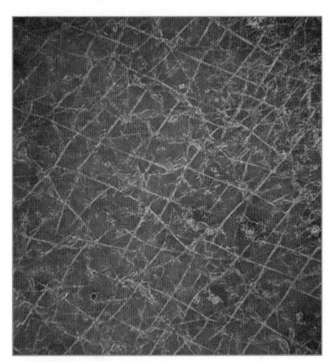

▲ **FIGURE 5-4** Darker, ashy, dry skin.

■ FIBROBLASTS

Fibroblasts make up the middle layer of the skin that lies over the muscle and fat layer. Fibroblasts are very important in skin aging because they are the cells that produce collagen, elastin, and hyaluronic acid (HA), which are all known to affect the skin's appearance. The fibroblast cell is responsible for the skin's thickness, volume, elasticity, and strength. This is because the fibroblast cell contains the "factory" or cellular organelles that produce key components of the skin: collagen, elastin, and HA.

Collagen

The main component of connective tissue, collagen is a family of proteins with a distinctive triple-helix structure. Of the 18 types of collagen, 11 are found in the dermis.[3] Type I is the most abundant protein in humans and types I, III, and VII are the most important forms of collagen in skin.[4] Collagen is excreted from the fibroblasts in a ready-to-go form that provides a scaffolding or structural framework that confers strength to the skin (Video 2). Aged skin contains less of types I and III collagen than young skin.[5] Several ingredients such as retinoids, glycolic acid, and ascorbic acid have been shown to increase the production of collagen. Lasers, light devices, and injectable HA products have also been shown to stimulate collagen production.[6–9]

Elastin

An essential component of the extracellular matrix of connective tissue, elastin is made up of two main constituents: fibrillin and tropoelastin.[10] These are secreted separately from the fibroblast. The skin must assemble them once they are secreted. Once these are assembled, the mature elastin fibril is rendered elastic and gives the skin its ability to bounce back. The complex assembly process makes it hard for the skin to produce functional elastin after puberty. This is why older skin sags and does not bounce back. Aged skin contains less functional elastin than young skin. At this point, no topical or injectable products have convincingly been able to induce skin to synthesize functional elastin.

Hyaluronic Acid

The most abundant glycosaminoglycans in the dermis, HA is a sugar that binds 1,000 times its weight in water. HA allows the joints to flow properly and helps the skin attract and hold onto water, giving the dermis its volume. In addition, HA plays an important role in cell growth, membrane receptor function, and cellular adhesion. Older people have less HA in their joints and skin. This is why a baby's skin is plump while an older person's skin is not. HA is the ingredient in dermal fillers such as Restylane and Juvéderm.

■ CONCLUSION

Aged skin has fewer fibroblasts than young skin. Topical cosmeceuticals have been developed to stimulate fibroblast production. To date, however, cosmeceuticals have only been successful in spurring fibroblasts to produce collagen. Elastin is associated with such a complex assembly process that no known topical formulations have been developed that undoubtedly increase the levels of functional elastin. There is some evidence that glucosamine supplementation can increase the production of HA but the evidence is weak.[11,12] Topical retinoids have been proven to increase HA production, though.[13] Many skin care products contain collagen, elastin, or HA in the preparation; however, these large structures do not penetrate into the dermis and are unable to replace lost collagen, elastin, and HA in the aged dermis despite the claims made by cosmetic product manufacturers.

Most products on the market, including cleansers, scrubs, antiaging products, and moisturizers, actually act on the epidermis and are unable to penetrate down into the dermis. These products can help temporarily improve cutaneous appearance by hydrating the skin, which diminishes fine lines and removes the desquamating keratinocytes. This smoothes the surface of the skin, allowing it to better reflect light and look "radiant." These products can also decrease skin pigmentation leading to a more even skin tone. Only a few ingredients are known to penetrate into and cause a long-lasting biological change in the dermis. Ingredients known to easily penetrate into the dermis include hormones such as estrogen, retinoids such as tretinoin, some growth factors, and immune response modifiers such as imiquimod. Proving that an ingredient penetrates into the dermis and causes a biologic change is a tricky proposition for a cosmetic company because of the way that cosmetic ingredients are regulated as compared to ingredients labeled as drugs.[14] If an ingredient is shown to penetrate into the dermis and produce a biologic change, then the Food and Drug Administration requires that the formulation enter the drug regulatory pathway, which is very expensive, can take years, and results in a product that is available only by prescription. For this reason, cosmetic companies are actually encouraged or incentivized not to do research, so that their product can be labeled as a "cosmetic" and be made available over the counter without required research trials. For more information about cosmetic claims, see Chapter 4, Cosmeceutical Marketing Claims.

REFERENCES

1. Sander CS, Chang H, Hamm F, et al. Role of oxidative stress and the antioxidant network in cutaneous carcinogenesis. *Int J Dermatol*. 2004;43:326.
2. De Graaf YG, Euvrard S, Bouwes Bavinck JN. Systemic and topical retinoids in the management of skin cancer in organ transplant recipients. *Dermatol Surg*. 2004;30(4 Pt 2):656.
3. Bornstein P, Sage H. Structurally distinct collagen types. *Annu Rev Biochem*. 1980;49:957.
4. Di Lullo GA, Sweeney SM, Korkko J, et al. Mapping the ligand-binding sites and disease-associated mutations on the most abundant protein in the human, type I collagen. *J Biol Chem*. 2002;277:4223.
5. Nelson B, Majmudar G, Griffiths C, et al. Clinical improvement following dermabrasion of photoaged skin correlates with synthesis of collagen I. *Arch Derm*. 1994;130:1136.
6. Skinner SM, Gage JP, Wilce PA, et al. A preliminary study of the effects of laser radiation on collagen metabolism in cell structure. *Aust Dent J*. 1996;41:188.
7. Orringer JS, Kang S, Johnson TM, et al. Connective tissue remodeling induced by carbon dioxide laser resurfacing of photodamaged human skin. *Arch Dermatol*. 2004;140:1326.
8. Weiss RA, Weiss MA, Beasley KL. Rejuvenation of photoaged skin: 5 years results with intense pulsed light of the face, neck, and chest. *Dermatol Surg*. 2002;28:1115.
9. Wang F, Garza LA, Kang S, et al. In vivo stimulation of de novo collagen production caused by cross-linked hyaluronic acid dermal filler injections in photodamaged human skin. *Arch Dermatol*. 2007;143:155.
10. Rosenbloom J, Abrams WR. Elastin and the microfibrillar apparatus. In: Royce PM, Steinmann B, eds. *Connective Tissue and Its Heritable Disorders: Molecular, Genetic, and Medical Aspects*. 2nd ed. Hoboken, NJ: Wiley-Liss; 2002:249–269.
11. Bissett DL. Glucosamine: An ingredient with skin and other benefits. *J Cosmet Dermatol*. 2006;5:309.
12. Murad H, Tabibian MP. The effect of an oral supplement containing glucosamine, amino acids, minerals, and antioxidants on cutaneous aging: A preliminary study. *J Dermatolog Treat*. 2001;12:47.
13. Tammi R, Tammi M. Influence of retinoic acid on the ultrastructure and hyaluronic acid synthesis of adult human epidermis in whole skin organ culture. *J Cell Physiol*. 1986;126:389.
14. Weisberg E, Baumann L. Cosmetic and drug regulation. In: Baumann L, Saghari S, Weisberg E, eds. *Cosmetic Dermatology: Principles and Practice*. 2nd ed. New York: McGraw-Hill; 2009:241.

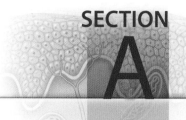

Cleansing Agents

C H A P T E R 6

Overview of Cleansing Agents

The primary purpose of cleansing is to remove oil, bacteria, sweat, dirt, and desquamated skin cells from the face and body. However, cleansers can react with lipids and proteins on the skin and incite keratinocytes to release cytokines, all of which can irritate or damage the skin's surface.[1,2] Surface-active substances, known as surfactants, work by reducing the surface tension on the skin and emulsifying dirt.[3] There are various kinds of surfactants found in cleansers.

ANIONIC (NEGATIVELY CHARGED) SURFACTANTS

Anionic surfactants form generous foam and have the highest cleansing power. Consequently, these compounds are often found as the primary surfactants in cleansers (Table 6-1). "Soap" contains the anionic surfactant alkyl carboxylate. These anionic agents are potent irritants to the skin,[4] and have been found to cause harmful swelling of cell membranes.[5,6] The well-known anionic agent (a type of alkyl sulfate) sodium lauryl sulfate (SLS), which strips lipids from the skin, is so irritating that it is used in the research setting to impair the skin barrier in order to test "barrier repair products." Sodium laureth sulfate (or sodium lauryl ether sulfate, also known as SLES) has good cleansing power but is less likely to provoke irritation than SLS.

TABLE 6-1

Anionic Agents used in Surfactants

Acyl glycinates
Acylglutamates
Alkyl acyl isethionates
Alkyl carboxylates
Alkyl ether sulfates
Alkyl ethoxy sulfates
Alkyl phosphates
Alkyl sulfates
Alkyl sulfonates
Alkyl sulfosuccinates
Alkyl taurates

CATIONIC (POSITIVELY CHARGED) SURFACTANTS

Cationic surfactants have lower detergent properties than anionic surfactants and are very irritating, but are typically used because of their antimicrobial properties. These surfactants often lead to the hand dermatitis seen in frequent hand washers. Cetrimide, chlorhexidine, and benzalkonium chloride are examples of cationic surfactants.

AMPHOTERIC SURFACTANTS

Amphoteric surfactants exhibit changing properties depending on the pH of the solution. Amphoterics are popular because they lather well, exhibit good cleansing power and compatibility with different pHs, display moderate antimicrobial activity, and cause minimal irritation. Examples include cocamidopropyl betaine, cocoamphoacetate, and cocoamphodiacetate.

NONIONIC SURFACTANTS

Nonionic agents have no electric charge. They are expensive and demonstrate poor cleansing characteristics but are believed to cause less irritation than anionic or cationic cleansers. Nonionic agents have been found to disrupt the skin barrier by solubilizing fatty acids and cholesterol.[2] Examples of nonionic surfactants include cocoglucoside, lauryl glucoside, decylglucoside, and coconut diethanolamine (cocamide DEA).

IRRITANCY

Several factors influence the irritancy potential of cleansers including the amount of time left on the skin, rinsability, pH, and the susceptibility of the skin to irritation. (Individuals with a Baumann Skin Type designated as S_4 are more susceptible to irritation because their skin barrier is impaired.) The surfactant type is the main influence on irritancy. Surfactants with C_{10}–C_{14} chain lengths are the most aggressive because they are the most active in solution.

NEWER CLASSES OF CLEANSERS

Attempts to diminish the irritancy of soaps through the addition of secondary components have led to the development of newer classes of cleansers such as superfatted soaps, transparent soaps, and combination bars (combars). Bars composed of synthetic surfactants are often referred to as "syndet bars." These surfactants have a neutral pH, and include ingredients such as alkyl glyceryl ether sulfonate, α-olefin sulfonates, betaines, sulfosuccinates, sodium cocoyl monoglyceride sulfate, and sodium cocoyl isethionate. Organic preparations are also available and include ingredients such as saponins and sucrose laurate.

NATURAL INGREDIENTS IN CLEANSERS

Saponins are a large family of structurally-related compounds derived from plants. The word "saponin" originates from the plant genus *Saponaria*. Many saponins manifest foaming characteristics that make them a good option for natural or organic cleansers. Saponins are composed of a steroid or triterpenoid aglycone (sapogenin) linked to one or more oligosaccharide moieties by glycosidic linkage.[7] The foaming action of saponins emerge by dint of the combination of the non-polar sapogenin and the water-soluble side chain. The *Sapindus mukorossi* (soapnut) plant has been used as a natural cleanser and displayed antimicrobial activity in one study.[8–11] *Camellia oleifera* has been shown to exhibit notable detergent abilities.[7] Several plants contain saponins, including alfalfa foliage, peas, chickpeas, horse chestnut trees, soybeans, and daisies. Desert plants, including *Yucca schidigera* and *Quillaja saponaria*, are good sources of saponins and are found in natural cleansers on the market.

CLEANSER CHOICE

The choice of cleanser is pivotal for individuals that suffer from excessively oily or dry skin. Oily skin benefits from foaming cleansers that can strip unwanted sebum lipids from the skin, while people with dry skin are better served with lipid-sparing gentle cleansers such as milks and creams.

REFERENCES

1. Bárány E, Lindberg M, Lodén M. Biophysical characterization of skin damage and recovery after exposure to different surfactants. *Contact Dermatitis.* 1999;40:98.
2. Ananthapadmanabhan KP, Moore DJ, Subramanyan K, et al. Cleansing without compromise: the impact of cleansers on the skin barrier and the technology of mild cleansing. *Dermatol Ther.* 2004;17(Suppl 1):16.
3. Corazza M, Lauriola MM, Zappaterra M, et al. Surfactants, skin cleansing protagonists. *J Eur Acad Dermatol Venereol.* 2010;24:1.
4. Effendy I, Maibach HI. Surfactants and experimental irritant contact dermatitis. *Contact Dermatitis.* 1995;33:217.
5. Wilhelm KP, Freitag G, Wolff HH. Surfactant-induced skin irritation and skin repair. Evaluation of the acute human irritation model by noninvasive techniques. *J Am Acad Dermatol.* 1994;30:944.
6. Froebe CL, Simion FA, Rhein LD, et al. Stratum corneum lipid removal by surfactants: Relation to in vivo irritation. *Dermatologica.* 1990;181:277.
7. Chen YF, Yang CH, Chang MS, et al. Foam properties and detergent abilities of the saponins from Camellia oleifera. *Int J Mol Sci.* 2010;11:4417.
8. Aneja KR, Joshi R, Sharma C. In vitro antimicrobial activity of Sapindus mukorossi and Emblica officinalis against dental caries pathogens. *Ethnobotanical Leaflets.* 2010;14:402.
9. Kamra DN, Patra AK, Chatterjee PN, et al. Effect of plant extracts on methanogenesis and microbial profile of the rumen of buffalo: A brief overview. *Austral J Exp Agric.* 2008;48:175.
10. Patra AK, Saxena J. The effect and mode of action of saponins on the microbial populations and fermentation in the rumen and ruminant production. *Nutr Res Rev.* 2009;22:204.
11. Rakesh M, Ashok K, Kumar S, et al. Formulation of herbal shampoos from Asparagus racemosus, Acacia concin, Sapindus mukorosii. *Int J Pharm Sci Rev Res.* 2010;4:39.

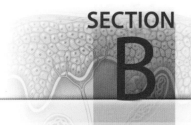

CHAPTER 7

Moisturizing Agents

In the 1950s, Blank demonstrated that low moisture content of the skin is a prime factor in dry skin conditions.[1] It is now known that the symptoms of dry skin can be treated by increasing the hydration state of the stratum corneum with occlusive or humectant ingredients; smoothing the rough surface with an emollient; restoring the integrity of the skin barrier; increasing natural moisturizing factor (NMF) or the activity of aquaporin; and controlling the calcium gradient. Choosing the correct cleanser is also crucial in the treatment of dry skin (see Chapter 6, Overview of Cleansing Agents).

Various types of moisturizers are combined to form the best strategy for treating the underlying issues leading to dry skin. Several factors should be taken into account when choosing the type of moisturizing ingredients. The first is the Baumann Skin Type (BST) (see Chapter 1, The Importance of Skin Type: The Baumann Skin Type System). The level of dryness determined by the Baumann Skin Typing System (BSTS), designated by D_1 D_2 D_3, gives information about the severity of skin dryness. A higher D score such as D_3 indicates that more than one defect is contributing to skin dryness and that multiple strategies should be chosen. If the BST also includes type 4 sensitive (S_4) skin, then there is evidence that the skin barrier is severely impaired and the barrier repair strategy should take top priority. If the Baumann Skin Type Indicator (BSTI) questionnaire that determines BST detects signs of increased sebum secretion, then an occlusive moisturizer would be unnecessary because sebum is a great occlusive moisturizer. Individuals who have dry skin with increased sebum secretion likely have defects such as impaired aquaporin function, decreased NMF, altered calcium channels, or they may be using barrier-disturbing cleansers that are leading to the dry skin. Noting the humidity level of the environment prior to choosing a moisturizer is important because humectant ingredients work better in a humid environment. Knowing habits such as increased sun exposure (which lowers NMF) and prolonged immersion in water (which disturbs the skin barrier) can also give clues about the causes of dry skin.

The ingredients in this chapter are divided into subsections according to their mechanism of action. Some ingredients have more than one mechanism of action. In that case, they will be discussed in the subsection that displays the unique characteristics of that ingredient and distinguishes it from others. For example, glycerin is a well-known and very effective humectant, but it has the unique property of being able to pass through the aquaporin channels so it will be discussed in the aquaporin subsection. The mechanisms will be briefly explained at the beginning of each subsection. For more detailed information on the causes of dry skin, see *Cosmetic Dermatology: Principles and Practice*, 2nd edition, McGraw-Hill (2009).

Emollients are substances added to cosmetics to soften and smooth the skin and are composed mainly of lipids and oil. They act by filling the spaces between desquamating corneocytes to create a smooth surface. Emollients provide increased cohesion of cells causing a flattening of the curled edges of the individual corneocytes and a smoother surface with less friction and greater light refraction. Most emollients function as occlusives but some exhibit humectant activity; therefore, they will be discussed in the corresponding subsections of this chapter. Lanolin, mineral oil, shea butter, safflower oil, and petrolatum are examples of occlusive ingredients that also confer an emollient effect. Long chain saturated fatty acids and fatty alcohols are often used as emollients, such as stearic, linoleic, linolenic, oleic, and lauric acids.

REFERENCE

1. Blank IH. Factors which influence the water content of the stratum corneum. *J Invest Dermatol*. 1952;18:433.

CHAPTER 8

Occlusives

Occlusive agents are usually oily substances that coat the stratum corneum (SC) rendering an emollient effect as well as the ability to decrease transepidermal water loss (TEWL). Two of the best occlusive ingredients currently available are petrolatum and mineral oil. Petrolatum, for example, has a water vapor loss resistance 170 times that of olive oil.[1] However, petrolatum and mineral oil have a greasy feeling on the skin, leaving them cosmetically undesirable, and have further lost popularity because of the greater awareness of the environmental effects of processing these products. Other synthetic agents commonly used as occlusive ingredients include paraffin, squalene, dimethicone, and propylene glycol.[2] Lanolin is an example of a natural occlusive ingredient. Organic occlusive ingredients have also become increasingly popular and include argan oil, beeswax, borage seed oil, safflower oil, olive oil, jojoba oil, and tamanu oil. Occlusive ingredients seem to be most effective when placed over damp skin and are only effective while present on the skin because once removed, TEWL returns to the normal level. Occlusives are usually combined with humectant ingredients.

INFLUENCES ON THE OCCLUSIVE EFFECT[3]

In order for an ingredient to impart an occlusive effect, the molecules in that ingredient must be able to align to form a tight barrier (or palisade). Short straight chains of the same length are the most efficient at aligning in this manner. When a product contains various compounds with diverse types of chains or with different chain lengths, it is inherently a less effective occlusive than an agent with a consistent type of molecule with a straight chain. An example of a well-structured occlusive is mineral oil, which contains straight alkyl chains but of varying lengths. This contributes to its ability to form a tight palisade on the skin and exhibit a strong occlusive effect (Figure 8-1). If mineral oil had straight alkyl chains of the same length, its occlusive effect would be even stronger. In contrast, the molecules in botanical oils can be extremely diverse, making it difficult for the molecules to tightly align. For this reason, many botanical oils make poor occlusive agents.

Another factor that determines occlusive ability is ingredient substantivity, or the ability of the ingredients to stay on the skin's surface. If the molecules rapidly penetrate into the SC, then the result is a weaker palisade or occlusive effect, which is known as lower substantivity. Therefore, ingredients with larger molecules and a comparatively lower capacity to penetrate the SC, thus higher substantivity, may display greater occlusive activity. Viscosity can also affect occlusive ability. For example, petrolatum has a higher viscosity than mineral oil and is a much better occlusive. In many cases, such as petrolatum, high viscosity corresponds with low spreadability. Therefore, ingredients with a very high viscosity may offer less cosmetic appeal to consumers because of their decreased spreadability. Viscosity also influences the occlusive effect insofar as in less viscous formulations, the ingredient diffuses laterally allowing the palisade to break down, which results in a less occlusive effect. The viscosity of a completed formulation can be adjusted with the addition of

Water vapor permeability of different emollients (conditions: 25°C, 35% rel. humidity, 24 hours)	
Emollient	*Water vapor permeability (%)*
Control	6.63
1. Isopropyl myristate	3.04
2. Ethyl oleate	2.84
3. Isopropyl palmitate	2.73
4. Isopropyl stearate	2.43
5. 2-ethyl-hexyl cocoate	2.07
6. 2-ethyl-hexyl palmitate	1.66
7. Decyl oleate	1.54
8. 2-ethyl-hexyl tallowate	1.51
9. 2-ethyl-hexyl stearate	1.47
10. Oleyl oleate	1.21
11. 2-octyl-dodecyl myristate	0.94
12. Oleyl erucate	0.93
13. 2-octyl-dodecyl palmitate	0.85
14. 2-octyl-dodecyl stearate	0.78
15. Mineral oil	0.30

▲ **FIGURE 8-1** Various ingredients were studied for effects on TEWL and mineral oil was found to be superior to the others tested. Reprinted with permission from Rawlings AV, Lombardi KJ. A review on the extensive skin benefits of mineral oil. *Int J Cosmet Sci* 2012;34:511.

hyaluronic acid, sugars, and various polymers that may positively or negatively impact the efficacy of the final product.

The concentration of ingredients also plays an important role in occlusive ability. There must be enough of the occlusive ingredient in a formula for it to be an active occlusive. Many cosmetic emollients are not included in a sufficient concentration to be effective. Other reasons that occlusives would lose efficacy include: they are not viscous enough to exhibit an adequate degree of substantivity; their components are not regularly shaped well enough to form a tight palisade; or their activity is diminished by other ingredients in the formulation. Therefore, when evaluating the occlusive aspects of a product, it is necessary to consider the final viscosity and physical characteristics of the formula and the interactions of major and minor ingredients.

REFERENCES

1. Spruitt D. The interference of some substances with the water vapor loss of human skin. *Dermatologica*. 1971;142:89.
2. Draelos Z. Moisturizers. In: *Atlas of Cosmetic Dermatology*. New York Churchill Livingstone; 2000:83.
3. Rawlings AV, Lombard KJ. A review on the extensive skin benefits of mineral oil. *Int J Cosmet Sci*. 2012;34:511.

CHAPTER 9

Oils

Oil is a substance that is liquid at room temperature and insoluble in water. Synthetic oils include mineral oil and petrolatum, which are derived from the distillation of petroleum in the production of gasoline. Vegetable oils are pressed out of seeds, and essential oils are steamed from several plant parts, including stems, leaves, and roots. The Cosmetic Ingredient Review (CIR) categorizes vegetable oils in the larger class of edible oils. Edible oils, such as peanut oil, are refined in a process that removes proteins that can cause sensitization in allergic individuals.[1] Manufacturers of animal-derived oils, such as lanolin, have to follow strictly certified processes in order to eliminate any risk of infectious agents.

TRIGLYCERIDES

Most oils and fats are triglycerides, which are composed of glycerol and fatty acids. Natural triglycerides contain the five most common fatty acids in various proportions: palmitic, stearic, oleic, linoleic, and linolenic acids.

FATTY ACIDS

Oils contain a large variety of fatty acids, with stearic, oleic, and linoleic acids among the most abundant.[2] The fatty acid profile for a certain oil helps to determine the oil's characteristics with respect to skin feel, substantivity, occlusive ability, penetration, biologic activity, and stability. Stability is influenced by susceptibility to oxidation: fatty acids with a higher degree of unsaturation are oxidized more easily. Essential fatty acids (EFAs) are those that the body cannot synthesize and, therefore, must be obtained topically or in the diet. Vegetable and fish oils contain EFAs such as ω-6 and ω-3 fatty acids. EFAs influence skin barrier function, membrane fluidity, cell signaling, and the inflammatory eicosanoid pathway. Nonessential fatty acids and EFAs play important roles in skin function.

Linoleic Acid

Linoleic acid is an EFA. Several edible oils contain linoleic acid. Linoleic acid is an unsaturated ω-6 fatty acid present in many oils including sunflower and safflower (Table 9-1). In addition to providing structural lipids needed for barrier integrity, linoleic acid is used by the body to produce γ-linolenic acid (GLA). GLA is a polyunsaturated essential cis-fatty acid important in the production of prostaglandins; therefore, it plays a role in the inflammatory process.

Oleic Acid

Oleic acid is technically not an EFA because the body can produce a small amount; however, it is a very important fatty acid for the skin. Oleic acid has a polar head group attached to a long alkyl chain.[3,4] This structure allows it to disrupt the

TABLE 9-1
Oils That Contain Linoleic Acid

OILS
Black currant
Borage
Chestnut
Coconut
Corn
Cotton seed
Evening primrose
Grape seed
Hemp
Macadamia
Olive
Palm
Peanut
Pistachio
Poppy seed
Rice bran
Safflower
Sesame
Soybean
Sunflower
Walnut
Wheat germ

barrier by inserting its alkyl chains into ceramides. In turn, this sets the stage for a phase separation to occur, leading to pools of oleic acid in the membrane, which is more fluid and easier for molecules to diffuse through than intact ceramides.[5] The result is barrier disruption and increased penetration of molecules. Oleic acid is found in high amounts in olive oil.

Stearic Acid

Stearic acid is made by the body, and therefore is not an EFA. It is very commonly seen in skin care products (see Chapter 23, Stearic Acid).

EDIBLE OILS VERSUS MINERAL OILS

Edible oils contain a wide variety of chemical components, such as unsaturated, aromatic groups and polyphenols, which affect its activity whereas mineral oil contains mainly straight-chain hydrocarbons. Edible oils can be used to deliver a specific effect or activity, such as anti-inflammatory or antioxidant, while mineral oils, which are inert, only provide an occlusive, softening effect. Some edible oils increase penetration of ingredients in other topically applied products while mineral oils seem to decrease penetration of ingredients.[6] Edible oils, including those in cosmetics,[7] may contain harmful aflatoxins that occur when the crops have an infestation of a type of fungus known as *Aspergillum*.[8] Aflatoxins are toxic and carcinogenic. In fact, aflatoxins have been used to induce skin cancer in the research setting.[9] High temperature and high humidity favor the growth of *Aspergillum*. The United States Food and Drug Administration (USFDA) has developed standards to protect crops from aflatoxin contamination, but not all countries have adopted this approach.[10] The risk of aflatoxins is an example that lends credence to the statement that "natural" products are not necessarily safer than synthetic products.[11]

SAFETY

Essential Oils

Essential oils have increased in popularity. However, it is crucial to realize that these products can act as allergens.[12] Massage therapists and others who are routinely exposed to essential oils are at risk for developing an allergy to the topically applied oil that can translate to an allergy to that oil in food products.[13]

The CIR report in December 2010 stated that edible oils are believed to be safe for use on the skin. Those with an allergy to a food are most likely allergic to the proteins in the food. This protein does not partition into the refined oil; therefore, someone with a peanut allergy likely will not react to peanut oil. Oils that have been associated with causing a contact allergy include soybean, sunflower seed, olive, avocado, sesame seed, cashew, and macadamia.[14]

TUMORIGENESIS

Published data provide substantial evidence that some vehicles, particularly the lighter oils, enhance penetration of ultraviolet radiation (UVR) into mouse skin, leading to a greater cutaneous response—sometimes nearly doubling the effectiveness of a UVR dose.[15] Heavier formulations, such as petrolatum and lanolin, were shown by Kligman and Kligman to prevent tumorigenesis.[16] Lu et al. demonstrated that certain moisturizing creams enhanced tumorigenesis in mice, but a formulation that excluded mineral oil did not.[17] It seems apparent that all oils have light-reflective properties and can allow more light to be absorbed into the skin; however, it is unknown at this time exactly what roles various oils play, if any, in skin cancer formation. Animal and human studies of mineral oil are conflicting. Botanical oils that contain antioxidants, for example, may be able to neutralize any damage caused by increased absorption of UV light.[18]

REFERENCES

1. Yunginger JW, Calobrisi SD. Investigation of the allergenicity of a refined peanut-oil-containing topical dermatologic agent in persons who are sensitive to peanuts. *Cutis*. 2001;68:153.
2. Lodén M. Role of topical emollients and moisturizers in the treatment of dry skin barrier disorders. *Am J Clin Dermatol*. 2003;4:771.
3. Naik A, Pechtold LA, Potts RO, et al. Mechanism of oleic acid-induced skin penetration enhancement in vivo in humans. *J Control Release*. 1995;37:299.
4. Ongpipattanakul B, Burnette RR, Potts RO, et al. Evidence that oleic acid exists in a separate phase within stratum corneum lipids. *Pharm Res*. 1991;8:350.
5. Hadgraft J. Modulation of the barrier function of the skin. *Skin Pharmacol Appl Skin Physiol*. 2001;14(Suppl 1):72.
6. Sahlin A, Edlund F, Lodén M. A double-blind and controlled study on the influence of the vehicle on the skin susceptibility to stinging from lactic acid. *Int J Cosmet Sci*. 2007;29:385.
7. Mahoney N, Molyneux RJ. Rapid analytical method for the determination of aflatoxins in plant-derived dietary supplement and cosmetic oils. *J Agric Food Chem*. 2010;58:4065.
8. Cavaliere C, Foglia P, Guarino C, et al. Determination of aflatoxins in olive oil by liquid chromatography-tandem mass spectrometry. *Anal Chim Acta*. 2007;596:141.
9. Rastogi S, Shukla Y, Paul BN, et al. Protective effect of Ocimum sanctum on 3-methylcholanthrene, 7,12-dimethylbenz(a) anthracene and aflatoxin B1 induced skin tumorigenesis in mice. *Toxicol Appl Pharmacol*. 2007;224:228.
10. el-Dessouki S. Aflatoxins in cosmetics containing substrates for aflatoxin-producing fungi. *Food Chem Toxicol*. 1992;30:993.
11. Antignac E, Nohynek GJ, Re T, et al. Safety of botanical ingredients in personal care products/cosmetics. *Food Chem Toxicol*. 2011;49:324.
12. Boonchai W, Iamtharachai P, Sunthonpalin P. Occupational allergic contact dermatitis from essential oils in aromatherapists. *Contact Dermatitis*. 2007;56:181.
13. Bleasel N, Tate B, Rademaker M. Allergic contact dermatitis following exposure to essential oils. *Australas J Dermatol*. 2002;43:211.
14. Cosmetic Ingredient Review: Draft report of the plant-derived edible oil group. http://www.cir-safety.org/sites/default/files/117_draft_oils.pdf. Washington, DC 2010. Accessed October 17, 2012.
15. Forbes PD. Moisturizers, vehicle effects, and photocarcinogenesis. *J Invest Dermatol*. 2009;129:261.
16. Kligman LH, Kligman AM. Petrolatum and other hydrophobic emollients reduce UVB-induced damage. *J Dermatolog Treat*. 1992;3:3.
17. Lu YP, Lou YR, Xie JG, et al. Tumorigenic effect of some commonly used moisturizing creams when applied topically to UVB-pretreated high-risk mice. *J Invest Dermatol*. 2009;129:468.
18. Perchellet JP, Perchellet EM, Belman S. Inhibition of DMBA-induced mouse skin tumorigenesis by garlic oil and inhibition of two tumor-promotion stages by garlic and onion oils. *Nutr Cancer*. 1990;14:183.

CHAPTER 10

Argan Oil

Activities:

Prostaglandin inhibition, antioxidant, barrier disruption and barrier repair, penetration enhancer

Important Chemical Components:

Major: Oleic acid, linoleic acid, palmitic acid, stearic acid[1]
Minor: Polyphenols (caffeic acid, vanillic acid, syringic acid, ferulic acid, tyrosol, catechol, resorcinol, (−)-epicatechin, (+)-catechin, p-hydroxybenzoic)
Sterols (stigmasta-8,22-diene-3-ol, spinasterol, schottenol, stigmasta, 7-24-diene-3-ol)
Tocopherols (α-, β-, γ-, and δ-tocopherols)
Squalene, carotenes, and triterpene alcohols[1-4]

Origin Classification:

This ingredient is considered natural. Organic forms are available.

Personal Care Category:

Antioxidant, moisturizing, anti-inflammatory

Recommended for the following Baumann Skin Types:

All dry types and sensitive types will benefit from this ingredient but it is best for DRNW, DRPW, DSNT, DSNW, DSPT, and DSPW.

SOURCE

Argan oil is derived from the fruit of *Argania spinosa*, which is a slow-growing tree native to the arid climate of southwestern Morocco (where it is the third most common tree regionally) as well as the Algerian province of Tindouf in the western Mediterranean area.[5,6]

HISTORY

For more than 800 years, native Moroccans and explorers to the region have cited the health benefits of argan oil consumption and topical use.[2] Traditionally, the vegetable oil has been prescribed for reputed cosmetic, bactericidal, and fungicidal properties and as a treatment for infertility and heart disease.[4,6] Argan oil has been used as a treatment for acne, dry skin, dry hair, hair loss, psoriasis, wrinkles, skin inflammation, and joint pain.[6,7]

CHEMISTRY

The ω-9 monounsaturated fatty acid known as oleic acid makes up a large proportion of the oil (43–49 percent) and has been found to be a penetration enhancer by disturbing the skin barrier.[8,9] An ω-6 polyunsaturated fatty acid known as linoleic acid (29–36 percent of the oil) is integral in the biosynthesis of inflammatory prostaglandins through the arachidonic acid pathway.[4,10] The

TABLE 10-1
Pros and Cons of Argan Oil

PROS	CONS
Polyphenol content supports antioxidant reputation	Oily, heavy texture
Use of argan forestry reforestation to stem desertification in Northern Africa	Very expensive, so often used in small amounts
Anecdotal experience has shown its usefulness in rosacea	

presence of linoleic acid may help prevent or decrease inflammation. Linoleic acid is also a component of ceramide 1 linoleate, which is decreased in dry skin. Topical application of linoleic acid can increase ceramide 1 linoleate levels in skin, thus reducing xerosis.[11] Argan oil also contains the saturated fatty acids palmitic acid (11–15 percent) and stearic acid (4–7 percent).[5]

Though argan oil is mainly composed of unsaturated fatty acids (80 percent), the unsaponifiable fraction (1 percent) is rife with antioxidants, including sterols, saponins, and polyphenols.[1,2,4,12] It is the polyphenolic constituents, mainly γ-tocopherol, that are thought to be primarily responsible for the antioxidant effects (Table 10-1).[1,2,12,13]

Olive and argan oils have been compared because of their similar roles in regional diets and their purported medical benefits. Though olive oil has been far more extensively studied, it is worth noting that both vegetable oils have oleic and linoleic acids as their primary constituents; both are also rich in vitamin E. However, argan oil contains two to three times the amount of tocopherol. The main form of vitamin E in olive oil is α-tocopherol. Argan oil contains γ-tocopherol, which is considered the most efficient among the tocopherols at scavenging free radicals.[1,5,14]

ORAL USES

Argan oil is available in edible and cosmetic grades. Argan fruit kernels are roasted in the preparation of edible argan oil. Virgin argan oil is higher in total antioxidant capacity than other vegetable oils.[3] Edible argan oil is known to have a taste similar to hazelnut. Argan oil used for cosmetic purposes is gold in color and has no taste. Given its abundant supply of fatty acids, phenolic constituents, squalene, sterols, and tocopherols, argan oil is also thought to be an important factor in enhancing the anticancer influences of the Moroccan diet.[12] Drissi and other colleagues involved in much of the published research on argan oil recently studied the effects of its regular consumption on the lipid profile and antioxidant status in healthy Moroccan subjects (62 consumers and 34 nonconsumers, of whom 76 were women and 20 were men). The researchers found that plasma low-density lipoprotein (LDL) cholesterol levels were lower in participants who regularly consumed virgin argan oil and their diets contained higher levels of polyunsaturated fats, as compared to the nonconsumers. They also investigated the *in vitro* effects of the tocopherols, sterols, and polyphenols in the herbal extract on LDL peroxidation, finding plasma lipoperoxides lower and the molar ratio of α-tocopherol/total cholesterol and concentration of α-tocopherol higher in the consumer group as compared to nonconsumers. LDL oxidation was found to be similar in the two groups, despite the fact that consumers had higher plasma antioxidant concentrations and lower lipoperoxide levels. The investigators concluded that their findings clearly established the antioxidant and cholesterol-lowering activity imparted by the regular consumption of virgin argan oil, suggesting the viability of this natural extract as a dietary adjunct for lowering the risk of cardiovascular events.[15]

TOPICAL USES

Unroasted kernels are used to produce cosmetic-grade argan oil. Cosmetic argan oil is used in moisturizing creams, body lotions, and shampoos. Although argan oil contains components that have antioxidant and anti-inflammatory features and there are many patents on the use of argan oil in skin care, there is a paucity of published research studies looking at the effects of argan oil-containing skin care products on aging, inflamed, or dry skin. In one study, Dobrev assessed the efficacy of a sebum control cream composed of saw palmetto extract, sesame seeds, and argan oil in 20 healthy volunteers, 16 with oily skin and 4 with combination skin. During the two test months in the winter, the test formulation was applied twice daily to the face over four weeks. The volunteers were assessed clinically and by instrumental measurement before and after the study period. Questionnaires were completed by participants for a subjective evaluation of efficacy, tolerance, and cosmetic qualities. Objective measurements were made using a Sebumeter, Sebufix, Visioscope and Surface Evaluation of the Living Skin (SELS) software. Results indicated that all volunteers tolerated the product. In 95 percent of the participants, a visible sebum-regulating or antisebum efficacy was observed. In addition, clinical evaluation scores, casual sebum levels, and areas covered by oily spots declined significantly after one month of treatment. Dobrev concluded that this argan oil-containing formulation was efficacious in mitigating the greasiness and ameliorating the appearance of oily facial skin.[16] The mechanism of the effects on sebum production is perplexing and questionable without further research looking at argan oil alone. In addition, this sole open-label study does not support the use of argan oil as an antiaging or anti-inflammatory product, as it is most frequently employed. There are no other published studies on topical argan oil listed in PubMed.

The presence of camphor and 1,8-cineole in the fruit pulp of the fruit of *A. spinosa* has led some researchers to conclude that there is potential of the essential oil for use as an insect repellent.[17] In spite of the dearth of research, anecdotal evidence abounds and argan oil is an expensive and popular cosmetic product.

The best use for argan oil is as a moisturizing anti-inflammatory serum. Although the oleic acid components can harm the skin barrier, this can allow penetration of other ingredients such as linoleic acid, which can help the skin form hydrating ceramides. The disruption of the barrier caused by oleic acid is likely counteracted by the occlusive properties of the oil that help prevent transepidermal water loss (TEWL) from the skin. In addition, linoleic acid may help increase ceramide 1, which in turn strengthens the skin barrier. More importantly, the linoleic acid in argan oil helps prevent the production of inflammatory prostaglandins. The polyphenols in this compound have an anti-inflammatory and antioxidant effect as well (see Chapter 46, Antioxidants, and Chapter 64, Anti-Inflammatory Agents).

SAFETY ISSUES

Argan oil has been used safely by the Amazigh population of southern Morocco for centuries as part of their diet and as a topical cosmetic agent for just as long. It is not believed to be associated with acute or chronic toxicity. One case of anaphylaxis was reported in 2010.[18]

ENVIRONMENTAL IMPACT

The argan tree is endangered by the harsh environment and overexploitation.[2] It was protected first by Moroccan law, then in 1998 by the United Nations Educational Scientific and Cultural Organization (UNESCO), and the tree was added to the World Heritage List in 1999 and designated as a bioreserve.[5,19] The trees are important to the region because the roots help prevent encroachment of the Sahara desert, the locals use the fruits, leaves, and wood for their own needs, and the oil extracted from the tree is used in cooking and sold for use in skin and hair care products providing much needed income for the local Berber women. A third of Morocco's argan forest has disappeared in the last 100 years. A local economic interest group for the development, preservation, and valorization of the forest has been created and collaborations have been formed to harvest argan oil in a sustainable fashion.[5,20] The "argan forest" in Morocco is considered to be a crucial factor in stemming desertification, with sustainable development of the forest dating to 1995.

FORMULATION CONSIDERATIONS

Virgin edible and beauty oils are produced only in Morocco, but industrially prepared cosmetic argan oil, which uses solvent extraction of imported kernels, occurs primarily in Europe.[5] Cosmetic argan oil is limited to inclusion in moisturizers, shampoos, and other cosmetic products.[5]

USAGE CONSIDERATIONS

Virgin edible argan oil has a longer shelf-life than virgin beauty argan oil. At 77°F (25°C), the edible variety can last as long as two years, whereas the topical oil has a notably brief shelf-life of three to four months.[5,21]

SIGNIFICANT BACKGROUND

Once prevalent in North Africa, the *A. spinosa* tree is cultivated only in Morocco presently,[20] and is considered to be endangered, so its oil, which is labor-intensive to obtain, is becoming more valuable, increasing the risk of overexploitation of the trees.

There is little research on this botanical compound, but the preponderance of recent investigations has focused on the cardiovascular benefits of virgin argan oil consumption. Specifically, antiatherogenic, cholesterol-lowering, antiproliferative, and antioxidant benefits have been observed.[22–26]

Argan oil may qualify as one of the latest in a long line of "flavors-of-the-month" in terms of so-called "miracle" ingredients in the beauty industry. It is quite popular in France, Japan, as well as North America, and English and French tourists have been known for several years to return with argan oil from vacations in Morocco.[1,19] In fact, argan oil was identified as the world's most expensive oil in 2009 and ranked by the public relations firm Pierce Mattei as the number one cosmetic ingredient.[2] As a cosmetic agent, argan oil is touted for hydrating and revitalizing the skin, treating acne, and making the hair shine. The reputed therapeutic activities of topical argan oil are characterized as antiacne, antisebum, antiaging, moisturizing, and wound healing, but such claims are based on traditional uses and are associated with minimal scientific evidence.[5]

CONCLUSION

The body of published research, particularly clinical data, on argan oil is scant. However, in the author's experience, it is very useful in rosacea and reduces redness better than licorice extract, feverfew, and prescription azelaic acid and metronidazole. Further study is warranted, and randomized controlled trials are necessary to establish the efficacy of the use of argan oil in inflammatory disorders such as rosacea. Argan oil is expensive and most products currently on the market contain such a small amount of the oil that efficacy is doubtful.

REFERENCES

1. Charrouf Z, Guillaume D. Should the amazigh diet (regular and moderate argan-oil consumption) have a beneficial impact on human health? *Crit Rev Food Sci Nutr.* 2010;50:473.
2. Monfalouti HE, Guillaume D, Denhez C, et al. Therapeutic potential of argan oil: a review. *J Pharm Pharmacol.* 2010;62:1669.
3. Cabrera-Vique C, Marfil R, Giménez R, et al. Bioactive compounds and nutritional significance of virgin argan oil – An edible oil with potential as a functional food. *Nutr Rev.* 2012;70:266.
4. Cherki M, Berrougui H, Drissi A, et al. Argan oil: Which benefits on cardiovascular diseases? *Pharmacol Res.* 2006;54:1.
5. Guillaume D, Charrouf Z. Argan oil. Monograph. *Altern Med Rev.* 2011;16:275.
6. Charrouf Z, Guillaume D. Ethnoeconomical, ethnomedical, and phytochemical study of Argania spinosa (L.) Skeels. *J Ethnopharmacol.* 1999;67:7.
7. El Babili F, Bouajila J, Fouraste I, et al. Chemical study, antimalarial and antioxidant, and cytotoxicity to human breast cancer cells (MCF7) of Argania spinosa. *Phytomedicine.* 2010;17:157.
8. Naik A, Pechtold LA, Potts RO, et al. Mechanism of oleic acid-induced skin penetration enhancement in vivo in humans. *J Control Release.* 1995;37:299.
9. Tanojo H, Bosvan Geest A, Bouwstra JA et al. In vitro human skin barrier perturbation by oleic acid: Thermal analysis and freeze fracture electron microscopy studies. *Thermochimica Acta.* 1997;293:77.
10. Das UN. Essential fatty acid metabolism in patients with essential hypertension, diabetes mellitus and coronary heart disease. *Prostaglandins Leukot Essent Fatty Acids.* 1995;52:387.
11. Conti A, Rogers J, Verdejo P, et al. Seasonal influences on stratum corneum ceramide 1 fatty acids and the influence of topical essential fatty acids. *Int J Cosmet Sci.* 1996;18:1.
12. Khallouki F, Younos C, Soulimani R, et al. Consumption of argan oil (Morocco) with its unique profile of fatty acids, tocopherols, squalene, sterols and phenolic compounds should confer valuable cancer chemopreventive effects. *Eur J Cancer Prev.* 2003;12:67.
13. Amzal H, Alaoui K, Tok S, et al. Protective effect of saponins from Argania spinosa against free radical-induced oxidative haemolysis. *Fitoterapia.* 2008;79:337.
14. Jiang Q, Christen S, Shigenaga MK, et al. Gamma-tocopherol, the major form of vitamin E in the US diet, deserves more attention. *Am J Clin Nutr.* 2001;74:714.
15. Drissi A, Girona J, Cherki M, et al. Evidence of hypolipemiant and antioxidant properties of argan oil derived from the argan tree (Argania spinosa). *Clin Nutr.* 2004;23:1159.
16. Dobrev H. Clinical and instrumental study of the efficacy of a new sebum control cream. *J Cosmet Dermatol.* 2007;6:113.
17. Harhar H, Gharby S, Ghanmi M, et al. Composition of the essential oil of Argania spinosa (Sapotaceae) fruit pulp. *Nat Prod Commun.* 2010;5:935.
18. Astier C, Benchad Yel A, Moneret-Vautrin DA, et al. Anaphylaxis to argan oil. *Allergy.* 2010;65:662.
19. Larocca A. Liquid Gold in Morocco. *The New York Times,* Travel, November 18, 2007. http://travel.nytimes.com/2007/11/18/travel/tmagazine/14get-sourcing-caps.html. Accessed June 13, 2008.
20. Stussi I, Henry F, Moser P, et al. Argania spinosa – How ecological farming, fair trade and sustainability can drive the research for new cosmetic active ingredients. *SÖFW-Journal.* 2005;131:35.
21. Harhar H, Gharby S, Kartah BE, et al. Long argan fruit drying time is detrimental for argan oil quality. *Nat Prod Commun.* 2010;5:1799.
22. Derouiche A, Cherki M, Drissi A, et al. Nutritional intervention study with argan oil in man: Effects on lipids and apolipoproteins. *Ann Nutr Metab.* 2005;49:196.
23. Cherki M, Derouiche A, Drissi A, et al. Consumption of argan oil may have an antiatherogenic effect by improving paraoxonase activities and antioxidant status: Intervention study in healthy men. *Nutr Metab Cardiovasc Dis.* 2005;15:352.
24. Samane S, Noël J, Charrouf Z, et al. Insulin-sensitizing and antiproliferative effects of Argania spinosa seed extracts. *Evid Based Complement Alternat Med.* 2006;3:317.
25. Drissi A, Bennani H, Giton, F, et al. Tocopherols and saponins derived from Argania spinosa exert an antiproliferative effect on human prostate cancer. *Cancer Invest.* 2006;24:588.
26. Bennani H, Drissi A, Giton F, et al. Antiproliferative effect of polyphenols and sterols of virgin argan oil on human prostate cancer cell lines. *Cancer Detect Prev.* 2007;31:64.

CHAPTER 11

Borage Seed Oil

Activities:

Blocks formation of leukotrienes, increases production of ceramide 1

Important Chemical Components:

γ-linolenic acid (GLA), which ranges from 20 to 27 percent in borage oil[1]
α-linolenic acid (10 percent)
Palmitic, stearic, oleic, linoleic, eicosenoic, and erucic acids

Origin Classification:

This ingredient is considered natural. Organic forms are available.

Personal Care Category:

Lipophilic, occlusive, emollient, anti-inflammatory, hydrating

Recommended for the following Baumann Skin Types:

All dry and sensitive types benefit from this ingredient. It is best for DSNT, DSPT, DSNW, and DSPW. This ingredient may feel too greasy to individuals with oily skin types.

SOURCE

Borage (*Borago officinalis*) is an annual herb native to Syria and grown now throughout the Mediterranean region, Middle East, North Africa, Europe, and South America (Figure 11-1). Derived from the seeds of the plant, borage seed oil is used in medical practice for its anti-inflammatory activity in the treatment of atopic dermatitis, rheumatoid arthritis, and other conditions.

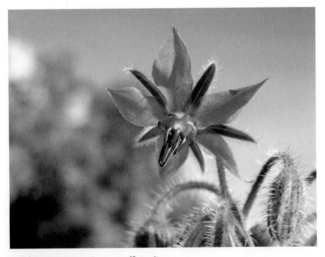

▲ **FIGURE 11-1** Borago officinalis.

HISTORY

B. officinalis, a wildflower also known as "starflower" for its star-shaped bright blue flowers, is a tall (average of 1.5 feet) herb used for over 1,500 years.[2] References to borage date back to the Roman historian Pliny the Elder and the Greek poet Homer, who cited the elixir "nepenthe," which is now believed to have been derived from borage leaves steeped in wine.[3] A medicinal tea made of borage leaves was frequently consumed in the Middle Ages.[2]

CHEMISTRY

Although human *skin* cannot synthesize GLA, it is produced elsewhere in the body but only in the presence of the fatty acid linoleic acid (LA). This is one of the main reasons why LA is a desirable ingredient in skin care products as well as oral supplements. LA also helps the body produce ceramide 1 (see Chapter 7, Moisturizing Agents). Because LA is not synthesized by the body, it must be consumed through the diet or absorbed topically. It is abundant in a wide range of vegetables, nuts, and seed oils.

The enzyme δ-6 desaturase (D6D), which is found in many cell types including fibroblasts and sebocytes, plays the crucial role of converting LA into GLA. GLA is subsequently metabolized into prostaglandin E_1 (PGE$_1$), which exhibits anti-inflammatory activity and aids in regulating transepidermal water loss (TEWL) and protecting the skin.[4] Borage seed oil has been shown to have two to three times more GLA than evening primrose oil, which itself is known to be a rich source of the essential acid.[5,6]

ORAL USES

Borage seed oil has been used for years to treat inflammatory conditions and dry skin (Table 11-1). Twenty years ago, Miller et al. fed guinea pigs borage oil containing 25 percent GLA or a control diet containing safflower oil (less than 0.5 percent GLA) for eight weeks. The goal of this study was to ascertain whether GLA could modulate cutaneous eicosanoids, which play an important role in inflammation. Examination of epidermal skin samples from the borage-treated animals revealed a significant increase in GLA and its product dihomo-γ-linolenic acid

TABLE 11-1
Pros and Cons of Borage Seed Oil

Pros	Cons
Potent anti-inflammatory agent	Greasy feel
Did not cause allergy in Cosmetic Ingredient Review studies	
May help increase ceramide production	
May help rosacea and other inflammatory skin conditions	
Does not inactivate retinoids or other ingredients	

(DGLA). A marked rise in the DGLA metabolites 15-hydroxy fatty acid (15-OH-20:3n-6) and (PGE_1), both of which exhibit anti-inflammatory potential, was also seen in the borage oil-fed guinea pigs. The investigators concluded that increased dietary GLA had the potential to produce local anti-inflammatory metabolites, thus warranting use to treat inflammatory skin disorders.[7]

Three years later, Miller et al. supplemented the diets of normal guinea pigs with either fish oil or GLA-rich borage oil, to determine the epidermal effects. Fish oil is rich in the ω-3 fatty acids eicosapentaenoic acid (EPA) and docosahexaenoic acid (DHA). The researchers found that fish oil and borage oil both inhibited production of leukotriene, which is a product of the arachidonic acid inflammatory cascade (see Chapter 64, Anti-inflammatory Agents). They concluded that the reported beneficial effects of fish and borage oils in treating chronic inflammatory skin disorders may be at least partly ascribed to the decreased production of leukotrienes.[8]

In 2000, Brosche and Platt assessed the effects of borage oil consumption on various skin parameters in 29 healthy elderly people (mean age 68.6 years). The subjects received a daily dose of borage oil in gelatin capsules for two months. A mean decrease of 10.8 percent was seen in TEWL. Although no significant changes in skin hydration were measured, the percentage of subjects that complained of dry skin dropped from 42 to 14 percent and complaints of itch dropped from 34 percent to none after treatment. The researchers concluded that consumption of borage oil improved the skin function of their healthy elderly study participants.[9] This study was not placebo controlled and changes in actual skin hydration were not seen in the measurements.

In early 2009, investigators tested the cutaneous effects of flaxseed oil and borage oil supplementation versus a medium-chain fatty acid placebo in a 12-week study of two groups of women. The flaxseed oil and borage seed oil groups experienced a decline in skin reddening and blood flow over the study. Skin hydration was increased in all groups, including the placebo group. After six weeks of supplementation, a 10 percent decrease in TEWL was noted in both the flaxseed and borage seed groups, with an additional reduction in TEWL after 12 weeks in the flaxseed group. Investigators found that skin roughness and scaling diminished significantly at week 12 as compared to baseline in both the flaxseed and borage seed groups.[10]

In 1999, Henz et al. conducted a 24-week double-blind, multicenter study with 160 adults with stable, moderately severe atopic eczema randomized to take daily a 500 mg borage oil capsule or a placebo. The researchers noted, though, that GLA metabolites increased in the borage oil-treated patients in this group, and serum IgE appeared to subside, and there was no improvement in eczema.[11] It is important to note that since the time of this trial, it has been discovered that eczema is caused by a genetic defect in filaggrin with a resulting decrease in natural moisturizing factor (NMF). Borage seed oil does not have any known effects on NMF, so studies looking at borage seed oil in subjects with eczema were really evaluating effects on inflammation rather than changes in the underlying problem of decreased NMF.

As an oral supplement, borage seed oil is believed to be useful in reducing skin inflammation and erythema. It may help improve the skin barrier and decrease TEWL by increasing ceramide levels. Studies have been conducted looking at borage seed oil in rheumatoid arthritis, where it seems to have an anti-inflammatory effect.[12] Borage seed oil may inhibit platelet function[13] and slow blood clotting, which would increase the risk of bruising.

TOPICAL USES

In 1993, Tollesson and Frithz studied the significance of TEWL and stratum corneum water content in disease and recovery in 37 patients with clinically diagnosed infantile seborrheic dermatitis and found that within 3 to 4 weeks of daily topical application of borage oil, all patients were symptom-free. The investigators concluded that GLA is key to maintaining normal TEWL and as a treatment for infantile seborrheic dermatitis.[14,15] It is likely that the anti-inflammatory properties of GLA rendered this treatment effective in seborrheic dermatitis.

The topical use of borage oil has demonstrated efficacy in the treatment of childhood eczema in small studies. In one study, the symptoms of childhood atopic dermatitis were relieved by undershirts coated with borage oil.[16–18] Borage seed oil cannot replace the missing NMF in eczema, but the hydrating and anti-inflammatory effects would explain the benefits seen in eczema. There are no published large, double-blinded, placebo-controlled trials looking at the effects of borage seed oil in non-eczematous dry skin or in inflammatory disorders like rosacea.

SAFETY ISSUES

No safety issues were found with borage seed oil in the plant-derived oils report by the Cosmetic Ingredient Review (CIR) on December 14, 2010.[19] The CIR report states that patch testing done by TKL labs and Clinique labs showed no irritation potential with topical borage seed oil.[20] WebMD states that borage seed oil is possibly safe for most adults and children as long as it is free of dangerous chemicals called pyrrolizidine alkaloids (PAs). They suggest that one should only use products that are certified and labeled PA-free.

ENVIRONMENTAL IMPACT

There are no known challenges or significant effects on the environment imposed by borage plant cultivation.

FORMULATION CONSIDERATIONS

Cold pressing borage oil extraction does not harm the final product quality, but its yield is lower than the yield of traditional oil extraction processes by solvent application. Using enzymes with pectinase and cellulase activities prior to the pressing stage can increase oil extraction yield.[21] Borage can be formulated with hydroxy acids and retinol and is thought to decrease the irritation that occurs from these compounds. A patent was filed on this by Chesebrough-Ponds in 1996. They stated that a preferred carrier is siloxane.

USAGE CONSIDERATIONS

Borage seed oil does not inactivate retinoids, antioxidants, or acids. Its effect on the absorption of other ingredients is unknown at this time.

SIGNIFICANT BACKGROUND

The use of borage oil has also been demonstrated as beneficial in treating rheumatoid arthritis, as indicated by recent double-blind studies.[22] It is believed that the GLA portion of borage oil raises PGE_1 levels that, in turn, augment cAMP levels, which inhibit the production of tumor necrosis factor-α, a central mediator in rheumatoid arthritis and other inflammatory processes.[23] Reviews of electronic database records by Cameron et al. in 2009 and 2011 of randomized controlled trials of herbal interventions to treat rheumatoid arthritis found moderate data that GLA-containing oils such as borage seed oil confer symptom relief.[24,25]

A 2010 review found 12 clinically controlled trials of oral or topical borage oil for the treatment of atopic dermatitis and one preventive trial. Though most were randomized and double-blind, they were typically small and otherwise limited methodologically, according to Foster et al. The results were mixed, with the effects of borage seed oil found to be significant in five studies, insignificant in five others, and inconclusive in two, though most studies indicated that at least a modest benefit was delivered by borage oil. Further, Foster and colleagues concluded that the studies suggested that a clinical effect from oral supplementation with borage seed oil is unlikely but may help a small percentage of patients with less severe atopic dermatitis.[5] Many of these trials were conducted before the filaggrin defect was identified as a cause of atopic dermatitis. It is likely that borage seed oil imparts a beneficial effect on non-eczematous dry skin, but the study data do not support this conclusion at this time.

CONCLUSION

As the greatest natural source of GLA, borage seed oil is an important ingredient for dry and inflamed skin types. Increasing evidence suggests that GLA-rich borage seed oil delivers anti-inflammatory activity in the treatment of various medical conditions, including several cutaneous ones. Anecdotal evidence suggests that borage seed oil would be useful in the treatment of eczema and rosacea. It likely has a hydrating effect by helping increase ceramide production and serving as an occlusive moisturizer; however, it does not repair the filaggrin defect in atopic dermatitis. Borage seed oil and GLA have been demonstrated to be effective through oral supplementation and topical administration. Much more research is necessary, though, to determine the extent to which borage seed oil can serve more than an adjuvant therapeutic role.

REFERENCES

1. Hoffmann D. *Medical Herbalism: The Science and Practice of Herbal Medicine.* Rochester, VT: Healing Arts Press; 2003:56.
2. Grieve M. *A Modern Herbal.* Vol 1. New York: Dover Publications; 1971:119.
3. Foster S. *An Illustrated Guide to 101 Medicinal Herbs: Their History, Use, Recommended Dosages, and Cautions.* Loveland, CO: Interweave Press; 1998:38.
4. Ziboh VA, Miller C. Essential fatty acids and polyunsaturated fatty acids: significance in cutaneous biology. *Annu Rev Nutr.* 1990;10:433.
5. Foster RH, Hardy G, Alany RG. Borage oil in the treatment of atopic dermatitis. *Nutrition.* 2010;26:708.
6. Melnik B, Plewig G. Atopic dermatitis and disturbances of essential fatty acid and prostaglandin E metabolism. *J Am Acad Dermatol.* 1991;25:859.
7. Miller CC, Ziboh VA. Gammalinolenic acid-enriched diet alters cutaneous eicosanoids. *Biochem Biophys Res Commun.* 1988;154:967.
8. Miller CC, Tang W, Ziboh VA, et al. Dietary supplementation with ethyl ester concentrates of fish oil (n-3) and borage oil (n-6) polyunsaturated fatty acids induces epidermal generation of local putative anti-inflammatory metabolites. *J Invest Dermatol.* 1991;96:98.
9. Brosche T, Platt D. Effect of borage oil consumption on fatty acid metabolism, transepidermal water loss and skin parameters in elderly people. *Arch Gerontol Geriatr.* 2000;30:139.
10. De Spirt S, Stahl W, Tronnier H, et al. Intervention with flaxseed and borage oil supplements modulates skin condition in women. *Br J Nutr.* 2009;101:440.
11. Henz BM, Jablonska S, van de Kerkhof PC, et al. Double-blind, multicentre analysis of the efficacy of borage oil in patients with atopic eczema. *Br J Dermatol.* 1999;140:685.
12. Macfarlane GJ, El-Metwally A, De Silva V, et al. Evidence for the efficacy of complementary and alternative medicines in the management of rheumatoid arthritis: A systematic review. *Rheumatology (Oxford).* 2011;50:1672.
13. Barre DE, Holub BJ. The effect of borage oil consumption on the composition of individual phospholipids in human platelets. *Lipids.* 1992;27:315.
14. Tollesson A, Frithz A. Transepidermal water loss and water content in the stratum corneum in infantile seborrheic dermatitis. *Acta Derm Venereol.* 1993;73:18.
15. Tollesson A, Frithz A. Borage oil, an effective new treatment for infantile seborrhoeic dermatitis. *Br J Dermatol.* 1993;129:95.
16. Kanehara S, Ohtani T, Uede K, et al. Undershirts coated with borage oil alleviate the symptoms of atopic dermatitis in children. *Eur J Dermatol.* 2007;17:448.
17. Kanehara S, Ohtani T, Uede K, et al. Clinical effects of undershirts coated with borage oil on children with atopic dermatitis: A double-blind, placebo-controlled clinical trial. *J Dermatol.* 2007;34:811.
18. Yates JE, Phifer JB, Flake D. Clinical inquiries. Do nonmedicated topicals relieve childhood eczema? *J Fam Pract.* 2009;58:280.
19. WebMD. Borage overview information. http://www.webmd.com/vitamins-supplements/ingredientmono-596-BORAGE.aspx?activeIngredientId=596&activeIngredientName=BORAGE. Accessed October 2, 2012.
20. Cosmetic Ingredient Review: Draft report of the plant-derived edible oil group. http://www.cir-safety.org/sites/default/files/117_draft_oils.pdf. Washington, DC 2010. Accessed October 2, 2012.
21. Soto CG, Chamy R, Zúñiga ME. Effect of enzymatic application on borage (Borago officinalis) oil extraction by cold pressing. *J Chem Eng Jpn.* 2004;37:326.
22. Belch JJ, Hill A. Evening primrose oil and borage oil in rheumatologic conditions. *Am J Clin Nutr.* 2000;71:352S.
23. Kast RE. Borage oil reduction of rheumatoid arthritis activity may be mediated by increased cAMP that suppresses tumor necrosis factor-alpha. *Int Immunopharmacol.* 2001;1:2197.
24. Cameron M, Gagnier JJ, Chrubasik S. Herbal therapy for treating rheumatoid arthritis. *Cochrane Database Syst Rev.* 2011;2:CD002948.
25. Cameron M, Gagnier JJ, Little CV, et al. Evidence of effectiveness of herbal products in the treatment of arthritis. Part 2: Rheumatoid arthritis. *Phytother Res.* 2009;23:1647.

CHAPTER 12

Jojoba Oil

Activities:

Anti-inflammatory, humectant, antiviral, antiacne, analgesic, antibacterial, antioxidant, antiparasitic, and antipyretic[1-4]

Important Chemical Components:

Triglycerides

Fatty acids (including linoleic, linolenic, oleic and arachidonic)

Triterpene alcohols (cycloartenol, cyclobranol, 24-methylenecyclobartenol)

4-demethylsterols (campesterol, stigmasterol, sitosterol, isofucosterol)

4-methylsterols (obtusifoliol, gramisterol, cycloeucalenol, citrostadeienol)[5]

Origin Classification:

This ingredient is considered natural. Organic forms are available. The natural form may undergo processing and there are also synthetic forms of jojoba oil.

Personal Care Category:

Emollient, occlusive

Recommended for the following Baumann Skin Types:

This ingredient is ideal for dry and sensitive types but is not recommended for acne types. Oily types may find it too sticky. Recommended for DRNT, DRNW, DRPT, DRPW, DSNT, DSNW, DSPT, and DSPW.

SOURCE

The jojoba (pronounced ho-ho-ba) plant (*Simmondsia chinensis* or *Buxus chinensis*) is a hardy perennial shrub endemic to the arid Sonoran Desert of northwest Mexico and adjacent areas in Arizona and southern California that grows up to 15 feet. The seeds of the plant, which are laden with a light yellow/gold, odorless liquid wax, were used by Native Americans for cosmetic and medical purposes to treat various conditions, including sores and wounds, sunburn, dry skin, hair loss, headaches, and renal colic.[2,5,6] Cosmetic products may contain various ingredient forms of this plant including *S. chinensis* (jojoba) seed oil, *S. chinensis* seed, and *S. chinensis* butter. Further processing yields other ingredients including: hydrogenated jojoba oil, hydrolyzed jojoba esters, isomerized jojoba oil, jojoba esters, and jojoba alcohol. Synthetic jojoba oil also is used in cosmetics. Jojoba seed oil is the most widely used type of *S. chinensis* derivative.

HISTORY

This evergreen plant, also known as goat nut, deer nut, pignut, wild hazel, quinine nut, coffeeberry, or gray box bush, can live up to 200 years. Native Americans are known to have eaten the smooth-skinned, odorless, oil-rich nuts or seeds of the jojoba. The oil from jojoba nuts or seeds has been used for centuries to promote hair growth and alleviate skin conditions.

As for modern medical applications, as early as 30 years ago, observers noted the increased use of the liquid wax derived from jojoba seeds in skin care formulations.[7] It is the oil of the plant (or liquid wax in this particular case), composed of straight chain monoesters of alcohols and fatty acids, that is of particular interest in the modern skin care industry as jojoba is one of the many popular botanical products available in cosmetics and cosmeceuticals. Indeed, jojoba is now cultivated for commercial purposes, including therapeutic options in Australia, Israel, several African countries, including Egypt, and India as well as throughout the Americas (including the United States, Mexico, Argentina, and Brazil).[2,6,8-10]

CHEMISTRY

Jojoba oil is derived by cold-pressing the seeds.[1] As noted above, it is actually a polyunsaturated liquid wax. Very similar in consistency to human sebum, jojoba oil is considered to be a natural moisturizer and thought to be highly conditioning, softening, and healing for skin.

ORAL USES

Jojoba seed extract is the source of simmondsin, a key dietary supplement used for weight loss. The meal that remains from the jojoba oil extraction process is approximately 30 percent protein and exhibits a significant appetite suppressant effect.[11] In 2006, Boozer and Herron tested the botanical ingredient over 8 weeks in lean Sprague-Dawley male rats and 16 weeks in obese rats and found dose-response effects in lowering food consumption and body weight at concentrations of 0.15 and 0.25 percent. Jojoba oil is not typically consumed in the diet as it is poorly digested.[5,12,13]

TOPICAL USES

In skin care products, jojoba oil is typically used as a humectant (Table 12-1). It also delivers a protective film over the skin that aids in retaining moisture, thus imparting occlusive properties.[14] The skin's natural sebum is readily compatible with the wide

TABLE 12-1

Pros and Cons of Jojoba Oil

Pros	Cons
Displays anti-inflammatory and humectant qualities	While results are promising, more research is necessary to establish a significant role in the dermatologic armamentarium
Stable	Expensive
Easy to formulate	Comedogenic (some forms)
Increased antioxidant value when combined with tocopherol	
Safe	

range of fatty acids (e.g., oleic, linoleic, linolenic, and arachidonic) and triglycerides that are key components of jojoba oil.[5,15] Some authors speculate that its efficacy as a nongreasy lubricant gives the oil, pure or in hydrogenated form, potential to be effective in various formulations (i.e., creams, lotions, soaps, lipsticks, etc.) intended for topical application on the skin or hair.[3] Jojoba oil has been found to confer a wide range of significant beneficial properties as an analgesic, antibacterial, anti-inflammatory, antioxidant, antiparasitic, and antipyretic agent.[1,3]

Human Studies

The inclusion of hydrolyzed jojoba esters in skin, hair, and nail products has been demonstrated to enhance cutaneous hydration and sensation for users.[9] In fact, jojoba has been reported to penetrate the outer layer of the stratum corneum and enhance hydration.[10] In 2008, Meyer et al. conducted a small pilot study of nine healthy women (between 22 and 55 years of age; six Caucasian, two Hispanic, one African American) to establish "proof of concept" that the combination of hydrolyzed jojoba esters (K-20W) and glycerol renders an additive skin moisturizing effect. The formulation was topically applied to the lower leg and investigators made baseline assessments as well as at eight and 24 hours after application. They found that transepidermal water loss values were significantly lower in association with the combination formula (containing 3.75 percent glycerol and 1.25 percent hydrolyzed jojoba esters) than with glycerol alone eight and 24 hours after treatment.[9]

In 2012, Meier et al. conducted an open, prospective, observational pilot study of 194 subjects (192 female, 2 male) with acne-prone skin with lesions in which participants completed questionnaires after using clay jojoba facial masks for six weeks (applying them two to three times weekly). The investigators noted that of the 133 individuals who also returned complete lesion counts, a 54 percent mean reduction in total lesions was calculated. Significant reductions in inflammatory and noninflammatory lesions from baseline were observed. The researchers concluded that clay jojoba facial masks exhibit the potential to successfully treat mild acne.[16]

SAFETY ISSUES

The Cosmetic Ingredient Review (CIR) safety report states that studies of the oral and topical forms of jojoba oil on animals were nontoxic in their effects.[17] It is important to realize that any plant-derived material can contain pesticide residues and/or heavy metals. The CIR stated, "The cosmetic industry should continue to limit pesticide and heavy metal impurities in the plant-derived ingredients before blending into cosmetic formulations." S. chinensis seed oil was neither a significant dermal irritant nor a sensitizer, according to the clinical test results reported in the CIR. In repeat insult patch tests, jojoba alcohol, jojoba esters, and hydrolyzed jojoba esters were not irritating during induction or sensitizing at challenge. Neither S. chinensis seed oil nor jojoba alcohol were phototoxic. None of the tested ingredients were genotoxic and there were no structural alerts for carcinogenicity. Some forms of jojoba can aggravate acne. S. chinensis seed wax was moderately comedogenic in tests using rabbits and jojoba esters were non-comedogenic to slightly comedogenic.

ENVIRONMENTAL IMPACT

Jojoba oil first gained industry interest and support for its viability as a replacement for sperm whale oil, the use of which was banned by the US government in the early 1970s as a result of the Endangered Species Act. It has been the primary natural source of wax esters for commercial use since then.[18] No significant environmental impact from jojoba harvesting has been reported. S. chinensis is a hardy, long-living perennial that revives or recovers well after fires.

FORMULATION CONSIDERATIONS

Jojoba oil is the primary biological source of wax esters, which have considerable commercial applications despite its high cost. In fact, the cost has prompted research into less expensive jojoba oil alternatives to be bioengineered using recombinant microorganisms.[18] S. chinensis seed oil forms stable emulsions in water with small particles,[19] and the emulsion of jojoba seed oil and water used for microcapsulization was found to be stable after freeze-drying and storage at room temperature for a year.[20] Seed oil is not easily oxidized and remains chemically unchanged for years.[17]

USAGE CONSIDERATIONS

Jojoba seed oil has been reported to readily penetrate nude mouse skin and to increase penetration of other agents such as aminophylline in clinical tests.[17] Its oxidative stability index decreases when exposed to zinc oxides and salicylic acid but increases with tocopherols, titanium dioxide, and kojic acid.[17]

SIGNIFICANT BACKGROUND

In Vitro

In 2010, Yarmolinsky et al. investigated the *in vitro* activity of purified fractions and aquatic and ethanol leaf extracts of *Callissia fragrans* and *S. chinensis* against herpetic viruses. They found that *S. chinensis* potently suppressed all of the herpetic viruses studied.[8]

In 2011, Ranzato et al. assessed, *in vitro*, the wound healing characteristics of jojoba liquid wax on HaCaT keratinocytes and human dermal fibroblasts. Cytotoxicity assays and scratch wound experiments respectively revealed that jojoba liquid wax displayed low toxicity while significantly accelerating wound closure. Jojoba was also determined to have promoted collagen I production in fibroblasts. Investigators concluded that jojoba liquid wax warrants consideration for a role in treatment options in the clinical environment.[6]

Animal Studies

In 2005, Habashy et al. used several experimental animal models to evaluate the anti-inflammatory potential of jojoba liquid wax. Their findings demonstrated that the botanical derivative diminished carrageenan-induced rat paw edema as well as prostaglandin E_2 (PGE_2) in inflammatory exudates; reduced croton oil-induced rat ear edema as well as neutrophil infiltration; improved histopathological alterations caused by croton oil; and decreased nitric oxide levels and tumor necrosis factor-α release. The investigators concluded that jojoba liquid wax exerted dynamic anti-inflammatory activity, without clearly identifying the components of the plant directly involved.[2]

CONCLUSION

The various forms of jojoba are mainly used to confer anti-inflammatory properties to cosmetics and cosmeceuticals. No studies could be found that looked at use in eczema or rosacea. The acne study discussed above likely revealed benefits due to the moisturizing and anti-inflammatory effects of jojoba but studies have demonstrated that moisturization alone can improve acne. Because *S. chinensis* seed wax has been shown to be comedogenic, jojoba would not be the best topical choice to relieve the inflammatory aspect of acne. The versatile botanical extract jojoba oil has not been shown to be harmful or to elicit significant adverse effects and is not phototoxic. Much research, in the form of randomized, placebo-controlled clinical trials, is necessary to compare jojoba-containing products with other formulations established as effective anti-inflammatory agents.

REFERENCES

1. Aburjai T, Natsheh FM. Plants used in cosmetics. *Phytother Res.* 2003;17:987.
2. Habashy RR, Abdel-Naim AB, Khalifa AE, et al. Anti-inflammatory effects of jojoba liquid wax in experimental models. *Pharmacol Res.* 2005;51:95.
3. Arquette DJ, Bailyn EM, Palenske J, et al. Non-comedogenic and hypoallergenic properties of jojoba oil and hydrogenated jojoba oil. *J Cosm Sci.* 1998;49:377.
4. Kampf A, Gringberg S, Galuun A. Oxidative stability of jojoba wax. *J Am Oil Chem Soc.* 1986;63:246.
5. Van Boven M, Daenens P, Maes K, et al. Content and composition of free sterols and free fatty alcohols in jojoba oil. *J Agric Food Chem.* 1997;45:1180.
6. Ranzato E, Martinotti S, Burlando B. Wound healing properties of jojoba liquid wax: an in vitro study. *J Ethnopharmacol.* 2011;134:443.
7. Yaron A, Samoiloff V, Benzioni A. Absorption and distribution of orally administered jojoba wax in mice. *Lipids.* 1982;17:169.
8. Yarmolinksy L, Zaccai M, Ben-Shabat S, et al. Anti-herpetic activity of Callissia fragrans and Simmondsia chinensis leaf extracts in vitro. *Open Virol J.* 2010;4:57.
9. Meyer J, Marshall B, Gacula M Jr, et al. Evaluation of additive effects of hydrolyzed jojoba (Simmondsia chinensis) esters and glycerol: a preliminary study. *J Cosmet Dermatol.* 2008;7:268.
10. Cummings M, Reinhart J, Lockhart L. Penetration effects of Jojoba. *Cosmet Toilet.* 2000;115:73.
11. Boozer CN, Herron AJ. Simmondsin for weight loss in rats. *Int J Obes (Lond).* 2006;30:1143.
12. Verschuren PM, Nutgeren DH. Evaluation of jojoba oil as a low-energy fat. 2. Intestinal transit time, stomach emptying and digestibility in short-term feeding studies in rats. *Food Chem Toxicol.* 1989;27:45.
13. Heise C, Decombaz J, Anantharaman K. Energy value of JO for the growing rat. *Int J Vitam Nutr Res.* 1982;52:216.
14. Dweck AC. Skin treatment with plants of the Americas. *Cosmet Toiletries.* 1997;112:47.
15. Van Boven M, Holser RA, Cokelaere M, et al. Characterization of triglycerides isolated from jojoba oil. *J Am Oil Chem Soc.* 2000;77:1325.
16. Meier L, Stange R, Michalsen A, et al. Clay jojoba oil facial mask for lesioned skin and mild acne – Results of a prospective, observational pilot study. *Forsch Komplementmed.* 2012;19:75.
17. Cosmetic Ingredient Review. Final report of the Cosmetic Ingredient Review Expert Panel: Safety assessment of Simmondsia chinensis (jojoba) seed oil, Simmondsia chinensis (jojoba) seed wax, hydrogenated jojoba oil, hydrolyzed jojoba esters, isomerized jojoba oil, jojoba esters, Simmondsia chinensis (jojoba) butter, jojoba alcohol, and synthetic jojoba oil. http://www.cir-safety.org/sites/default/files/115_buff3f_suppl.pdf. Washington, DC 2008. Accessed October 5, 2012.
18. Kalscheuer R, Stöveken T, Luftmann H, et al. Neutral lipid biosynthesis in engineered Escherichia coli: jojoba oil-like wax esters and fatty acid butyl esters. *Appl Environ Microbiol.* 2006;72:1373.
19. Chung H, Kim TW, Kwon M, et al. Oil components modulate physical characteristics and function of the natural oil emulsions as drug or gene delivery system. *J Controlled Release.* 2001;71:339.
20. Esquisabel A, Hernandez RM, Igartua M, et al. Preparation and stability of agarose microcapsules containing BCG. *J Microencapsul.* 2002;19:237.

CHAPTER 13

Mineral Oil

Activities:

Inert substance

Important Chemical Components:

Highly refined saturated hydrocarbons[1] such as:
paraffins
naphthenes (cycloalkanes)

Origin Classification:

Mineral oil is derived from petroleum, and is considered synthetic because solvents and other chemicals are used during the refining process.

Personal Care Category:

Emollient, occlusive

Recommended for the following Baumann Skin Types:

Best for dry skin types because oily ones will not like the greasiness. Does not have any anti-inflammatory properties. Best for DRNT, DRNW, DRPT, and DRPW.

SOURCE

Mineral oil (also known as liquid petrolatum, heavy mineral oil, light mineral oil, liquid paraffin, mineral oil mist, paraffin oil, paraffinum liquidum, petrolatum liquid, petroleum oil, white mineral oil, and white oil)[1] is a complex mixture of highly refined saturated hydrocarbons derived from the distillation of petroleum in the production of gasoline.[2] Along with petrolatum, lanolin, and silicones, mineral oil is among the most effective of occlusive ingredients used in skin care products (Table 13-1).[3] As such, it is a popular cosmetic ingredient in moisturizers, creams, and baby lotions.

HISTORY

The use of petrolatum dates back to its discovery in 1872 by Robert A. Chesebrough.[4] The cosmetic use of mineral oil followed shortly thereafter, incorporated in such agents since the 1880s, and remains one of the most frequently used oils in skin care formulations.[2] A notable study in the more recent history of mineral oil showed, in 1989, that an emulsion

TABLE 13-1
Pros and Cons of Mineral Oil

PROS	CONS
One of the most effective occlusive ingredients	Requires repeated applications
Inexpensive	May increase susceptibility to UV damage
Stable	Inert, so it confers no biologic activity
	Greasy

containing mineral oil was more effective than various linoleic acid emulsions in reducing skin vapor loss in volunteers who received topical applications of sodium lauryl sulfate solution.[5]

CHEMISTRY

Mineral oil is a byproduct of the process of converting petroleum to gasoline. Petroleum itself is composed of fossil plankton and algae-derived substances largely made up of hydrocarbons.[1] It is refined using solvents and other methods to produce mineral oil. Refined mineral oil is composed of two hydrocarbon types: paraffinics, which are branched-chain alkanes, and naphthenics, which are alkanes containing one or more saturated cyclic structures.[1] The ratio of paraffinics to naphthenics and their respective molecular weight determines the physical properties of the resulting oil. Mineral oils are classified by their viscosities. "Light" mineral oil has low viscosity. "Heavy" mineral oil has a high viscosity.

Mineral oil is known to have strong occlusive properties, and is one of the best occlusive ingredients known (second to petrolatum). It is able to form a tight barrier that prevents the passage of other molecules because it has straight alkyl chains that easily align to form the occlusive palisade. The highly variable chain length of the alkyl chains keeps mineral oil from being a perfect occlusive, because short straight chains of the same length represent the ideal structure for an occlusive ingredient (see Chapter 8, Occlusives). As compared to heavy mineral oil, light mineral oil contains more cyclic (saturated) molecules that prevent the consistent build-up of the palisade; therefore, heavy mineral oil is a better occlusive than light mineral oil.[1]

ORAL USES

Cosmetic mineral oil is not to be taken internally. A food grade mineral oil exists, but is beyond the scope of this chapter.

TOPICAL USES

In 1989, investigators found that a topical emulsion containing mineral oil was more effective than several linoleic acid emulsions in diminishing skin vapor loss in volunteers with an iatrogenically-induced impaired skin barrier.[5] Since then, many studies have demonstrated the occlusive and skin-softening benefits of mineral oil.[6,7] One reason that mineral oil is such a good occlusive is that it is poorly absorbed into the skin;[8,9] therefore, it exhibits high substantivity, which is one of the hallmarks of a good occlusive ingredient. Conversely, when mineral oil is placed in water dispersions, such as when used as a bath oil, it is better absorbed into the skin than vegetable oils. This absorptive ability varies with oil concentration and bath water temperature.[10] The viscosity of the mineral oil also affects its occlusive abilities.

Mineral oil can decrease the penetration of other ingredients. Sahlin et al. showed that increasing the concentration of mineral oil from 10 to 50 percent in formulations containing the same concentration of lactic acid tended to decrease the stinging effect of lactic acid. They surmised that this was because the increased concentrations of mineral oil diminished the penetration of lactic acid.[11]

When used for its primary purpose, as a moisturizer, mineral oil has been shown to be safe and effective. In 2004, a randomized double-blind controlled trial demonstrated that mineral oil and extra virgin coconut oil were equally efficacious and safe as moisturizers in treating mild-to-moderate dry skin in 34 patients, with surface lipid levels and skin hydration significantly enhanced in both groups.[12]

SAFETY ISSUES

Because of its source, several criticisms have emerged regarding mineral oil. The mineral oil used in cosmetic products, USP or BP grade, is highly refined and purified but industrial grade petroleum may contain benzene and has been associated with formation of cancer.[13] In fact, a 1997 epidemiologic review of the relationship between mineral oil exposure and cancer revealed several associations,[14] but these were cases of protracted exposure to *industrial* grade mineral oil. Cosmetic grade mineral oil has never been associated with cancer etiology.

Mineral oil has also been blamed for causing blocked pores (comedones) and acne and playing a role in the etiology of "acne cosmetica." In 1989, Fulton published a list of comedogenic ingredients that included mineral oil.[15] Conflicting results were published by Mills and Kligman, who found no comedogenicity in human and rabbit models.[16] A 2005 study suggested that even though industrial grade mineral oil may be comedogenic, cosmetic grade mineral oil is not.[2] Certainly the viscosity and purity of the mineral oil, the study subject susceptibility, and combination with other ingredients and products could affect the results of these studies. Actual use patterns and environmental factors could also influence the incidence of comedogenicity (e.g., ambient humidity; light exposure; stress levels; combination with other products, drugs, or devices; and diet).

Mineral oil has strong light-reflective properties and allows more light to be absorbed into skin.[1] Studies in humans have shown that typical moisturizers containing 10 percent mineral oil or glycerol make the skin slightly more sensitive to turning red upon ultraviolet (UV) light exposure. One study showed that these moisturizers decreased the minimal erythema dose of skin to UVB irradiation by 5 to 7.6 percent.[17]

ENVIRONMENTAL IMPACT

Mineral oil, or liquid petrolatum, as stated above, is derived from the distillation of petroleum in the production of gasoline. Many consumers who favor organic products may opt against mineral oil because of the deleterious effects of its production process on the environment. It is important to remember that mineral oil is a byproduct and not the primary goal of the petroleum extraction process. Many benefits are derived, clearly, but the cost/benefit debate on this issue is beyond the purview of this text. Mineral oil is certainly not considered a natural or organic product and its disposal in the environment and dispersal in the human body have not been examined. Similarly, the long-term outcomes or effects of mineral oil have not been compared with the long-term outcomes from the use of natural oils.

FORMULATION CONSIDERATIONS

Mineral oil is inert and thus insensitive to light and resistant to oxidation, which gives it a long shelf life.[1,4]

USAGE CONSIDERATIONS

Mineral oil may decrease the skin penetration of other ingredients.

SIGNIFICANT BACKGROUND

Mineral oil became a popular addition to skin care products because the low cost, bulk availability, reproducible quality, as well as affluence and influence of the petrochemical industry all played a role in increasing the usage of this raw material.[18] The mild backlash against mineral oil preceded the current environmental reawakening by several decades. That is, mineral oil was one of the products associated with "acne cosmetica," an expression that emerged in the early 1970s to describe cosmetics-related acne breakouts. Notably, mineral oil was not found to be as comedogenic as some other agents, but Fulton did identify mineral oil as one of the culprits in his study using rabbits.[15] However, Mills and Kligman had previously found no comedogenic association for mineral oil in rabbit and human models.[16] The DiNardo report in 2005 finally brought some resolution to this subject, concluding that mineral oil is not comedogenic.[2]

CONCLUSION

Mineral oil is one of the most effective occlusive ingredients in moisturizers. There is some question about the safety of mineral oil in those with significant sun exposure and more studies are needed to determine the safety of its use during UV light exposure. The occlusive properties of mineral oil lead to the retention of stratum corneum water content by reducing or preventing TEWL in people with dry skin. Individuals with sensitive skin also benefit from using mineral oil. Although popular claims suggest that mineral oil clogs pores or contributes to acne, there is no evidence to support such myths. Repeated application is necessary to provide or maintain cutaneous benefits.

REFERENCES

1. Rawlings AV, Lombard KJ. A review on the extensive skin benefits of mineral oil. *Int J Cosmet Sci*. 2012; 34:511.
2. DiNardo JC. Is mineral oil comedogenic? *J Cosmet Dermatol*. 2005;4:2.
3. Kraft JN, Lynde CW. Moisturizers: What they are and a practical approach to product selection. *Skin Therapy Lett*. 2005;10:1.
4. Lodén M. Role of topical emollients and moisturizers in the treatment of dry skin barrier disorders. *Am J Clin Dermatol*. 2003;4:771.
5. Blanken R, van Vilsteren MJ, Tupker RA, et al. Effect of mineral oil and linoleic-acid-containing emulsions on the skin vapour loss of sodium-lauryl-sulphate-induced irritant skin reactions. *Contact Dermatitis*. 1989;20:93.
6. Overgaard Olsen L, Jemec GB. The influence of water, glycerin, paraffin oil and ethanol on skin mechanics. *Acta Derm Venereol*. 1993;73:404.
7. Maes D, Short J, Turek BA, et al. In vivo measuring of skin softness using the Gas Bearing Electrodynamometer. *Int J Cosmet Sci*. 1983;5:189.
8. Brown EB, Diembeck W, Hoppe U, et al. Fate of topical hydrocarbons in the skin. *J Soc Cosmet Chem*. 1995;46:1.
9. Stamatas GN, de Sterke J, Hauser M, et al. Lipid uptake and skin occlusion following topical application of oils on adult and infant skin. *J Dermatol Sci*. 2008;50:135.
10. Taylor EA. Oil adsorption: A new method to determine the affinity of skin to adsorb oil from aqueous dispersions of water-dispensable oil preparations. *J Invest Dermatol*. 1961;37:69.
11. Sahlin A, Edlund F, Lodén M. A double-blind and controlled study on the influence of the vehicle on the skin susceptibility to stinging from lactic acid. *Int J Cosmet Sci*. 2007;29:385.

12. Agero AL, Verallo-Rowell VM. A randomized double-blind controlled trial comparing extra virgin coconut oil with mineral oil as a moisturizer for mild to moderate xerosis. *Dermatitis.* 2004;15:109.

13. Cruickshank CN, Squire JR. Skin cancer in the engineering industry from the use of mineral oil. *Br J Ind Med.* 1950;7:1.

14. Tolbert PE. Oils and cancer. *Cancer Causes Control.* 1997;8:386.

15. Fulton JE. Comedogenicity and irritancy of commonly used ingredients in skin care products. *J Soc Cosmet Chem.* 1989;40:321.

16. Mills OH Jr, Kligman AM. A human model for assessing comedogenic substances. *Arch Dermatol.* 1982;118:903.

17. Forbes PD. Moisturizers, vehicle effects, and photocarcinogenesis. *J Invest Dermatol.* 2009;129:261.

18. Barton S. Formulation of skin moisturizers. In: Leyden J, Rawlings A, (eds), *Skin Moisturization.* New York: Marcel Dekker Inc.; 2002:552.

CHAPTER 14

Olive Oil

Activities:

Anti-inflammatory, antioxidant

Important Chemical Components:

Polyphenols
squalene
fatty acids (predominantly oleic acid with some stearic and linoleic)
triglycerides
tocopherols
carotenoids
sterols (mainly β-sitosterol, avenasterol, and campesterol)
chlorophylls[1–3]

Origin Classification:

This ingredient is natural, but organic forms are available.

Personal Care Category:

Occlusive and emollient, anti-inflammatory, antioxidant

Recommended for the following Baumann Skin Types:

DRNW, DRNT, DRPT, and DRPW

SOURCE

Olive oil is derived from the olive tree (*Olea europaea*) and has long been considered one of the most significant of the natural essential oils. In the Mediterranean diet, known as one of the world's healthiest diets, it is the primary source of fat. It was also used for dermatologic purposes among ancient Egyptians, Greeks, and Romans.

Olive oil is an effective hydrating agent and has been shown to confer anti-inflammatory and anticarcinogenic properties.[1,4,5] In fact, topically applied olive oil has been reportedly used successfully to treat xerosis, pruritus, rosacea, psoriasis, atopic dermatitis, contact dermatitis (particularly in the diaper area), eczema (including severe cases on the hands and feet), seborrhea, and various inflammations, burns and other skin damage.[1] In terms of additional potential cutaneous applications, olive oil has demonstrated promise as a photoprotective agent.[5]

HISTORY

Olive oil has been used for dermatologic purposes for thousands of years, since the times of the ancient Egyptians, Greeks, and Romans. A staple of the Mediterranean diet, known to be one of the healthiest around the world, olive oil has long been considered one of the most important of the natural essential oils. For as long as it has been a component in the human diet, people have also used olive oil for its beneficial effects on the skin. Ancient Greeks bathed with olive oil,[1] and the essential oil was also used in various ways – food, cosmetic, massage oil

for athletes, anointing oil, salve for soothing wounds – by ancient Egyptians and Romans. In an interesting historical study, Nomikos et al. used a comprehensive study of Greek and world literature, including works attributed to Hippocrates and Aristotle, as a portal through which to assess the use of olive oil for the prevention and treatment of sports injuries in the ancient world. They found that olive oil was used in massage to diminish muscle fatigue, eliminate lactic acid, and promote flexibility, thus possibly preventing the occurrence of injury. The authors also noted that the ancient world openly acknowledged the therapeutic use of oils, which were distributed freely to athletes at sporting events.[6]

In contemporary times, the topical application of olive oil has reportedly been successful in treating xerosis, rosacea, psoriasis, atopic dermatitis, contact dermatitis (especially in the diaper area), eczema (including severe cases on the hands and feet), seborrhea, and various inflammations, burns and other skin damage.[1]

CHEMISTRY

Various potent compounds, many of which display antioxidant properties, are found in olive oil, including polyphenols, squalene, fatty acids (notably oleic acid), triglycerides, tocopherols, carotenoids, sterols, and chlorophylls (Table 14-1).[1,7] The primary phenolic compounds found in olive oil are simple phenols (hydroxytyrosol and tyrosol), secoiridoids (oleuropein, the aglycone of ligstroside, and their respective decarboxylated dialdehyde derivatives), and the lignans [(+)-]-acetoxypinoresinol and pinoresinol.[8] The polar fraction of olive oil is composed primarily of the polyphenols oleuropein, tyrosol, hydroxytyrosol, and caffeic acid.[9] The antioxidant characteristics of these phenolic compounds are well established.[7] Studies have also demonstrated that these polyphenolic compounds in olive oil yield protective effects against inflammation.[1,4] (See the introduction to the Polyphenols section.) Lignans are also considered strong antioxidants.[10]

The main components of the unsaponifiable fraction of virgin olive oil include erythrodiol, β-sitosterol, and squalene. Olive oil contains much more squalene than other edible oils.[5,11,12] Assays evaluating the unsaponifiable and polar fractions of olive oil have revealed anti-inflammatory effects exhibited by both groups.[9]

ORAL USES

Olive oil is one of the primary and most nutritional cooking oils in current use. Olives and olive oil contain high levels of monounsaturated fats, which are believed to be important in ameliorating xerosis.

TABLE 14-1
Pros and Cons of Olive Oil

Pros	Cons
Readily available	May impair skin barrier
Rich in antioxidants	Greasy feel

In 2001, Moreno et al. examined the effect of a diet rich in olive oil on key inflammation mediators, specifically oxidative stress and prostaglandin production. The investigators compared the effects on rats of an olive oil-rich diet to those of corn-oil rich and fish oil-rich diets. Both olive and fish oils were found to reduce arachidonic acid (AA) release and the ensuing synthesis of AA metabolites, but olive oil was more efficient in reducing oxidative stress. Prostaglandin E_2 levels were found to be lower in the rats fed the olive oil or fish oil diets as compared to the corn oil diet.[13] A different 2001 study, by Purba et al., also found that the high consumption of olive oil, along with vegetables and legumes, imparted protection against actinic damage.[14] Indeed, the high consumption of extra virgin olive oil, which is laden with antioxidants from these polyphenols as well as other compounds, is thought to protect against oxidative stress and some of its manifestations, such as skin and other cancers as well as aging.[8]

Of note, the study by Purba et al. implied that diets high in monounsaturated acids may raise the levels of monounsaturated fatty acids in the epidermis, which resist oxidative damage, unlike epidermal polyunsaturated fatty acids, which are more vulnerable to oxidation.[15] They theorized that this may explain their observed association between monounsaturated olive oil and less wrinkling as well as the higher level of wrinkling linked to the consumption of polyunsaturated margarine.[14]

In 2012, Latreille et al. conducted a cross-sectional survey of 1,264 women and 1,655 men between the ages of 45 and 60 years to ascertain a link between the risk of photoaging and monounsaturated fatty acids intake. Using estimates of dietary monounsaturated fatty acid consumption in at least ten 24-hour diet records completed during the first 2.5 years of the follow-up period, and baseline facial skin photoaging assessments by trained investigators, the researchers found that higher consumption of olive oil, in both sexes, was linked to lower risk of severe photoaging.[16]

TOPICAL USES

Olive oil is currently used in topical applications for the treatment of several skin conditions, including xerosis, pruritus, and inflammation as well as disorders such as rosacea. A study by de la Puerta et al. in 2000 of the effects of topically applied virgin olive oil on edema in mice induced by AA or 12-O-tetradecanoylphorbol acetate (TPA) revealed that the unsaponifiable fraction of the oil more strongly inhibited AA, and oleuropein was found to be a strong inhibitor among the polar components. The researchers concluded that the anti-inflammatory activity attributed to both groups of compounds may be important in delivering the health benefits ascribed to virgin olive oil.[9] The polyphenolic components of olive oil have been shown in other studies to play a role in protecting against inflammation,[1,4] which is a key mediator in dermatologic disorders, not to mention other conditions.

In a 2012 randomized controlled clinical trial of 100 nulliparous pregnant women conducted at various health care centers and hospitals affiliated with Tehran University of Medical Sciences, Soltanipoor et al. evaluated the effects of olive oil in preventing striae gravidarum (stretch marks). The treatment group, to which 50 women were randomized, received 1 cc of topical olive oil for twice daily gentle application to abdominal skin, not massaging it into the skin until after delivery. The control group of 50 women received no treatment. The investigators did not find a statistically significant difference between the groups, though they noted that olive oil lowered the incidence of severe striae gravidarum but was associated with an increase in the incidence of mild striae.[17]

Although olive oil is increasingly considered an anti-inflammatory agent, it is also considered to be a weak irritant. There have been occasional reports of adverse side effects to its topical use, and it is considered unsuitable or contraindicated in patients with venous insufficiency and related eczema on the lower extremities.[18] In a recent study, Danby et al. recruited 19 adults with and without a history of atopic dermatitis (AD) into two randomized forearm-controlled mechanistic studies. One group was instructed to apply, twice daily, six drops of olive oil to one forearm for five weeks. Over a four-week period, the second group applied, twice daily, the same amount of olive oil to one forearm along with six drops of sunflower seed oil. The investigators found that olive oil precipitated a decline in stratum corneum (SC) integrity as well as well mild erythema in the subjects regardless of AD history. Conversely, sunflower seed oil supported SC integrity, improved hydration, and did not provoke erythema. In light of these results, the investigators concluded that olive oil exhibits the potential to aggravate AD and they recommend against its use for dry skin or infant massage.[19]

SAFETY ISSUES

Olive oil is generally recognized as safe, but as a weak irritant.[18] It has a high content of oleic acid, which likely accounts for the "decrease in SC integrity" reported in studies.

ENVIRONMENTAL IMPACT

As in the case with any plant that is cultivated for food and industrial uses, positive and negative effects on the environment are not uncommon. Considerable care must be taken to ensure environmental sustainability, which has become increasingly important to growers particularly in the European Union and the four main olive-producing countries (i.e., Greece, Italy, Spain, and Portugal).[20] Optimal disposal of olive mill waste water is a key consideration.[21] It is also necessary to monitor the impact on olive cultivation of European Union subsidies leading to the intensification of olive production.[22]

FORMULATION CONSIDERATIONS

Olive oil is lipophilic. It can be successfully made into stable oil-in-water emulsions or used as a pure oil.[23]

USAGE CONSIDERATIONS

Olive oil has significant amounts of oleic acid, which has been shown to increase skin penetration by disturbing the barrier.[24,25] Its use may increase penetration of other ingredients. Extra virgin olive oil is the product obtained from the first olive pressings and is much higher in polyphenols than the oil obtained during further pressings.

SIGNIFICANT BACKGROUND

Olive oil has been found to be an important ingredient in some botanical combination therapies and for various conditions.

Combination Therapy

In multiple studies, Al-Waili has shown that a honey, olive oil, and beeswax mixture (1:1:1) can be used effectively for multiple conditions, including AD, diaper dermatitis, psoriasis, anal fissures, and fungal as well as bacterial infections. In 2003, Al-Waili performed a partially controlled, single-blind study to evaluate the effects of the mixture on 21 patients with AD and 18 patients with psoriasis. Most of the AD patients exhibited significant improvement in the evaluated symptoms (i.e., erythema, scaling, lichenification, excoriation, indurations, oozing, and pruritus) after two weeks as did a majority of the psoriasis patients (i.e., redness, scaling, thickening, and pruritus).[26] In 2004, Al-Waili tested the same ointment in 37 patients as treatment for the cutaneous fungal infections pityriasis versicolor, tinea cruris, tinea corporis, and tinea faciei. Three daily applications on the lesions for up to four weeks resulted in observed clinical responses (i.e., reductions in erythema, scaling, and itching) in 86 percent of pityriasis versicolor patients, 78 percent of tinea cruris patients, and 75 percent of tinea corporis patients, with mycological resolution achieved in a significant percentage of patients (75 percent, 71 percent, and 62 percent of patients with pityriasis versicolor, tinea cruris, and tinea corporis, respectively).[27]

In 2005, Al-Waili evaluated the effects of the honey/olive oil/beeswax mixture on the growth of *Staphylococcus aureus* and *Candida albicans* isolated from humans and found that while the mixture as well as honey alone were effective in inhibiting bacterial growth, mild-to-moderate growth occurred on media containing olive oil or beeswax.[28] Also that year, Al-Waili assessed the mixture for its effects on 12 infants with diaper dermatitis. Four daily treatments for seven days yielded significant declines in mean lesion scores. Further, *Candida albicans* was isolated in four patients before treatment began, but only two patients after the one week of treatment, leading to Al-Waili's conclusion that the honey/olive/beeswax ointment is safe as well as clinically and mycologically effective for treating diaper dermatitis.[29] The ointment was found to be clinically effective in a pilot study to treat anal fissures and hemorrhoids in 2006.[30]

In 2008, Kiechl-Kohlendorfer et al. reported on their randomized controlled trial to test the cutaneous effects of two topical ointments on the skin of 173 premature infants conducted between October 2004 and November 2006. Researchers prospectively enrolled the infants (between 25 and 36 weeks of gestation) admitted into a neonatal intensive care unit, and randomly scheduled them for daily treatment with a water-in-oil emollient cream, an olive oil cream (70 percent lanolin, 30 percent olive oil), or a control ointment. Statistically less dermatitis was noted in the infants treated with the olive oil cream after four weeks as compared to the emollient cream and control.[31]

In 2012, Panahi et al. conducted a randomized double-blind clinical trial in 67 Iranian injured war veterans to determine the clinical efficacy of a topical cream combining *Aloe vera* and olive oil in comparison to β-methasone 0.1 percent cream. Thirty-one out of 34 subjects randomized to the botanical combination completed the regimen of twice daily application for six weeks and 32 out of the 33 randomized to β-methasone

finished the trial. A pruritic score questionnaire and visual analog scale were used for assessment. Significant decreases in pruritus frequency, burning, scaling, and xerosis by the end of the trial were seen in both groups. The rate of amelioration in pruritus severity was comparable between the groups; reductions in fissures and excoriations were observed only in the *A. vera*/olive oil group. The investigators concluded that the botanical cream was as effective as β-methasone 0.1 percent in treating sulfur mustard-induced chronic skin complications and displays potential as a therapeutic option for such patients.[32]

Antifungal Activity

In 2006, Battinelli et al. found that the aliphatic aldehydes in olives [hexanal, nonanal, (E)-2-hexenal, (E)-2-heptenal, (E)-2-octenal, and (E)-2-nonenal] exhibited antifungal effects against *T. mentagrophytes* and *M. canis* and concentration-dependently inhibited elastase activity.[33]

Cancer

Data over the last decade suggest the potential of anticarcinogenic properties in olive oil. In 2000, the topical application of olive oil following ultraviolet (UVB) exposure was found to be effective against photocarcinogenesis in mouse skin models.[5] That same year, Ichihashi et al. found that topically applied extra virgin olive oil may diminish the formation of the free radical-induced 8-hydroxy-deoxyguanosine (8-OHdG), which is known to be involved in gene mutation, and thus has the potential to slow the development of UV-induced skin cancer in humans as it appears to do in mice.[34] In a more recent study in humans on the effects of various topical agents on the transmission of UVB radiation therapy, Fetil et al. found that olive oil did not affect the minimal erythema dose and was therefore appropriate to use before phototherapy.[35] Olive oil may also exhibit activity against UVA. Hydroxytyrosol, one of the key polyphenolic components of the polar fraction of olive oil, has displayed a capacity to suppress cell proliferation in human leukemia (HL60) cells,[36] and to prevent UVA-induced protein damage in melanoma cells.[37]

CONCLUSION

Various compounds in olive oil with known antioxidant activity, as well as evidence suggesting anti-inflammatory and anti-carcinogenic properties, suggest reasons to consider further research to establish what appears to be an important ingredient in skin care formulations. That said, the salutary effects of dietary olive oil are much better researched and understood. There is a paucity of evidence, particularly from randomized, double-blind, controlled trials, establishing the efficacy of topically applied olive oil. While there appears to be emerging data suggesting a role for olive oil in the topical dermatologic armamentarium, particularly in relation to photoprotective, anti-inflammatory, and antioxidant activity, more research is necessary to elucidate whether the increasing inclusion of olive oil in over-the-counter products is warranted and, if so, whether the botanical can be harnessed for more effective use in dermatologic treatments. The high amounts of oleic acid in olive oil can disturb the skin barrier, which would affect the efficacy of olive oil in dry skin conditions. It seems certain that the utility of olive oil in treating dry skin conditions depends upon the other ingredients with which it is combined.

REFERENCES

1. Aburjai T, Natsheh FM. Plants used in cosmetics. *Phytother Res.* 2003;17:987.
2. Charrouf Z, Guillaume D. Should the amazigh diet (regular and moderate argan-oil consumption) have a beneficial impact on human health? *Crit Rev Food Sci Nutr.* 2010;50:473.
3. Cunha SS, Fernandes JO, Oliveira MB. Quantification of free and esterified sterols in Portuguese olive oils by solid-phase extraction and gas chromatography-mass spectrometry. *J Chromatogr A.* 2006;1128:220.
4. Martínez-Domínguez E, de la Puerta R, Ruiz-Gutiérrez V. Protective effects upon experimental inflammation models of a polyphenol-supplemented virgin olive oil diet. *Inflamm Res.* 2001;50:102.
5. Budiyanto A, Ahmed NU, Wu A, et al. Protective effect of topically applied olive oil against photocarcinogenesis following UVB exposure of mice. *Carcinogenesis.* 2000;21:2085.
6. Nomikos NN, Nomikos GN, Kores DS. The use of deep friction massage with olive oil as a means of prevention and treatment of sports injuries in ancient times. *Arch Med Sci.* 2010;6:642.
7. de la Puerta R, Martínez Domínguez ME, Ruíz-Gutíerrez V, et al. Effects of virgin olive oil phenolics on scavenging of reactive nitrogen species and upon nitrergic neurotransmission. *Life Sci.* 2001;69:1213.
8. Owen RW, Giacosa A, Hull WE, et al. Olive-oil consumption and health: the possible role of antioxidants. *Lancet Oncol.* 2000;1:107.
9. de la Puerta R, Martínez-Domínguez E, Ruíz-Gutiérrez V. Effect of minor components of virgin olive oil on topical anti-inflammatory assays. *Z Naturforsch C.* 2000;55:814.
10. Owen RW, Mier W, Giacosa A, et al. Identification of lignans as major components in the phenolic fraction of olive oil. *Clin Chem.* 2000;46:976.
11. Newmark HL. Squalene, olive oil, and cancer risk: A review and hypothesis. *Cancer Epidemiol Biomarkers Prev.* 1997;6:1101.
12. Kohno Y, Egawa Y, Itoh S, et al. Kinetic study of quenching reaction of singlet oxygen and scavenging reaction of free radical by squalene in n-butanol. *Biochim Biophys Acta.* 1995;1256:52.
13. Moreno JJ, Carbonell T, Sánchez T, et al. Olive oil decreases both oxidative stress and the production of arachidonic acid metabolites by the prostaglandin G/H synthase pathway in rat macrophages. *J Nutr.* 2001;131:2145.
14. Purba MB, Kouris-Blazos A, Wattanapenpaiboon N, et al. Skin wrinkling: Can food make a difference? *J Am Coll Nutr.* 2001;20:71.
15. Baumann LS, Weisberg EM. Olive oil in botanical cosmeceuticals. In: Preedy VR, Weston R, (eds), *Olives and Olive Oil in Health and Disease Prevention.* New York: Academic Press; 2010: 1117-1124.
16. Latreille J, Kesse-Guyot E, Malvy D, et al. Dietary monounsaturated fatty acids intake and risk of skin photoaging. *PLoS One.* 2012;7:e44490.
17. Soltanipoor F, Delaram M, Taavoni S, et al. The effect of olive oil on prevention of striae gravidarum: A randomized controlled clinical trial. *Complement Ther Med.* 2012;20:263.
18. Kränke B, Komericki P, Aberer W. Olive oil – Contact sensitizer or irritant? *Contact Dermatitis.* 1997;36:5.
19. Danby SG, Alenezi T, Sultan A, et al. Effect of olive and sunflower seed oil on the adult skin barrier: implications for neonatal skin care. *Pediatr Dermatol.* 2013; 30:42.
20. Camarsa G, Gardner S, Jones W, et al. LIFE ("The Financial Instrument for the Environment") among the olives: Good practice in improving environmental performance in the olive sector. In: Martin H, ed. Brussels: European Union; 2010.
21. Topi D, Thomaj F, Beqiraj I, et al. The environmental implications from olive industry in Albania. BALWOIS (Water Observation and Information System for Balkan Countries). 28 May–2 June 2012.
22. Allen HD, Randall RE, Amable GS, et al. The impact of changing olive cultivation practices on the ground flora of olive groves in the Messara and Psiloritis regions, Crete, Greece. *Land Degrad Develop.* 2006;17:249.
23. Smaoui S, Ben Hlima H, Jarraya R, et al. Cosmetic emulsion from virgin olive oil: Formulation and bio-physical evaluation. *Afr J Biotechnol.* 2012;11:9664.
24. Naik A, Pechtold LA, Potts RO, et al. Mechanism of oleic acid-induced skin penetration enhancement in vivo in humans. *J Control Release.* 1995;37:299.
25. Ongpipattanakul B, Burnette RR, Potts RO, et al. Evidence that oleic acid exists in a separate phase within stratum corneum lipids. *Pharm Res.* 1991;8:350.
26. Al-Waili NS. Topical application of natural honey, beeswax and olive oil mixture for atopic dermatitis or psoriasis: Partially controlled, single-blinded study. *Complement Ther Med.* 2003;11:226.
27. Al-Waili NS. An alternative treatment for pityriasis versicolor, tinea cruris, tinea corporis and tinea faciei with topical application of honey, olive oil and beeswax mixture: an open pilot study. *Complement Ther Med.* 2004;12:45.
28. Al-Waili NS. Mixture of honey, beeswax and olive oil inhibits growth of Staphylococcus aureus and Candida albicans. *Arch Med Res.* 2005;36:10.
29. Al-Waili NS. Clinical and mycological benefits of topical application of honey, olive oil and beeswax in diaper dermatitis. *Clin Microbiol Infect.* 2005;11:160.
30. Al-Waili NS, Saloom KS, Al-Waili TN, et al. The safety and efficacy of a mixture of honey, olive oil, and beeswax for the management of hemorrhoids and anal fissure: A pilot study. *ScientificWorldJournal.* 2006;6:1998.
31. Kiechl-Kohlendorfer U, Berger C, Inzinger R. The effect of daily treatment with an olive oil/lanolin emollient on skin integrity in preterm infants: a randomized controlled trial. *Pediatr Dermatol.* 2008;25:174.
32. Panahi Y, Davoudi SM, Sahebkar A, et al. Efficacy of Aloe vera/ olive oil cream versus betamethasone cream for chronic skin lesions following sulfur mustard exposure: A randomized double-blind clinical trial. *Cutan Ocu Toxicol.* 2012;31:95.
33. Battinelli L, Daniele C, Cristiani M, et al. In vitro antifungal and anti-elastase activity of some aliphatic aldehydes from Olea europaea L. fruit. *Phytomedicine.* 2006;13:558.
34. Ichihashi M, Ahmed NU, Budiyanto A, et al. Preventive effect of antioxidant on ultraviolet-induced skin cancer in mice. *J Dermatol Sci.* 2000;23(Suppl 1):S45.
35. Fetil E, Akarsu S, Ilknur T, et al. Effects of some emollients on the transmission of ultraviolet. *Photodermatol Photoimmunol Photomed.* 2006;22:137.
36. Fabiani R, De Bartolomeo A, Rosignoli P, et al. Cancer chemoprevention by hydroxytyrosol isolated from virgin olive oil through G1 cell cycle arrest and apoptosis. *Eur J Cancer Prev.* 2002;11:351.
37. D'Angelo S, Ingrosso D, Migliardi V, et al. Hydroxytyrosol, a natural antioxidant from olive oil, prevents protein damage induced by long-wave ultraviolet radiation in melanoma cells. *Free Radic Biol Med.* 2005;38:908.

CHAPTER 15

Safflower Oil

Activities:

Anti-inflammatory, hydrating, increases ceramide 1 production

Important Chemical Components:

Linoleic acid
Oleic acid
Palmitic acid
Arachidonic acid (trace amounts)
Polyphenols[1]

Origin Classification:

This ingredient is considered natural. Organic forms are available.

Personal Care Category:

Occlusive, barrier repair

Recommended for the following Baumann Skin Types:

It is useful in dry and inflamed skin types (S_2, S_3, S_4) but should not be used in S_1 (acne type) sensitive skin. Best for DRNT, DRPT, DRNW, DRPW, DSNT, DSPT, DSNW, and DSNT.

SOURCE

Safflower (*Carthamus tinctorius*) is a thistle-like annual plant with many branches that belongs to the Asteraceae or Compositae family. Plants range in height from 1 to almost 5 feet with yellow, orange, or red flowers. Safflower oil is obtained by pressing the seeds of the plant. The fatty acid composition of safflower oil can be experimentally manipulated and varies depending on the geographical location of the plants.[2]

HISTORY

Safflower is one of the oldest cultivated crops, its use dating back 4,000 years to ancient Egypt, though its native country is not known.[3,4] The plant was traditionally grown for its seeds, which were used in foods and folk medicine. The plant is now globally cultivated, in regions with long dry seasons, for its vegetable oil. The oil has been found to exert notable health benefits when consumed through the diet and also when used in topical formulations. The flower of *C. tinctorius* has been used for laxative and diaphoretic purposes as well as for skin eruptions, fevers, and measles in children.[3] In traditional Chinese medicine (TCM), *C. tinctorius* has been associated with uterostimulant activity.[5] In addition, there is a lengthy history of safflower seed use in the clinical setting in Korea to prevent osteoporosis, to foster bone development, and to treat rheumatism.[6]

CHEMISTRY

Linoleic acid (LA) is a primary constituent of safflower seeds and the ingredient typically cited for providing its cutaneous benefits (Table 15-1). In fact, safflower oil is one of the richest sources of LA, which is essential for the endogenous production of ceramides, important components of the epidermal layer that play a crucial role in barrier function and cutaneous water retention. LA is not produced by the body and, therefore, must be obtained through the diet. LA applied to skin has been shown to strengthen the skin barrier and lower transepidermal water loss.[7]

LA is also a critical component in the systemic synthesis of γ-linolenic acid (GLA), which plays an important role in the control of inflammation. See Chapter 11, Borage Seed Oil, for the significance of LA metabolism in the production of inflammatory eicosanoids (i.e., prostaglandins, thromboxanes, and leukotrienes).

ORAL USES

Odorless and tasteless safflower oil is one of several plant-based oils available on the market. It is also marketed in dietary supplement capsule form. Safflower oil is used clinically as a source for LA and has been used to treat essential fatty acid deficiency (EFAD), Friedreich's ataxia, and hangovers.[2]

Diabetes

Safflower oil has been found to impart dietary benefits to diabetic pregnant rats and their embryos, preventing diabetes-induced developmental harm during early organogenesis.[8] Supplementation has also been demonstrated to prevent excessive activity by matrix metalloproteinases (specifically MMP-2 and MMP-9) in the placenta of diabetic rats.[9] In addition, in a recent study, safflower oil and folic acid supplementations were demonstrated to interact, protecting rat embryos from diabetes-induced harm through diminished proinflammatory mediators.[10]

TABLE 15-1
Pros and Cons of Safflower Oil

Pros	Cons
Rich in linoleic acid	Mildly comedogenic
Stable unless prolonged exposure to air	Minimal data on efficacy
Nontoxic	Greasy, so individuals with oily skin will not like it
Anti-inflammatory properties	
Penetrates into skin	
Useful for rosacea	
Does not inactivate other ingredients	

Menopause

In addition, Asp et al. recently completed a randomized, double-blinded crossover study of 55 postmenopausal women with type 2 diabetes (with 35 completing the study), which revealed that the daily consumption of 8 g of safflower oil improved glycemia, inflammation, and blood lipids.[11] A study by Kim et al. in 2002 in female Sprague-Dawley rats provided evidence that safflower seeds exert protection against bone loss due to estrogen deficiency.[6]

TOPICAL USES

When applied topically, safflower oil is absorbed into skin as evidenced by studies on rodents with EFAD.[7] Safflower oil is incorporated in moisturizing agents for its emollient, occlusive, and anti-inflammatory properties. Its high concentration of LA, and its stability make it an important ingredient in personal care products. LA gives safflower oil its anti-inflammatory properties.[12,13] Pure safflower oil is a mild-to-moderate comedogenic agent,[2] so it is not the best choice of products for acne patients.

Inflammation/Tumorigenesis

In an early study on the antiproliferative potential of *C. tinctorius* extracts, Yasukawa et al., in 1996, applied the tumor-promoting agent 12-O-tetradecanoylphorbol-13-acetate (TPA) to the ears of mice (1 μg/ear) to induce inflammation. The investigators then isolated erythro-alkane-6,8-diols from the flowers of *C. tinctorius* and applied the extract to the same area. They reported that the alkane-6,8-diols suppressed inflammation and significantly inhibited TPA-induced skin tumor formation in mice.[14]

Pigmentation

In 2004, Roh et al. investigated potential melanogenesis-suppressing activity of safflower seeds to develop a novel skin-whitening agent. They reported that an 80 percent aqueous methanol extract and ethyl acetate fraction from the seeds significantly inhibited mushroom tyrosinase, and identified three active constituents [N-feruloylserotonin, N-(p-coumaroyl)serotonin, and acacetin]. Of these, N-feruloylserotonin and N-(p-coumaroyl)serotonin were found to more potently suppress the melanin synthesis of *Streptomyces bikiniensis* and B16 melanoma cells than arbutin, a well-known inhibitor of melanogenesis.[15] There are no published *in vivo* studies on the use of topical safflower oil in pigmentation disorders.

SAFETY ISSUES

Safflower oil is nontoxic when ingested. There are no reports of significant adverse side effects to its topical usage. Given its membership in the Asteraceae or Compositae family, known to be associated with contact dermatitis, topical safflower oil should be considered to have the potential to elicit such a reaction. Safflower oil comes from the seeds of plants; therefore, contamination from pesticides could occur. Although aflatoxin contamination of safflower seeds has been reported in India, this is unlikely in seeds from plants grown in the United States.[2] Undiluted safflower oil can cause skin irritation as seen in repeat open patch tests, but contact dermatitis to products containing safflower oil is very unlikely.[2] Safflower oil does not appear to be phototoxic.[2] The Cosmetic Ingredient Review panel considers safflower oil to be a safe ingredient.[2]

ENVIRONMENTAL IMPACT

Safflower is cultivated in several countries, but is considered a minor crop. Its environmental impact is minimal. The plant is susceptible to frost and to developing fungal diseases in rainy conditions.[16]

FORMULATION CONSIDERATIONS

Safflower oil is liquid at room temperature and soluble in fats and oil solvents. It is relatively resistant to oxidation unless exposure to air has been prolonged, in which case the product becomes thickened and rancid. The stability of safflower oil or its resistance to oxidation increases as its oleic acid concentration increases.

USAGE CONSIDERATIONS

Safflower oil may affect penetration of other ingredients both positively and negatively depending on its fatty acid composition and concentration.

SIGNIFICANT BACKGROUND

In 2005, Solanki et al. conducted a short randomized controlled study in a tertiary care neonatal intensive care unit of a large teaching hospital to assess the transcutaneous absorption of oil traditionally used in massage of newborns and to compare the effects of safflower oil and coconut oil on fatty acid profiles of massaged babies. The investigators randomly assigned 120 babies to three groups – safflower oil, coconut oil, or no oil controls (40 in each group). Oil (5 mL) was massaged four times daily for five days. Triglyceride levels were significantly elevated in all groups, though much more so in the non-control groups. Significant increases in essential fatty acids (linolenic and arachidonic) were seen in the safflower oil group and similar increases in saturated fats were seen in the coconut oil group, with changes more evident in term babies. The researchers concluded that topically applied oil is absorbed in neonates and is likely available nutritionally. Consequently, they deemed the fatty acid constituents of the massage oils significant in potentially impacting the fatty acid profiles of patients.[17] Safflower oil is rich in essential fatty acids and coconut oil is rife with saturated fat.

CONCLUSION

Safflower oil, rich in linoleic acid, can be used to strengthen the skin barrier, hydrate skin through occlusion, and decrease inflammation. It is used topically and as a dietary supplement. There are many studies in the literature investigating the benefits of linoleic acid on skin but there is a paucity of trials looking at safflower oil to treat dry, irritated skin. However, in the author's experience, it joins borage seed oil and argan oil as the best oils to use for dry and inflamed skin including rosacea. More controlled studies are needed to examine its role in rosacea and other disorders that cause skin redness. Although some trials described above considered safflower oil as an anticancer treatment, the larger dietary trials have been inconclusive.[2] Only one trial in the literature discussed the tyrosinase inhibitory effect of safflower oil, so this claim is poorly founded and not supported by data.

REFERENCES

1. Cho SH, Lee HR, Kim TH, et al. Effects of defatted safflower seed extract and phenolic compounds in diet on plasma and liver lipid in ovariectomized rats fed high-cholesterol diets. *J Nutr Sci Vitaminol (Tokyo)*. 2004;50:32.

2. Elder RL. Final report on the safety assessment of safflower oil. *Int J Toxicol*. 1985;4:171.

3. Grieve M. *A Modern Herbal*. Vol 1. New York Dover Publications; 1971:698.

4. Smith Joseph R. Safflower. Champaign, IL: AOCS Press; 1996:2.

5. Mills S, Bone K. *Principles and Practice of Phytotherapy: Modern Herbal Medicine*. London: Churchill Livingstone; 2000:240.

6. Kim HJ, Bae YC, Park RW, et al. Bone-protecting effect of safflower seeds in ovariectomized rats. *Calcif Tissue Int*. 2002;71:88.

7. Hartop PJ, Prottey C. Changes in transepidermal water loss and the composition of epidermal lecithin after applications of pure fatty acid triglycerides to skin of essential fatty acid-deficient rats. *Br J Dermatol*. 1976;95:255.

8. Higa R, White V, Martínez N, et al. Safflower and olive oil dietary treatments rescue aberrant embryonic arachidonic acid and nitric oxide metabolism and prevent diabetic embryopathy in rats. *Mol Hum Reprod*. 2010;16:286.

9. Martinez N, Sosa M, Higa R, et al. Dietary treatments enriched in olive and safflower oils regulate seric and placental matrix metalloproteinases in maternal diabetes. *Placenta*. 2012;33:8.

10. Higa R, Kurtz M, Mazzucco MB, et al. Folic acid and safflower oil supplementation interacts and protects embryos from maternal diabetes-induced damage. *Mol Hum Reprod*. 2012; 18:253.

11. Asp ML, Collene AL, Norris LE, et al. Time-dependent effects of safflower oil to improve glycemia, inflammation and blood lipids in obese, post-menopausal women with Type 2 diabetes: a randomized, double-masked, crossover study. *Clin Nutr*. 2011;30:443.

12. Letawe C, Boone M, Piérard GE. Digital image analysis of the effect of topically applied linoleic acid on acne microcomedones. *Clin Exp Dermatol*. 1998;23:56.

13. Darmstadt GL, Mao-Qiang M, Chi E, et al. Impact of topical oils on the skin barrier: Possible implications for neonatal health in developing countries. *Acta Paediatr*. 2002;91:546.

14. Yasukawa K, Akihisa T, Kasahara Y, et al. Inhibitory effect of alkane-6,8-diols, the components of safflower, on tumor promotion by 12-O-tetradecanoylphorbol-13-acetate in two-stage carcinogenesis in mouse skin. *Oncology*. 1996;53:133.

15. Roh JS, Han JY, Kim JH, et al. Inhibitory effects of active compounds isolated from safflower (Carthamus tinctorius L.) seeds for melanogenesis. *Biol Pharm Bull*. 2004;27:1976.

16. Smith Joseph R. *Safflower*. Champaign, IL: AOCS Press; 1996:2.

17. Solanki K, Matnani M, Kale M, et al. Transcutaneous absorption of topically massaged oil in neonates. *Indian Pediatr*. 2005; 42:998.

CHAPTER 16

Tamanu Oil

Activities:

Anti-inflammatory, analgesic, antibacterial, antioxidant, antiviral, ultraviolet (UV) radiation absorption, anticancer

Important Chemical Components:

Major: Dipyranocoumarins (including 4-phenylcoumarins, calanolides, inocalophyllins);
Oleic acid
Linoleic acid
Palmitic acid
Stearic acid
Glycolipids, phospholipids;
Inophyllum B and P;
Phytosterols (β-sitosterol, stigmasterol, campesterol)
Tocotrienols (δ-tocotrienol, γ-tocotrienol)[1-4]
Terpenoids
Minor: Triterpenes (friedelin, friedelan-3-β-ol), steroids, benzodipyranones, xanthones, flavonoids, tocopherols[5-7]

Origin Classification:

This ingredient is considered natural. Organic forms are available.

Personal Care Category:

Anti-inflammatory, occlusive, emollient, sun protective, antioxidant, scar treatment, and first aid for burns

Recommended for the following Baumann Skin Types:

Perfect for dry, sensitive S_1 (acne) type skin. May be too greasy for individuals with oily skin types. Best for DSNT, DSNW, DSPT, and DSPW.

SOURCE

Calophyllum inophyllum, a member of the mangosteen family (Clusiaceae, also known as Guttiferae), is a large, nondeciduous tree native to Africa, South India, Southeast Asia, Polynesia, the Philippines, and Australia.[1] *C. inophyllum* ranges from nearly 25 to 75 feet high and is found in the high plateaus of Madagascar as well as the shores throughout the Philippines and India, and is characterized as a tropical evergreen shrub that grows along the southern coast of Taiwan.[4,6-8] It is rumored that the trees that grow along the coastal shore provide a better oil for use in cosmetics than the inland trees, but there have been no scientific studies to support this claim.[9]

C. inophyllum is now cultivated in much of the tropical world. The oil derived from this abundant plant, known by a wide variety of names, including Alexandrian laurel, Domba oil, beach mahogany, beauty leaf, beach calophyllum, dilo, and kamani, but perhaps best known by the French Polynesian term *tamanu*, is a cold-pressed vegetable oil extracted from the fruit and seeds of the plant. The leaves, bark, and seeds (almonds) of *C. inophyllum* are widely used in traditional medicine in most

Pacific islands as well as the regions mentioned above.[10] The fruits contain a nut kernel, which has little oil. However, if it is dried on racks for a month, a chocolate brown, rich oil forms. Mechanical pressing results in a greenish yellow oil, similar to olive oil, with an aromatic odor and an insipid taste.

HISTORY

C. inophyllum has been used for hundreds of years in cuisine and as an ornamental plant because of its beauty and sweet fragrance. Its name comes from Greek – *kalos* (beautiful) and *phullon* (leaf). The wood is hard and is used in construction and canoe building. The seeds are the source of the oil, which is used for cosmetic and medicinal purposes and was once used as a lamp oil. Polynesians considered tamanu trees as sacred,[8] and the wood was used to carve idols. The trees were planted inside the royal marae (sacred areas) and it was believed that the gods would hide in tamanu trees and watch human sacrifices without being seen.

The leaves and wood of the trees have been used for various purposes but it is the oil that is used for cosmetic and dermatologic purposes.[8,10] Ocular burn and cutaneous wound healing are distinct conditions for which the oil of *C. inophyllum* has long been used in traditional folk medicine.[8,11] Several medical conditions have also been treated with *C. inophyllum* in traditional Chinese medicine (TCM), including skin infections, wounds, inflammation, rheumatism, leprous nephritis, pain, and eye disorders.[6] *C. inophyllum* was used for centuries in Madagascar to treat skin infections, facial neuralgia, hair loss, and wounds; in modern times, the herb has been used there to treat abrasions, burns, impetigo, insect bites, rashes, psoriasis, and as an antirheumatic agent.[7,8,12] Tamanu oil is also considered a historical beauty secret of the women of Tahiti.[8]

CHEMISTRY

The *C. inophyllum* constituents to which wound-healing activity have been attributed include calophyllolide, calophyllic acid, and inophyllum as well as various polyphenols, many of which exert antioxidant effects.[8] *C. inophyllum* also contains δ-tocotrienol, a form of vitamin E that acts as an antioxidant.[1,2] Calophyllolide and calophyllic acid are coumarin derivatives found in tamanu oil with antibacterial and anti-inflammatory properties. A wide variety of phospholipids are found in the oil (Table 16-1).[13-15]

ORAL USES

Tamanu oil is for external use only, though the oleoresin of the oil can be taken orally for pulmonary conditions.[8]

TOPICAL USES

Although the bark and leaves have been used topically, this chapter will be confined to the uses of the oil. Several health benefits have been attributed to tamanu oil and the ingredient is found in an increasing number of topical products. It is thought to impart anti-inflammatory, antioxidant, antibacterial, antiviral, and photoprotective activity (Table 16-2). Although the

TABLE 16-1
Lipid Contents of Tamanu Oil[13–15]

LIPID COMPOSITON OF TAMANU OIL
The oil of tamanu contains basic classes of lipids (fats), enumerated below.

GENERAL LIPID COMPOSITION	
Neutral lipids	92.0%
Glycolipids	6.4%
Phospholipids	1.6%
NEUTRAL LIPIDS	
Monoacylglycerols	1.8%
sn -1,3 – Diaglycerides	2.4%
sn -1,2 (2,3) – Diaglycerides	2.6%
Free fatty acids	7.4%
Triacylglycerols	82.3%
Sterols, sterolesters, and hydrocarbons	3.5%
GLYCOLIPIDS	
Monogalactosyldiacylglycerol	11.4%
Acylated sterolglucoside	13.1%
Monogalactosylmonoacylglycerol	22.2%
Acylmonogalactosyldiacylglycerol	53.3%
PHOSPHOLIPIDS	
Phosphatidylethanolamine	46.3%
Phosphatidylcholine	33.8%
Phosphatidic acid	8.1%
Phosphatidylserine	6.1%
Lysophosphatidylcholine	5.7%

Source: References 2, 15, 22.

TABLE 16-2
Pros and Cons of Tamanu Oil

PROS	CONS
Provides UV protection	Insufficient research to establish potential in the dermatologic armamentarium
Anti-inflammatory and antimicrobial	Parts of the plant are poisonous
Possible benefit in wound healing	
May play a role in the treatment of acne in dry skin patients	Feels greasy

scientific data are sparse, tamanu oil are recommended throughout the world for treating abrasions, acne, anal fissures, blisters, burns (chemical, sun, X-ray), chilblains, diabetic sores, eczema, hair loss, herpes lesions, psoriasis, scars, and xerosis as well as to diminish foot and body odor.[4,8] The best published data support the anti-inflammatory properties of the oil.

Anti-inflammatory Activity

In 2012, Tsai et al. investigated the anti-inflammatory properties of an acetone extract of *C. inophyllum* leaves using lipopolysaccharide (LPS)-induced RAW 264.7 cells to assess the impact of the extract on nitric oxide (NO) expression and inducible nitric oxide synthase (iNOS). They found that *C. inophyllum* significantly inhibited, in dose-dependent fashion, the LPS-induced synthesis of NO in addition to the expression of iNOS, cyclooxygenase (COX)-2 and nuclear factor-κB (NF-κB). This suggested that the leaf extracts had components with anti-inflammatory activity, but this study did not evaluate tamanu oil.[11]

The oil contains coumarin derivatives including calophyllolide and calophyllic acid. Coumarin derivatives have been shown to function as nonsteroidal anti-inflammatory drugs (NSAIDs) because of their ability to inhibit synthesis of prostaglandins and leukotrienes.[16] Calophyllolide has been shown to decrease capillary permeability, which decreases inflammation and edema.[17] Another study showed that this effect is likely due, in part, to a decrease in the release of histamine.[8] The antioxidants in the oil likely play a role in decreasing inflammation as does the presence of linoleic acid (see Chapter 64, Anti-Inflammatory Agents).

Photoprotection

In 2007, Said et al. investigated the anti-UV activity of tamanu oil for eye protection. *C. inophyllum* oil, even at low concentration (1/10,000, v/v), exhibited significant UV absorption properties (maximum at 300 nm) and was associated with an important sun protection factor.[18–22] Tamanu oil appeared to act as a cytoprotective agent against oxidative stress and DNA damage (85 percent of the DNA damage induced by UV was inhibited with 1 percent tamanu oil).[7] Given the apparent antioxidant and cytoprotective effects displayed by the oil in the study, the researchers concluded that tamanu oil has potential as a natural UV filter in ophthalmic formulations.[7]

Wounds and Burns

Modern research supports the use of tamanu oil for corneal protection from burns. In 2009, Said et al. performed *in vitro*, *in vivo*, and *ex vivo* studies to evaluate the effects of different rinsing and healing protocols for alkali-induced ocular burn and inflammation in rabbits. NaOH was used to induce corneal reactions in rabbits, followed by rinses with NaCl 0.9 percent or controlled ionization marine formula combined with N-acetylcysteine or vegetable oils (from *C. inophyllum* and *Aleurites moluccana*). The investigators used confocal microscopy to assess corneal epithelium regeneration and inflammatory cell infiltration *in vivo* and *ex vivo* histological cuts. They found that the combination of controlled ionization marine solution with 10 percent *C. inophyllum* oil and 90 percent *A. moluccana* oil spurred corneal epithelium regeneration while decreasing inflammatory cells, suggesting its suitability as ocular burn therapy.[18]

Scars

In a nine-week open-label noncontrolled study in 2002, six subjects were given tamanu oil to apply to their scars twice a day. The scars were at least one year old. The appearance of the scars was found to significantly improve, and a decreased length and overall size was noted.[8] It is important to realize that this study did not utilize a placebo and the improvement in scars could be due to the natural healing process by which scars improve over time; however, the use of old scars gives some credibility to this trial.

Antimicrobial Activity

As early as 1954, Bhat et al. showed that *C. inophyllum* has activity against gram-positive bacteria.[12] Fifty years later, Yimdjo et al. investigated the chemical constituents of the root bark and nut of *C. inophyllum*, resulting in the isolation of the xanthone derivative inoxanthone, as well as several other compounds and the discovery... of antibacterial activity against several microbes.[19] Canophyllic acid has also been demonstrated to exhibit potent antimicrobial properties.[20]

C. inophyllum leaf extracts from the islands of French Polynesia have also been touted for several constituents that hold promise as anti-HIV-1 agents, including inophyllum B and P.[5] In addition, quantitative high-performance liquid chromatography (HPLC) analysis of callus cultures of *C. inophyllum* has revealed the anti-HIV activity of the dipyranocoumarins inophyllum B and P.[3]

Moisturizing Activity

Tamanu oil contains oleic acid, linoleic acid, and other fatty acids, as do most oils. These fatty acids provide occlusive and emollient benefits (see Chapter 7, Moisturizing Agents). There are no published studies evaluating the effects of tamanu oil on dry skin; however, the data suggest that there would be a positive benefit in dry, inflamed skin.

SAFETY ISSUES

One case of allergic contact dermatitis has been reported in association with tamanu oil.[4] The plant, including the mature fruit, kernel seed, sap, and milky juice, are virulent poisons.[8] Samoans use the sap as an arrow poison.[8] The milky juice causes blindness when it comes into contact with the eye.[20]

ENVIRONMENTAL IMPACT

C. inophyllum is abundant in tropical regions worldwide and its harvesting is not known to damage the local environment. It is rated as lower risk/least concern on the International Union for Conservation of Nature and Natural Resources (IUCN) Red List of Threatened Species because its timber is cut in fairly large amounts and sold as "beach calophyllum."[21]

FORMULATION CONSIDERATIONS

Tamanu oil is extracted from the seeds or raw fruits, filtered, and stabilized with vitamin E.[4] Tamanu oil is thought to have a shelf life of approximately five years if stored in a cool, dry location.

USAGE CONSIDERATIONS

Currently, tamanu oil is sometimes used in lomi lomi massage and can be formulated to make soap as well as various topical skin care formulations.

SIGNIFICANT BACKGROUND

In 2011, Ayyanar et al. concluded a four-year study intended to identify the herbs used in traditional medicine practiced by the Kani tribes in the Tirunelveli hills of Western Ghats, India. The researchers identified 90 species of plants used traditionally as ethnomedicinal treatments, with 65 different indications reported, particularly dermatologic conditions and gastrointestinal illnesses. Based on their study, they identified 16 species, including *C. inophyllum*, for additional ethnopharmacological investigation as potential sources of new drug agents.[22]

Anticancer activity has been exhibited by *C. inophyllum* according to some recent studies. Just over a decade ago, Itogawa et al. examined the potential inhibitory effects of *C. inophyllum* 4-phenylcoumarin isolates on Epstein-Barr virus early antigen (EBV-EA) activation caused by 12-*O*-tetradecanoylphorbol-13-acetate in Raji cells. All 10 of the isolates displayed inhibitory activity against EBV and no cytotoxicity. The strongest compound tested was calocoumarin-A [5], which also demonstrated a significant capacity to suppress murine skin tumor promotion in a two-stage cancer model. The investigators concluded that some 4-phenylcoumarin constituents of *C. inophyllum* warrant further study as possible antitumor agents.[23]

C. inophyllum was one of among 155 extracts from 93 plant species found on peninsular Malaysia screened by Ong et al. in 2009 for *in vitro* photocytotoxic activity using human leukemia cells (cell line HL-60). Further, *C. inophyllum* was among the 29 plants to lower the *in vitro* cell viability by more than 50 percent after exposure to 9.6 J/cm^2 of a broad-spectrum light tested at a concentration of 20 µg/mL.[24] In addition, Li et al. isolated one new friedelane-type triterpene and seven previously discovered triterpenoids from the stems and leaves of *C. inophyllum* and found that the compounds demonstrated growth-inhibitory activity against human leukemia HL-60 cells.[25]

In 2008, Xiao et al. isolated a new prenylated xanthone (caloxanthone) as well as two previously known xanthones from the ethanolic extract of *C. inophyllum* twigs and reported that two of the constituents (including the new xanthone) demonstrated cytotoxicity against myelogenous leukemia (cell line K562).[26]

Tamanu oil has the potential to treat many topical inflammatory diseases but data are lacking. The myriad uses for tamanu oil are quite amazing, though. It has even demonstrated potential use for humans and domestic animals as an insect repellent, specifically against *Stomoxys calcitrans* (stable fly).[27,28]

CONCLUSION

The oil of *C. inophyllum* has been used in traditional societies in the mainly eastern and southern hemispheres for medicinal and culinary purposes for centuries. There are sparse data in the form of randomized, placebo-controlled clinical trials to establish the effectiveness and appropriate role(s) of *C. inophyllum* within the topical dermatologic arsenal. However, the fact that tamanu oil contains fatty acids, coumarin derivatives, and antioxidant abilities in addition to antimicrobial properties makes it quite unique and worthy of further study. In the author's experience, this oil is a useful moisturizing ingredient in dry skin types that suffer from acne.

REFERENCES

1. Crane S, Aurore G, Joseph H, et al. Composition of fatty acids triacylglycerols and unsaponifiable matter in Calophyllum calaba L. oil from Guadeloupe. *Phytochemistry*. 2005;66:1825.
2. He L, Mo H, Hadisusilo S, et al. Isoprenoids suppress the growth of murine B16 melanomas in vitro and in vivo. *J Nutr*. 1997;127:668.
3. Pawar KD, Joshi SP, Bhide SR, et al. Pattern of anti-HIV dipyranocoumarin expression in callus cultures of Calophyllum inophyllum Linn. *J Biotechnol*. 2007;130:346.
4. Le Coz CJ. Allergic contact dermatitis from tamanu oil (Calophyllum inophyllum, Calophyllum tacamahaca). *Contact Dermatitis*. 2004;51:216.
5. Laure F, Raharivelomanana P, Butaud JF, et al. Screening of anti-HIV-1 inophyllums by HPLC-DAD of Calophyllum inophyllum leaf extracts from French Polynesia Islands. *Anal Chim Acta*. 2008;624:147.
6. Shen YC, Hung MC, Wang LT, et al. Inocalophyllins A, B and their methyl esters from the seeds of Calophyllum inophyllum. *Chem Pharm Bull (Tokyo)*. 2003;51:802.
7. Said T, Dutot M, Martin C, et al. Cytoprotective effect against UV-induced DNA damage and oxidative stress: Role of new biological UV filter. *Eur J Pharm Sci*. 2007;30:203.
8. Dweck AC, Meadows T. Tamanu (Calophyllum inophyllum) – The African, Asian, Polynesian and Pacific Panacea. *Int J Cosmet Sci*. 2002;24:341.
9. Kilham C. Tamanu oil: A tropical topical remedy. *Herbal Gram*. 63. Austin, TX: American Botanical Council. www.herbalgram.org; 2004:10–15.

10. Leu T, Raharivelomanana P, Soulet S, et al. New tricyclic and tetracyclic pyranocoumarins with an unprecedented C-4 substituent. Structure elucidation of tamanolide, tamanolide D and tamanolide P from Calophyllum inophyllum of French Polynesia. *Magn Reson Chem*. 2009;47:989.

11. Tsai SC, Liang YH, Chiang JH, et al. Anti-inflammatory effects of Calophyllum inophyllum L. in RAW 264.7 cells. *Oncol Rep*. 2012;28:1096.

12. Bhat SG, Kane JG, Sreenivasan A. The in vitro evaluation of the antibacterial activity of undi oil (Calophyllum inophyllum Linn.). *J Am Pharm Assoc Am Pharm Assoc (Baltim)*. 1954;43:543.

13. Petard P. Tahiti-Polynesian medicinal plants and Tahitian remedies. Noum!a, New Caledonia: South Pacific Commission; 1972.

14. Hemavathy J, Prabhakar JV. Lipid composition of Calophyllum inophyllum kernel. *J Am Oil Chem Soc*. 1990;67:955.

15. Lederer E, Dietrich P, Polonsky J. On the chemical constitution of calophylloide and calophyllic acid from the nuts of Calophyllum inophyllum. *Bull Fr Chem Soc*. 1953;5:546.

16. Fylaktakidou KC, Hadjipavlou-Litina DJ, Litinas KE, et al. Natural and synthetic coumarin derivatives with anti-inflammatory/antioxidant activities. *Curr Pharm Des*. 2004;10(30):3813.

17. Saxena RC, Nath R, Palit G, et al. Effect of calophyllolide, a nonsteroidal anti-inflammatory agent, on capillary permeability. *Planta Med*. 1982;44:246.

18. Said T, Dutot M, Labbé A, et al. Ocular burn: rinsing and healing with ionic marine solutions and vegetable oils. *Ophthalmologica*. 2009;223:52.

19. Yimdjo MC, Azebaze AG, Nkengfack AE, et al. Antimicrobial and cytotoxic agents from Calophyllum inophyllum. *Phytochemistry*. 2004;65:2789.

20. Lim TK. Calophyllum inophyllum. In: *Edible Medicinal and Non-Medicinal Plants*. Vol 2. Fruits. New York: Spring; 2012: 7–19.

21. International Union for Conservation of Nature and Natural Resources (IUCN). The Red List of Threatened Species. www.iucnredlist.org. Accessed October 25, 2012.

22. Ayyanar M, Ignacimuthu S. Ethnobotanical survey of medicinal plants commonly used by Kani tribals in Tirunelveli hills of Western Ghats, India. *J Ethnopharmacol*. 2011;134:851.

23. Itoigawa M, Ito C, Tan HT, et al. Cancer chemopreventive agents, 4-phenylcoumarins from Calophyllum inophyllum. *Cancer Lett*. 2001;169:15.

24. Ong CY, Ling SK, Ali RM, et al. Systematic analysis of in vitro photo-cytotoxic activity in extracts from terrestrial plants in Peninsula Malaysia for photodynamic therapy. *J Photochem Photobiol B*. 2009;96:216.

25. Li YZ, Li ZL, Yin SL, et al. Triterpenoids from Calophyllum inophyllum and their growth inhibitory effects on human leukemia HL-60 cells. *Fitoterapia*. 2010;81:586.

26. Xiao Q, Zeng YB, Mei WL, et al. Cytotoxic prenylated xanthones from Calophyllum inophyllum. *J Asian Nat Prod Res*. 2008;10:993.

27. Hieu TT, Kim SI, Lee SG, et al. Repellency to Stomoxys calcitrans (Diptera: Muscidae) of plant essential oils or in combination with Calophyllum inophyllum nut oil. *J Med Entolmol*. 2010;47:575.

28. Hieu TT, Kim SI, Kwon HW, et al. Enhanced repllency of binary mixtures of Zanthoxylum piperitum pericarp steam distillate or Zanthoxylum armamatum seed oil constituents and Calophyllum inophyllum nut oil and their aerosols to Stomoxys calcitrans. *Pes Manag Sci*. 2010;66:1191.

CHAPTER 17

Petrolatum

Activities:

Hydrating, protecting

Important Chemical Components:

Aliphatic hydrocarbons

Origin Classification:

Petrolatum is derived from petroleum, and is considered synthetic because solvents and other chemicals are used during the refining process.

Personal Care Category:

Emollient, occlusive

Recommended for the following Baumann Skin Types:

All 16 skin types can use this ingredient but it is most useful for dry and S_4 sensitive (allergic) skin types.

SOURCE

Petrolatum is a byproduct of the process of converting petroleum to gasoline. Petroleum itself is composed of fossil plankton and algae-derived substances largely made up of hydrocarbons.[1] Mineral oil and petrolatum are similar but not identical compounds. Both are produced from petroleum but through different complex processes resulting in substances made with hydrocarbons but with very different characteristics. Confusion occurs among many people regarding mineral oil and petrolatum because mineral oil is sometimes referred to as "liquid petrolatum" or "petrolatum liquid." Mineral oil is a mixture of alkanes in the C_{18}–C_{24} range while petrolatum is a mixture of C_{24}–C_{30} alkanes.[2]

HISTORY

Industrial drilling for petroleum started in 1852.[1] The legend goes that Robert A. Chesebrough, a kerosene dealer in the Brooklyn borough of New York City at the time, went to the Titusville, Pennsylvania oil strike to buy cheap kerosene. He heard the men talking about a fatty grease that would accumulate on the drill rods that could cure all kinds of ailments.[3] He developed a way to produce petrolatum from raw crude oil, filed US Patent number 127,568 and Vaseline Petroleum Jelly was born in 1872 as a skin care product.[4] Petrolatum has long been considered by many, including Kligman, to be one of the best moisturizers.[5] It is recognized by the United States Food and Drug Administration (USFDA) as an over-the-counter skin protectant and there is a monograph on its use. Petrolatum is regarded as the most effective of the best occlusive ingredients, which include lanolin, silicones, and mineral oil (Table 17-1).[6] As such, it is a popular cosmetic ingredient in moisturizers, creams, and baby lotions.

TABLE 17-1
Pros and Cons of Petrolatum

PROS	CONS
Considered the most effective occlusive ingredient	Cosmetically inelegant (greasy feeling)
Inexpensive	May increase susceptibility to UV damage
Extremely stable	Effects reverse once ingredient is removed
Does not inactivate other ingredients	May prevent penetration of other ingredients

CHEMISTRY

Petrolatum is a hydrophobic mixture of long-chain aliphatic hydrocarbons with a melting point of 37°C (99°F). Aliphatic hydrocarbons are thought to protect terrestrial plants and insects.[7] Studies have shown that petrolatum confers a protective effect on human skin.[8] It is used to prevent diaper rash and chapped lips as well as to protect wounds while they heal.

Petroleum jelly for cosmetic use comes in the following grades: United States Pharmacopeia (USP), British Pharmacopeia (BP), or European Pharmacopeia (Ph. Eur.) grade. These grades are assigned according to the purity of the raw materials and how the petroleum jelly is processed and intended for medical and personal care, with methods and ranges for physical tests varying by regulatory body.

The Environmental Protection Agency's Toxic Substances Control Act (TSCA) Inventory Number for Petrolatum, 8009-03-8, officially defines petrolatum as "A complex combination of hydrocarbons obtained as a semi-solid from dewaxing paraffinic residual oil. It consists predominantly of saturated crystalline and liquid hydrocarbons having carbon numbers predominately greater than C_{25}."[9] This definition gives no information about the processing or purity of the petrolatum.

Petrolatum is a superior occlusive, and is thought by many to have the best occlusive effects of any substance, because it has the proper alkyl chain lengths that stack up and align to form a tight palisade. Its high viscosity, which prevents the substance from spreading laterally, allows petrolatum to stay in a thick layer at the spot of application. The high viscosity accounts in part for its superior occlusive abilities but causes low spreadability, which makes petrolatum less cosmetically elegant than other ingredients. Occlusive membranes applied to the surface of the skin inhibit lipid synthesis and barrier repair by blocking the many steps in barrier repair linking increased cholesterol and lipid synthesis and lamellar body formation and DNA synthesis. Although it displays occlusive properties, topical petrolatum does not impair barrier function or any of these processes.[10]

ORAL USES

Petrolatum is not to be taken internally.

TOPICAL USES

Petrolatum, when applied topically, has been shown to penetrate into all layers of the stratum corneum (SC). It has also been demonstrated to impart an occlusive effect and to improve barrier function. Grubauer has shown that vapor-impermeable membranes impede barrier recovery, while vapor-permeable ones do not (although they do slow lipid biosynthetic rates).[11] Petrolatum does not interfere with barrier recovery and may actually improve barrier repair.[12] One study by Loden compared barrier recovery in tape-stripped skin in subjects treated with either skin lipids or petrolatum and found that petrolatum performed as well as lipids.[13] However, in this study, oleic acid was used as one of the lipids, even though it is not the ideal lipid choice for barrier repair.

The hydration effect of petrolatum is well established and has been demonstrated using capacitance, conductance, optothermal infrared spectrometry, and transepidermal water loss.[14–17] Ghadially et al. showed that topically applied petrolatum accumulates intercellularly in a nonlamellar manner.[12]

SAFETY ISSUES

Because of its source, several concerns have emerged regarding petrolatum, particularly regarding its potential for toxicity or provoking unwanted side effects. The main purity test for petrolatum is the analytical procedure for polynuclear aromatic hydrocarbons. In animals as well as humans, particular condensed polynuclear aromatic (PNA) compounds have been demonstrated to cause cancer. The FDA and others developed a method in the 1960s that minimized the PNA content of petrolatum and petroleum wax.[9] It is also worth noting that several years of animal feeding studies have yielded no evidence that petrolatum plays a role in carcinogenesis.[9] In some feeding studies, very small portions of petrolatum hydrocarbons have been shown to be absorbed by Fisher 344 rats. The liver and mesenteric lymph nodes were the sites of hydrocarbon accumulation, leading to the typical immune response that any foreign body would provoke. All of the animals successfully eliminated the oil from their systems when petrolatum was removed from their diets.[9]

Notably, petrolatum is well known for being noncomedogenic.[18] Although extremely rare, allergic contact dermatitis to petrolatum has been reported in the literature.[19,20] The possibility of an individual being allergic to petrolatum is so infrequent that most dermatologists believe it to be a nonsensitizing agent.[21] Formulations that contain petrolatum have demonstrated excellent stability with minimal chemical degradation and minor alterations in incorporated compound concentrations.[22,23]

ENVIRONMENTAL IMPACT

See Chapter 13, Mineral Oil.

FORMULATION CONSIDERATIONS

Petrolatum used in drug products is either an active or non-active (excipient) ingredient. It can also serve as the "carrier" or "vehicle" for the active ingredient. In addition, petrolatum can be deemed the active ingredient in over-the-counter (OTC) products.[9] Petrolatum has a markedly long shelf life because of its oxidation-resistant qualities and the fact that it undergoes minimal chemical degradation.[24] It can be used as a delivery system for lipophilic agents and in liposomal formulations.[25] The USP sets a range for consistency, melting point, and maximum color in the two monographs for petrolatum: White Petrolatum USP and Petrolatum USP. The basic difference between these categories is the maximum color. White Petrolatum USP can have some yellow coloring but Petrolatum USP has a definite yellow tint.

USAGE CONSIDERATIONS

Petrolatum displays a water vapor loss resistance 170 times that of olive oil.[26] However, petrolatum is associated with a greasy feeling on the skin that may render agents containing it cosmetically unacceptable. Other commonly used occlusive ingredients include paraffin, squalene, dimethicone, soybean oil, grapeseed oil, propylene glycol, lanolin, and beeswax.[27]

SIGNIFICANT BACKGROUND

Petrolatum is a purified mixture of hydrocarbons that is derived from petroleum (crude oil). The hydrocarbon molecules present in petrolatum prevent oxidation, giving petrolatum a long shelf life. In a 1995 study comparing the capacity of physiologic lipid mixtures to petrolatum in providing barrier repair showed that petrolatum remains limited to the SC whereas physiologic lipids (cholesterol, free fatty acids, and ceramides) penetrate the barrier and are incorporated into organelles.[10] Importantly, though, exogenously applied petrolatum improves the skin barrier within minutes, while exogenously applied physiologic lipids take around two hours to improve the skin barrier. This is likely due to the fact that considerable time is elapsed as keratinocytes absorb the lipids and process them into lamellar bodies. Petrolatum provides immediate barrier recovery even in cold-exposed skin (which experiences slower lamellar body formation), whereas physiologic lipids take longer to repair the barrier.[10] Because petrolatum is one of the most occlusive moisturizing ingredients known, it is often the gold standard to which other occlusive ingredients are compared.[23] However, when used alone, many find the greasy, oily texture cosmetically inelegant. Therefore, petrolatum is often combined with other ingredients to minimize the greasy feeling.

CONCLUSION

Petrolatum is the most effective occlusive ingredient, but is significantly undermined as a popular choice by its uncomfortable feeling on the skin.

REFERENCES

1. Rawlings AV, Lombard KJ. A review on the extensive skin benefits of mineral oil. *Int J Cosmet Sci.* 2012;34:511.
2. Stoker S. Chemical properties of alkanes and cycloalkanes. In: *General, Organic, and Biological Chemistry.* 6th ed. Stamford, Brooks/Cole: Cengage Learning; 2012:369.
3. Goodrum C, Dalrymple H. Cosmetics – How to attract the opposite sex. In: *The First 200 Years: Adverting in America.* New York: Harry Abrams Inc.; 1990:125.
4. Lodén M. Role of topical emollients and moisturizers in the treatment of dry skin barrier disorders. *Am J Clin Dermatol.* 2003;4771.
5. Kligman A. Regression method for assessing the efficacy of moisturizers. *Cosm Toiletr.* 1978;93:27.

6. Kraft JN, Lynde CW. Moisturizers: What they are and a practical approach to product selection. *Skin Therapy Lett*. 2005;10:1.

7. Hadley NF. Lipid water barriers in biological systems. *Prog Lipid Res*. 1989;28:1.

8. Wigger-Alberti W, Elsner P. Petrolatum prevents irritation in a human cumulative exposure model in vivo. *Dermatology*. 1997;194:247.

9. Faust HR, Casserly EW. Petrolatum and Regulation Requirements. Penreco, 2004.

10. Mao-Qiang M, Brown BE, Wu-Pong S, et al. Exogenous nonphysiologic vs physiologic lipids. Divergent mechanisms for correction of permeability barrier dysfunction. *Arch Dermatol*. 1995;131:809.

11. Grubauer G, Feingold KR, Elias PM. Relationship of epidermal lipogenesis to cutaneous barrier function. *J Lipid Res*. 1987;28:746.

12. Ghadially R, Halkier-Sorensin L, Elias P. Effects of petrolatum on stratum corneum structure and function. *J Am Acad Dermatol*. 1992;26:387.

13. Lodén M, Bárány E. Skin identical lipids versus petrolatum in the treatment of tape stripped and detergent perturbed human skin. *Acta Derm Venereol*. 2000;80:412.

14. Skin Moisturization. In: Leyden JJ, Rawlings AV, eds. Zug, Switzerland: Informa Healthcare; 2002:229.

15. Jemee GB, Wulf HC. Correlation between the greasiness and the plasticizing effect of moisturizers. *Acta Derm Venereol*. 1999;79:115.

16. Petersen EN. The hydrating effect of a cream and white petrolatum measured by optothermal infrared spectrophotometry in vivo. *Acta Derma Venereol*. 1991;71:373.

17. Lodén M, Lindberg M. The influence of a single application of different moisturizers on the skin capacitance. *Acta Derm Venereol*. 1991;71:79.

18. American Academy of Dermatology Invitational Symposium on Comedogenicity. *J Am Acad Dermatol*. 1989;20:272.

19. Tam CC, Elston DM. Allergic contact dermatitis caused by white petrolatum on damaged skin. *Dermatitis*. 2006;17:201.

20. Ulrich G, Schmutz JL, Trechot P et al. Sensitization to petrolatum: an unusual cause of false-positive drug patch-tests. *Allergy*. 2004;59:1006.

21. Schnuch A, Lessmann H, Geier J et al. White petrolatum (Ph. Eur.) is virtually non-sensitizing. Analysis of IVDK data on 80 000 patients tested between 1992 and 2004 and short discussion of identification and designation of allergens. *Contact Dermatitis*. 2006;54:338.

22. Fluhr J, Holleran WM, Berardesca E. Clinical effects of emollients on skin. In: Leyden JJ, Rawlings AV, eds. *Skin Moisturization*. New York: CRC Press; 2002:232.

23. Morrison DS. Petrolatum. In: Lodén M, Maibach H, eds. *Dry Skin and Moisturizers*. Boca Raton: CRC;2000:251–257.

24. Fluhr J, Holleran WM, Berardesca E. Clinical effects of emollients on skin. In: Leyden JJ, Rawlings AV, eds. *Skin Moisturization*. New York: CRC Press; 2002:229.

25. Foldvari M. Effect of vehicle on topical liposomal drug delivery: petrolatum bases. *J Microencapsul*. 1996;13:589.

26. Spruitt D. The interference of some substances with the water vapor loss of human skin. *Dermatologica*. 1971;142:89.

27. Draelos Z. Moisturizers. In: *Atlas of Cosmetic Dermatology*. New York: Churchill Livingstone; 2000:83.

CHAPTER 18

Dimethicone and Silicones

Activities:

Occlusive, emollient, skin protectant, antifoaming agent

Important Chemical Components:

The chemical formula for dimethicone (also known as polydimethylsiloxane or PDMS) is $CH_3[Si(CH_3)_2O]n$ $Si(CH_3)_3$ where n is the number of repeating monomer units [molecular formula = $(C_2H_6OSi)_n$]. Silicon dioxide (silica) is the base material from which silicones are derived. Silicon is element number 14 on the atomic chart (see Figure 18-1).

Origin Classification:

Laboratory made from natural ingredients

Personal Care Category:

Hair conditioner, moisturizer

Recommended for the following Baumann Skin Types:

All 16 skin types can use these ingredients.

SOURCE

Dimethicone is derived from silicon. It is a hypoallergenic, noncomedogenic, and nonacnegenic silicone-based polymer second only to petrolatum in terms of frequency of use as an ingredient in moisturizers.[1] Silicones are derived from silica (silicon dioxide), found in sandstone, beach sand, granite, and quartz, and represent the source of all oil-free moisturizers.[2]

HISTORY

Silicon was discovered by the Swedish chemist Jöns Jacob Berzelius in 1824. Today it is produced by heating sand (SiO_2) with carbon to temperatures approaching 2200°C. For this reason it is difficult to categorize silicones as natural or laboratory made. Dimethicone was suggested as a protective ingredient for the skin barrier as early as the late 1950s, and is covered in the United States Food and Drug Administration (USFDA) monograph for skin protectants.[3–5]

CHEMISTRY

According to Nair, "Dimethicone is a fluid mixture of fully methylated linear siloxane polymers end-blocked with trimethylsiloxy units."[6] The potent siloxane bonds that unite

silica and oxygen in these compounds account for the noted thermal and oxidizing stability of silicones.[7] The silicone used in topical skin care products is odorless, colorless, as well as nontoxic and is ideal for water-resistant formulations because it is also immiscible and insoluble in water.[2]

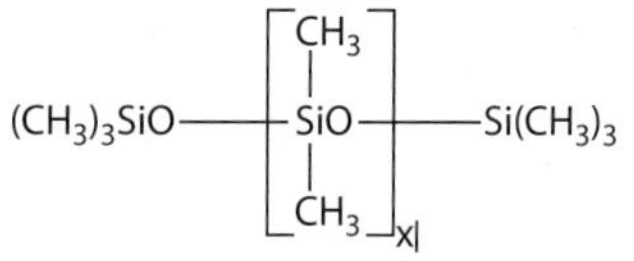

ORAL USES

Dimethicone and silicone products are found in some foods and are not considered to be toxic when taken orally. However, they have no oral activity that would justify their use for skin conditions.[6]

TOPICAL USES

Dimethicone and silicones exert a protective effect on the skin by forming a barrier that hinders the penetration of irritants and allergens. They also decrease transepidermal water loss (TEWL), but not as effectively as petrolatum (Table 18-1). Whereas petrolatum lowers TEWL by 98 percent, dimethicone and other silicones typically reduce TEWL by 20 to 30 percent.[8–10]

The permeability of dimethicone to water vapor makes it an attractive ingredient in facial products because it allows sweat to evaporate off of the skin, but it is insoluble in water and does not mix well with sebum, which gives it staying power on the skin.[2] Dimethicone is commonly used in primers and makeup foundations because its emollient characteristics allow it to fill in surface imperfections, creating a "smoother canvas" for makeup application. It is often found in "long wearing," "oil control," and "waterproof" skin care formulations. Dimethicone coats the hair shaft, smoothing irregularities, so it is found in hair products that condition and add shine to the hair.

In 2000, Fowler enrolled 31 subjects with chronic hand dermatitis lasting at least one year and strongly linked to their work in a study over two months (including a two-week observation period prior to treatment) to determine if a protective foam containing dimethicone and glycerin could mitigate the condition. Twenty-eight patients completed the study, with 21 experiencing significant improvement. The tested foam

$$(CH_3)_3SiO \underset{\underset{\text{Dimethicone}}{}}{-\!\!\left[\begin{array}{c} CH_3 \\ | \\ SiO \\ | \\ CH_3 \end{array}\right]_{x|}\!\!-} Si(CH_3)_3$$

▲ **FIGURE 18-1** Chemical structure of dimethicone.

TABLE 18-1
Pros and Cons of Dimethicone and Silicones

PROS	CONS
Prevents some TEWL	Inert
Inexpensive	Less effective than petrolatum
Less greasy than petrolatum	May hold sebum on the skin's surface
Insoluble in water	May clog pores if used over uncleansed skin
Water permeable	
Hypoallergenic	
Does not mix with sebum	
Has an FDA monograph	

product was indeed found to be protective as subjects continued in their occupations while reporting favorable effects.[11]

Earlier that year, Zhai et al. assessed the efficacy of a dimethicone skin protectant lotion against sodium lauryl sulfate (SLS)-induced irritant contact dermatitis in 12 healthy subjects. The flexor aspects of both forearms of each individual were pretreated with the test formulation or vehicle control 30 minutes before exposure to SLS (0.2 mL of 0.5 percent SLS). A third test site, serving as positive control, received only the irritant. Investigators evaluated the test sites for five days based on visual scoring, TEWL, skin color, and cutaneous blood flow volume. Although they found no statistical differences in treatment sites in terms of cutaneous blood flow and skin color, the researchers noted a significant reduction on the site pretreated with dimethicone as compared to the SLS-only and control vehicle sites in terms of visual score. In addition, TEWL values were significantly lower in the dimethicone lotion-treated sites as compared to the SLS-only sites. The investigators concluded that the appropriate use of dimethicone products can prevent irritant contact dermatitis.[12]

SAFETY ISSUES

Dimethicone and other silicones are unlikely to be absorbed systemically when used topically according to the Cosmetic Ingredient Review (CIR) because of their large molecular weight.[6] Specific silicones found to be safe for use in cosmetic formulations by the CIR include stearoxy dimethicone, dimethicone, methicone (a linear monomethyl polysiloxane), amino bispropyl dimethicone, aminopropyl dimethicone, amodimethicone, amodimethicone hydroxystearate, behenoxy dimethicone, C_{24}–C_{28} alkyl methicone, C_{30}–C_{45} alkyl methicone, C_{30}–C_{45} alkyl dimethicone, cetearyl methicone, cetyl dimethicone, dimethoxysilyl ethylenediaminopropyl dimethicone, hexyl methicone, hydroxypropyldimethicone, stearamidopropyl dimethicone, stearyl dimethicone, stearyl methicone, and vinyldimethicone.[6]

Dimethicone and other silicones have not been found to be comedogenic or to cause contact dermatitis, but are mild ocular irritants.[6] Dimethicone was negative in all genotoxicity assays.

ENVIRONMENTAL IMPACT

Dimethicone and cyclotetrasiloxane degrade into the environment with dimethicone settling into the soil and cyclotetrasiloxane dissipating into the atmosphere. Both are degraded to inorganic constituents, carbon dioxide, silicic acid, and water with no noted ill effects on the environment.[13]

FORMULATION CONSIDERATIONS

Dimethicone comes in various viscosities and is known to add slip and glide to formulations. It is popular in hair conditioning products as well as many skin care products including moisturizers and sunscreens. Dimethicone is often found in "oil-free" personal care products. It is covered by an FDA monograph as a skin care protectant so it does not have to be declared as an active ingredient on product labels.

USAGE CONSIDERATIONS

Dimethicone has not been found to alter drug penetration rates.[14]

SIGNIFICANT BACKGROUND

Combination Treatments

In 2007, Short et al. evaluated the effects of a moisturizer containing dimethicone and glycerin on 15 women with moderately photoaged forearms treated twice daily for four weeks. The investigators noted increases in epidermal thickness, barrier function improvement as evidenced by 13 percent reduction in TEWL, a decline in melanin intensity, and increased keratinocyte proliferation, suggesting structural and functional enhancement via daily use of a dimethicone- and glycerin-containing moisturizer.[15]

Dimethicone, along with glycerin, has also been shown to be an important added ingredient for providing moisturization in an acne formulation that combines clindamycin and benzoyl peroxide in a water-based gel. The same formulation that lacked dimethicone and glycerin was less satisfying and tolerable for patients.[16]

A 2011 randomized, controlled clinical trial with 141 patients in 11 nursing home wards in 4 nursing homes in Belgium showed that a washcloth treated with a 3 percent dimethicone formula significantly outperformed standard of care (water and pH-neutral soap) for incontinence-associated dermatitis. The dimethicone-treated washcloth also significantly lowered the prevalence of incontinence-associated dermatitis, and was linked to a trend toward reduced severity.[17]

CONCLUSION

As the second most used ingredient in moisturizers, dimethicone plays an important role in the topical skin care arsenal. It is an oil-free moisturizing alternative; therefore, it is often used in oil control products because it helps hold the sebum to the surface of the skin, preventing facial shine. However, dimethicone gives the product a slippery feel that some individuals with oily skin types find objectionable. Many studies have shown that dimethicone is not comedogenic. In the author's experience, though, when dimethicone-containing ingredients are not washed off at night, they may contribute to dirt and sebum clogging the pores by holding this debris close to the skin's surface. It is recommended to thoroughly cleanse the dirt and sebum from the face before applying products containing this ingredient and to cleanse the face again at night. It is acceptable to reapply a silicone-containing product to a cleansed face at night. Dimethicone is a safe and useful ingredient in thousands of skin care products when combined with proper cleansing techniques.

REFERENCES

1. Nolan K, Marmur E. Moisturizers: Reality and the skin benefits. *Dermatol Ther*. 2012;25:229.
2. Draelos ZD. Active agents in common skin care products. *Plast Reconstr Surg*. 2010;125:719.
3. Carter BN 2nd, Sherman RT. Dimethicone (silicone) skin protection in surgical patients. *AMA Arch Surg*. 1957;75:116.
4. Banerjee BN, Chakrabarty J. Dimethicone 20 B.P.C. (SILOCERM) – A new multipurpose skin protective barrier ointment as prophylaxis in skin disease, a preliminary report. *Indian J Dermatol*. 1969;14:133.
5. Johnson AW. The skin moisturizer marketplace. In: Leyden JJ, Rawlings AV, eds. *Skin Moisturization*. New York: CRC Press; 2002:20.
6. Nair B. Final report on the safety assessment of dimethicone. Cosmetic Ingredients Review Expert panel. *Int J Toxicol*. 2003;22(Suppl 2):11.

7. Draelos ZD. New treatments for restoring impaired epidermal barrier permeability: Skin barrier repair creams. *Clin Dermatol.* 2012;30:345.

8. Kraft JN, Lynde CW. Moisturizers: What they are and a practical approach to product selection. *Skin Therapy Lett.* 2005;10:1.

9. Lynde CW. Moisturizers: What they are and how they work. *Skin Therapy Lett.* 2001;6:3.

10. Ghadially R, Halkier-Sorensen L, Elias PM. Effects of petrolatum on stratum corneum structure and function. *J Am Acad Dermatol.* 1992;26(3 Pt 2):387.

11. Fowler JF Jr. Efficacy of a skin-protective foam in the treatment of chronic hand dermatitis. *Am J Contact Dermat.* 2000;11:165.

12. Zhai H, Brachman F, Pelosi A, et al. A bioengineering study on the efficacy of a skin protectant lotion in preventing SLS-induced dermatitis. *Skin Res Technol.* 2000;6:77.

13. Stevens C. Environmental fate and effects of dimethicone and cyclotetrasiloxane from personal care applications. *Int J Cosmet Sci.* 1998;20:296.

14. Leopold CS, Maibach HI. Effect of lipophilic vehicles on in vivo skin penetration of methyl nicotinate in different races. *Int J Pharm.* 1996;139:161.

15. Short RW, Chan JL, Choi JM, et al. Effects of moisturization on epidermal homeostasis and differentiation. *Clin Exp Dermatol.* 2007;32:88.

16. Del Rosso JQ. The role of the vehicle in combination acne therapy. *Cutis.* 2005;76(Suppl 2):15.

17. Beeckman D, Verhaeghe S, Defloor T, et al. A 3-in-1 perineal care washcloth impregnated with dimethicone 3% versus water and pH neutral soap to prevent and treat incontinence-associated dermatitis: a randomized, controlled clinical trial. *J Wound Ostomy Continence Nurs.* 2011;38:627.

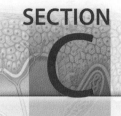

SECTION C

Barrier Repair Ingredients

CHAPTER 19

Barrier Repair Ingredients

The skin barrier is a watertight seal around the keratinocytes in the upper levels of the epidermis. It prevents evaporation of water from the surface of the skin, which is known as transepidermal water loss (TEWL). It is important to note that TEWL is not the same as sweating or perspiration. Increased TEWL occurs when a defect in the permeability barrier allows excessive water to be lost to the atmosphere. The skin barrier decreases TEWL and helps keep unwanted compounds out of the skin, such as allergens and irritants. Skin with an injured barrier is more susceptible to contact and irritant dermatitis as well as infection. Skin barrier perturbation can be caused by many different factors such as detergents, acetone, friction, ultraviolet exposure, prolonged or frequent water immersion, cholesterol-lowering drugs, low-fat diets, and genetic predisposition (e.g., to disorders of filaggrin).

The extracellular lipid mixture surrounding keratinocytes in the upper layer of the epidermis (stratum corneum or SC) is well known to be responsible for that layer's water barrier function.[1] This lipid mixture, which is synthesized by lamellar bodies in the lower levels of the epidermis, is composed of 50 percent ceramides, about 25 percent cholesterol, and about 15 percent fatty acids.[2] Many studies have considered the effect of topically applying these important skin barrier lipids to improve skin barrier function and, thus, skin hydration. These investigations have demonstrated that the exogenously applied lipids must be in the proper ratio to form the correct three-dimensional structure of the skin barrier. When the correct ratios of ceramides, fatty acids, and cholesterol were used, the barrier recovered.[3] Application of a mixture of cholesterol, ceramides, and the essential/nonessential free fatty acids palmitate and linoleate in an equimolar ratio allows normal barrier recovery, whereas a 3:1:1:1 ratio of these four ingredients accelerates barrier recovery.[4] Today, the goal of the best barrier repair moisturizers is to provide these vital components in a 3:1:1:1 ratio.

AGE AND THE SKIN BARRIER

Older skin displays increased drug penetration, dryness, and other signs that the skin barrier may be impaired. Ghadially et al. showed that although the composition, dimensions, and lamellar structure of the bilayer lipids were normal in older individuals (80+ years), their skin had 30 percent less lipids than younger people (20–30 years old) and the number of focal SC lamellar bilayers was decreased. In addition, the barrier recovery time was much longer in older individuals.[5] Waller and Maibach reviewed studies on lipids in aged skin and deemed the findings to be conflicting, with no consensus on whether or not older skin displays a different lipid composition as compared to younger skin.[6]

EXOGENOUSLY APPLIED LIPIDS

Topically applied lipids are transported to the nucleated layers of the SC (such as the spinous layer), internalized, and transported to the distal Golgi apparatus where they are incorporated into lamellar bodies.[7] These lamellar bodies are present in the granular layer of the epidermis and are secreted (containing the newly synthesized lipids) into the intercellular space between the keratinocytes, thus contributing to the lipid bilayer membrane. This *de novo* synthesis of lipids is a crucial mechanism involved in barrier recovery.[8]

The lamellar or Odland bodies play an important role in barrier function, because they deliver enzymes that metabolize lipid hydrolases and lipids to the intercellular spaces of the SC. The lipid hydrolases metabolize lipid precursors such as cholesterol sulfate, phospholipids, sphingomyelin, and glycosylceramides into nonpolar products, which form the extracellular lamellar membrane.[1,9] This lipid processing cascade is affected by changes in pH and other metabolic activity that remains to be elucidated.[10,11] The presence of cholesterol seems to be important in the normal function of lamellar bodies in barrier repair.[12] When cholesterol levels are low, peroxisome proliferator-activated receptors (PPARs) and retinoid X receptors increase expression of ATP-binding cassette transporter A1 (ABCA1), a membrane transporter that regulates cholesterol efflux,[13] resulting in increased transport of cholesterol across keratinocyte cell membranes. It is important to note that replacement of only one of the three primary components of the extracellular matrix (cholesterol, ceramides, or fatty acids) impairs the barrier, while replacement in a 1:1:1 ratio of all of these three classes of compounds repairs the barrier.[3]

ENDOGENOUSLY SYNTHESIZED LIPIDS

Basal cells are capable of absorbing cholesterol from the circulation; however, most lipids are synthesized in cells such as the keratinocytes. Exogenously applied lipids are incorporated into the keratinocytes and lamellar bodies in the granular layer of the SC.[3,8]

There are three rate-limiting enzymes involved in the production of the main lipids of epidermal skin. They include 3-hydroxy-3-methylglutaryl coenzyme A (HMG-CoA) reductase (the rate-limiting enzyme in cholesterol synthesis), acetyl Co-A carboxylase (ACC), and the fatty acid synthase involved in the synthesis of free fatty acids and serine palmitoyl transferase (SPT), which is the regulatory enzyme for the synthesis of ceramides.[14,15] As expected, when skin barrier disruption occurs, the activity of these enzymes is enhanced in order to compensate for barrier dysfunction.[16,17] In addition, a group of transcription factors known as sterol regulatory element-binding proteins (SREBPs) regulate cholesterol and fatty acid synthesis. When epidermal sterols are decreased, the SREBPs are activated via proteolytic processes, enter the cell nucleus and activate genes, leading to increased production of cholesterol and fatty acid synthesis enzymes.[18,19] There are three known types of SREBPs: SREBP-1a, -1c, and SREBP-2. In human keratinocytes, SREBP-2 has been shown to be the predominant form and is involved in regulating cholesterol and fatty acid synthesis.[18] Interestingly, the ceramide pathway is not affected by SREBPs.

FATTY ACIDS

Fatty acids play a crucial role in conferring hydrophobic characteristics to the epidermis. Their addition to cream formulations makes them slightly alkaline with a pH of 7.5 to 9.5.[20] The properties of the fatty acids, and the lipids derived from them, are markedly dependent on chain length and degree of saturation.[21] Fatty acids that have double bonds are known as unsaturated while fatty acids without double bonds are known as saturated. Fatty acids are divided into categories depending on the length of their aliphatic tail chain. Short-chain fatty acids are fatty acids with aliphatic tails of fewer than six carbons, medium-chain fatty acids have 6 to 12 carbons, long-chain fatty acids have 13 to 21 carbons, and very long-chain fatty acids have aliphatic tails longer than 22 carbons. Unsaturated fatty acids found in skin include oleic acid, linoleic acid, α-linolenic acid, and arachidonic acid. Saturated fatty acids found in skin include palmitic and stearic acids. Studies investigating the use of fatty acids to repair the skin barrier have shown that linoleic, palmitic, and stearic acids can repair the barrier within two hours when applied exogenously.[22]

A few notable fatty acids play an important role in inflammation. Linoleic acid, found in corn oil, sunflower seed oil, sesame oil, and safflower oil, forms a prostaglandin known as PGE_1, which exhibits anti-inflammatory and immune-enhancing properties. The fatty acid arachidonic acid forms PGE_2 and leukotrienes, which are highly inflammatory substances. Arachidonic acid is found rarely in plant oils but is abundantly present in animal-derived products such as meat, eggs, and dairy.

CERAMIDES

Ceramide 1 is the most important type of ceramide in skin. It is composed partially of linoleic acid. Because ceramides are expensive additions to skin care formulations, a less costly alternative is to use ingredients that contain linoleic acid, which may help the skin increase production of certain ceramides. Linoleic acid is found in vegetable oils, rapeseed, walnuts, soybeans, and flaxseed. Applying ceramide alone to the skin (without the proper ratio of fatty acids and cholesterol) disrupts the skin barrier and increases TEWL.[22]

CHOLESTEROL

Cholesterol is found in the diet and is included in some moisturizers; however, most of the cholesterol found in the skin is produced by keratinocytes. Cholesterol is synthesized in the keratinocytes by the enzyme cholesterol sulfotransferase type 2B isoform 1b, abbreviated as SULT2B1b. The rate-limiting enzyme in this process is HMG-CoA reductase (see Chapter 21, Cholesterol). Cholesterol esters added to skin moisturizers without the presence of the correct ratio of ceramides and fatty acids have been shown to disrupt barrier function.[1]

BARRIER DISRUPTION

Barrier disruption is caused when alterations occur in the ceramides, cholesterol, and fatty acids that constitute the bilamellar membrane that renders the SC watertight. The three-dimensional structure of this bilayer is important and many factors can affect its shape and function. Cholesterol levels can be reduced by cholesterol-lowering drugs such as statins, leading to decreased cholesterol in the bilamellar membrane. All three components can be damaged or diminished by surfactants, friction, ultraviolet light, prolonged water immersion, immersion in chlorine, and application of moisturizers. Stress and increased cortisol levels have been shown to damage the skin barrier.[23,24]

Certain ingredients can negatively impact the skin's barrier. Solvents such as propylene glycol can cause lipid fluidization or extraction that can alter the barrier.[25] Ingredients with a polar head group attached to alkyl chain lengths of around C_{10}–C_{12} yield a potent penetration enhancer, for example, oleic acid,[26,27] which disrupts the barrier by inserting alkyl chains into ceramides. This leads to pools of oleic acid in the membrane, which becomes more fluid and easier for molecules to diffuse through than intact ceramides.[25] Other ingredients containing unsaturated alkyl chains can also enhance penetration but, in this case, C_{18} appears near optimum. For such unsaturated compounds, the bent *cis* configuration disturbs intercellular lipid packing more so than the *trans* arrangement, which differs little from the saturated analogue.[28] Fatty acid analogues have been developed to function as penetration enhancers.[29]

In summary, the epidermis and surrounding lipid barrier have been described as having a brick-and-mortar structure, with the keratinocytes as the bricks and the cholesterol, ceramides, and fatty acids representing the mortar. Many well-controlled intricate processes govern the formation of this brick-and-mortar structure and much can go awry that impairs its function. Skin care products can significantly influence the formation and proper functioning of this structure as has been shown by a multitude of studies.

REFERENCES

1. Elias PM, Menon GK. Structural and lipid biochemical correlates of the epidermal permeability barrier. *Adv Lipid Res*. 1991;24:1.
2. Feingold KR. Thematic review series: Skin lipids. The role of epidermal lipids in cutaneous permeability barrier homeostasis. *J Lipid Res*. 2007;48:2531.
3. Man MQ, Feingold KR, Elias PM. Exogenous lipids influence permeability barrier recovery in acetone-treated murine skin. *Arch Dermatol*. 1993;129:728.
4. Zettersten EM, Ghadially R, Feingold KR, et al. Optimal ratios of topical stratum corneum lipids improve barrier recovery in chronologically aged skin. *J Am Acad Dermatol*. 1997;37(3 Pt 1):403.

5. Ghadially R, Brown BE, Sequeira-Martin SM, et al. The aged epidermal permeability barrier. Structural, functional, and lipid biochemical abnormalities in humans and a senescent murine model. *J Clin Invest*. 1995;95:2281.

6. Waller J, Maibach H. Age and skin structure and function, a quantitative approach (II): protein, glycosaminoglycan, water, and lipid content and structure. *Skin Res Technol*. 2006;12:145.

7. Madison KC, Howard EJ. Ceramides are transported through the Golgi apparatus in human keratinocytes in vitro. *J Invest Dermatol*. 1996;106:1030.

8. Mao-Qiang M, Brown BE, Wu-Pong S, et al. Exogenous nonphysiologic vs physiologic lipids. Divergent mechanisms for correction of permeability barrier dysfunction. *Arch Dermatol*. 1995;131:809.

9. Elias PM. The epidermal permeability barrier: from the early days at Harvard to emerging concepts. *J Invest Dermatol*. 2004;122:xxxvi.

10. Behne MJ, Meyer JW, Hanson KM, et al. NHE1 regulates the stratum corneum permeability barrier homeostasis. Microenvironment acidification assessed with fluorescence lifetime imaging. *J Biol Chem*. 2002;277:47399.

11. Fluhr JW, Kao J, Jain M et al. Generation of free fatty acids from phospholipids regulates stratum corneum acidification and integrity. *J Invest Dermatol*. 2001;117:44.

12. Feingold KR, Man MQ, Menon GK, et al. Cholesterol synthesis is required for cutaneous barrier function in mice. *J Clin Invest*. 1990;86:1738.

13. Proksch E, Jensen J-M. Skin as an organ of protection. In: Wolff K, Goldsmith LA, Katz SI, Gilchrest BA, Paller AS, Leffell DJ, eds. *Fitzpatrick's Dermatology in General Medicine*. 7th ed. New York: McGraw-Hill; 2007:386–387.

14. Bigby M, Corona R, Szklo M. Evidence-based dermatology. In: Wolff K, Goldsmith LA, Katz SI, Gilchrest BA, Paller AS, Leffell DJ, eds. *Fitzpatrick's Dermatology in General Medicine*. 7th ed. New York: McGraw-Hill; 2007:13.

15. Holleran WM, Feingold KR, Man MQ et al. Regulation of epidermal sphingolipid synthesis by permeability barrier function. *J Lipid Res*. 1991;32:1151.

16. Brown MS, Goldstein JL. Sterol regulatory element binding proteins (SREBPs): Controllers of lipid synthesis and cellular uptake. *Nutr Rev*. 1998;56:S1.

17. Wertz PW. Biochemistry of human stratum corneum lipids. In: Elias PM, Feingold KR, eds. *Skin Barrier*. New York: Taylor & Francis; 2006:33–42.

18. Elias PM. Stratum corneum defensive functions: An integrated view. *J Invest Dermatol*. 2005;125:183.

19. Harris IR, Farrell AM, Holleran WM et al. Parallel regulation of sterol regulatory element binding protein-2 and the enzymes of cholesterol and fatty acid synthesis but not ceramide synthesis in cultured human keratinocytes and murine epidermis. *J Lipid Res*. 1998;39:412.

20. Cosmetic Ingredient Review. Final Report on the Safety Assessment of Oleic Acid, Lauric Acid, Palmitic Acid, Myristic Acid, and Stearic Acid. *J Am Col Toxicol*. 1987;6:321. http://www.cir-safety.org/sites/default/files/115_draft_steary_suppl3.pdf. Accessed November 1, 2012.

21. Berg JM, Tymoczko JL, Stryer L. Lipids and Cell Membranes. In: *Biochemistry*. 5th ed. New York: WH Freeman; 2002:321.

22. Man MQ M, Feingold KR, Thornfeldt CR, et al. Optimization of physiological lipid mixtures for barrier repair. *J Invest Dermatol*. 1996;106:1096.

23. Altemus M, Rao B, Dhabhar FS, et al. Stress-induced changes in skin barrier function in healthy women. *J Invest Dermatol*. 2001;117:309.

24. Denda M, Tsuchiya T, Elias PM, et al. Stress alters cutaneous permeability barrier homeostasis. *Am J Physiol Regul Integr Comp Physiol*. 2000;278:R367.

25. Hadgraft J. Modulation of the barrier function of the skin. *Skin Pharmacol Appl Skin Physiol*. 2001;14(Suppl 1):72.

26. Naik A, Pechtold LA, Potts RO et al. Mechanism of oleic acid-induced skin penetration enhancement in vivo in humans. *J Control Release*. 1995;37:299.

27. Ongpipattanakul B, Burnette RR, Potts RO, et al. Evidence that oleic acid exists in a separate phase within stratum corneum lipids. *Pharm Res*. 1991;8:350.

28. Williams AC, Barry BW. Penetration enhancers. *Adv Drug Deliv Rev*. 2004;56:603.

29. Takahashi K, Sakano H, Numata N, et al. Effect of fatty acid diesters on permeation of anti-inflammatory drugs through rat skin. *Drug Dev Ind Pharm*. 2002;28:1285.

CHAPTER 20

Ceramides

Activities:

Barrier integrity, cell signaling, anti-inflammatory, cellular differentiation and apoptosis,[1] intermediate in sphingomyelin synthesis (effects on cell membranes)[2,3]

Important Chemical Components:

Sphingolipids (sphingosine, phytosphingosine, or 6-hydroxysphingosine)
Linoleic acid

Origin Classification:

Ceramides are naturally occurring but synthetic forms and pseudoceramides are also available.

Personal Care Category:

Barrier repair moisturizer

Recommended for the following Baumann Skin Types:

DRNT, DRNW, DRPT, DRPW, DSNT, DSNW, DSPT, and DSPW. Important to use in all S_4 (allergic) sensitive skin types.

■ SOURCE

Ceramides are derived from the precursor glucosylceramides (GC), which is formed in large quantities by the epidermis and stored in lamellar granules. The enzyme responsible for GC synthesis has been localized to the golgi apparatus and is called ceramide glucosyltransferase.[4] Structured in lamellar sheets, the primary lipids of the epidermis – ceramides, cholesterol, and free fatty acids – play a crucial role in the barrier function of the skin (see Chapter 19, Barrier Repair Ingredients). The intercellular lipids of the SC are composed of approximately equal proportions of ceramides (which may constitute up to 40 percent),[5] cholesterol, and fatty acids.[6] Ceramides are found in the upper levels of the stratum corneum (SC) but are not found in significant supply in the lower levels of the epidermis such as the stratum granulosum or basal layer. This is simply because ceramides are produced in the lamellar bodies in the granular layer of the SC.

There are several ways to generate ceramides in mammalian cells[7–9]:

1. Catabolism of sphingomyelin by the enzyme sphingomyelinase, which is coded by the gene SMPD1. (This is the most important pathway because sphingomyelin is abundant in most cell membranes.)

2. *De novo* synthesis from palmitate and serine by the enzyme serine palmitoyltransferase (SPT), which is coded in part by the gene SPTLC1.[10]

3. Hydrolysis of glucosylceramides by β-glucocerebrosidase.

4. Hydrolysis of galactosylceramides by galactoceramidase.

5. Synthesis from sphinogosine and fatty acid.

6. Dephosphorylation of ceramide 1-phosphate.

Ceramide Synthesis

Production of ceramides is affected by many processes. Exposure to ultraviolet B (UVB) radiation and cytokines has been associated with an increase in the regulatory enzyme for ceramide synthesis, SPT and increased sphingolipid synthesis at the mRNA and protein levels.[11] Stress and other causes of increased cortisol and exposure to glucocorticoids affect barrier function, but the mechanism has not yet been delineated.[12] Dexamethasone stimulates ceramide biosynthesis by upregulating gene expression of SPT.[13] Ceramide production has been shown to be increased by 1,25-dihydroxyvitamin D_3, retinoic acid, ursolic acid, and lactic acid.[14–17] An alkaline pH suppresses β-glucocerebrosidase and acid sphingomyelinase activity (these enzymes need an acidic pH).[18] This is one of the reasons that alkaline soaps can result in poor barrier formation. In addition, a low or neutral pH is associated with poor barrier recovery.[19]

Cytokines may also play a role in ceramide synthesis. TNF and interleukin-1 alpha (IL-1α) stimulate ceramide synthesis and SPT levels.[20] Imiquimod, a TLR-7 receptor agonist, is known to increase IL-1α levels and has been shown to improve the skin's barrier. IL-4 inhibits the production of ceramides.[21]

UV radiation has been shown to increase the amount of intracellular ceramides,[22–24] and UV-damaged skin has been reported to exhibit increased barrier function that renders it less susceptible to damage from irritants.[25] A study by Kim et al. showed that UV radiation induces ceramide production by activation of sphingomyelinase.[23]

Enchanced Ceramide Synthesis Using Precursors

Topical formulations containing linoleic acid such as safflower oil have been shown to increase the formation of Ceramide 1.[26] Nicotinamide applied topically has been shown to increase ceramide synthesis and decrease transepidermal water loss (TEWL).[27] N-acetyl-L-hydroxyproline topically applied to a synthetic skin model resulted in increased ceramide synthesis through its actions on SPT.[28] Topical lactic acid, especially the L-isomer, can increase ceramides.[17]

■ HISTORY

Ceramide 1 was the first natural ceramide identified, in 1982. Synthetic ceramides, studied since the 1950s, are increasingly sophisticated because they are easier to formulate (Table 20-1). Ceramides have come to be known as a complex family of lipids (sphingolipids – a sphingoid base and a fatty acid) involved in cell signaling in addition to their role in barrier homeostasis and water-holding capacity. In fact, they are known to play a critical role in cell proliferation, apoptosis, cell growth, senescence, and cell cycle control differentiation.[29,30]

TABLE 20-1
Pros and Cons of Synthetic Ceramides

Pros	Cons
Improves skin barrier when formulated properly	Must be used in combination with fatty acids and cholesterol or the barrier is impacted negatively
Hydrates and decreases sensitivity to irritant agents	Expensive
	Some forms are derived from animal CNS tissue

CHEMISTRY

Ceramides can be free lipids but in most cases are found as the hydrophobic backbone of a sphingolipid. Ceramides have been classified as Ceramides 1 to 9, along with two protein-bound ceramides labeled as Ceramides A and B, which are covalently bound to cornified envelope proteins (e.g., involucrin).[31] (See Figure 20-1.) All epidermal ceramides are produced from a lamellar body-derived glucosylceramide (GC) precursor.

Ceramides are named based on the polarity and composition of the molecule. As suggested above, the foundational ceramide structure is an amide-linked free fatty acid covalently bound to a long-chain amino alcohol sphingoid base.[32] The various classes of ceramides are grouped according to the arrangements of sphingosine (S), phytosphingosine (P), or 6-hydroxysphingosine (H) bases, to which an α-hydroxy (A) or nonhydroxy (N) fatty acid is attached, in addition to the presence or absence of a discrete ω-esterified linoleic acid residue.[33]

Ceramide 1 is unique insofar as it is nonpolar and contains the fatty acid linoleic acid. The unique structure of Ceramide 1 allows it to act as a molecular rivet, binding the multiple bilayers of the SC together,[5] and contributing to the stacking of lipid bilayers in the intercellular lamellar sheets. Ceramides 1, 4, and 7 exhibit critical functions in terms of epidermal integrity and by serving as the primary storage areas for linoleic acid, an essential fatty acid with significant roles in the epidermal lipid barrier[34] (see Chapter 15, Safflower Oil, and Chapter 19 Barrier Repair Ingredients). The sphingomyelin-derived ceramides (Ceramides 2, 5) are essential for maintaining the integrity of the SC.[35]

Synthetic ceramides, or pseudoceramides, contain hydroxyl groups, two alkyl groups, and an amide bond – the same key structural components of natural ceramides. Consequently, various synthetic ceramides including N-(3-hexadecyloxy-2-hydroxypropyl)-N-2-hydroxyethylhexadecanamide (PC-104) and N-(2-hydroxyethyl)-2-pentadecanolylhexadecanamide (Bio391) have been reported to form the multilamellar structure observed in the intercellular spaces of the SC.[36,37]

ORAL USES

Synthetic ceramides have no effect on skin condition when taken internally because they are broken down by stomach acids. However, oral ingestion of precursors such as linoleic acid may, according to the sparse studies available, help facilitate ceramide production. One study looked at oral administration of glucosylceramides in mice and found that proinflammatory cytokines and scratching were suppressed in an irritant contact dermatitis model.[38]

TOPICAL USES

Ceramides are popular ingredients in skin care preparations. They have been shown to be able to penetrate into the skin when exogenously applied.[39,40] Several derivatives of ceramides

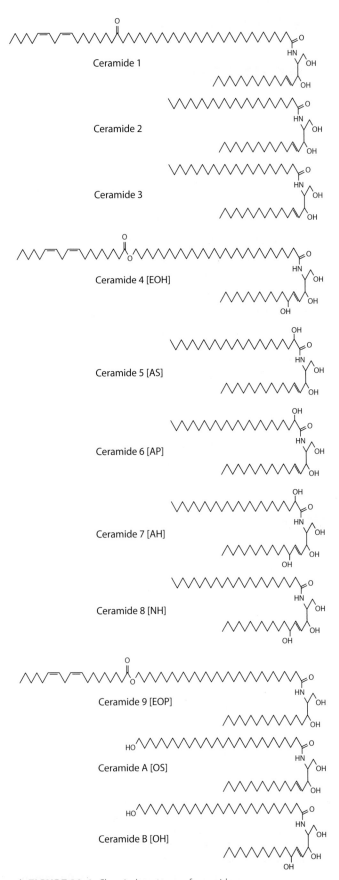

▲ **FIGURE 20-1** Chemical structures of ceramides.

are currently being studied in the dermatology field. Skin conditions such as atopic dermatitis (AD), psoriasis, contact dermatitis, and some genetic disorders have been associated with depleted ceramide levels,[41] but can be ameliorated through the use of exogenous ceramides or their synthetic analogues.

Atopic Dermatitis

AD is known to be a multifactorial disorder recently found to be related to a defect in the filaggrin gene. Prior to the discovery of the role of the filaggrin defect in AD, many studies evaluated the role of barrier lipids in the disease. In 1991, Imokawa reported that subjects with AD had a significantly decreased amount of ceramides in the skin, with Ceramide 1 being the most significantly reduced compared to normal subject skin ceramide content.[42] In addition, the activities of enzymes that break down ceramides and other important lipids in the SC, particularly ceramidase, sphingomyelin deacylase, and glucosylceramide deacylase, have been shown to be elevated in epidermal AD.[41] In a 2004 study published in the *Journal of Investigative Dermatology*, AD skin was found to have less sphingomyelinase activity than normal skin.[43]

Kang et al. conducted studies using synthetic ceramide derivatives of PC-9S (N-Ethanol-2-mirystyl-3-oxo-stearamide), which have been shown to be effective in atopic and psoriatic patients. Both mice studies demonstrated that the topical application of the derivatives K6PC-9 and K6PC-9p resulted in the reduction of skin inflammation and AD symptoms.[44,45] Subsequently, Kang et al. studied the effects of another ceramide derivative, K112PC-5 (2-Acetyl-N-(1,3-dihydroxyisopropyl)-tetradecanamide), on immune cell function, skin inflammation, and AD in mice. Among several findings, the investigators noted that K112PC-5 suppressed AD induced by extracts of dust mites and exhibited *in vitro* and *in vivo* anti-inflammatory activity. They concluded that K112PC-5 is another synthetic ceramide derivative with potential as a topical agent for the treatment of AD.[46]

Frankel et al. compared the short-term effectiveness and desirability of a ceramide-hyaluronic acid emollient to pimecrolimus cream 1 percent in treating AD. Both agents displayed efficacy in mild-to-moderate AD across a broad age range of patients over four weeks. Target lesions were deemed "clear" or "almost clear" in 82 percent of the cases using the ceramide foam and in 71 percent of lesions treated with pimecrolimus, with no reported adverse reactions.[47]

In 2011, Kircik et al. conducted a multicenter, open-label, interventional study to assess the clinical efficacy of a topical emulsion containing ceramides, cholesterol, and fatty acids in a 3:1:1 ratio in 207 patients with mild-to-moderate AD over a three-week period. The formulation was used as single therapy or in combination with another AD medication. The investigators reported that about half of participants received clear or almost clear investigator global assessment scores after monotherapy or combination therapy. A majority (75 percent) of patients reported satisfaction with the treatment as pruritus was diminished and quality of life improved. The authors concluded that the ceramide-containing lipid-based formulation was effective in treating mild-to-moderate AD.[48]

That same year, Miller et al. compared the efficacy of three formulations, including a glycyrrhetinic acid-containing barrier repair cream (BRC-Gly, Atopiclair®), a ceramide-dominant, triple-lipid barrier repair cream (BRC-Cer, EpiCeram™),[49] and a petroleum-based skin protectant moisturizer (OTC-Pet, Aquaphor Healing Ointment®). The study looked at mild-to-moderate AD in 39 children aged 2 to 17 years old randomized 1:1:1 to receive one of the three treatments three times daily for three weeks. Investigators evaluated disease severity and improvement at baseline and days 7 and 21, finding no statistically significant difference in efficacy between the three groups at each time point.[50]

In 2012, Simpson et al. conducted a randomized, intra-individual study to examine the effects of a new moisturizer containing a ceramide precursor on barrier function in patients with controlled AD over a four-week period. In this investigator-blinded study, the cream was applied to one lower leg for 27 days while the other leg served as the untreated control. Researchers took readings at baseline and day 28 on TEWL, skin hydration, and xerosis severity, reporting that after four weeks, significant reductions in TEWL and clinical dryness scores were observed along with increased skin hydration in the areas treated with ceramide cream. In addition, no adverse events were reported.[51] In another study of pseudoceramide formulations and patients with AD, the use of a ceramide complex that also included eucalyptus leaf extract dose-dependently reduced erythema and improved TEWL in comparison to a control vehicle and also increased endogenous SC ceramide levels.[52]

Diminution of Effects from Steroids

Corticosteroids are well known to cause atrophy of the skin with prolonged use. They also cause a defect in the barrier function of the skin demonstrated by increased TEWL.[53] Studies have shown that they disrupt epidermal differentiation resulting in deceased keratohyaline granule formation and a disruption of the lamellar lipid bilayers.[54] A study by Ahn showed that a pseudoceramide containing multilamellar emulsion (MLE) reduced the atrophy resulting from topical steroid use.[55] In addition, the MLE cream when applied after the steroid cream prevented the increase in TEWL normally associated with steroid use and preserved the normal structure of the lamellar lipid bilayers.

Dry Non-Atopic Skin

Ceramide deficiency leads to increased TEWL. Subjects that do not have a history of AD or inflammation can still suffer dry skin due to a ceramide deficiency. In the Baumann Skin Typing system, these subjects would be classified as "Dry, Resistant" types, because they exhibit dry skin without underlying inflammation.

Keratinocyte Differentiation

While extracellular ceramides play important roles in skin hydration, intracellular ceramides found in keratinocytes affect differentiation of keratinocytes.[6,56] In 2007, Kwon et al. generated multiple ceramide derivatives and assessed their impact on keratinocyte differentiation. They found that K6PC-4 [N-(2,3-dihydroxypropyl)-2-hexyl-3-oxo-decanamide], K6PC-5, [N-(1,3-dihydroxypropyl-2-hexyl-3-oxo-decanamide] and K6PC-9 (N-ethanol-2-hexyl-3-oxo-decanamide) spurred a fleeting increase in intracellular calcium levels, incited the phosphorylation of p42/44 extracellular signal-regulated kinase and c-Jun N-terminal kinase, and, in the suprabasal layer of a reconstituted epidermis model, significantly enhanced keratin 1 expression. The investigators concluded that synthetic ceramide derivatives exhibit potential for treating skin diseases involving abnormal keratinocyte differentiation.[57] Ceramides have also been shown to induce phosphorylation of the epidermal growth factor receptor, possibly by activating a protein kinase.[58]

Inflammation

For years, the deficit of ceramides in AD was thought to be the cause of the disorder, leading to many studies examining the effects of ceramides on inflammation. Some studies have shown ceramides to have proinflammatory properties while others emphasize its anti-inflammatory properties.[59,60] For example, in 1996 Di Nardo et al. demonstrated that skin with low ceramide levels was characterized by increased cutaneous inflammation while other studies have shown that ceramides lead to eicosanoid synthesis.[61,62] Sallusto et al. showed that ceramides inhibit the uptake and presentation of antigens by dendritic cells in a murine model.[63] Ceramides seem to modulate inflammation through prostaglandins and by modulation of cytokines such as IL-1, and interferon-γ.[64–66] However, the role of ceramides in inflammation is not completely understood. It may be that the amount of ceramide present influences the inflammatory pathways.[21] Ceramide 1-phosphate may be a more important form of ceramide with respect to its purported proinflammatory activity.[67–69] Ceramide 1-phosphate plays a role in activation of degranulation in mast cells and stimulation of macrophage migration.[70,71]

SAFETY ISSUES

Early forms of ceramides were obtained from animal brains and spinal cords such as cows. The fear of mad cow disease led to the development of laboratory-made ceramides; however, these were initially very expensive. New forms derived from wheat germ and other sources provide a more natural option.

Excess amounts of intracellular ceramides can be toxic to cells, inhibiting growth and causing apoptosis.[22,37,72] Synthetic pseudoceramides differ in structure from naturally occurring ceramides, which raises concerns about their safety.[37]

In 2009, Morita et al. conducted a study evaluating potential adverse effects of the synthetic pseudoceramide SLE66 and showed that the tested product failed to provoke cutaneous irritation or sensitization in animal and human studies. In addition, no phototoxicity or photosensitization was observed and they established 1,000 mg/kg/day (the highest level tested) as the no-observed-adverse-effect (NOAEL) for systemic toxicity after oral administration or topical application.[73] In a related rat study on the potential maternal and fetal effects of SLE66, Morita et al. observed no clinical or internal impact from the orally-administered pseudoceramide across multiple metrics, including fetal malformations.[29]

EpiCeram™ was used in a 2012 study by Lowe et al. to test safety and compliance in a six-week, open-label, phase one trial that found 80 percent of mothers daily applied the cream to their infants (0–4 weeks of age) on 80 percent or more of the days of the study.[49] The investigators concluded that EpiCeram is sufficiently safe and demonstrated satisfactory parental compliance to prevent eczema.[74]

In light of the uncertainty regarding the metabolic impact of pseudoceramides, in 2008 Uchida et al. compared the effects of two chemically unrelated commercially available products to exogenous cell-permeant or natural ceramide on cell growth and apoptosis thresholds in cultured human keratinocytes and found that commercial ceramides did not suppress keratinocyte growth or increase cell toxicity, as did the cell-permeant. The investigators suggested that these findings buttress the preclinical studies indicating that these pseudoceramides are safe for topical application.[37]

ENVIRONMENTAL IMPACT

Now that ceramides can be made in the lab and derived from plants such as wheat germ the environmental impact as was seen when these were sourced from animals is considerably blunted.

FORMULATION CONSIDERATIONS

Natural vs. Synthetic

Identical synthetic ceramides are very expensive ($2,000–$10,000/kg).[37] Less expensive naturally occurring ceramides are derived from the bovine central nervous system, which raises the concern of transmission of bovine spongiform encephalopathy (also known as mad cow disease). For these reasons, synthetic pseudoceramides are often used in skin care products.[37]

Ceramides and pseudoceramides are very hydrophobic and tend to crystallize, thus are difficult to formulate.[75] Organic solvents have been used but tend to dry the skin. Liposomes are often unstable. Oil-in-water emulsions are often used.

Linoleic acid, an important component of ceramides, is very susceptible to oxidation.[76]

USAGE CONSIDERATIONS

Ceramides alone will impair the skin barrier. They must be combined with the proper ratio of cholesterol and fatty acids to improve the skin barrier (see Chapter 19 Barrier Repair Ingredients).

SIGNIFICANT BACKGROUND

Coderch et al., in a review of ceramides and skin function, endorsed the potential of topical therapy for several skin conditions using complete lipid mixtures and some ceramide supplementation, as well as the topical delivery of lipid precursors.[6] And, in fact, the topical application of synthetic ceramides has been shown to speed up the repair of impaired SC.[77,78] Recent reports by Tokudome et al. also indicate that the application of sphingomyelin-based liposomes effectively augments the levels of various ceramides in cultured human skin models.[79,80] It is important to note that ceramides applied topically without the proper equimolar ratio of cholesterol and fatty acids will actually delay barrier recovery in perturbed skin and amplify TEWL[81] (see Chapter 19 Barrier Repair Ingredients).

In 2005, de Jager et al. used small-angle and wide-angle X-ray diffraction to show that lipid mixtures prepared with well-defined synthetic ceramides are very similar to the lamellar and lateral SC lipid organization and lipid phase behavior and can be used to further elucidate the molecular structure and roles of individual ceramides.[82] Previously, stress-induced ceramide accumulation had been shown to result in plasma membrane reorganization and development of ceramide-laden structures known as "rafts," which attract and cluster receptors as well as signaling molecules at the cell membrane to promotesignal transduction cascades.[9] Interestingly, the pathogenesis of various common disorders has been ascribed to raft-related signaling processes, primarily through ceramide accumulation and activation of apoptotic signaling pathways.[83]

Effects of Ceramides on Collagen Production and Degradation

Type I collagen levels in the skin have been shown to be important in the appearance of skin.[84] Antiaging strategies are aimed at: 1) Increasing the amount of collagen produced in the skin and 2) Decreasing the amount of collagen breakdown by collagenase and other matrix metalloproteinases (MMPs).

Ceramides have been shown to play a role in both of these processes and, therefore, likely play an important role in photoaging. Kim demonstrated that UV radiation induces ceramide production by activation of sphingomyelinase.[23] The increased ceramide levels led to increased production of MMP-1, which is known to degrade collagen and facilitate photoaging of the skin.[85] Reunanen showed that ceramide induces collagenase synthesis and that Ceramide 2 inhibits collagen synthesis when added to fibroblast cultures.[86] It is unknown at this time if including ceramides in topical skin formulations can lead to increased induction of MMP-1 mRNA expression because such studies have not been done. However, one study revealed that when linoleic acid was applied to skin and then irradiated with UV, MMP-1 expression was increased,[87] which may have been caused by the oxidation of linoleic oxide to linoleic hyperoxide by the UV.[39] MMP-1 expression also increased when the synthetic ceramide N-oleoyl-phytosphingosine was applied. However, when cholesterol was applied alone, MMP-1 expression was decreased.[39] A small German study (10 human subjects) showed that when jojoba oil and jojoba oil with vitamins were placed on human skin and irradiated with UVA, downregulation of collagen genes resulted.[88] However, when the same oils were combined with phytosterols and ceramides, less downregulation occurred. It is possible that the phytosterols had a protective effect. Antioxidants (such as phytosterols) that block the ERK1/2 pathway may also help inhibit the downregulation of collagen genes. In the case of Ceramide 2 downregulation of collagen synthesis, the downregulation was dependent upon activation of the ERK1/2 pathway, p38 MAPK pathway, and PKC.[86] In the author's opinion, antioxidants may help mitigate the deleterious effects of ceramides on collagen in the skin, especially in the presence of UV radiation.

CONCLUSION

Ceramides are among the primary lipid constituents, along with cholesterol and fatty acids, of the lamellar sheets found in the intercellular spaces of the SC. Together, these lipids maintain the water permeability barrier role of the skin. Ceramides also play an important role in cell signaling. Research over the last 20 years, in particular, indicates that topically applied synthetic ceramide agents, so-called topical ceramide-dominant creams, can effectively compensate for diminished ceramide levels associated with various skin disorders. These products appear to restore barrier integrity and are considered safe and associated with minimal side effects. Ceramides are a crucial component in the skin care regimen of all dry skin types and sensitive skin types (S_4) susceptible to irritant and allergic dermatitis.

REFERENCES

1. Kolesnick RN, Krönke M. Regulation of ceramide production and apoptosis. *Annu Rev Physiol.* 1998;60:643.
2. Hannun YA. The sphingomyelin cycle and the second messenger function of ceramide. *J Biol Chem.* 1994;269:3125.
3. Ruiz-Argüello MB, Basáñez G, Goñi FM, et al. Different effects of enzyme-generated ceramides and diacylglycerols in phospholipid membrane fusion and leakage. *J Biol Chem.* 1996;271:26616.
4. Madison KC, Howard EJ. Ceramides are transported through the Golgi apparatus in human keratinocytes in vitro. *J Invest Dermatol.* 1996;106:1030.
5. Downing DT, Stewart ME, Wertz PW, et al. Skin lipids: An update. *J Invest Dermatol.* 1987;88:2s.
6. Coderch L, López O, de la Maza A, et al. Ceramides and skin function. *Am J Clin Dermatol.* 2003;4:107.
7. Holleran WM, Gao WN, Feingold KR, et al. Localization of epidermal sphingolipid synthesis and serine palmitoyl transferase activity: alterations imposed by permeability barrier requirements. *Arch Dermatol Res.* 1995;287:254.
8. Jensen JM, Schütze S, Förl M, et al. Roles for tumor necrosis factor receptor p55 and sphingomyelinase in repairing the cutaneous permeability barrier. *J Clin Invest.* 1999;104:1761.
9. He X, Schuchman EH. Potential role of acid sphingomyelinase in environmental health. *Zhong Nan Da Xue Xue Bao Yi Xue Ban.* 2012;37:109.
10. Elias PM. Stratum corneum defensive functions: An integrated view. *J Invest Dermatol.* 2005;125:183.
11. Farrell AM, Uchida Y, Nagiec MM, et al. UVB irradiation up-regulates serine palmitoyltransferase in cultured human keratinocytes. *J Lipid Res.* 1998;39:2031.
12. Altemus M, Rao B, Dhabhar FS, et al. Stress-induced changes in skin barrier function in healthy women. *J Invest Dermatol.* 2001;117:309.
13. Holland WL, Brozinick JT, Wang LP, et al. Inhibition of ceramide synthesis ameliorates glucocorticoid-, saturated-fat-, and obesity-induced insulin resistance. *Cell Metab.* 2007;5:167.
14. Geilen CC, Bektas M, Wieder T, et al. The vitamin D3 analogue, calcipotriol, induces sphingomyelin hydrolysis in human keratinocytes. *FEBS Lett.* 1996;378:88.
15. Kalén A, Borchardt RA, Bell RM. Elevated ceramide levels in GH4C1 cells treated with retinoic acid. *Biochim Biophys Acta.* 1992;1125:90.
16. Both DM, Goodtzova K, Yarosh DB, et al. Liposome-encapsulated ursolic acid increasea ceramides and collagen in human skin cells. *Arch Dermatol Res.* 2002;293:569.
17. Rawlings AV, Davies A, Carlomusto M, et al. Effect of lactic acid isomers on keratinocyte ceramide synthesis, stratum corneum lipid levels and stratum corneum barrier function. *Arch Dermatol Res.* 1996;288:383.
18. Hachem JP, Man MQ, Crumrine D, et al. Sustained serine proteases activity by prolonged increase in pH leads to degradation of lipid processing enzymes and profound alterations of barrier function and stratum corneum integrity. *J Invest Dermatol.* 2005;125:510.
19. Hachem JP, Crumrine D, Fluhr J, et al. pH directly regulates epidermal permeability barrier homeostasis, and stratum corneum integrity/cohesion. *J Invest Dermatol.* 2003;121:345.
20. Barland CO, Zettersten E, Brown BS, et al. Imiquimod-induced interleukin-1 alpha stimulation improves barrier homeostasis in aged murine epidermis. *J Invest Dermatol.* 2004;122:330.
21. Hatano Y, Terashi H, Arakawa S, et al. Interleukin-4 suppresses the enhancement of ceramide synthesis and cutaneous permeability barrier functions induced by tumor necrosis factor-alpha and interferon-gamma in human epidermis. *J Invest Dermatol.* 2005;124:786.
22. Geilen CC, Wieder T, Orfanos CE. Ceramide signaling: Regulatory role in cell proliferation, differentiation and apoptosis in human epidermis. *Arch Dermatol Res.* 1997;289:559.
23. Kim S, Kim Y, Lee Y, et al. Ceramide accelerates ultraviolet-induced MMP-1 expression through JAK1/STAT-1 pathway in cultured human dermal fibroblasts. *J Lipid Res.* 2008;49:2571.
24. Grether-Beck S, Timmer A, Felsner I, et al. Ultraviolet A-induced signaling involves a ceramide-mediated autocrine loop leading to ceramide de novo synthesis. *J Invest Dermatol.* 2005;125:545.
25. Lehmann P, Hölzle E, Melnik B, et al. Effects of ultraviolet A and B on the skin barrier: a functional, electron microscopic and lipid biochemical study. *Photodermatol Photoimmunol Photomed.* 1991;8:129.
26. Prottey C, Hartop PJ, Press M. Correction of the cutaneous manifestations of essential fatty acid deficiency in man by application of sunflower-seed oil to the skin. *J Invest Dermatol.* 1975;64:228.
27. Tanno O, Ota Y, Kitamura N, et al. Nicotinamide increases biosynthesis of ceramides as well as other stratum corneum lipids to improve the epidermal permeability barrier. *Br J Dermatol.* 2000;143:524.
28. Hashizume E, Nakano T, Kamimura A, et al. Topical effects of N-acetyl-L-hydroxyproline on ceramides synthesis and alleviation of pruritus. *Clin Cosmet Investig Dermatol.* 2013;6:43.
29. Morita O, Knapp JF, Tamaki Y, et al. Safety studies of pseudo-ceramide SLE66. Part 3: Effects on embryo/fetal development in rats. *Food Chem Toxicol.* 2009;47:681.
30. Sawai H, Domae N, Okazaki T. Current status and perspectives in ceramide targeting molecular medicine. *Curr Pharm Des.* 2005;11:2479.

31. Bouwstra JA, Pilgrim K, Ponec M. Structure of the skin barrier. In: Elias PM, Feingold KR, eds. *Skin Barrier*. New York: Taylor and Francis; 2006:65.

32. Sajić D, Asiniwasis R, Skotnicki-Grant S. A look at epidermal barrier function in atopic dermatitis: physiologic lipid replacement and the role of ceramides. *Skin Therapy Lett*. 2012;17:6.

33. de Jager MW, Gooris GS, Dolbnya IP, et al. Novel lipid mixtures based on synthetic ceramides reproduce the unique stratum corneum lipid organization. *J Lipid Res*. 2004;45:923.

34. Elias PM, Brown BE, Ziboh VA. The permeability barrier in essential fatty acid deficiency: Evidence for a direct role for linoleic acid in barrier function. *J Invest Dermatol*. 1980;74:230.

35. Uchida Y, Hara M, Nishio H, et al. Epidermal sphingomyelins are precursors for selected stratum corneum ceramides. *J Lipid Res*. 2000;41:2071.

36. Mizushima H, Fukasawa J, Suzuki T. Phase behavior of artificial stratum corneum lipids containing a synthetic pseudo-ceramide: A study of the function of cholesterol. *J Lipid Res*. 1996;37:361.

37. Uchida Y, Holleran WM, Elias PM. On the effects of topical synthetic pseudoceramides: Comparison of possible keratinocyte toxicities provoked by the pseudoceramides, PC104 and BIO391, and natural ceramides. *J Dermatol Sci*. 2008;51:37.

38. Yeom M, Kim SH, Lee B, et al. Oral administration of glucosylceramide ameliorates inflammatory dry-skin condition in chronic oxazolone-induced irritant contact dermatitis in the mouse ear. *J Dermatol Sci*. 2012;67:101.

39. Byun HJ, Cho KH, Eun HC, et al. Lipid ingredients in moisturizers can modulate skin responses to UV in barrier-disrupted human skin in vivo. *J Dermatol Sci*. 2012;65:110.

40. Mao-Qiang M, Brown BE, Wu-Pong S, et al. Exogenous nonphysiologic vs physiologic lipids. Divergent mechanisms for correction of permeability barrier dysfunction. *Arch Dermatol*. 1995;131:809.

41. Choi MJ, Maibach HI. Role of ceramides in barrier function of healthy and diseased skin. *Am J Clin Dermatol*. 2005;6:215.

42. Imokawa G, Abe A, Jin K, et al. Decreased level of ceramides in stratum corneum of atopic dermatitis: An etiologic factor in atopic dry skin? *J Invest Dermatol*. 1991;96:523.

43. Jensen JM, Fölster-Holst R, Baranowsky A, et al. Impaired sphingomyelinase activity and epidermal differentiation in atopic dermatitis. *J Invest Dermatol*. 2004;122:1423.

44. Kang JS, Youm JK, Jeong SK, et al. Topical application of a novel ceramide derivative, K6PC-9, inhibits dust mite extract-induced atopic dermatitis-like skin lesions in NC/Nga mice. *Int Immunopharmacol*. 2007;7:1589.

45. Kang JS, Yoon WK, Youm JK, et al. Inhibition of atopic dermatitis-like skin lesions by topical application of a novel ceramide derivative, K6PC-9p, in NC/Nga mice. *Exp Dermatol*. 2008;17:958.

46. Kang JS, Lee CW, Lee K, et al. Inhibition of skin inflammation and atopic dermatitis by topical application of a novel ceramide derivative, K112PC-5, in mice. *Arch Pharm Res*. 2008;31:1004.

47. Frankel A, Sohn A, Patel RV, et al. Bilateral comparison study of pimecrolimus cream 1% and a ceramide-hyaluronic acid emollient foam in the treatment of patients with atopic dermatitis. *J Drugs Dermatol*. 2011;10:666.

48. Kircik LH, Del Rosso JQ, Aversa D. Evaluating clinical use of a ceramide-dominant, physiologic lipid-based topical emulsion for atopic dermatitis. *J Clin Aesthet Dermatol*. 2011;4:34.

49. Draelos ZD. New treatments for restoring impaired epidermal barrier permeability: Skin barrier repair creams. *Clin Dermatol*. 2012;30:345.

50. Miller DW, Koch SB, Yentzer BA, et al. An over-the-counter moisturizer is as clinically effective as, and more cost-effective than, prescription barrier creams in the treatment of children with mild-to-moderate atopic dermatitis: a randomized, controlled trial. *J Drugs Dermatol*. 2011;10:531.

51. Simpson E, Böhling A, Bielfeldt S, et al. Improvement of skin barrier function in atopic dermatitis patients with a new moisturizer containing a ceramide precursor. *J Dermatolog Treat*. 2013;24:122.

52. Ishikawa J, Shimotoyodome Y, Chen S, et al. Eucalyptus increases ceramide levels in keratinocytes and improves stratum corneum function. *Int J Cosmet Sci*. 2012;34:17.

53. Kolbe L, Kligman AM, Schreiner V, et al. Corticosteroid-induced atrophy and barrier impairment measured by non-invasive methods in human skin. *Skin Res Technol*. 2001;7:73.

54. Radoja N, Komine M, Jho SH, et al. Novel mechanism of steroid action in skin through glucocorticoid receptor monomers. *Mol Cell Biol*. 2000;20:4328.

55. Ahn SK, Bak HN, Park BD, et al. Effects of a multilamellar emulsion on glucocorticoid-induced epidermal atrophy and barrier impairment. *J Dermatol*. 2006;33:80.

56. Geilen CC, Barz S, Bektas M. Sphingolipid signaling in epidermal homeostasis. Current knowledge and new therapeutic approaches in dermatology. *Skin Pharmacol Appl Skin Physiol*. 2001;14:261.

57. Kwon YB, Kim CD, Youm JK, et al. Novel synthetic ceramide derivatives increase intracellular calcium levels and promote epidermal keratinocyte differentiation. *J Lipid Res*. 2007;48:1936.

58. Raines MA, Kolesnick RN, Golde DW. Sphingomyelinase and ceramide activate mitogen-activated protein-kinase in myeloid HL-60 cells. *J Biol Chem*. 1993;268:14572.

59. Hayakawa M, Jayadev S, Tsujimoto M, et al. Role of ceramide in stimulation of the transcription of cytosolic phospholipase A2 and cyclooxygenase 2. *Biochem Biophys Res Commun*. 1996;220:681.

60. Masini E, Giannini L, Nistri S, et al. Ceramide: A key signaling molecule in a Guinea pig model of allergic asthmatic response and airway inflammation. *J Pharmacol Exp Ther*. 2008;324:548.

61. di Nardo A, Sugino K, Wertz P, et al. Sodium lauryl sulfate (SLS) induced irritant contact dermatitis: A correlation study between ceramides and in vivo parameters of irritation. *Contact Dermatitis*. 1996;35:86.

62. Lamour NF, Stahelin RV, Wijesinghe DS, et al. Ceramide kinase uses ceramide provided by ceramide transport protein: Localization to organelles of eicosanoid synthesis. *J Lipid Res*. 2007;48:1293.

63. Sallusto F, Nicolò C, De Maria R, et al. Ceramide inhibits antigen uptake and presentation by dendritic cells. *J Exp Med*. 1996;184:2411.

64. Kirtikara K, Laulederkind SJ, Raghow R, et al. An accessory role for ceramide in interleukin-1beta induced prostaglandin synthesis. *Mol Cell Biochem*. 1998;181:41.

65. Ballou LR, Chao CP, Holness MA, et al. Interleukin-1-mediated PGE2 production and sphingomyelin metabolism. Evidence for the regulation of cyclooxygenase gene expression by sphingosine and ceramide. *J Biol Chem*. 1992;267:20044.

66. Wakita H, Nishimura K, Tokura Y, et al. Inhibitors of sphingolipid synthesis modulate interferon (IFN)-gamma-induced intercellular adhesion molecule (ICAM)-1 and human leukocyte antigen (HLA)-DR expression on cultured normal human keratinocytes: Possible involvement of ceramide in biologic action of IFN-gamma. *J Invest Dermatol*. 1996;107:336.

67. Pettus BJ, Bielawska A, Spiegel S, et al. Ceramide kinase mediates cytokine- and calcium ionophore-induced arachidonic acid release. *J Biol Chem*. 2003;278:38206.

68. Wijesinghe DS, Lamour NF, Gomez-Munoz A, et al. Ceramide kinase and ceramide-1-phosphate. *Methods Enzymol*. 2007;434:265.

69. Chalfant CE, Spiegel S. Sphingosine 1-phosphate and ceramide 1-phosphate: Expanding roles in cell signaling. *J Cell Sci*. 2005;118:4605.

70. Mitsutake S, Kim TJ, Inagaki Y, et al. Ceramide kinase is a mediator of calcium-dependent degranulation in mast cells. *J Biol Chem*. 2004;279:17570.

71. Granado MH, Gangoiti P, Ouro A, et al. Ceramide 1-phosphate (C1P) promotes cell migration involvement of a specific C1P receptor. *Cell Signal*. 2009;21:405.

72. Hannun YA, Obeid LM. The Ceramide-centric universe of lipid-mediated cell regulation: Stress encounters of the lipid kind. *J Biol Chem*. 2002;277:25847.

73. Morita O, Ogura R, Hayashi K, et al. Safety studies of pseudo-ceramide SLE66: Acute and short-term toxicity. *Food Chem Toxicol*. 2009;47:669.

74. Lowe AJ, Tang ML, Dharmage SC, et al. A phase I study of daily treatment with a ceramide-dominant triple lipid mixture commencing in neonates. *BMC Dermatol*. 2012;12:3.

75. Park BD, Kim Y, Lee M-J, et al. Properties of a pseudoceramide multilamellar emulsion in vitro and in vivo. *Cosm Toiletr*. 2001;116:65.

76. Spiteller G. The relation of lipid peroxidation processes with atherogenesis: A new theory on atherogenesis. *Mol Nutr Food Res*. 2005;49:999.

77. Imokawa G, Yada Y, Higuchi K, et al. Pseudo-acylceramide with linoleic acid produces selective recovery of diminished cutaneous barrier function in essential fatty acid-deficient rats and has an inhibitory effect on epidermal hyperplasia. *J Clin Invest*. 1994;94:89.

78. Takagi Y, Nakagawa H, Higuchi K, et al. Characterization of surfactant-induced skin damage through barrier recovery induced by pseudoacylceramides. *Dermatology*. 2005;211:128.

79. Tokudome Y, Jinno M, Todo H, et al. Increase in ceramide level after application of various sizes of sphingomyelin liposomes to

TABLE 21-2
Pros and Cons of Cholesterol

Pros	Con
Endogenous synthesis	Topical application alone (without ceramides or fatty acids) delays barrier repair
Key regulator of membrane fluidity and keratinization	

Leaders of the research in this field include Elias, Feingold, Menon, and Ghadially. Their work showed that cholesterol, fatty acids, and ceramides must all be replaced in the skin in an equivalent ratio (1:1:1) in order for barrier repair to occur. Topically placing only cholesterol on the skin leads to *delayed* barrier repair.

Research in the ensuing years has examined the process by which cholesterol is synthesized and released into the space between skin cells providing a watertight barrier. Ceramides, cholesterol, and fatty acids are synthesized by keratinocytes and packaged in lamellar bodies, which carry them until they are extruded into the intracellular space where they form the "skin barrier" that helps prevent TEWL from the epidermis (see Chapter 19, Barrier Repair Ingredients). When the skin barrier is disturbed by detergents, friction, prolonged water immersion, and other insults, keratinocytes repair it by synthesizing more lipids. Cholesterol plays a crucial role in the early stages of barrier repair as shown in a 1990 study that demonstrated that when cholesterol synthesis is inhibited, lamellar secretion is impaired and lamellar body internal structure is altered, leading to delayed barrier repair.[19] Studies have shown that delivery of circulating sterols does not increase after barrier disruption, implying that locally derived sterol from cholesterol is necessary for the synthesis of lipids in lamellar bodies.[13,20,21] It is now known that in the early stages of barrier repair, cholesterol is essential to contribute to the free sterol that is packaged into lamellar bodies. In fact, the topical application of lovastatin, a competitive inhibitor of HMG-CoA reductase that is known to block cholesterol synthesis, delays barrier recovery.[12]

CHEMISTRY

Cholesterol is a lipid but it differs in structure from other lipids because of its steroid nucleus. A hydrocarbon tail is linked to the steroid nucleus at one end and a hydroxyl group is attached at the

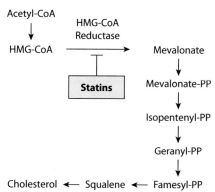

▲ **FIGURE 21-1** Cholesterol Synthesis. Cholesterol is synthesized from Acetyl Co A. The rate-limiting enzyme is HMG-CoA reductase, which is the enzyme that statin cholesterol-lowering drugs block.

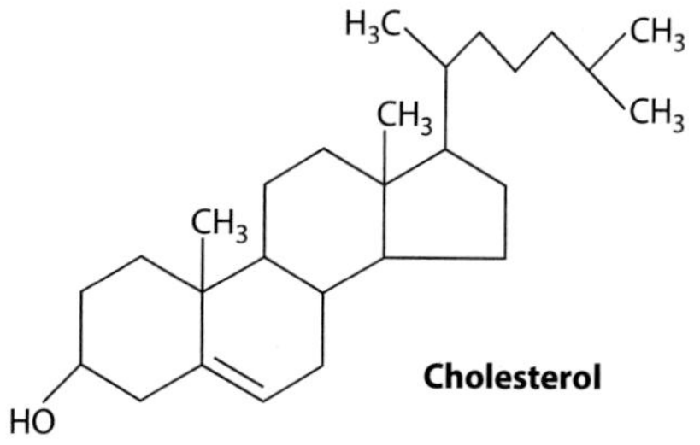

▲ **FIGURE 21-2** A hydrocarbon tail is linked to a steroid nucleus at one end and a hydroxyl group is attached at the other end.

other end (Figure 21-2). The hydroxyl group (polar head) in position 3 causes cholesterol to be roughly perpendicular to the bilayer membrane surface. This structure allows cholesterol to be a key regulator of membrane fluidity, plasticity, and rigidity.[22,23]

In the biosynthetic pathway of endogenous cholesterol synthesis, the conversion of HMGCoA to mevalonic acid is an early rate-limiting step. Cholesterol-lowering drugs such as lovastatin block this enzyme, leading to a decrease in serum cholesterol but also to a decrease in barrier recovery.[19]

ORAL USES

Cholesterol in the diet has been associated with an increased risk of cardiovascular disease, but dietary cholesterol does not necessarily correlate with serum cholesterol levels or increases in LDL, the so-called "bad" cholesterol. This is a complex topic a thorough discussion of which is beyond the scope of this book, however.

TOPICAL USES

Barrier Repair

Topically applied cholesterol can penetrate into the nucleated layers of the SC and be taken up into the cytosol, where its components are broken down and packaged into lamellar bodies.[12] Exogenously applied cholesterol does not downregulate cholesterol synthesis in the skin.[24] For these reasons, cholesterol is an important and popular additive to barrier repair creams. Cholesterol is required for the permeability barrier to function normally (see Chapter 19 Barrier Repair Ingredients). Aged skin shows a decreased ability for lipid synthesis, particularly cholesterol synthesis, which leads to a delayed barrier recovery response in older individuals. Ghadially reported that topical application of cholesterol after perturbation of the skin barrier accelerated barrier repair in aged mice skin and, in a different study a year later with Zettersten, was able to accelerate barrier repair using a mixture containing cholesterol/ceramide/palmitate and linoleate at a ratio of 3:1:1:1.[25,26] Topically applied lovastatin, a drug that inhibits HMG-CoA reductase and prevents cholesterol synthesis, delayed barrier recovery in mice by 50 percent. Addition of cholesterol to the skin of these same mice normalized barrier recovery, showing the importance of cholesterol in barrier recovery and function.[19]

Keratinization

In order for keratinocytes to develop the permeability barrier, they must first undergo differentiation and maturation, which culminates in the formation of the outermost layer of the skin – the SC. This process is known as *keratinization*. Keratinization affects the skin barrier and skin moisturization for two main reasons: 1) Keratinocyte maturation allows formation of the lamellar bodies in which cholesterol, phospholipids, and glucosylceramides are synthesized and stored prior to being released into the extracellular space; 2) Keratinocyte maturation leads to the production of structural proteins such as loricrin and involucrin that provide scaffolding needed for the development of lamellar bodies.[5,27,28]

Cholesterol plays a crucial role in regulating the keratinization process, through various mechanisms.[29,30] In cell membranes, cholesterol is organized into "lipid rafts,"[4] which modulate the activation of epidermal stem cells into amplifying keratinocytes by regulating specific enzymes and influencing various signaling processes.[4,29,31] Many pathways affect the keratinization process in the skin. A few that are known to alter keratinization by affecting cholesterol synthesis include:

1. SULT2B1b is the key enzyme in the synthesis of cholesterol sulfate.
2. HMG-CoA reductase is the rate-limiting step in the production of cholesterol.
3. Activation of PPARα, PPAR β/Δ, and PPAR-γ increases cholesterol synthesis.[32]
4. SREBPs also regulate cholesterol and fatty acid synthesis.
5. Liver X receptors (LXR) and PPARs regulate the expression of SULT2B1b.[33–36]

Cholesterol sulfate is important for cell-to-cell cohesion. The removal of sulfate by steroid sulfatase is required for desquamation of the SC.[23] Alterations in cholesterol sulfate result in impaired epidermal differentiation and corneocyte desquamation.[36] For example, X-linked ichthyosis (also known as steroid sulfatase deficiency), a skin disease caused by a deficiency of cholesterol sulfate, is characterized by abnormal corneocyte retention, resulting in rough, dry, "fish-like" skin. Ichthyosis has also been reported in patients on cholesterol-lowering drugs.[37]

SAFETY ISSUES

There are no studies that demonstrate that topically applied cholesterol raises serum cholesterol levels.

ENVIRONMENTAL IMPACT

None

FORMULATION CONSIDERATIONS

Applying topical cholesterol alone is known to impair the skin barrier. It must be combined with an equimolar amount of ceramides and fatty acids as discussed above and in Chapter 19.[38]

USAGE CONSIDERATIONS

One intriguing aspect about cholesterol is that it need not be applied to the skin. The skin cells can be prompted to synthesize cholesterol. For example, cytokines such as interleukin-1α and interferon-γ increase cholesterol synthesis.[39]

SIGNIFICANT BACKGROUND

Cholesterol and Photoaging

Ultraviolet A has been shown to engender peroxidation of cholesterol to cholesterol hydroperoxides (Chol-OOHs),[40] which can cause damage to cell membranes and become even more deleterious when further reduced to oxylradicals.[41] Oxylradicals are free radicals that lead to a cascade of chain peroxidation reactions, thus elevating matrix metalloproteinase-9 MMP-9 levels,[41] collagenase expression, and other harmful effects (see Chapter 2, Basic Cosmetic Chemistry, and Chapter 46, Antioxidants). Notably, Chol-OOHs have been used as a biomarker of physiological aging in the skin.[42]

CONCLUSION

Cholesterol is a fascinating skin care ingredient because of its effects on the skin barrier and the keratinization process. Cholesterol may play a role in skin care even when it is not included in the actual skin care product, because other ingredients can influence or spur cholesterol production.

REFERENCES

1. Herchi W, Harrabi S, Sebei K, et al. Phytosterols accumulation in the seeds of Linum usitatissimum L. *Plant Physiol Biochem.* 2009;47:880.
2. Ros E. Health benefits of nut consumption. *Nutrients.* 2010;2:652.
3. Gniadecki R, Christoffersen N, Wulf HC. Cholesterol-rich plasma membrane domains (lipid rafts) in keratinocytes: Importance in the baseline and UVA-induced generation of reactive oxygen species. *J Invest Dermatol.* 2002;118:582.
4. Simons K, Toomre D. Lipid rafts and signal transduction. *Nat Rev Mol Cell Biol.* 2000;1:31.
5. Feingold KR, Jiang YJ. The mechanisms by which lipids coordinately regulate the formation of the protein and lipid domains of the stratum corneum: Role of fatty acids, oxysterols, cholesterol sulfate and ceramides as signaling molecules. *Dermatoendocrinol.* 2011;3:113.
6. Proksch E, Jensen J-M. Skin as an organ of protection. In: Wolff K, Goldsmith LA, Katz SI, Gilchrest BA, Paller AS, Leffell DJ, eds. *Fitzpatrick's Dermatology in General Medicine.* 7th ed. New York: McGraw-Hill; 2007:386–387.
7. Jackson SM, Wood LC, Lauer S, et al. Effect of cutaneous permeability barrier disruption on HMG-CoA reductase, LDL receptor, and apolipoprotein E mRNA levels in the epidermis of hairless mice. *J Lipid Res.* 1992;33:1307.
8. Fenjves ES, Gordon DA, Pershing LK, et al. Systemic distribution of apolipoprotein E secreted by grafts of epidermal keratinocytes: implications for epidermal function and gene therapy. *Proc Natl Acad Sci U S A.* 1989;86:8803.
9. Mommaas-Kienhuis AM, Grayson S, Wijsman MC, et al. Low density lipoprotein receptor expression on keratinocytes in normal and psoriatic epidermis. *J Invest Dermatol.* 1987;89:513.
10. Elias PM. Stratum corneum defensive functions: an integrated view. *J Invest Dermatol.* 2005;125:183.
11. Harris IR, Farrell AM, Holleran WM, et al. Parallel regulation of sterol regulatory element binding protein-2 and the enzymes of cholesterol and fatty acid synthesis but not ceramide synthesis in cultured human keratinocytes and murine epidermis. *J Lipid Res.* 1998;39:412.
12. Menon GK, Feingold KR, Mao-Qiang M, et al. Structural basis for the barrier abnormality following inhibition of HMG CoA reductase in murine epidermis. *J Invest Dermatol.* 1992;98:209.
13. Grubauer G, Feingold KR, Elias PM. Relationship of epidermal lipogenesis to cutaneous barrier function. *J Lipid Res.* 1987;28:746.
14. Wertz PW. Biochemistry of human stratum corneum lipids. In Elias PM, Feingold KR, eds. *Skin Barrier.* New York: Taylor and Francis; 2006:33–42.

15. Ponec M, Havekes L, Kempenaar J, et al. Calcium-mediated regulation of the low density lipoprotein receptor and intracellular cholesterol synthesis in human epidermal keratinocytes. *J Cell Physiol.* 1985;125:98.

16. Proksch E, Elias PM, Feingold KR. Regulation of 3-hydroxy-3-methylglutaryl-coenzyme A reductase activity in murine epidermis: Modulation of enzyme content and activation state by barrier requirements. *J Clin Invest.* 1990;85:874.

17. Feingold KR, Man MQ, Proksch E, et al. The lovastatin-treated rodent: A new model of barrier disruption and epidermal hyperplasia. *J Invest Dermatol.* 1991;96:201.

18. Elias PM. The epidermal permeability barrier: From the early days at Harvard to emerging concepts. *J Invest Dermatol.* 2004;122:xxxvi.

19. Feingold KR, Man MQ, Menon GK, et al. Cholesterol synthesis is required for cutaneous barrier function in mice. *J Clin Invest.* 1990;86:1738.

20. Feingold KR, Brown BE, Lear SR, et al. Effect of essential fatty acid deficiency on cutaneous sterol synthesis. *J Invest Dermatol.* 1986;87:588.

21. Grubauer G, Elias PM, Feingold KR. Transepidermal water loss: the signal for recovery of barrier structure and function. *J Lipid Res.* 1989;30:323.

22. Berg JM, Tymoczko JL, Stryer L. Lipids and cell membranes. In *Biochemistry.* 5th ed. New York: WH Freeman and Co.; 2002:338.

23. Choi MJ, Maibach HI. Role of ceramides in barrier function of healthy and diseased skin. *Am J Clin Dermatol.* 2005;6:215.

24. Menon GK, Feingold KR, Moser AH, et al. De novo sterologenesis in the skin. II. Regulation by cutaneous barrier requirements. *J Lipid Res.* 1985;26:418.

25. Ghadially R, Brown BE, Hanley K, et al. Decreased epidermal lipid synthesis accounts for altered barrier function in aged mice. *J Invest Dermatol.* 1996;106:1064.

26. Zettersten EM, Ghadially R, Feingold KR, et al. Optimal ratios of topical stratum corneum lipids improve barrier recovery in chronologically aged skin. *J Am Acad Dermatol.* 1997;37:403.

27. Elias PM, Schmuth M, Uchida Y, et al. Basis for the permeability barrier abnormality in lamellar ichthyosis. *Exp Dermatol.* 2002;11:248.

28. Schmuth M, Fluhr JW, Crumrine DC, et al. Structural and functional consequences of loricrin mutations in human loricrin keratoderma (Vohwinkel syndrome with ichthyosis). *J Invest Dermatol.* 2004;122:909.

29. Jans R, Atanasova G, Jadot M, et al. Cholesterol depletion upregulates involucrin expression in epidermal keratinocytes through activation of p38. *J Invest Dermatol.* 2004;123:564.

30. Schmidt R, Parish EJ, Dionisius V, et al. Modulation of cellular cholesterol and its effect on cornified envelope formation in cultured human epidermal keratinocytes. *J Invest Dermatol.* 1991;97:771.

31. Gniadecki R, Bang B. Flotillas of lipid rafts in transit amplifying cell-like keratinocytes. *J Invest Dermatol.* 2003;121:522.

32. Man MQ, Choi EH, Schmuth M, et al. Basis for improved permeability barrier homeostasis induced by PPAR and LXR activators: liposensors stimulate lipid synthesis, lamellar body secretion and post-secretory lipid processing. *J Invest Dermatol.* 2006;126:386.

33. Kömüves LG, Schmuth M, Fowler AJ, et al. Oxysterol stimulation of epidermal differentiation is mediated by liver X receptor-beta in murine epidermis. *J Invest Dermatol.* 2002;118:25.

34. Jiang YJ, Lu B, Kim P, et al. PPAR and LXR activators regulate ABCA12 expression in human keratinocytes. *J Invest Dermatol.* 2008;128:104.

35. Rivier M, Castiel I, Safonova I, et al. Peroxisome proliferator-activated receptor-alpha enhances lipid metabolism in a skin equivalent model. *J Invest Dermatol.* 2000;114:681.

36. Jiang YJ, Kim P, Elias PM, et al. LXR and PPAR activators stimulate cholesterol sulfotransferase type 2 isoform 1b in human keratinocytes. *J Lipid Res.* 2005;46:2657.

37. Williams ML, Feingold KR, Grubauer G, Elias PM. Ichthyosis induced by cholesterol-lowering drugs. Implications for epidermal cholesterol homeostasis. *Arch Dermatol.* 1987;123:1535.

38. Madison KC. Barrier function of the skin: "la raison d'être" of the epidermis. *J Invest Dermatol.* 2003;121:231.

39. Grunfeld C, Soued M, Adi S, et al. Evidence for two classes of cytokines that stimulate hepatic lipogenesis: Relationships among tumor necrosis factor, interleukin-1 and interferon-alpha. *Endocrinology.* 1990;127:46.

40. Girotti AW. Photosensitized oxidation of cholesterol in biological systems: Reaction pathways, cytotoxic effects and defense mechanisms. *J Photochem Photobiol* B. 1992;13:105.

41. Minami Y, Kawabata K, Kubo Y, et al. Peroxidized cholesterol-induced matrix metalloproteinase-9 activation and its suppression by dietary β-carotene in photoaging of hairless mouse skin. *J Nutr Biochem.* 2009;20:389.

42. Tahara S, Matsuo M, Kaneko T. Age-related changes in oxidative damage to lipids and DNA in rat skin. *Mech Ageing Dev.* 2001;122:415.

CHAPTER 22

Lanolin

Activities:

Occlusive, emollient

Important Chemical Components:

Lanolin contains long-chain waxy esters many of which have not yet been characterized. It is thought of as a highly complex combination of esters, di-esters, and hydroxyl esters of high molecular weight lanolin alcohols (i.e., aliphatic alcohols, sterols, including cholesterol, and trimethyl sterols) as well as high molecular weight lanolin acids (i.e., normal, iso-, anteiso-, and hydroxyl acids).[1,2]

Origin Classification:

This ingredient is considered natural. It is animal derived.

Personal Care Category:

Lipophilic

Recommended for the following Baumann Skin Types:

DRNW, DRNT, DRPT, and DRPW

SOURCE

Lanolin is a greasy yellow substance derived from the sebaceous secretions of sheep and other wool-bearing animals. Most lanolin used in skin care products is obtained from domesticated sheep.

HISTORY

Lanolin has been used for thousands of years by human beings for its emollient qualities, and for hundreds of years as an ingredient in skin care ointments (Table 22-1).[3]

CHEMISTRY

Lanolin shares two important features with stratum corneum (SC) lipids: 1) lanolin contains cholesterol, an essential constituent of SC lipids, and 2) lanolin and SC lipids can coexist as solids and liquids at physiologic temperatures. Lanolin is characterized by a very different composition than human sebum, though.[4] This is also the case for commercial lanolin products.

TABLE 22-1
Pros and Cons of Lanolin

PRO	CONS
Effective emollient	Is a chemical sensitizer
	Is unsuitable for those who are opposed to using animal products

Significantly, the method used to refine the compound determines the quality and composition of the resulting formulation; therefore, not all lanolin products exhibit the same activity.[5] Unfortunately, a small percentage of individuals who use lanolin develop contact sensitization to the occlusive/emollient agent. Consequently, lanolin has developed a reputation as a sensitizer that, according to some, may not be deserved.[3,6] Nevertheless, manufacturers have responded to such claims and many moisturizing products are now touted as "lanolin free." Another response to the notion that lanolin provokes allergic reactions has spurred the development of an ultrapure hypoallergenic medical grade lanolin formulation such as Medilan™.

ORAL USES

Lanolin is not to be taken internally.

TOPICAL USES

Lanolin is one among several commonly used occlusive agents and is effective as an ingredient in skin care products for its ability to treat dry skin, delivering an emollient effect and reducing TEWL.

SAFETY ISSUES

Lanolin had long been thought of as a sensitizer given reports beginning several decades ago of links to contact dermatitis. However, lanolin is no longer considered a common allergen so much as one affecting compromised or high-risk populations, such as elderly individuals with chronic xerosis, dermatitis, or venous stasis dermatitis.[7–9] In a 2008 study of 276 moisturizers, lanolin, found in 10 percent of products, was the ninth most common allergen, far behind fragrance, parabens, vitamin E, and essential oils and biologic additives.[9]

In 2008, investigators sought to identify the frequency of positive patch test reactions to common allergens in leg ulcer or venous disease patients by using a case series of 100 consecutive consenting subjects suffering from chronic venous disease and other leg ulcer etiologies. At least one positive patch test was observed in 46 percent of patients, with multiple reactions in the same subject frequently seen. Of the 38 common allergens tested, lanolin was identified among the most frequent sensitizers, which also included fragrances, antibacterial agents, and rubber-related compounds.[10] Of course, these results suggest that lanolin may be contraindicated in patients with leg ulcers, but are not generalizable to a healthy population.

ENVIRONMENTAL IMPACT

The impact on the environment of lanolin cultivation is directly related to the effects of sheep farming on land and air quality as well as water run-off. As an animal-derived product, lanolin is not an option for vegan or vegetarian patients.

FORMULATION CONSIDERATIONS

Although a plant-derived substitute has been recently produced, lanolin itself is a complex natural product that cannot be synthesized. It is also a commonly used occlusive ingredient, along with products or compounds such as paraffin, squalene, dimethicone, soybean oil, grapeseed oil, propylene glycol, and beeswax.[11] Importantly, though, lanolin, like mineral oil and petrolatum, is known for its dual activity exerting both occlusive and emollient effects.

USAGE CONSIDERATIONS

Lanolin is typically used to moisturize and smooth the skin and is generally considered safe in noncompromised skin. It is easily absorbed through the skin and is thus conducive to delivering medicinal chemicals in an ointment.[9]

SIGNIFICANT BACKGROUND

In 2003, Dodd and Chalmers led a multicenter, prospective, randomized controlled clinical trial to compare the effects of hydrogel dressings to lanolin ointment for the prevention and treatment of nipple soreness in 106 lactating mothers. A board-certified lactation specialist provided breastfeeding guidance at the beginning of the study. During the first 12 days of the study, participants, who were randomized to either of the two groups, were instructed to rate pain intensity according to a numeric pain intensity scale as well as a verbal description scale. Patients then forwarded self-reported skin assessments of the bilateral breasts, nipples, and areolae to investigators. A significantly greater reduction in pain score mean values was identified in the hydrogel group at baseline, day 10, and day 12, as compared to the lanolin group, and the hydrogel group discontinued treatment earlier than the participants using lanolin. Overall, researchers found hydrogel to be superior to lanolin ointment for the management of nipple soreness.[12]

Additional evidence that lanolin is not the optimal therapeutic option for sore or cracked nipples came four years later when investigators conducted a randomized double-blind clinical trial to compare a peppermint gel formulation, modified lanolin, and a placebo control ointment for the treatment of nipple fissures related to breastfeeding. Two hundred and sixteen primiparous mothers were randomly assigned to the three groups, comparable in mean age, and were instructed to apply their selected formulation on both breasts for 14 days. Patients were seen for up to four follow-up visits as well as a final visit at week 6. Researchers found that nipple and areola cracks were less frequent in the peppermint gel group as compared to the lanolin or placebo groups.[13]

Nevertheless, such results do not detract from the appropriateness of lanolin for other dry skin indications. In 2003, investigators conducted a four-week double-blind, randomized-comparison clinical trial to assess the effectiveness of pure lanolin as compared to ammonium lactate 12 percent cream in the treatment of moderate to severe xerosis on the feet. Fifty-one patients, of the original 92 enrolled, completed the study. Both treatment groups exhibited significant improvement in xerosis scores after two and four weeks of treatment, with no statistically significant differences identified between the groups. The researchers concluded that pure lanolin as well as ammonium lactate cream used twice daily for a month were effective in ameliorating moderate to severe dry skin.[14]

In 2008, authors reported on a comparison of two different topical ointments used in cutaneous therapy on 173 prospectively enrolled infants between 25 and 36 weeks of gestation admitted to a neonatal intensive care unit from October 2004 and November 2006. Each infant was treated for up to four weeks after being randomly assigned to daily treatment with water-in-oil emollient cream (Bepanthen), olive oil cream (70 percent lanolin, 30 percent olive oil), or a topical control. Skin was evaluated weekly. Investigators found that while both treatment groups exhibited greater improvement than the control group, with enduring treatment effects, infants in the lanolin/olive oil group experienced statistically less dermatitis than the water-in-oil emollient group.[15]

CONCLUSION

Through the last several decades, only a small proportion of the population has been found to be allergic to lanolin. Although allergic responses have not been reported in association with the use of more modern, medical grade, or other highly refined lanolin products, the author has seen several patients with lanolin allergy. To patients who demur to use lanolin due to the animal origin of the substance, it is important to at least address this argument by noting that while lanolin is secreted by the sebaceous glands of sheep and then obtained from their shorn wool and refined, the process is conducted without harming the animal. Lanolin, particularly in the newest formulations, is an effective first-line occlusive and emollient agent for various xerotic conditions.

REFERENCES

1. Barnett G. Lanolin and derivatives. *Cosm Toiletr.* 1986;101:21.
2. Clark EW. A brief history of lanolin. *Pharm Hist.* 1980;10:5.
3. Stone L. Medlian: A hypoallergenic lanolin for emollient therapy. *Br J Nurs.* 2000;9:54.
4. Proserpio G. Lanolides: Emollients or moisturizers? *Cosm Toiletr.* 1978;93:45.
5. Harris I, Hoppe U. Lanolins. In: Loden M, Maibach H, eds. *Dry Skin and Moisturizers.* Boca Raton: CRC Press; 2000:259.
6. Kligman AM. The myth of lanolin allergy. *Contact Dermatitis.* 1998;39:103.
7. White-Chu EF, Reddy M. Dry skin in the elderly: complexities of a common problem. *Clin Dermatol.* 2011;29:37.
8. Lee B, Warshaw E. Lanolin allergy: History, epidemiology, responsible allergens, and management. *Dermatitis.* 2008;19:63.
9. Zirwas MJ, Stechschulte SA. Moisturizer allergy: Diagnosis and management. *J Clin Aesthet Dermatol.* 2008;1:38.
10. Smart V, Alavi A, Coutts P, et al. Contact allergens in persons with leg ulcers: A Canadian study in contact sensitization. *Int J Low Extrem Wounds.* 2008;7:120.
11. Draelos Z. Moisturizers. In: Draelos Z, ed. *Atlas of Cosmetic Dermatology.* New York: Churchill Livingstone; 2000:83.
12. Dodd V, Chalmers C. Comparing the use of hydrogel dressings to lanolin ointment with lactating mothers. *J Obstet Gynecol Neonatal Nurs.* 2003;32:486.
13. Melli MS, Rashidi MR, Nokhoodchi A, et al. A randomized trial of peppermint gel, lanolin ointment, and placebo gel to prevent nipple crack in primiparous breastfeeding women. *Med Sci Monit.* 2007;13:CR406.
14. Jennings MB, Alfieri DM, Parker ER, et al. A double-blind clinical trial comparing the efficacy and safety of pure lanolin versus ammonium lactate 12% cream for the treatment of moderate to severe foot xerosis. *Cutis.* 2003;71:78.
15. Kiechl-Kohlendorfer U, Berger C, Inzinger R. The effect of daily treatment with an olive oil/lanolin emollient on skin integrity in preterm infants: a randomized controlled trial. *Pediatr Dermatol.* 2008;25:174.

CHAPTER 23

Stearic Acid

Activities:

Emulsifying, hydrating, barrier repair, surfactant

Important Chemical Components:

Saturated fatty acid containing long alkyl chains.
The International Union of Pure and Applied Chemistry (IUPAC) name is octadecanoic acid and its chemical formula is $CH_3(CH_2)_{16}CO_2H$. Its molecular formula is $C_{18}H_{36}O_2$.

Origin Classification:

Stearic acid is a naturally occurring fatty acid found in many natural and organic moisturizers and soaps.

Personal Care Category:

Cleanser, moisturizer

Recommended for the following Baumann Skin Types:

DRNT, DRNW, DRPT, DRPW, DSNT, DSNW, DSPT, and DSPW or any skin types with allergic type sensitive skin (S_4)

SOURCE

Stearic acid, a waxlike saturated fatty acid also known as octadecanoic acid, is an important naturally occurring component of stratum corneum (SC) lipids. Besides being synthesized by human beings, stearic acid is also found in butter, cocoa butter, shea butter, vegetable fats, and animal tallow. It is found in many oils but the highest concentrations are in cocoa butter (chocolate), butter, and shea butter. The nonanimal-derived oil with one of the highest amounts of stearic acid is argan oil, which has a concentration of 4 to 7 percent.[1] Stearic acid is found in all cosmetic product categories including soaps, syndet bars, body oils, moisturizers, color cosmetics, and perfumes.

HISTORY

Stearic acid is one of the most common fatty acids found in nature. It is one of the oldest cosmetic ingredients because it is a component of vegetable and animal oils that have been used on the skin for centuries. Historically it has not been used as a singular ingredient, but is found as a component of many popular ingredients such as cocoa butter and various oils.

Stearic acid plays an important role in the skin's permeability barrier along with linoleic acid and palmitic acid (from palm oil). Palmitic and stearic acids are both saturated fatty acids. Linoleic acid is an unsaturated fatty acid and displays anti-inflammatory properties that stearic acid does not exhibit. Stearic acid has been incorporated into many personal care products because of its safety profile, ubiquity, and inexpensive cost in addition to its surfactant and hydrating abilities. It is found in many "hydrating" body washes and bars that deposit stearic acid on the skin. Stearic acid is found in argan oil, the world's most expensive oil, at a concentration of 4 to 7 percent.[1]

CHEMISTRY

Stearic acid is a saturated long-chain fatty acid with the chemical formula $CH_3(CH_2)_{16}CO_2H$ (see Figure 23-1). The International Union of Pure and Applied Chemistry (IUPAC) name is octadecanoic acid. It is also known as cetylacetic acid and stearophanic acid.

Stearic acid is the saturated form of oleic acid, a monounsaturated ω-9 fatty acid (see Figure 23-2). While stearic acid helps improve the skin's barrier function, oleic acid impairs it.

ORAL USES

Stearic acid can be safely taken as an ingredient in dietary supplements; however, it is the most poorly absorbed of the fatty acids.[2]

Stearic acid gives food a desirable taste and texture. It makes up about 9 to 12 percent of total calories in beef, pork, lamb, and veal and about 6 percent of calories in poultry. Although it is a saturated fatty acid, it may be associated with fewer health risks than other saturated fatty acids in the diet. Studies in humans and animals suggest that it has a neutral effect on plasma cholesterol levels in contrast to lauric, myristic, and palmitic acids.[3] Stearic acid makes up about 2 to 4 percent of calories in most cooking oils.[4]

TOPICAL USES

As a Food and Drug Administration (FDA)-approved ingredient in several cosmetic products, it is used as a surfactant and emulsifying agent, for fragrance, and as the base for other fatty acid ingredients that are synthesized into emollients and lubricants (Table 23-1). Specifically, it is used most often to retain the shape of, and as a thickener in, soaps (indirectly, through saponification of triglycerides composed of stearic acid esters) as well as in shampoos, shaving creams, and detergents.

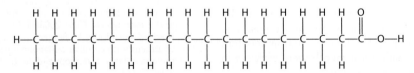

▲ **FIGURE 23-1** Stearic acid is a saturated fatty acid with an 18-carbon chain.

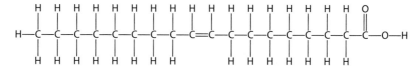

▲**FIGURE 23-2** Oleic acid is an unsaturated fatty acid with an 18-carbon chain.

TABLE 23-1
Pros and Cons of Stearic Acid

Pros	Con
Effective as an emulsifier and surfactant	Oral use is controversial because saturated fatty acids increase risk of heart disease, although this has been shown not to be the case with stearic acid. Thus, this issue is a source of confusion.
Use in cleansers allows deposition on the skin even after rinsing	
Found in inexpensive products such as cocoa butter	
Repairs skin barrier when used in combination with ceramide and cholesterol	
More stable than unsaturated fatty acids	

SAFETY ISSUES

Stearic acid is approved by the FDA for use in topical skin care formulations and is generally considered safe. Evaluation by the Cosmetic Ingredient Review (CIR) showed no phototoxicity, minimal to no skin irritation, no tumorigenicity, and no comedogenicity. Stearic acid was labeled as "safe" by the CIR.

ENVIRONMENTAL IMPACT

Stearic acid is found abundantly in animals and plants, more so in the fat of animals. Individuals concerned about harming animals are advised to delve more deeply into the origins of the stearic acid used in products that they might consider. A significant environmental impact is not exerted in culling and processing stearic acid.

FORMULATION CONSIDERATIONS

Stearic acid is used to thicken and stabilize formulations. Its high amount of saturation makes it more solid at room temperature and gives it a waxy consistency. The acid can be neutralized with triethanolamine and other alkalis to form soap (sodium stearate), which acts as an emulsifier.[5]

USAGE CONSIDERATIONS

Saturated fats such as stearic acid are more stable than unsaturated fatty acids. This is important because oxygen and heat can degrade fatty acids, rendering them rancid. Combination with antioxidants can slow the degradation process. Notably, stearic acid may decrease penetration of other ingredients by strengthening the skin barrier.

SIGNIFICANT BACKGROUND

In 2000, Khalil et al. studied the effects of cream formulations on chemically-induced burns in mice based on reports that the

ingredients, docosanol or stearic acid, were associated with antiviral and anti-inflammatory activity. Burns were engendered by painting murine abdomens with a chloroform solution of phenol. Researchers then topically applied the test formulations 0.5, 3, and 6 hours after injury. They found that the docosanol- and stearic acid-containing creams significantly lessened the severity and progression of skin lesions compared to untreated sites, yielding, respectively, 76 and 57 percent declines in mean lesion scores.[6]

In 2001, Fluhr et al., in a study of the effects of the free fatty acid pool on SC acidification and function, topically applied two phospholipase inhibitors, bromphenacylbromide and 1-hexadecyl-3-trifluoroethylglycero-sn-2-phosphomethanol, for three days to murine skin. This raised skin pH and yielded permeability barrier abnormality, altered SC integrity, and reduced SC cohesion. All malfunctions were normalized, including SC pH, with the coapplication of either palmitic, stearic, or linoleic acids along with the inhibiting agents.[7]

In 2010, Mukherjee et al. evaluated a recently-marketed mild moisturizing body wash, with stearic acid and emollient soybean oil, to determine the location and amount of stearic acid deposited in the SC after *in vivo* usage of the product. They conducted clinical cleansing studies using the soybean product or petroleum jelly. The deuterated variant of stearic acid replaced the free stearic acid in the soybean formulation. The investigators detected deuterated stearic acid in all 10 consecutive layers of SC, with a total stearic acid level measured at 0.33 μg/cm² after five washes with the soybean oil product. They concluded that the estimated total fatty acid delivered to the skin from cleansing, probably incorporated into the SC lipid phase, is comparable to the fatty acid level in an SC layer.[8]

CONCLUSION

Stearic acid is an important component in stratum corneum lipids, but it is rarely used alone. Therefore, there is a paucity of research to consider its individual attributes. Most studies use stearic acid-containing substances, such as argan oil or shea butter, that are not purely stearic acid so other components also play a role in the results seen. Although it is difficult to tease out the individual role of stearic acid, it seems certain that its presence affects skin penetration and barrier function and is a superior moisturizing ingredient when combined in the proper ratio with cholesterol and ceramides (see Chapter 19, Barrier Repair Ingredients). Much more research is necessary, then, to determine just how significant stearic acid is as a therapeutic agent.

REFERENCES

1. Guillaume D, Charrouf Z. Argan oil. Monograph. *Altern Med Rev.* 2011;16:275.
2. Cosmetic Ingredient Review. Final Report on the Safety Assessment of Oleic Acid, Lauric Acid, Palmitic Acid, Myristic Acid, and Stearic Acid.

J Am Col Toxicol. 1987;6:321. http://www.cir-safety.org/sites/default/files/115_draft_steary_suppl3.pdf. Accessed November 14, 2012.

3. Monsma CC, Ney DM. Interrelationship of stearic acid content and triacylglycerol composition of lard, beef tallow and cocoa butter in rats. *Lipids.* 1993;28:539.

4. Beef Facts: Nutrition, Stearic Acid—A Unique Saturated Fat. Website: www.beefnutrition.org. Accessed November 14, 2012.

5. Website: http://www.lotioncrafter.com/stearic-acid-nf.html. Accessed November 14, 2012.

6. Khalil MH, Marcelletti JF, Katz LR, et al. Topical application of docosanol- or stearic acid-containing creams reduces severity of phenol burn wounds in mice. *Contact Dermatitis.* 2000;43:79.

7. Fluhr JW, Kao J, Jain M, et al. Generation of free fatty acids from phospholipids regulates stratum corneum acidification and integrity. *J Invest Dermatol.* 2001;117:44.

8. Mukherjee S, Edmunds M, Lei X, et al. Stearic acid delivery to corneum from a mild and moisturizing cleanser. *J Cosmet Dermatol.* 2010;9:202.

CHAPTER 24

Humectants

Humectants are water-soluble materials with high water absorption capabilities. They are hygroscopic and therefore able to attract water from the atmosphere (if atmospheric humidity is greater than 80 percent) and from the underlying epidermis. Although humectants may draw water from the environment to help hydrate the skin, in low-humidity conditions they may take water from the deeper epidermis and dermis, resulting in increased skin dryness.[1] For this reason, they work better when combined with occlusives. Humectants are also popular additives to cosmetic moisturizers for many reasons. They prevent product evaporation and thickening, which increases the shelf life of formulations, and some humectants help prevent bacterial growth in products.[2] Humectants can cause an almost immediate improvement in skin texture because they draw water into the skin, causing a slight swelling of the stratum corneum (SC) that gives the perception of smoother skin with fewer wrinkles. Humectants, by inducing swelling, can temporarily give the user the perception of increased skin firmness. Humectants have been shown to enhance the penetration of other ingredients by causing swelling of keratinocytes,[3] and disruption of the skin barrier by loosening the closely packed SC cells.[4] Propylene glycol enhances penetration of minoxidil and steroids,[5] while hyaluronic acid increases drug delivery in prescription medications such as Diclofenac.[4] Examples of commonly used humectants include glycerin, sorbitol, sodium hyaluronate (hyaluronic acid), urea, propylene glycol, α-hydroxy acids, and sugars.

REFERENCES

1. Idson B. Dry skin: moisturizing and emolliency. *Cosmet Toiletr.* 1992;107:69.
2. Mitsui T, ed. *New Cosmetic Science.* New York: Elsevier; 1997:134.
3. Warner RR, Stone KJ, Boissy YL. Hydration disrupts human stratum corneum ultrastructure. *J Invest Dermatol.* 2003;120:275.
4. Brown MB, Jones SA. Hyaluronic acid: A unique topical vehicle for the localized delivery of drugs to the skin. *J Eur Acad Dermatol Venereol.* 2005;19:308.
5. Hannuksela M. Glycols. In: Loden M, Maibach H. eds. *Dry Skin and Moisturizers.* Boca Raton: CRC Press; 2000:413–415.

CHAPTER 25

Glycerin

Activities:

Anti-inflammatory, barrier recovery

Important Chemical Components:

Simple polyol with three hydroxyl groups derived from triglycerides

Origin Classification:

Glycerin is a natural ingredient and organic forms are available. Synthetic, laboratory-made forms are also used.

Personal Care Category:

Humectant, moisturizer

Recommended for the following Baumann Skin Types:

Is a superior choice for dry skin types but is appropriate for all 16 types (DRNT, DRNW, DRPT, DRPW, DSNT, DSNW, DSPT, DSPW, ORNT, ORNW, ORPT, ORPW, OSPT, OSPW, OSNT, and OSNW).

SOURCE

Glycerol provides the molecular skeleton of all animal and vegetable fats known as triglycerides. It is derived from the saponification of fats. Throughout this chapter, the terms "glycerol" and "glycerin" (also spelled as glycerine and referred to more often in the literature as glycerol) will be used interchangeably; glycerin is the designation most familiar to consumers (and the one used here more often in relation to topical products). Glycerol is a potent, nonvolatile trihydroxylated humectant. When the body consumes fat stores (triglycerides) to produce energy, glycerol and fatty acids are released into the bloodstream. The glycerol component is converted to glucose in the liver, thus providing energy for cellular metabolism. Natural glycerol is obtained hydrolytically from fats and oils during soap and fatty acid manufacturing, and by transesterification (an interchange of fatty acid groups with another alcohol) during the production of biodiesel fuel.[1] Synthetic glycerol refers to material obtained from nontriglyceride sources.

Glycerin exhibits hygroscopic ability very similar to that associated with natural moisturizing factor (NMF).[2] NMF is found within keratinocytes in the stratum corneum (SC) and is composed of amino acids, lactate, urea, citrate, and sugars. It can absorb large quantities of water (i.e., hygroscopic) even when humidity levels are low. This allows the SC to maintain a sufficient hydration level even in dry environments. Numerous ingredients have been used in moisturizing products to mimic NMF activity; glycerin is one of the primary ones.

The topical application of glycerin is considered a useful component in treatment regimens for various cutaneous conditions, including bedsores, bites, burns, calluses, cuts, rashes and, occasionally, psoriasis. It is well known to protect against cutaneous irritation.

HISTORY

The name glycerol is derived from the Greek word *glyko*, meaning "sweet." Carl Wilhelm Scheele discovered glycerol in 1779. Since then it has been included and used widely in topical skin cosmetics, with approximately 160,000 tons of glycerol sold annually in the United States alone.[3,4] Glycerol is one of the most versatile and valuable chemical substances known and is considered the most effective humectant ingredient in the personal care industry (Table 25-1).[5,6] It has long been used as an active as well as excipient ingredient in skin care products. Procter and Gamble (P&G) started producing glycerin around 1858, about the time they started producing consumer products. Today, P&G Chemicals is one of the largest manufacturers of glycerin in the world.

CHEMISTRY

Glycerol contains three hydrophilic alcoholic hydroxyl groups, which are responsible for its solubility in water and its hygroscopic nature (Figure 25-1). It is a highly flexible molecule forming both intra- and intermolecular hydrogen bonds. There are 126 possible conformers of glycerol.[7]

TABLE 25-1
Pros and Cons of Glycerin

Pros	Cons
Contributes to barrier repair	May feel sticky
One of the most effective humectant ingredients	Individuals with oily skin may object to the feel of the product
Useful in prolonging product shelf life	More data needed
Inexpensive	
Nonallergenic	
Transverses aquaporin-3 channels	
Helps skin retain water for over 24 hours	

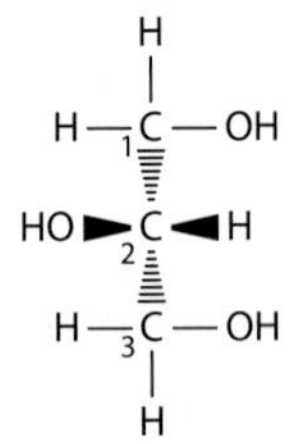

▲ **FIGURE 25-1** Glycerol has three hydroxyl groups.

ORAL USES

Glycerin has been shown to display some antibacterial properties and is useful in treating halitosis. It is commonly used as an artificial sweetener. Its oral use has no known role in skin care.

TOPICAL USES

Glycerin, which helps condition the skin, is the most widely used hydrating agent and, consequently, a common ingredient in skin cleansers, creams, and lotions. In addition to its well-established hygroscopic activity and solubility similar to water, glycerin is characterized by the ability to prevent freezing and prolong the shelf life of a product.[3] Glycerin is one of the best moisturizing ingredients because of its strong humectant (hygroscopic) properties. It is often combined with occlusive agents to impart a synergistic improvement in dry skin disorders.[6,8] Glycerin may also play a role in increasing desquamation because it facilitates corneocyte maturation by spurring the activity of residual transglutaminase in the SC.[6,9]

In addition to its humectant properties, glycerol is a unique ingredient because it is able to transverse between keratinocytes via aquaporin-3 (AQP-3) channels, which allows the movement from cell to cell[10] (see Chapter 29, Aquaporin).

SAFETY ISSUES

Glycerin has a long track record of safety with no risk of allergic reactions. Some Internet sites state that glycerin will dry out the skin; however, this occurs when it is used in a dry environment without an occlusive ingredient, a setting in which the glycerin pulls water fom the skin. When glycerin is formulated properly it gives the skin sustained moisturization.[11]

ENVIRONMENTAL IMPACT

The synthesis of glyercin poses no environmental risk. It is naturally occurring in plants and animals.

FORMULATION CONSIDERATIONS

Glycerin is soluble in water. Its versatility makes it easy to formulate.

USAGE CONSIDERATIONS

Glycerin can be used in conjunction with other ingredients. It is known to enhance the skin barrier but has also been shown to enhance skin penetration of some other ingredients.[12]

SIGNIFICANT BACKGROUND

In Vitro Studies

Xerosis, or dry skin, is associated with incomplete desmosome degradation. In a 1995 *in vitro* study of moisturizers facilitating the process of desmosome digestion, investigators observed via electron microscopy that desmosomes treated with glycerol were in more advanced stages of degradation than control tissue. In two other *in vitro* models evaluated by the same team, glycerol raised the corneocyte loss rate from the superficial surface of human skin biopsies and significantly lowered inter-corneocyte forces.[13] Since then, it has been established that by inducing activity of residual transglutaminase in the SC, glycerol accelerates corneocyte maturation.[6,9] In addition, glycerol diminishes xerotic scaling by contributing to desmosome digestion and then enhancing desquamation.[6,13] These studies show that glycerol can function as an aid to skin exfoliation.

Animal Studies

In a 2003 study in which mice deficient in the epidermal water/glycerol transporter AQP-3 exhibited diminished SC hydration and skin elasticity, as well as poor barrier recovery after SC removal, investigators showed that glycerol replacement ameliorated each defect in AQP-3-null mice. Notably, SC water content, which was measured as threefold lower in AQP-3-null mice than wild-type mice, was restored via topical or systemic glycerol administration, but administration of glycerol-like osmolytes (e.g., xylitol, erythritol, and propanediol) was unsuccessful. In addition to concluding that glycerol is an important determinant of SC water retention, investigators suggested that their data provide a strong scientific foundation for the centuries-old practice of including glycerol in skin formulations for medicinal as well as cosmetic purposes.[4] Further, the authors noted that when added to SC lipids *in vitro*, glycerol is thought to combine with lipid lamellae and foster water absorption and hinder the conversion of lipid lamellar structures from liquid to solid crystal, thereby inhibiting or preventing water loss.[4,14] This hypothesis, the data from this study, and the fact that in three days pure glycerol absorbs its own weight in water,[15] led the authors to speculate that glycerol likely improves SC water absorption and retention.[4]

Also in 2003, a study of asebia mice with profound sebaceous gland hypoplasia revealed that the topical application of glycerol, which, endogenously, is believed to be the result of triglyceride hydrolysis in sebaceous glands, restored normal SC hydration whereas the endogenous humectant urea did not. Further, the investigators showed that glycerol from triglycerides in sebaceous glands contributes significantly to SC hydration.[16]

Human Studies

In a five-year study in which two high-glycerin moisturizers were compared to 16 other popular moisturizers in 394 patients with severe xerosis, the high-glycerin products were found to perform better than all other products tested throughout the period by more rapidly restoring normal hydration and preventing the resumption of dryness for a longer period, longer even than petrolatum.[17] According to ultrastructural analysis of skin treated with high-glycerin formulations, glycerin expands the space between layers of corneocytes and the thickness of corneocytes, which results in the expansion of the SC.[18] These findings indicate that glycerin gives the skin the capacity to hold a reservoir of moisture that renders it more resistant to drying. In addition, glycerin stabilizes and fluidizes cell membranes as well as hydrates enzymes required for desmosome degradation.[17]

In 1999, Fluhr et al. conducted two studies to examine the capacity of glycerol as a barrier stabilizer and moisturizing compound. In the first study, barrier repair was found to be more rapid in glycerol-treated sites; significant differences were noted three days after treatment between glycerol open vs. untreated and glycerol occluded vs. untreated, and SC hydration was superior in the glycerol plus occlusion sites. In the second study, barrier repair was again more rapid in areas treated by glycerol, with significant differences compared to untreated and base-treated areas at day 7, and after three days of treatment, SC hydration was superior in areas treated by glycerol. The authors concluded that glycerol promotes barrier repair, notably after acute exogenous disturbance, and enhances SC hydration.[2]

In a study on dermatologic vehicles and their effect on the horny layer, investigators found that adding glycerol to oil-in-water (O/W) emulsions eliminated the barrier-damaging effect of such formulations. Glycerol added to O/W emulsions also decreased horny layer damage in stress tests with wash solutions. O/W emulsions that contain glycerol are also appropriate in atopic dermatitis therapy.[19]

In 2005, investigators found that endogenous glycerol from circulation into the epidermis via AQP-3 and from triglyceride hydrolysis in sebaceous glands is associated with SC hydration in humans. Indeed, they observed glycerol from both sources forms a water reservoir that affects such hydration. The authors also noted that other findings in their study support the use of therapeutic moisturizers that contain glycerol.[20]

Also, in 2008, a small pilot study with nine healthy women supported the "proof of concept" that hydrolyzed jojoba esters combined with glycerol produces an additive effect, enhancing moisturization for at least 24 hours.[21]

In a 2010 study of the effects of glycerol on human skin impaired by acute irritation induced by sodium lauryl sulfate (SLS), Atrux-Tallau et al. found that glycerol seems to serve the same function as natural moisturizing factors eliminated by the detergent action of SLS. This leads to improving skin hydration. The investigators concluded that the inclusion of glycerol in topical formulations intended to treat irritated skin is warranted.[22]

CONCLUSION

Glycerin is an important ingredient in skin care products, cosmetics, and cosmeceuticals because of its efficacy, safety, low cost, long history of use, and pervasiveness in the skin care product market. Recent research has indicated that glycerin displays several mechanisms of action and its efficacy depends on the choice of vehicle and emulsifying agent.

REFERENCES

1. Pagliaro M, Ross M. *The future of glycerol: New uses of a versatile raw material (RSC Green Chemistry Series)*. London: Royal Society of Chemistry; 2008:10.
2. Fluhr JW, Gloor M, Lehmann L, et al. Glycerol accelerates recovery of barrier function in vivo. *Acta Derm Venereol*. 1999;79:418.
3. Thau P. Glycerin (glycerol): Current insights into the functional properties of a classic cosmetic raw material. *J Cosmet Sci*. 2002;53:229.
4. Hara M, Verkman AS. Glycerol replacement corrects defective skin hydration, elasticity, and barrier function in aquaporin-3-deficient mice. *Proc Natl Acad Sci U S A*. 2003;100:7360.
5. Bonnardeaux J. Glycerin Overview, report for the Western Australia Department of Agriculture and Food, Novemeber 2006. http://www.agric.wa.gov.au/content/sust/biofuel/glycerinoverview.pdf. Accessed July 5, 2013.
6. Kraft JN, Lynde CW. Moisturizers: What they are and a practical approach to product selection. *Skin Therapy Lett*. 2005;10:1.
7. Callam CS, Singer Sj, Lowary TL, et al. Computational analysis of the potential energy surfaces of glycerol in thegas and aqueous phases: Effects of level of theory, basis set, and solvation on strongly intramolecularly hydrogen-bonded systems. *J Am Chem Soc*. 2001;123:11743.
8. Summers RS, Summers B, Chandar P, et al. The effect of lipids with and without humectant on skin xerosis. *J Soc Cosmet Chem*. 1996;47:39.
9. Harding CR, Long S, Richardson J, et al. The cornified cell envelope: An important marker of stratum corneum maturation in healthy and dry skin. *Int J Cosmet Sci*. 2003;25:157.
10. Hara M, Ma T, Verkman AS. Selectively reduced glycerol in skin of aquaporin-3-deficient mice may account for impaired skin hydration, elasticity, and barrier recovery. *J Biol Chem*. 2002;277:46616.
11. Lodén M, Wessman W. The influence of a cream containing 20% glycerin and its vehicle on skin barrier properties. *Int J Cosmet Sci*. 2001;23:115.
12. Bettinger J, Gloor M, Peter C, et al. Opposing effects of glycerol on the protective function of the horny layer against irritants and on the penetration of hexyl nicotinate. *Dermatology*. 1998;197:18.
13. Rawlings A, Harding C, Watkinson A, et al. The effect of glycerol and humidity on desmosome degradation in stratum corneum. *Arch Dermatol Res*. 1995;287:457.
14. Froebe CL, Simion FA, Ohlmeyer H, et al. Prevention of stratum corneum lipid phase transitions in vitro by glycerol: An alternative mechanism for skin moisturization. *J Soc Cosmet Chem*. 1990;41:51.
15. Rieger MM, Deem DE. Skin moisturizers II. The effects of cosmetic ingredients on human stratum corneum. *J Soc Cosmet Chem*. 1974;25:253.
16. Fluhr JW, Mao-Qiang M, Brown BE, et al. Glycerol regulates stratum corneum hydration in sebaceous gland deficient (asebia) mice. *J Invest Dermatol*. 2003;120:728.
17. Orth D, Appa Y. Glycerine: A natural ingredient for moisturizing skin. In: Loden M, Maibach H, eds. *Dry Skin and Moisturizers*. Boca Raton, FL: CRC Press; 2000:217.
18. Orth D, Appa Y, Contard E, et al. Effect of high glycerin therapeutic moisturizers on the ultrastructure of the stratum corneum. Poster presentation at the 53rd annual meeting of the American Academy of Dermatology, New Orleans, LA, February 1995.
19. Gloor M. How do dermatological vehicles influence the horny layer? *Skin Pharmacol Physiol*. 2004;17:267.
20. Choi EH, Man MQ, Wang F, et al. Is endogenous glycerol a determinant of stratum corneum hydration in humans? *J Invest Dermatol*. 2005;125:288.
21. Meyer J, Marshall B, Gacula M Jr, et al. Evaluation of additive effects of hydrolyzed jojoba (Simmondsia chinensis) esters and glycerol: A preliminary study. *J Cosmet Dermatol*. 2008;7:268.
22. Atrux-Tallau N, Romagny C, Padois K, et al. Effects of glycerol on human skin damaged by acute sodium lauryl sulphate treatment. *Arch Dermatol Res*. 2010;302:435.

CHAPTER 26

Hyaluronic Acid

Activities:

Humectant, antiaging

Important Chemical Components:

Hyaluronic acid (HA) is formed by repeating units of the disaccharides D-glucuronic acid and D-N-acetylglucosamine, which are linked to each other by alternating β-1,4 and β-1,3 glycosidic bonds. HA is composed of carbon, hydrogen, nitrogen, and oxygen (molecular formula: $C_{14}H_{21}NO_{11}$). See Figure 26-1.

Origin Classification:

HA is isolated from bacterial or yeast cultures, so it is considered natural but laboratory made. It is not considered organic.

Personal Care Category:

Humectant, moisturizer

Recommended for the following Baumann Skin Types:

DRNT, DRNW, DRPT, DRPW, DSNT, DSNW, DSPT, and DSPW, but only if used in a humid environment or with an occlusive ingredient. ORNW, ORPW, OSNW, and OSPW in any environment.

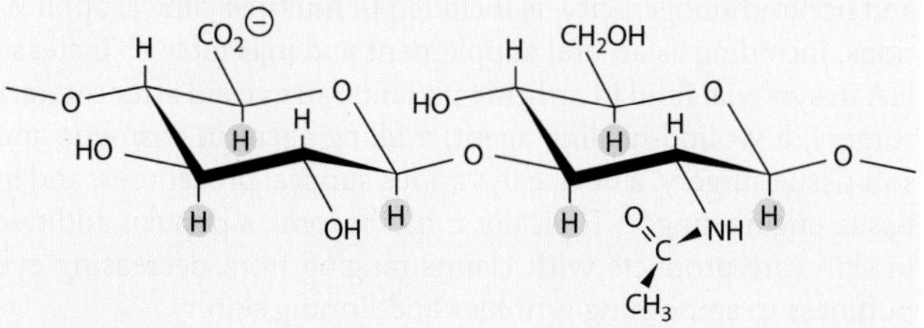

▲ **FIGURE 26-1** Hyaluronic acid is composed of repeating dimers of glucuronic acid and N-acetyl glucosamine assembled into long chains.

SOURCE

Hyaluronic acid (HA), or hyaluronan, is the most abundant glycosaminoglycan (GAG) found in the human dermis (Table 26-1). GAGs are polysaccharide chains made up of repeating disaccharide units linked to a core protein. Together the GAGs

TABLE 26-1
Pros and Cons of Hyaluronic Acid

Pros	Cons
Strong humectant	Penetration into skin depends on size
Nonimmunogenic	Does not penetrate into the dermis
Forms reservoirs in the epidermis	High consumer recognition
May effect cytokines	Dehydrates skin in a dry environment
Enhances drug delivery	
Various biological/medical applications	

(HA, dermatan sulfate, heparin, heparin sulfate, keratin sulfate, chondroitin-4, and chondroitin-6-sulfate) and attached core proteins form proteoglycans. The only nonsulfated GAG and the only one not synthesized on a core protein, HA is produced by an enzyme complex of the plasma membrane.[1] In addition, HA is a hygroscopic sugar that can bind over 1,000 times its weight in water. It is responsible for giving skin its plumpness and volume. HA is made by fibroblasts and broken down by the enzyme hyaluronidase.

The HA used in skin care products and injectables was originally harvested from rooster combs but now most HA in skin care products is derived from a bacterial origin and produced in the laboratory setting. The molecular weight of the HA varies according to its source and chain length. The HA isolation process can be adjusted to determine its corresponding molecular weight, altering its physiochemical properties.

Uncrosslinked chains of HA in the skin are broken down by hyaluronidase and free radicals in approximately 24 to 36 hours. Chemical modifications, such as crosslinking HA chains with 1,4-butanediol diglycidyl ether (BDDE), can increase the amount of time that HA resides in the skin. Dermal fillers such as Restylane are crosslinked with BDDE so that the HA lasts in the skin for six or more months; however, these crosslinked HA chains are too large to penetrate into the skin and must be injected.[2] Topical forms of HA must have a small enough molecular weight to pass into the skin, thus obviating the use of crosslinked HA.

HISTORY

HA was discovered in bovine vitreous humor by Meyer and Palmer in 1934.[3] It was named based on its glassy appearance (the Greek word for glass is *hyalos*) and the presence of a sugar known as uronic acid. HA, which appears freely in the dermis and is more concentrated in areas where cells are less densely packed, is an important dermal component responsible for attracting water and giving the dermis its volume. The popularity of HA fillers for injection into the dermis to correct wrinkles emerged in the 1990s and available products now include the Juvéderm line, Belotero, Restylane, Perlane, and Voluma. HA is also a popular ingredient in cosmetic products because of its humectant activity. However, traditionally, the HA found in many moisturizers, because of its large size, could not penetrate the epidermis and enter the dermis when topically applied, despite the claims of manufacturers.[4] Conflicting reports claim that smaller sizes of HA may penetrate into the epidermis when used in the proper formulations. In the author's knowledge, there are no published studies demonstrating the penetration of topical HA into the dermis.

CHEMISTRY

HA is a linear, naturally occurring polyanionic polysaccharide that consists of repeating disaccharide units of N-acetyl-D-glucosamine and β-glucuronic acid (D-glucuronate).[5,6]

Present in most biologic fluids and tissues (notably, most vertebrate connective tissue), it is most abundant, and an important component, in the extracellular matrix of soft connective tissues, particularly skin, where it plays a protective, shock-absorbing role.[5,6] Although it can be derived from humans, animals, or bacterial cultures, the structure of HA is identical among all of these species. HA exhibits key functions in cell growth and signaling, membrane receptor function, and adhesion, as well as wound repair and regeneration, morphogenesis, matrix organization, and pathobiology.[6] In young skin, HA is present at the periphery of collagen and elastin fibers and where these fibers interface. Such connections with HA are absent in aged skin.[7] In addition, HA appears to play a role in keratinocyte differentiation and lamellar body formation through its interaction with CD44,[8] a cell surface glycoprotein receptor with HA binding sites.[9–11] It is also thought to foster neutrophil migration, fibroblast proliferation, and neoangiogenesis.[12] In 2000, Sakai et al. used high performance liquid chromatography to show that HA is delivered by keratinocytes and is present in the normal stratum corneum (SC) of mice. Further, they speculated that HA contributes to moisturizing the SC and/or regulating its mechanical properties.[13]

ORAL USES

HA is available in oral supplement form, but the stomach breaks it down rendering it worthless to the skin when taken in an oral form. Glucosamine supplements, however, may help skin increase its production of HA.

TOPICAL USES

HA is the main ingredient in the barrier repair products Bionect and Hylatopic to impart water retention. Bionect contains 0.2 percent HA sodium salt, which acts as a humectant, with other humectant ingredients (e.g., glycerin) and a 70 percent sorbitol solution. Hylatopic combines HA sodium salt with the humectant glycerin in a foam preparation along with occlusive ingredients such as dimethicone and petrolatum.[14] Notably, the Food and Drug Administration (FDA) has approved the barrier repair products Atopiclair and Hylatopic, in which HA is the main ingredient.[14] Topical medications such as 3 percent Diclofenac have HA as an additive in the formulation.[5]

The humectant properties of HA allow it to bind 1,000 times its weight in water. Topical use of HA has been shown to improve skin hydration.[15] It functions as a skin-hydrating agent best when used in a humid environment. In a dry environment, it can draw water from the skin into the HA, thus dehydrating the skin. For this reason, HA should be used in combination with an occlusive ingredient in a dry environment. Individuals with oily skin types have sufficient sebum to impart occlusive properties. Therefore, those with oily skin types can use HA in any environment but people with dry skin should not use it in a dry environment unless the HA is combined with an occlusive agent. Applying HA to the skin in a humid environment attracts water to the skin and can result in immediate improvement of wrinkles. The effect is lessened in a low-humidity environment because there is less water in the atmosphere to draw to the skin. In one study, subjects saw improvement within minutes after using a face product with HA.[16]

SAFETY ISSUES

Studies that considered HA for drug delivery have shown that it can facilitate drug penetration into the epidermis and prevent it from entering the dermis as well as the blood stream.[5]

ENVIRONMENTAL IMPACT

No significant environmental impact is likely due to the production of topical HA products.

FORMULATION CONSIDERATIONS

Although HA is a very important skin component, its topical utility is thwarted by its large size and inability to pass into the dermis. However, if the proper size of HA is used, it can penetrate into the epidermis causing a rapid, if short-lived, improvement of fine lines through its effects on skin hydration. It is important to realize that the process of isolating and chemically processing HA greatly impacts its biological activity so that "not all HA is created equal."

USAGE CONSIDERATIONS

HA can enhance drug penetration, an important consideration when designing a skin care regimen and designating the order in which products will be applied. For example, applying a retinol after using a product with HA could theoretically increase absorption of retinol.[17]

SIGNIFICANT BACKGROUND

HA, in large part due to its viscoelastic nature, biocompatibility, and nonimmunogenicity, is included in multiple clinical applications, including as an oral supplement and injectable to increase HA in synovial fluid in arthritic patients, an eye aid after cataract surgery, a wound-healing agent, a filling agent in cosmetic and soft tissue surgery, a device in various surgical procedures, and in tissue engineering.[5,6] Topically it has become a popular additive in skin care products with claims ranging from decreasing eye puffiness to smoothing wrinkles and firming skin.

Wound Healing

In a small prospective study of 27 patients delivering by cesarean section and 20 patients delivering vaginally with episiotomy, researchers assessed the effects of an HA sodium salt (Bionect) in 15 subjects from the cesarean group and 10 from the episiotomy group (with standard wound care applied to the remaining patients) and found that daily application of the HA treatment yielded a lower incidence of edema, infiltration, and wound exudates compared to standard treatment. One case of wound dehiscence in each standard treatment group occurred, but none in the HA groups.[12]

In a recent 60-day, double-blind, randomized, controlled superiority trial intended to examine the efficacy and safety of a gauze pad containing HA in local treatment of venous leg ulcers in 89 patients, Humbert et al. found that ulcer surface was diminished significantly in the HA group compared to the neutral control group at day 45. In addition, at days 45 and 60, the number of healed ulcers was significantly higher in the HA treatment group. Notably, pain intensity was significantly lower in the HA group at day 30.[18]

Topical Antiaging Activity

In 2011, Pavicic et al. studied the efficacy of topically applied 0.1 percent HA formulations of various molecular weights (50, 130, 300, 800, and 2,000 kDa) in the periocular area to treat wrinkles in 76 randomized females ranging in age from 30 to 60 years. Subjects applied one of the preparations twice daily around one eye and a vehicle control cream around the other eye. Investigators measured skin hydration and elasticity at baseline as well as 30 and 60 days posttreatment. They observed significant improvement in skin hydration and elasticity in association with all of the HA-based creams in comparison to placebo. Wrinkle depth measurements indicated significant improvement in the periocular areas treated with 50 and 130 kDA HA as compared to areas treated with placebo. The researchers concluded that lower molecular weight HA formulations were linked to greater wrinkle depth reduction due likely to deeper penetration capacity.[15] This study controlled room humidity at 50 percent during wrinkle assessment, which is an important aspect to consider when using HA for antiaging.

Anti-inflammatory Activity

In 2012, Schlesinger et al. conducted, in an outpatient setting, a small prospective, observational, nonblinded safety and efficacy study of a topical anti-inflammatory formulation containing low-molecular weight HA (HA sodium salt gel 0.2 percent) to treat facial seborrheic dermatitis in 15 subjects ranging in age from 18 to 75 years. The hypothesis was that low-molecular weight HA would have an anti-inflammatory effect because of its actions on the immune system and cytokine formation.[19] Although immune system effects and cytokines were not measured in this study, interim data for seven of the 15 patients showed that HA treatment resulted in improvement of all measured endpoints, including erythema, pruritus, and scaliness.[20] This is the only published study looking at the use of HA in inflammatory skin disorders. Most of the literature on this topic is in the treatment of osteoarthritis.

Combination Therapy

HA has been shown to be effective in several combination products. In 2010, Guevara et al. evaluated the safety and efficacy of a new cream for treating melasma that contains hydroquinone, glycolic acid, and HA. In this small, open, uncontrolled 12-week study, 15 Latin American women applied the formulation to both sides of their face twice daily. Fourteen of the patients improved, with a significant reduction in melasma area and severity index (MASI) scores of 64 percent. After eight weeks of treatment, 53 percent of the subjects needed to use a moisturizer. Most reported adverse events were mild.[21]

In 2011, Cordero et al. conducted a three-month, open, multicentered, international study of 1,462 subjects to evaluate a cream combining retinaldehyde and HA fragments for treating photoaging. Participants were instructed to daily apply either retinaldehyde 0.05 percent-HA fragments 0.5 percent (Eluage® cream), retinaldehyde 0.05 percent-HA fragments 1 percent (Eluage® antiwrinkle concentrate) or both products. Dermatologists evaluated photoaging severity at baseline as well as days 30 and 90 using Larnier's scale. Significant improvement was observed by the investigators, with reduction in Larnier scores in all three groups. Wrinkles (i.e., on the forehead, nasolabial folds, crow's feet, and perioral) were significantly ameliorated in subjects using Eluage antiwrinkle concentrate as well as both formulations. Both products were well tolerated by subjects and clinical signs of photoaging diminished significantly in the Eluage cream and the group using both products in terms of elasticity, hyperpigmentation, and ptosis.[22]

In 2011, Frankel et al. conducted a bilateral comparison investigation of pimecrolimus cream 1 percent and a ceramide-HA emollient foam for the treatment of mild-to-moderate atopic dermatitis, and reported that both products displayed efficacy. After four weeks of treatment, 82 percent of target lesions treated with the ceramide-HA foam were scored "clear" or "almost clear" compared to 71 percent of lesions treated with pimecrolimus.[23]

Later that year, Gazzabin et al. evaluated a spray product combining colloidal silver and HA in 54 patients, 30 with chronic wounds and 24 with superficial traumatic wounds. Patients were instructed to apply treatments at intervals of three to seven days based on lesion traits. Investigators found that chronic lesions healed by week 12 (70 percent closure rate at six weeks) and traumatic wounds healed at six weeks (80 percent substantial closure at three weeks). They also noted satisfactory microbial contamination control in treated ulcers and concluded that the HA and silver combination spray was effective in spurring re-epithelialization of superficial cutaneous wounds of various origins.[24]

In 2012, Joksimovic et al. conducted a small double-blind, placebo-controlled clinical trial with 36 hemorrhoid patients to assess the efficacy and tolerability of a gel medical device containing HA, tea tree oil, and methyl-sulfonyl-methane. Findings from the 14-day treatment regimen showed statistically significant reductions in all symptoms as compared to placebo. The HA-containing gel was also found to be safe and tolerable in this small sample.[25] HA is also being used in combination with an iodine complex to achieve measurable clinical benefits in various wound types.[26]

CONCLUSION

HA is a ubiquitous and versatile component of the extracellular matrix and a key constituent of the dermis, contributing significantly to skin hydration, skin volume, and a youthful appearance. HA is known to diminish as one ages. Aside from its role in popular dermal filling agents, HA has also been used in exogenous topical products as a moisturizing agent. Its utility in a topical formulation is determined by several factors including the ambient humidity, the molecular weight of the HA, and what chemical alterations have been made to the HA molecule. Topically delivered HA may not be able to penetrate into the skin at all due to its large size. If it does penetrate, it remains localized in the epidermis forming reservoirs,[27] and does not penetrate into the dermis. This makes it a popular ingredient to enhance drug delivery to the epidermis but impairs its ability to add volume to a photoaged dermis like an injectable form of HA would do. For this reason, much of the marketing of HA in skin care products is misleading. Topically delivered HA should be considered as a humectant skin moisturizer when used in a normal or humid environment. Any antiaging properties it demonstrates would be based on skin hydration alone and the effects are temporary. Injectable HA is a different topical agent altogether and is covered thoroughly in Chapter 2, Basic Science of the Dermis in *Cosmetic Dermatology: Principles and Practice*, 2nd ed. (McGraw-Hill, 2009).

REFERENCES

1. Uitto J, Chu M, Gallo R, et al. Collagen, elastic fibers, and extracellular matrix of the dermis. In: Wolff K, Goldsmith L, Katz S, Gilchrest B, Paller A, Leffell D, eds. *Fitzpatrick's Dermatology in General Medicine*. 7th ed. New York: McGraw-Hill; 2008:539.
2. Baumann L, Saghari S. Basic science of the dermis. In: Baumann L, Saghari S, Weisberg E, eds. *Cosmetic Dermatology: Principles and Practice*. 2nd ed. New York: McGraw-Hill; 2009:11.
3. Meyer K, Palmer JW. The polysaccharide of the vitreous humor. *J Biol Chem*. 1934;107:629.
4. Rieger M. Hyaluronic acid in cosmetics. *Cosm Toiletr*. 1998;113:35.
5. Brown MB, Jones SA. Hyaluronic acid: A unique topical vehicle for the localized delivery of drugs to the skin. *J Eur Acad Dermatol Venereol*. 2005;19:308.
6. Volpi N, Schiller J, Stern R, et al. Role, metabolism, chemical modifications and applications of hyaluronan. *Curr Med Chem*. 2009;16:1718.
7. Ghersetich I, Lotti T, Campanile G, et al. Hyaluronic acid in cutaneous intrinsic aging. *Int J Dermatol*. 1994;33:119.
8. Bourguignon LY, Ramez M, Gilad E, et al. Hyaluronan-CD44 interaction stimulates keratinocyte differentiation, lamellar body formation/secretion, and permeability barrier homeostasis. *J Invest Dermatol*. 2006;126:1356.
9. Aruffo A, Stamenkovic I, Melnick M, et al. CD44 is the principal cell surface receptor for hyaluronate. *Cell*. 1990;61:1303.
10. Culty M, Miyake K, Kincade PW, et al. Thy hyaluronate receptor is a member of the CD44 (H-CAM) family of cell surface glycoproteins. *J Cell Biol*. 1990;111:2765.
11. Underhill C. CD44: the hyaluronan receptor. *J Cell Sci*. 1992;103:293.
12. Ivanov C, Mochova M, Russeva R, et al. Clinical application of Bionect (Hyaluronic Acid Sodium Salt) in wound care by cesarean section and episiotomy. *Akush Ginekol (Sofia)*. 2007;46:20.
13. Sakai S, Yasuda R, Sayo T, et al. Hyaluronan exists in the normal stratum corneum. *J Invest Dermatol*. 2000;114:1184.
14. Draelos ZD. New treatments for restoring impaired epidermal barrier permeability: skin barrier repair creams. *Clin Dermatol*. 2012;30:345.
15. Pavicic T, Gauglitz GG, Lersch P, et al. Efficacy of cream-based novel formulations of hyaluronic acid of different molecular weights in anti-wrinkle treatment. *J Drugs Dermatol*. 2011;10:990.
16. Trookman NS, Rizer RL, Ford R, et al. Immediate and long-term clinical benefits of a topical treatment for facial lines and wrinkles. *J Clin Aesthet Dermatol*. 2009;2:38.
17. Jenning V, Gysler A, Schäfer-Korting M, et al. Vitamin A loaded solid lipid nanoparticles for topical use: Occlusive properties and drug targeting to the upper skin. *Eur J Pharm Biopharm*. 2000;49:211.
18. Humbert P, Mikosinki J, Benchikhi H, et al. Efficacy and safety of a gauze pad containing hyaluronic acid in treatment of leg ulcers of venous or mixed origin: a double-blind, randomised, controlled trial. *Int Wound J*. 2013;10:159.
19. Wang CT, Lin YT, Chiang BL, et al. High molecular weight hyaluronic acid down-regulates the gene expression of osteoarthritis-associated cytokines and enzymes in fibroblast-like synoviocytes from patients with early osteoarthritis. *Osteoarthritis Cartilage*. 2006;14:1237.
20. Schlesinger T, Rowland Powell C. Efficacy and safety of a low-molecular weight hyaluronic acid topical gel in the treatment of facial seborrheic dermatitis. *J Clin Aesthet Dermatol*. 2012;5:20.
21. Guevara IL, Werlinger KD, Pandya AG. Tolerability and efficacy of a novel formulation in the treatment of melasma. *J Drugs Dermatol*. 2010;9:215.
22. Cordero A, Leon-Dorantes G, Pons-Guiraud A, et al. Retinaldehyde/hyaluronic acid fragments: a synergistic association for the management of skin aging. *J Cosmet Dermatol*. 2011;10:110.
23. Frankel A, Sohn A, Patel RV, et al. Bilateral comparison study of pimecrolimus cream 1% and a ceramide-hyaluronic acid emollient foam in the treatment of patients with atopic dermatitis. *J Drugs Dermatol*. 2011;10:666.
24. Gazzabin L, Bucalossi M, Mariani F, et al. Spray formulation of silver and hyaluronic acid in the treatment of superficial cutaneous ulcers of different etiopathogenesis: Analysis of fifty-four clinical cases. *Panminerva Med*. 2011;53:185.
25. Joksimovic N, Spasovski G, Joksimovic V, et al. Efficacy and tolerability of hyaluronic acid, tea tree oil and methyl-sulfonyl-methane in a new gel medical device for treatment of haemorrhoids in a double-blind, placebo-controlled clinical trial. *Updates Surg*. 2012;64:195.
26. Cutting KF. Wound healing through synergy of hyaluronan and an iodine complex. *J Wound Care*. 2011;20:424.
27. Brown MB, Ingham S, Moore A, et al. A preliminary study of the effect of hyaluronan in drug delivery. In: Willoughby DA, ed. *Hyaluronan in Drug Delivery*. London: Royal Society of Medicine Press; 1995:48–52.

CHAPTER 27

Vitamin B₅ (Pantothenic Acid/Dexpanthenol)

Activities:

Hydration, barrier protection, reduction of transepidermal water loss (TEWL), fibroblast stimulation, re-epithelialization.

Important Chemical Components:

Pantothenic acid ($C_9H_{17}O_5N$): chemically known as 3-[(2,4-Dihydroxy-3,3-dimethylbutanoyl) amino] propanoic acid

Dexpanthenol (D-panthenol): chemically known as (+)-2,4-dihydroxy-N-(3-hydroxypropyl)-3,3-dimethylbutyramide

Origin Classification:

Pantothenic acid is natural and found throughout the plant and animal kingdoms. Dexpanthenol is synthetic and, therefore, not considered organic or natural.

Personal Care Category:

Humectant, emollient, anti-inflammatory

Recommended for the following Baumann Skin Types:

DRNT, DRNW, DRPT, DRPW, DSNT, DSNW, DSPT, and DSPW

SOURCE

Present in all living cells, pantothenic acid is a precursor for the production of acetyl coenzyme A, an essential substrate for acetylcholine synthesis. Pantothenic acid, or vitamin B₅, belongs to the water-soluble B vitamin family and is also an essential ingredient in the enzymes necessary for metabolizing carbohydrates and fats. Proper growth and development depends partly on this vitamin as does the maintenance of normal epithelial function, including skin regrowth.[1] Among the best sources of pantothenic acid (PA) are fish, beef, whole grains, dairy, eggs, mushrooms, peanuts and other legumes, cashews, broccoli, soybeans, and avocados, but most whole foods contain some PA. In fact, deficiency of PA is virtually unknown because of its broad availability in food sources.

HISTORY

The word "pantothenic" is derived from the Greed word *pantos* ("everywhere"), suggesting the omnipresence of the vitamin in the plant and animal world. Dexpanthenol (provitamin B₅) is the stable alcohol form of pantothenic acid. It is popular and well regarded in the treatment of various skin conditions.[2]

CHEMISTRY

Not found naturally, synthetic dexpanthenol is converted to PA in the skin, stimulating skin regeneration in a fashion comparable to vitamin A. This process of cell division and formation of new skin tissue restores skin elasticity and promotes wound healing. In fact, both *in vitro* and *in vivo*, dexpanthenol has been shown to promote fibroblast proliferation.[1] Therefore, water-soluble dexpanthenol has been used topically to foster wound healing. Formulations containing dexpanthenol have exhibited a capacity to stimulate epithelialization and granulation while imparting an antipruritic, anti-inflammatory effect on experimental ultraviolet-induced erythema.[1] In an early study, treatment with dexpanthenol over a three- to four-week period resulted in significant improvement in skin-irritation symptoms such as xerosis, pruritus, erythema, roughness, scaling, and fissures.[1] Several other benefits to the skin have been associated with provitamin B₅. In a randomized, double-blind, placebo-controlled study, treatment with topical dexpanthenol over a seven-day period resulted in enhanced stratum corneum (SC) hydration and decreased TEWL.[3]

Dexpanthenol is used in a wide range of cosmetic products, typically to moisturize the skin, and formulated in some intramuscular and intravenous products. Topically applied provitamin B₅ also acts to prevent TEWL while moisturizing the skin. It is well tolerated and poses minimal risk of irritation or sensitivity.

ORAL USES

Vitamin B₅ is available in various foods. Dexpanthenol can also be taken orally, and is metabolized into pantothenic acid.

TOPICAL USES

Topical dexpanthenol is well established as an effective moisturizer, enhancing SC hydration and decreasing TEWL in healthy skin, protecting against irritation as a pretreatment, and facilitating wound healing (Table 27-1).[1]

TABLE 27-1
Pros and Cons of Vitamin B₅

Pros	Cons
Found in many products	Should not be combined or layered with oil-containing vehicles because penetration is decreased
Decent data demonstrate healing, anti-inflammatory, and hydrating activity	No organic forms
Safe	

Human Studies

Proksch and Nissen, in 2002, conducted a study with 20 subjects (12 women, 8 men) to identify the effects of a dexpanthenol-containing cream, applied twice daily, on skin barrier repair, SC hydration, skin roughness, and inflammation after irritation induced by sodium lauryl sulfate (SLS). The investigators found that the dexpanthenol-containing cream significantly increased the pace of skin barrier repair compared with placebo or untreated skin. SC hydration was enhanced and skin roughness reduced by both the dexpanthenol cream and placebo, but significantly more by the cream containing dexpanthenol. The test cream also significantly diminished erythema, whereas the placebo had no impact on skin redness.[4] A different study in 2002, a prospective, randomized, double-blind trial, demonstrated that the prophylactic and consistent use of an emollient containing dexpanthenol ameliorated the effects of radiation dermatitis, though it was less effective than topical corticosteroid (0.1 percent methylprednisolone).[5]

In 2003, Biro et al. conducted a prospective, randomized, double-blind, placebo-controlled study of 25 healthy volunteers (21 of whom completed the trial) to study the efficacy of dexpanthenol in protecting against skin irritation. For 26 days, the patients (between 18 and 45 years old) twice daily applied either Bepanthol Handbalsam containing 5 percent dexpanthenol or placebo to the inner part of both forearms. Twice daily from days 15 to 22, SLS 2 percent was applied. The investigators reported that intraindividual comparisons revealed better results in areas treated with dexpanthenol in 11 cases as compared to one placebo site. Irritant contact dermatitis was reported by six patients, with greater severity associated with the placebo site in five of the cases.[2]

In 2009, Radtke et al. conducted a prospective observational study in 392 networked pharmacies, consecutively recruiting 1,886 patients with irritated skin to determine the patient-relevant benefit of dexpanthenol treatment. They found that 94.7 percent achieved successful results and all symptoms of irritated skin improved significantly independent of age, gender, and underlying cutaneous disease.[6]

Dexpanthenol is firmly established enough as a therapeutic option for irritant dermatitis and cutaneous inflammation to have allowed Wolff and Kieser to use it as a comparison standard in an observational study to gauge the effectiveness of hamamelis (better known as witch hazel) for children with minor skin disorders. They treated 309 children (231 with hamamelis and 78 with dexpanthenol) and found statistically significant improvements in both groups, with both products equally effective and hamamelis slightly better tolerated.[7]

In 2011, Camargo et al. studied the skin moisturizing capacity of formulations including 0.5, 1.0, or 5.0 percent panthenol topically applied daily to the forearms of healthy subjects over 15- and 30-day periods. They found that use of the 1.0 and 5.0 percent formulations yielded significant reductions in TEWL after application for 30 days. To assess the immediate effects on TEWL and skin moisture, the research protocol also included using the formulations after skin washing with sodium laureth sulfate (SLES). The investigators noted significant TEWL decreases two hours after using the panthenol formulations in comparison to control and vehicle.[8]

Early in 2012, a small comparative pilot study, completed by 26 children (mean age 7.19 years), revealed that 5 percent dexpanthenol was equally effective as 1 percent hydrocortisone ointment in treating mild-to-moderate childhood atopic dermatitis.[9]

Also in 2012, Heise et al. set out to correlate *in vitro* findings of a stimulatory effect rendered by pantothenate on migration, proliferation, and gene regulation in cultured human dermal fibroblasts to the *in vivo* wound healing environment. Their clinical data resulting from comparisons of dexpanthenol-treated skin and placebo-treated skin were analyzed at the molecular level and revealed that the provitamin B modulated gene expression in cutaneous wound healing (upregulating IL-6, IL-1β, CYP1B1, CXCL1, CCL18 and KAP 4-2 gene expression and downregulating psorasin mRNA and protein expression).[10]

Combination Therapy

Over a decade ago, dexpanthenol was used effectively in combination therapy with xylometazoline for the treatment of rhinitis.[11] Dexpanthenol has also been shown, in combination with zinc oxide, to be effective in treating irritant diaper dermatitis, as demonstrated in a prospective, block randomized, investigator-blinded study of 46 children.[12]

In 2008, Abdelatif et al. assessed the safety and effectiveness of an ointment combining royal jelly and panthenol (PEDYPHAR) in 60 patients with limb-threatening diabetic foot infections. Patients were divided into three treatment groups, based on lesion severity. After irrigation and cleansing with normal saline, as well as surgical debridement if necessary, patients were treated with the combination ointment. Lesions were then covered with dressings and the patients were followed up for six months or until full healing, with clinical response checked at weeks 3, 9, and 24. By week 9 and through the follow-up period, 96 percent of the patients in groups 1 and 2 [Group 1: full-thickness skin ulcer (Wagner grades 1 and 2); group 2: deep tissue infection and suspected osteomyelitis (Wagner grade 3)] were deemed to have been cured, with all ulcers in group 1 patients healed and 92 percent among group 2 patients. Group 3 patients [gangrenous lesions (Wagner grades 4 and 5)] healed after surgery, debridement, and conservative therapy with PEDYPHAR. The investigators concluded that the ointment appears promising but additional randomized, double-blind trials are necessary to bear this out.[13]

In a 2011 prospective open pilot trial conducted over 28 days, Castello and Milani evaluated the effect of topically applied 10 percent Urea ISDIN® plus dexpanthenol lotion in the treatment of xerosis and pruritus in 15 hemodialyzed patients (12 women, 3 men, mean age 66 years). The results of twice-daily application on arms and legs were assessed after two and four weeks of treatment and measured against baseline scores for itch, scaling, roughness, redness, and cracks. Significant reductions were observed in all parameters through two, and especially four, weeks of treatment. One patient experienced a mild burning sensation, but the urea and dexpanthenol lotion was found to be effective in ameliorating xerosis and pruritus in hemodialysis patients.[14]

Further, in a 2011 study using Wistar rats, Guimarães et al. found that the combination of ultrasound and dexpanthenol (10 percent) sped up the production and organization of collagen in the early phases of wound healing.[15]

SAFETY ISSUES

Dexpanthenol confers soothing effects to formulations for the treatment of sunburn and other types of burn. Topically applied dexpanthenol is considered safe, with minimal association with local skin reactions or sensitization. Products with a high concentration of dexpanthenol may be contraindicated in people with hemophilia. Despite its frequency of use in topical products, contact allergy is rare. There is one report of one case of allergic contact dermatitis to panthenol combined with cocamidopropyl PG dimonium chloride phosphate in a facial hydrating lotion.[16]

ENVIRONMENTAL IMPACT

There is no measureable environmental impact from the vitamin pantothenic acid, found throughout nature, or the synthetic dexpanthenol.

FORMULATION CONSIDERATIONS

Water-in-oil topical emulsions are the best vehicle to deliver sufficient skin penetration and local concentrations of dexpanthenol.[1]

USAGE CONSIDERATIONS

Pantothenic acid is not well absorbed into skin but dexpanthenol is well absorbed through the skin and is rapidly converted to pantothenic acid.[1] Absorption into skin was found to be reduced when dexpanthenol is combined with olive oil, highlighting the relevance of the vehicle.[17] One study used a perfused skin udder model and demonstrated that the rate and extent of penetration of dexpanthenol is much lower in an oil/water formulation.[18] Therefore, panthenol-containing formulations should not be layered over oil-containing preparations if maximal dexpanthenol absorption is desired.

SIGNIFICANT BACKGROUND

Dexpanthenol is included as an ingredient in various topical skin formulations and shampoos. In fact, this form of vitamin B₅ has long been considered an effective ingredient in cosmetic products. The foundation for the use of dexpanthenol in shampoo – and anecdotal reports that its use restores color to gray hair – stems from a study several years ago evaluating dexpanthenol deficiency in rats. Deficiency was correlated with hair turning gray or falling out. Pantothenic acid deficiency in humans is exceedingly rare, though, and is not likely associated with hair changes in humans.[19] Clearly, the etiologies of graying of hair and baldness are not related to this vitamin. Also, no oral or topical formulations containing pantothenic acid or dexpanthenol as the main active ingredient have been shown to prevent gray hair or balding in humans. Nevertheless, it is believed that dexpanthenol penetrates well into the hair shaft, promotes luster and elasticity, and leaves the hair easier to comb.

CONCLUSION

Dexpanthenol is a versatile compound suitable for use in treating various dermatoses and its topical application is employed broadly in clinical practice to enhance wound healing. Few controlled clinical trials have been conducted evaluating the efficacy of topical formulations containing dexpanthenol intended for skin care. Despite a dearth of randomized, double-blind, case-controlled studies establishing the efficacy of such products, current data warrant further study and support the conclusion that dexpanthenol as an active ingredient at least confers some benefit as a humectant.

There is an increasing body of anecdotal, empirical evidence also suggesting significant potential contributions by provitamin B₅ as an ingredient in topical formulations.

REFERENCES

1. Ebner F, Heller A, Rippke F, et al. Topical use of dexpanthenol in skin disorders. *Am J Clin Dermatol.* 2002;3:427.
2. Biro K, Thaçi D, Ochsendorf FR, et al. Efficacy of dexpanthenol in skin protection against irritation: A double-blind, placebo-controlled study. *Contact Dermatitis.* 2003;49:80.
3. Gehring W, Gloor M. Effect of topically applied dexpanthenol on epidermal barrier function and stratum corneum hydration. Results of a human in vivo study. *Arzneimittelforschung.* 2000;50:659.
4. Proksch E, Nissen HP. Dexpanthenol enhances skin barrier repair and reduces inflammation after sodium lauryl sulphate-induced irritation. *J Dermatolog Treat.* 2002;13:173.
5. Schmuth M, Wimmer MA, Hofer S, et al. Topical corticosteroid therapy for acute radiation dermatitis: A prospective, randomized, double-blind study. *Br J Dermatol.* 2002;146:983.
6. Radtke MA, Lee-Seifert C, Rustenbach SJ, et al. Efficacy and patient benefit of treatment of irritated skin with ointments containing dexpanthenol: Health services research (observational study) on self-medication in a pharmaceutical network. *Hautarzt.* 2009;60:414.
7. Wolff HH, Kieser M. Hamamelis in children with skin disorders and skin injuries: Results of an observational study. *Eur J Pediatr.* 2007;166:943.
8. Camargo FB Jr, Gaspar LR, Maia Campos PM. Skin moisturizing effects of panthenol-based formulations. *J Cosmet Sci.* 2011;62:361.
9. Udompataikul M, Limpa-o-vart D. Comparative trial of 5% dexpanthenol in water-in-oil formulation with 1% hydrocortisone ointment in the treatment of childhood atopic dermatitis: a pilot study. *J Drugs Dermatol.* 2012;11:366.
10. Heise R, Skazik C, Marquardt Y, et al. Dexpanthenol modulates gene expression in skin wound healing in vivo. *Skin Pharmacol Physiol.* 2012;25:241.
11. Kehrl W, Sonnemann U. Improving wound healing after nose surgery by combined administration of xylometazoline and dexpanthenol. *Laryngorhinootologie.* 2000;79:151.
12. Wananukul S, Limpongsanuruk W, Singalavanija S, et al. Comparison of dexpanthenol and zinc oxide ointment with ointment base in the treatment of irritant diaper dermatitis from diarrhea: a multicenter study. *J Med Assoc Thai.* 2006;89:1654.
13. Abdelatif M, Yakoot M, Etmaan M. Safety and efficacy of a new honey ointment on diabetic foot ulcers: A prospective pilot study. *J Wound Care.* 2008;17:108.
14. Castello M, Milani M. Efficacy of topical hydrating and emollient lotion containing 10% urea ISDIN® plus dexpanthenol (Ureadin Rx 10) in the treatment of skin xerosis and pruritus in hemodialyzed patients: an open prospective pilot trial. *G Ital Dermatol Venerol.* 2011;146:321.
15. Guimarães GN, Pires-De-Campos MS, Leonardi GR, et al. Effect of ultrasound and dexpanthenol on collagen organization in tegumentary lesions. *Rev Bras Fisioter.* 2011;15:227.
16. Roberts H, Williams J, Tate B. Allergic contact dermatitis to panthenol and cocomidopropyl PG dimonium chloride phosphate in a facial hydrating lotion. *Contact Dermatitis.* 2006;55:369.
17. Stuettgen G, Krause H. Percutaneous absorption of tritium-labelled panthenol in man and animal. *Arch Klin Exp Dermatol.* 1960;209:578.
18. Förster T, Pittermann W, Schmitt M, et al. Skin penetration properties of cosmetic formulations using a perfused bovine udder model. *J Cosmet Sci.* 1999;50:147.
19. Plesofsky-Vig N. Pantothenic acid. In: Ziegler EE, Filer LJ Jr, eds. *Present Knowledge in Nutrition.* 7th ed. Washington, DC: ILSI Press; 1996:210–211.

CHAPTER 28

Urea

Activities:

Anti-inflammatory, hydrating, keratolytic

Important Chemical Components:

The chemical formula of urea (or carbamide) is $CO(NH_2)_2$. Its molecular formula is CH_4N_2O.

Origin Classification:

Urea is a natural organic compound.

Personal Care Category:

Humectant, emollient

Recommended for the following Baumann Skin Types:

DRNT, DRNW, DRPT, and DRPW

SOURCE

Urea, the primary nitrogen-containing substance found in mammalian urine, is among the most commonly used humectant ingredients, along with glycerin, sorbitol, sodium hyaluronate, propylene glycol, α-hydroxy acids, and sugars (Table 28-1). It is a component of the natural moisturizing factor (NMF) and also exhibits a mild antipruritic effect.[1] Urea in high concentrations (e.g., 40 percent) is effective as a hydrating and keratolytic agent in various cutaneous conditions including xerosis, psoriasis, onychomycosis and other nail disorders, ichthyosis, eczema, calluses, and corns.

HISTORY

Urea was first discovered in the 1700s in Europe. Its discovery is most often attributed to French chemist Hilaire Rouelle's work in 1773, though Dutch scientist Herman Boerhaave is said to have first identified the compound as a major constituent of mammalian urine in 1727.[2,3] German physician and chemist Friedrich Wöhler discovered, in 1828, that urea could be synthesized *in vitro* by combining the inorganic materials cyanic acid and ammonium without using any organic substances.[2] This was the first credited laboratory synthesis of a naturally occurring organic compound.[2] Interestingly, the chemical synthesis reported by Wöhler is not the chain of events that occurs in the mammalian liver to produce urea;

TABLE 28-1
Pros and Cons of Urea

PROS	CONS
Strong humectant activity	Occasional contact allergy
Inexpensive	Mild odor
Easy to find brands that contain it	

the "urea cycle" was identified by German physician Hans A. Krebs and his medical student Kurt Henseleit in 1932.[2] Urea has been used in hand creams since the 1940s.[4] Thirty years later, urea in 20 percent concentrations was found to be effective in treating pruritus.[5]

CHEMISTRY

The urea molecule has two NH_2 groups united with a carbonyl functional group. It acts as a physiological NMF.[6]

ORAL USES

Oral urea is used for some medical indications and has a long history of traditional folk medicine use, but this mode of administration is not thought to have appreciable cutaneous benefits.

TOPICAL USES

Twenty years ago, a double-blind, randomized comparison of two urea-containing creams revealed that 3 and 10 percent urea cream were equally effective in treating aspects of dry skin, particularly increasing hydration and decreasing scaling, and more effective than the vehicle control. Transepidermal water loss (TEWL) was unchanged after treatment with the 3 percent urea cream, but the 10 percent urea cream reduced TEWL. Use of the 3 percent cream resulted in a slightly golden tint to the skin color.[7]

In 1998, Jennings et al. conducted a double-blind, randomized paired comparison of the keratolytic effects of 5 percent salicylic acid and 10 percent urea ointment (Kerasal) on one foot and 12 percent ammonium lactate lotion (Lac-Hydrin) on the other foot in 70 patients with mild-to-moderate xerosis. After two weeks of treatment, 54 patients were evaluated, 39 of whom were evaluated after four weeks of treatment. There were no significant differences in the treatment arms, but after four weeks of treatment, both yielded significant reductions in xerosis severity.[8]

Urea in high concentrations is also a useful adjuvant, as is salicylic acid, in the keratolytic phase of psoriasis treatment.[9] In 10 percent creams, urea is used to treat ichthyosis and hyperkeratotic skin conditions;[10] in lower concentrations, it is employed to treat mild xerosis.[6]

In 2002, Ademola et al. conducted a randomized, double-blind, bilateral study with 25 women and men to compare the clinical effectiveness and tolerability of a 40 percent urea topical cream (Carmol 40) and 12 percent ammonium lactate topical lotion (Lac-Hydrin 12 percent) used to treat moderate-to-severe xerosis. Patients were assessed at baseline as well as two and four weeks after the initiation of therapy. Ratings by the 18 patients who completed the study as well as investigators revealed that xerosis symptoms were reduced in less time in the urea group. Further, instrumental and clinical measurements showed that by day 14, 40 percent urea cream was associated with less skin roughness, fissures, thickness, and dryness than 12 percent ammonium lactate lotion.[11]

In 2008, Stebbins et al. performed a single-blind pilot study with 12 trained female panelists to evaluate the acceptability (spreadability, odor, and postapplication residue) of six 40 to 50 percent urea preparations. They compared the composite scores of the five older formulations with that of new emollient product, and found that the novel preparation (U-Kera E) was the most cosmetically acceptable (most spreadable and left less residue). Odor scores were low overall and comparable among the six preparations. The investigators noted that while all urea-based creams exhibited a detectable odor, it was usually fleeting and often such products are used in areas furthest from the nose (i.e., legs and feet).[12]

In 2010, Lodén et al. randomized 53 patients with successfully treated hand eczema to compare the time to relapse when using a barrier-strengthening urea (5 percent) preparation or receiving no treatment. They observed that the median time to relapse was two days in the no treatment group and 20 days in the urea-containing moisturizer group. At the time of relapse, there were no noted variations in severity. The investigators concluded that the barrier-strengthening moisturizer containing urea successfully acted to extend the remission of controlled hand eczema.[13]

SAFETY ISSUES

Cases of contact allergy from urea-containing products are rare. In one instance, at least, the reaction may have been due to ingredients other than urea.[14] However, urea is considered generally safe and nontoxic. Urea is contraindicated in neonates due to the risk of systemic absorption.[15]

ENVIRONMENTAL IMPACT

Used widely in fertilizer as well as cosmetic products, urea is produced in copious amounts on an industrial scale from liquid ammonia and liquid carbon dioxide, with global production in 2012 estimated at 184 million tons.[16] The inclusion of urea in topical products, thus, certainly exerts some kind of impact on the environment, primarily in fuel transportation costs.

FORMULATION CONSIDERATIONS

There are many different types of formulations using urea as discussed in this chapter that are beyond the scope of this book. (Please see the NWU Institutional Repository website, http://dspace.nwu.ac.za/handle/10394/251, for more information on urea product formulations.)

USAGE CONSIDERATIONS

The combination of urea with hydrocortisone, retinoic acid, and other agents has been shown to enhance the penetration of these agents.[17,18] Urea has also been combined with several other compounds in recent years to achieve significant clinical effects.

SIGNIFICANT BACKGROUND

In 2009, Amichai and Gunwald conducted a three-week randomized, double-blind study with 36 males and females with mild-to-moderate atopic dermatitis, ranging in age from 3 to 40 years, to ascertain the efficacy of liquid soap containing 12 percent ammonium lactate and 20 percent urea. Investigator and patient assessment indicated that significant improvements were observed, specifically reductions in erythema, scaling, and xerosis, in the active soap group (24 patients) compared to results in the 12-person control group.[19]

In 2010, Pardo Masferrer led a prospective observational study in 98 breast cancer patients to investigate the intensive use of a hydrating lotion containing 3 percent urea, polidocanol and hyaluronic acid to treat and mitigate the severity of radiodermatitis. The investigators monitored patients weekly for skin toxicity and compared the incidence and grade of toxicity with a control sample from 174 breast cancer patients whose skin was treated at radiotherapy initiation in 2006 or upon the emergence of radiodermatitis. They found the incidence of radiodermatitis lower in the intensive use group. In addition, intensive use of the combination lotion was also associated with a lower grade of toxicity.[20]

The use of urea in combination with other ingredients in the Ureadin line of products has garnered recent attention. In 2011, Castello and Milani found, in a prospective open pilot trial with 15 patients, that the twice-daily application of topical 10 percent urea plus dexpanthenol (Ureadin Rx 10) significantly reduced itching scores as well as scores along the SRRC (scaling, roughness, redness, and cracks) Index, indicating that the formulation was effective in treating xerosis and pruritus in such patients.[21]

Later that year, Tadini et al. studied the keratolytic and moisturizing activity of Ureadin Rx10 in a four-week randomized, controlled, single-blind, two-center, intra-patient trial with 30 ichthyosis vulgaris patients ranging in age between 8 and 56 years. In a right-vs.-left study design, patients were treated with 10 percent urea-based Ureadin Rx 10 lotion on one side and the glycerol-based emollient cream Dexeryl on the other side. Patients were assessed at baseline as well as two and four weeks after treatment initiation. Twenty-seven participants completed the study, in which the researchers found that both topical formulations were clinically effective after four weeks and well tolerated. SRRC scores significantly fell from 9.5 to 3.3 (65 percent decline) in association with Ureadin use and from 9.5 to 5.7 (40 percent decline) in Dexeryl-treated areas. Mean global efficacy scores were significantly higher in areas treated with Ureadin (8.9) as compared to Dexeryl (7.3). The investigators concluded that Ureadin is a more effective option than Dexeryl for reducing the hyperkeratosis and xerosis associated with ichthyosis, but larger sample sizes would be necessary in future research to establish safety and tolerability for the urea-based lotion in these patients.[22]

In 2012, Federici et al. conducted a 28-day, randomized, evaluator-blinded, comparative study in 40 type 2 diabetics, aged 40 to 75 years, to assess the efficacy of a topical preparation containing urea 5 percent, arginine, and carnosine (Ureadin) as compared to the glycerol-based emollient Dexeryl. Twice-daily application of the urea-based product resulted in significantly more hydration as compared to the glycerol-based emollient. Visual Analogue Scores increased in both groups, but were significantly higher in the Ureadin group. The investigators concluded that the urea/arginine/carnosine cream enhanced skin hydration while lessening xerosis in type 2 diabetic patients more efficiently than the glycerol-based control formulation.[23]

Also in 2012, Emtestam et al. led a 24-week, randomized, double-blind, placebo-controlled multicenter study of 493 patients ($n = 346$; placebo = 147) to test the efficacy, safety, and tolerability of a novel topical preparation (K101) combining urea, propylene glycol, and lactic acid for treating distal subungual onychomycosis. Patients were stratified based on level of nail involvement, with investigators finding that 27.2 percent of patients with ≤ 50 percent nail involvement treated with K101 achieved the primary endpoint and 10.4 percent in the placebo group. Among the patients with 51 to 75 percent nail involvement, 19.1 percent achieved the primary endpoint as compared to 7.0 percent in the placebo group (not a significant difference). The investigators noted that the antifungal topical preparation was safe and imparted clinically significant as well as visible nail improvements. Further, they noted that when applied in concentrations greater than 20 percent, urea displays nail-dissolving properties.[24–26] Others have noted a concentration-dependent keratolytic effect of softening and macerating the nail with 30 to 50 percent concentrations of urea.[14]

Ciammaichella et al. reported at the end of that year on a pilot registry study of the effects of twice-daily application of Ureadin for four weeks in diabetic patients with microangiopathy and mild-to-moderate xerosis of the foot. A reduction in skin breaks was associated with Ureadin treatment as compared to controls. Improvements were also linked to Ureadin use along various other parameters in comparison to controls (i.e., greater skin thickness, favorable investigator global assessments and subject assessments, no new skin lesions vs. four lesions in the control group). The researchers concluded that given the good level of diabetes control prior to inclusion in the study and no such changes after four weeks, the improvements seen in the study could be attributed to the topical application of Ureadin and not to systemic diabetes management.[27]

CONCLUSION

Urea has long been used in dermatology for its well-established activity as a hydrating and moisturizing agent. It remains as one of the most effective humectant agents.

REFERENCES

1. Kligman AM. Dermatologic uses of urea. *Acta Derm Venereol.* 1957;37:155.
2. Kinne-Saffran E, Kinne RK. Vitalism and synthesis of urea. From Friedrich Wöhler to Hans A. Krebs. *Am J Nephrol.* 1999;19:290.
3. Kurzer F, Sanderson PM. Urea in the history of organic chemistry: Isolation from natural sources. *J Chem Educ.* 1956;33:452.
4. Harding C, Bartolone J, Rawlings A. Effects of natural moisturizing factor and lactic acid isomers on skin function. In: Lodén M, Maibach H, eds. *Dry Skin and Moisturizers.* Boca Raton, FL: CRC Press; 2000:236.
5. Swanbeck G, Rajka G. Antipruritic effect of urea solutions. An experimental and clinical study. *Acta Derm Venereol.* 1970;50:225.
6. Lodén M. The clinical benefit of moisturizers. *J Eur Acad Dermatol Venereol.* 2005;19:672.
7. Serup J. A double-blind comparison of two creams containing urea as the active ingredient. Assessment of efficacy and side-effects by non-invasive techniques and a clinical scoring scheme. *Acta Derm Venereol Suppl.* 1992;177:34.
8. Jennings MB, Alfieri D, Ward K, et al. Comparison of salicylic acid and urea versus ammonium lactate for the treatment of foot xerosis. A randomized, double-blind, clinical study. *J Am Podiatr Med Assoc.* 1998;88:332.
9. Fluhr JW, Cavallotti C, Berardesca E. Emollients, moisturizers, and keratolytic agents in psoriasis. *Clin Dermatol.* 2008;26:380.
10. Rosten M. The treatment of ichthyosis and hyperkeratotic conditions with urea. *Australas J Dermatol.* 1970;11:142.
11. Ademola J, Frazier C, Kim SJ, et al. Clinical evaluation of 40% urea and 12% ammonium lactate in the treatment of xerosis. *Am J Clin Dermatol.* 2002;3(3):217.
12. Stebbins W, Alexis A, Levitt J. Cosmetic acceptability of six 40–50% urea preparations: a single-blind, pilot study. *Am J Clin Dermatol.* 2008;9:319.
13. Lodén M, Wirén K, Smerud K, et al. Treatment with a barrier-strengthening moisturizer prevents relapse of hand-eczema. An open, randomized, prospective, parallel group study. *Acta Derm Venereol.* 2010;90:602.
14. Piraccini BM, Alessandrini A, Bruni F, et al. Acute periungueal dermatitis induced by application of urea-containing cream under occlusion. *J Dermatol Case Rep.* 2012;6:18.
15. Oji V, Traupe H. Ichthyosis: Clinical manifestations and practical treatment options. *Am J Clin Dermatol.* 2009;10:351.
16. Ceresana Market Intelligence Consulting. http://www.ceresana.com/en/market-studies/agriculture/urea/. Accessed June 9, 2013.
17. Wohlrab W. The influence of urea on the penetration kinetics of topically applied corticosteroids. *Acta Derm Venereol.* 1984;64:233.
18. Wohlrab W. Effect of urea on the penetration kinetics of vitamin A acid into human skin. *Z Hautkr.* 1990;65:803.
19. Amichai B, Gunwald MH. A randomized, double-blind, placebo-controlled study to evaluate the efficacy in AD of liquid soap containing 12% ammonium lactate + 20% urea. *Clin Exp Dermatol.* 2009;34:e602.
20. Pardo Masferrer J, Murcia Mejía M, Vidal Fernández M, et al. Prophylaxis with a cream containing urea reduces the incidence and severity of radio-induced dermatitis. *Clin Transl Oncol.* 2010;12:43.
21. Castello M, Milani M. Efficacy of topical hydrating and emollient lotion containing 10% urea ISDIN® plus dexpanthenol (Ureadin Rx 10) in the treatment of skin xerosis and pruritus in hemodialyzed patients: An open prospective pilot trial. *G Ital Dermatol Venereol.* 2011;146:321.
22. Tadini G, Giustini S, Milani M. Efficacy of topical 10% urea-based lotion in patients with ichthyosis vulgaris: A two-center, randomized, controlled, single-blind, right-vs.-left study in comparison with standard glycerol-based emollient cream. *Curr Med Res Opin.* 2011;27:2279.
23. Federici A, Federici G, Milani M. An urea, arginine and carnosine based cream (Ureadin Rx Db ISDIN) shows greater efficacy in the treatment of severe xerosis of the feet in Type 2 diabetic patients in comparison with glycerol-based emollient cream. A randomized, assessor-blinded, controlled trial. *BMC Dermatol.* 2012;12:16.
24. Emtestam L, Kaaman T, Rensfeldt K. Treatment of distal subungual onychomycosis with a topical preparation of urea, propylene glycol and lactic acid: Results of a 24-week, double-blind, placebo-controlled study. *Mycoses.* 2012;55:532.
25. South DA, Farber EM. Urea ointment in the nonsurgical avulsion of nail dystrophies – A reappraisal. *Cutis.* 1980;25:609.
26. Farber EM, South DA. Urea ointment in the nonsurgical avulsion of nail dystrophies. *Cutis.* 1978;22:689.
27. Ciammaichella G, Belcaro G, Dugall M, et al. Product evaluation of Ureadin Rx Db (ISDIN) for prevention and treatment of mild-to-moderate xerosis of the foot in diabetic patients. Prevention of skin lesions due to microangiopathy. *Panminerva Med.* 2012;54:35.

CHAPTER 29

Aquaporin

Aquaporins (AQPs) are integral membrane proteins that form a water channel and facilitate water transport in various organs such as the skin, renal tubules, eyes, the digestive tract, and the brain. In 2003, Peter Agre received the Nobel Prize in chemistry for discovering AQPs. There are 13 isoforms of AQPs found in mammals classified as types 1 to 13. Functionally, they can be classified into two subtypes: AQPs 1, 2, 4, 5, and 8, which only transport water, and AQPs 3, 7, 9, and 10, which can conduct other substances such as glycerol (also known as glycerin) or urea in addition to water.[1] AQP-3 is the predominant water channel found in human epidermis, and is permeable to both water and glycerin. For years scientists have known that glycerin plays a superior role in hydrating skin,[2] but the reasons for this became more clear when AQP-3 was discovered. Studies have shown that defects in AQP-3 in mice models result in epidermal dryness as well as decreased stratum corneum hydration and glycerin content of the epidermis, followed by reduced elasticity and impaired skin barrier recovery.[3,4] Aquaporin facilitates the transport of water, glycerin, and solutes between keratinocytes.

AQPs are transmembrane structures arranged as homotetramers in the cell membrane. Each subunit of the tetramer consists of six α-helical domains and contains a distinct aqueous pore. The intricate shape and the transmembrane position make it impossible to exogenously add aquaporin to skin as the marketing claims of some cosmetic products imply. Ultraviolet light has been shown to diminish the expression of AQP-3, likely through MAP kinase pathways.[5] Free radicals have also been demonstrated to decrease AQP-3 expression.[5] This is one of the reasons that sun-exposed skin becomes dehydrated.[5]

In addition, aquaporin performance can be affected by topical ingredients that can increase the opening and closing of the aquaporin pore or upregulate AQP-3 expression. *Ajuga turkestanica* has been shown to increase AQP-3 function.[6] Retinol and the antioxidant n-acetyl cysteine both have been shown to inhibit the downregulation of AQP-3 upon UV exposure.[5] AQPs are intriguing water channels that allow water and glycerin to flow from cell to cell. In the next few years, many more facets of their dynamic mechanisms of action will be elucidated.

REFERENCES

1. Takata K, Matsuzaki T, Tajika Y. Aquaporins: Water channel proteins of the cell membrane. *Prog Histochem Cytochem.* 2004;39:1.
2. Choi EH, Man MQ, Wang F, et al. Is endogenous glycerol a determinant of stratum corneum hydration in humans? *J Invest Dermatol.* 2005;125:288.
3. Hara M, Ma T, Verkman AS. Selectively reduced glycerol in skin of aquaporin-3-deficient mice may account for impaired ski hydration, elasticity, and barrier recovery. *J Biol Chem.* 2002;277:46616.
4. Hara M, Verkman AS. Glycerol replacement corrects defective skin hydration, elasticity, and barrier function in aquaporin-3-deficient mice. *Proc Natl Acad Sci USA.* 2003;100:7360.
5. Cao C, Wan S, Jiang Q, et al. All-trans retinoic acid attenuates ultraviolet radiation-induced down-regulation of aquaporin-3 and water permeability in human keratinocytes *J Cell Physiol.* 2008;215:506.
6. Dumas M, Gondran C, Barré P, et al. Effect of an Ajuga turkestanica extract on aquaporin 3 expression, water flux, differentiation and barrier parameters of the human epidermis. *Eur J Dermatol.* 2002;12:XXV.

CHAPTER 30

Ajuga Turkestanica

Activities:

Activation of aquaporin
Antimicrobial, antiviral, antitumor, antibiotic
Anabolic steroidal

Important Chemical Components:

Clerodane diterpenes
Phytoecdysteroids, including α-ecdysone, 2-desoxy-ecdysterone, ecdysterone, sileneoside A, and turkesterone
Iridoid glycosides

Origin Classification:

This ingredient is considered natural, but was not certified by the Natural Products Association (NPA) when this book went to press.

Personal Care Category:

Skin hydration, skin conditioning

Recommended for the following Baumann Skin Types:

DRNT, DRPT, DRNW, DRPW, DSNT, DSNW, DSPT, and DSPW

SOURCE

Ajuga turkestanica is a perennial herb and member of the mint family Lamiaceae. There are over 300 species of the genus *Ajuga* found throughout Europe, Asia, Africa, Australia, and North America. *A. turkestanica* is indigenous to Uzbekistan. It derives its name from the fact that it contains a powerful ecdysteroid called turkesterone. Ecdysterones are a group of plant sterols that have a steroid-like effect on the human body.

HISTORY

This plant has been used in traditional medicine to treat fevers, toothaches, dysentery, malaria, high blood pressure, diabetes, and gastrointestinal disorders, as well as antifungal, antihelminthic, anti-inflammatory, antimycobacterial, and diuretic agents.[1] Athletes and body builders have used *A. turkestanica* as an anabolic steroid because it contains phytoecdysteroids.[2] Many bodybuilding supplements containing turkesterone can be found on the Internet. *A. turkestanica* is known to contain several bioactive compounds and has been used in traditional medical approaches to heart disease as well as stomach and muscle aches.[3,4] In addition, it is one of the many species of *Ajuga* gaining attention for demonstrating medicinal properties with the potential for commercial applications.[5] In November 2000, US Patent Number 7060693 was filed for the cosmetic use of *A. turkestanica* (awarded in 2006) by scientists at Dior Research.

CHEMISTRY

There are three classes of potentially bioactive compounds found in the *Ajuga* genus[5]:

1. Clerodane diterpenes are recognized sources of antimicrobial, antiviral, antitumor, antibiotic, and amoebicidal activities.[6]
2. Phytoecdysteroids have anabolic steroid activity. *A. turkestanica* reportedly contains several phytoecdysteroids (turkesterone, 20-hydroxyecdysone, cyasterone, cyasterone 22-acetate, ajugalactone, ajugasterone B, α-ecdysone and ecdysone 2, 3-monoacetonide) as well as the iridoids harpagide and harpagide 8-acetate.[5,7–12]
3. Iridoid glycosides, especially abundant in *Ajuga decumbens*, have exhibited anticancer activity.[13]

ORAL USES

A. turkestanica extract is included in some anabolic muscle growth supplements.

TOPICAL USES

Patented extracts of *A. turkestanica* were shown in 2006 to have sufficient ecdysteroids and other active ingredients to improve the differentiation of keratinocytes, thus facilitating skin hydration and yielding antiaging effects (Table 30-1).[14,15] The patent inventors observed that the extracts are especially effective in regulating epidermal water and glycerol transport, achieving improved hydration of the basal layer by working in concert with or enhancing aquaporin-3 (AQP-3).[14,16] AQP-3 is a water transport channel known to transport water and glycerol between cells.[17] The function of AQP-3 was shown to be increased by *A. turkestanica* extract.[18]

SAFETY ISSUES

A. turkestanica has not been reviewed for safety by the Cosmetic Ingredient Review (CIR) panel.

TABLE 30-1
Pros and Cons of *Ajuga Turkestanica*

Pros	Cons
The only agent known and commercially available to play a role in regulating AQP-3[25]	Limited number of brands contain this extract
Unique and proven mechanism of action	Expensive
Proven efficacy	
Can be combined with other ingredients	
Good shelf stability	

ENVIRONMENTAL IMPACT

A. turkestanica hairy root cultures have been developed as a sustainable alternative to wild-harvesting.[19]

FORMULATION CONSIDERATIONS

The only considerations that have been made public are disclosed in US Patent Number 7060693.

USAGE CONSIDERATIONS

There are no known restrictions. *A. turkestanica* can be used in the morning or at night and can be used in combination with other skin care products.

SIGNIFICANT BACKGROUND

Aquaporins

Aquaporins (AQPs) are integral membrane proteins that facilitate water transport in several organs, including the skin, brain, renal tubules, eyes, and digestive tract. Thirteen isoforms of aquaporins (AQP 0–12) are found in mammals. Of these, there are two functional subtype classifications: AQPs 1, 2, 4, 5, and 8 conduct only water, and AQPs 3, 7, 9, and 10 transport water and other substances including glycerol and urea.[20] **AQP-3, permeable to water and glycerol, is the main water channel in human epidermis.** Glycerol acts as an endogenous humectant thereby facilitating hydration of the stratum corneum (SC).[21] Defects in AQP-3 in mice models have been demonstrated to lead to epidermal xerosis, reduced SC hydration and epidermal glycerol content, followed by diminished elasticity and impaired skin barrier recovery.[22,23] Such findings underscore the important role of glycerol in cutaneous hydration. AQP-3 contributes to the transport of water, glycerol and solutes between keratinocytes.

Dumas et al. note that the role of AQPs in hydrating the living layers of the epidermis where keratinocyte differentiation occurs and in barrier development and recovery suggests that they are significant protein targets for improving the quality and resistance of the skin surface as well as ameliorating aging- and UV-induced xerosis.[18]

Ajuga Turkestanica and Aquaporins

In 2007, Dumas et al. conducted *in vitro* and *in vivo* studies of active ingredients capable of raising AQP-3 levels to enhance hydration in human skin keratinocytes, with the understanding that improving hydration in human keratinocytes would ultimately improve epidermal hydration.[24] They used an ethanolic/water (70/30 v/v) extract of *A. turkestanica* as the hydrating agent (2.5 μg/mL) and found that after 17 days of *in vitro* treatment every 2 days in human reconstructed epidermis, AQP-3 expression measured at the protein level was significantly elevated. Increased epidermal proliferation and differentiation was also noted. Electron microscopy showed a significantly thicker, compact SC and more clearly differentiated desmosomes.[18]

The investigators prepared an oil-water emulsion infused with *A. turkestanica* extract (0.3 percent w/w) for an *in vivo* study in which 15 healthy female volunteers (between 22 and 56 years old)

applied the formulation twice daily to their forearms for 21 days. Significant reductions in TEWL were seen in the treated area compared to the control at days 7 and 21. The researchers concluded that the tested *A. turkestanica* extract formulation enhanced AQP-3 expression and human epidermal differentiation *in vitro* and ameliorated epidermal barrier structure and human skin recovery *in vivo*.[15,18]

CONCLUSION

The *Ajuga turkestanica* story is a very interesting one because the cosmetic scientists Dumas, Bonté, and Gondran were the first to identify AQP-3 in skin cells. They published this information, sharing it with other scientists rather than keeping the information hidden and proprietary. Several compounds were tested with *A. turkestanica* found to affect water flux through the AQP channels. They filed patents to protect this technology. This is a great example of scientific discovery leading to new technologies. Unfortunately, many companies have started to claim that their products "contain aquaporin," which is misleading. If AQP was included in a formulation, it would not be able to penetrate into the skin and span the lipid bilayer in the manner that is necessary to affect water flux (Figure 30-1). The only way that is proven to affect water flux between cells is for an ingredient to act upon AQP in the manner that *Ajuga turkestanica* does. The discovery of AQP-3 as well as the understanding of its significance and how to harness its power to improve skin appearance occurred over a span of two decades. The scientists should be congratulated for their perseverance.

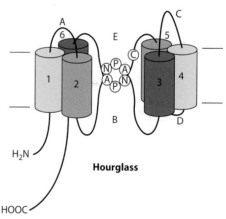

▲ **FIGURE 30-1** Hourglass model for aquaporin-1 membrane topology. Reprinted with permission from Borgnia M, Nielsen S, Engel A, et al. Cellular and molecular biology of the aquaporin water channels. *Annu Rev Biochem* 1999;68:425. Copyright © 1999, Annual Reviews.

REFERENCES

1. Israili ZH, Lyoussi B. Ethnopharmacology of the plants of genus Ajuga. *Pak J Pharm Sci*. 2009;22:425.
2. Cheng DM, Yousef GG, Grace MH, et al. In vitro production of metabolism-enhancing phytoecdysteroids from Ajuga turkestanica. *Plant Cell Tiss Organ Cult*. 2008;93:73.
3. Mamatkhanov AU, Yakubova MR, Syrov VN. Isolation of turkesterone from the epigeal part of Ajuga turkestanica and its anabolic activity. *Chem Nat Compd*. 1998;34:150.
4. Abdukadirov IT, Khodzhaeva MA, Turakhozhaev MT, et al. Carbohydrates from Ajuga turkestanica. *Chem Nat Compd*. 2004;40:85.
5. Grace MH, Cheng DM, Raskin I, et al. Neo-Clerodane Diterpenes from Ajuga turkestanica. *Phytochem Lett*. 2008;1:81.
6. Coll J, Tandron YA. Neo-Clerodane diterpenoids from Ajuga: structural elucidation and biological activity. *Phytochem Rev*. 2008;7:25.

7. Ramazanov NS. Phytoecdysteroids and other biologically active compounds from plants of the genus Ajuga. *Chem Nat Compd.* 2005;41:361.

8. Baltaev UA. Phytoecdysteroids: Structure, sources, and biosynthesis in plants. *Russ J Bioorg Chem.* 2000;26:799.

9. Usmanov VZ, Rashkes YV, Abubakirov NK. Phytoecdysones of Ajuga turkestanica VI. 22-acetylcyasterone. *Chem Nat Compd.* 1978;2:215.

10. Usmanov VZ, Gorovits MB, Abubakirov NK. Phytoecdysones of Ajuga turkestanica III. *Chem Nat Compd.* 1975;4:466.

11. Usmanov VZ, Gorovits MB, Abubakirov NK. Phytoecdysones of Ajuga turkestanica II. *Chem Nat Compd.* 1973;1:125.

12. Usmanov VZ, Gorovits MB, Abubakirov NK. Phytoecdysones of Ajuga turkestanica. *Chem Nat Compd.* 1971;4:535.

13. Konoshima T, Takasaki M, Tokuda H, et al. Cancer chemopreventive activity of an iridoid glycoside, 8-acetylharpagide, from Ajuga decumbens. *Cancer Lett.* 2000;157:87.

14. Brewster B. Aquaporins: stimulation by vitamins, steroids and sugar alcohols. *Cosmet Toil.* 2008;123:20.

15. Dumas M, Bonté F, Gondran C, inventors. LVMH Recherche, assignee. Ajuga turkestanica extract and its cosmetic uses. US Patent 7,060,693 B1, June 13, 2006.

16. WIPO Patent Application WO/1994/004132. Use of an ecdysteroid in cosmetics or dermatology.

17. Bonté F. Skin moisturization mechanisms: New data. *Ann Pharm Fr.* 2011;69:135.

18. Dumas M, Sadick NS, Noblesse E, et al. Hydrating skin by stimulating biosynthesis of aquaporins. *J Drugs Dermatol.* 2007;6:s20.

19. Cheng DM, Yousef GG, Grace MH, et al. In vitro production of metabolism-enhancing phytoecdysteroids from Ajuga turkestanica. *Plant Cell Tiss Organ Cult.* 2008;93:73.

20. Takata K, Matsuzaki T, Tajika Y. Aquaporins: water channel proteins of the cell membrane. *Prog Histochem Cytochem.* 2004;39:1.

21. Choi EH, Man MQ, Wang F, et al. Is endogenous glycerol a determinant of stratum corneum hydration in humans? *J Invest Dermatol.* 2005;125:288.

22. Hara M, Ma T, Verkman AS. Selectively reduced glycerol in skin of aquaporin-3-deficient mice may account for impaired skin hydration, elasticity, and barrier recovery. *J Biol Chem.* 2002;277:46616.

23. Hara M, Verkman AS. Glycerol replacement corrects defective skin hydration, elasticity, and barrier function in aquaporin-3-deficient mice. *Proc Natl Acad Sci U S A.* 2003;100:7360.

24. Dumas M, Gondran C, Barré P, et al. Effect of an Ajuga turkestanica extract on aquaporin 3 expression, water flux, differentiation and barrier parameters of the human epidermis. *Eur J Dermatol.* 2002;12:XXV.

25. Baumann L. Cosmetics and skin care in dermatology. In: Goldsmith LA, Katz SI, Gilchrest BA, et al. *Fitzpatrick's Dermatology in General Medicine.* 8th ed. Vol. 2. New York: McGraw-Hill; 2012:3010.

CHAPTER 31

Natural Moisturizing Factor

Natural moisturizing factor (NMF) is found inside keratinocytes and helps regulate stratum corneum (SC) hydration. NMF is a mixture of amino acids including pyrrolidone carboxylic and urocanic acids,[1,2] which are water-soluble byproducts of filaggrin.

Filaggrin, also known as filament aggregating protein, has two different cutaneous functions. In lower levels of the skin, filaggrin plays a structural role; however, higher up in the skin, it is broken down into amino acids that are hygroscopic and strongly bind water. Histidine, glutamine, and arginine are metabolites of filaggrin in the SC that are metabolized into trans-urocanic acid, pyrrolidone carboxylic acid, and citrulline, respectively. They create the osmotically active component that regulates skin hydration known as NMF.[1,3] Other constituents of NMF include lactic acid, urea, and inorganic ions such as sodium, potassium, calcium, and chloride, all of which contribute to epidermal hydration. The osmotically active and humectant properties of NMF allow the epidermis to retain hydration even in dry environments. Extraction of NMF components results in a decrease in the moisture accumulation rate (MAT) of the epidermis,[4] emphasizing the importance of NMF in skin hydration. Interestingly, NMF constituents undergo seasonal changes: the breakdown of filaggrin and production of NMF increase in low humidity and decrease in high humidity. NMF is intracellular and at this time it is not known if exogenously applied NMF or its precursors would result in increased NMF levels.

Patients with atopic dermatitis exhibit a reduction in NMF and have been found to have mutations in the filaggrin gene.[6,7] A defect in filaggrin also results in a structural impairment that is seen in atopic dermatitis because filaggrin plays a structural role in lower levels of the epidermis.[8] NMF levels are decreased by ultraviolet exposure, surfactants, and prolonged water immersion.

REFERENCES

1. Scott IR, Harding CR, Barrett JG. Histidine-rich protein of the keratohyalin granules. Source of the free amino acid, urocanic acid and pyrrolidone carboxylic acid in the stratum corneum. *Biochim Biophys Acta*. 1982;719:110.
2. Horii I, Kawasaki K, Koyama J, et al. Histidine-rich protein as a possible origin of free amino acids of stratum corneum. *Curr Probl Dermatol*. 1983;11:301.
3. Elias PM. Stratum corneum defensive functions: an integrated view. *J Invest Dermatol*. 2005;125:183.
4. Visscher MO, Tolia GT, Wickett RR, et al. Effect of soaking and natural moisturizing factor on stratum corneum water-handling properties. *J Cosmet Sci*. 2003;54:289.
5. Nakagawa N, Sakai S, Matsumoto M, et al. Relationship between NMF (lactate and potassium) content and the physical properties of the stratum corneum in healthy subjects. *J Invest Dermatol*. 2004;122:755.
6. Weidinger S, Illig T, Baurecht H, et al. Loss-of-function variations within the filaggrin gene predispose for atopic dermatitis with allergic sensitizations. *J Allergy Clin Immunol*. 2006;118:214.
7. Irvine AD, McLean WH. Breaking the (un)sound barrier: Filaggrin is a major gene for atopic dermatitis. *J Invest Dermatol*. 2006;126:1200.
8. Chu DH. Development and structure of skin. In: Goldsmith LA, Katz SI, Gilchrest BA, et al. *Fitzpatrick's Dermatology In General Medicine*. 8th ed. New York: McGraw-Hill Medical; 2012:62.

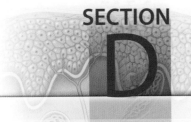

SECTION D

Skin Lightening Agents

CHAPTER 32

Overview of the Pigmentation Process

Skin color results from the incorporation of melanin-containing melanosomes, produced by the melanocytes, into the keratinocytes in the epidermis and their ensuing degradation. Although other factors contribute to skin color, such as carotenoids or hemoglobin,[1] the amount, quality, and distribution of melanin present in the epidermis represent the primary sources of human skin color. The number of melanocytes in human skin is equal across humanity, thus, their activity and interaction with the keratinocytes emerge as the accountable factors for skin color.[2]

Melanin pigment is produced in the melanosome, an organelle located in the cytoplasm of melanocytes. When excess melanin is produced, disorders of pigmentation or dyschromia can result. Melanin production is stimulated by several factors including ultraviolet light, estrogen, melanocyte-stimulating hormones (MSH), stress, inflammation, injury, infrared light, and heat. The most common forms of dyschromia are melasma, solar lentigos, postinflammatory hyperpigmentation, and dark circles under the eyes.

Melasma, also known as chloasma or "mask of pregnancy," refers to a very common condition that is usually seen in women of childbearing age. It is a chronic disorder that can be frustrating to patients and physicians because it often recurs, especially due to exposure to the sun or estrogen. Melasma presents as irregularly shaped, but often distinctly defined, blotches of light- to dark-brown pigmentation. These patches are usually seen on the upper lip, nose, cheeks, chin, arms, forehead, and neck.

Solar lentigos are caused by both acute and chronic exposure and manifest as macular brown lesions usually 1 cm in diameter. The face, shoulders, chest, back, and hands are the areas typically affected because they receive the most sun exposure.

Postinflammatory hyperpigmentation, also known as postinflammatory pigment alteration (PIPA), can present as a result of various skin disorders. Occasionally, therapies for skin disease can cause or exacerbate dyschromia, such as resurfacing lasers or chemical peels. This occurs more commonly in people with darker skin types.

The cause of dark circles under the eyes is poorly understood. Many believe that the thin skin in this area allows the blood vessels to become more visible. Any inflammation or vasodilation in this region may manifest as darkening.[3] However, there also seems to be a pigmentary component that may be caused by excessive melanin production or deposition of the iron-storage complex hemosiderin from sluggish blood flow in the area. Unfortunately, there is no consensus about the best treatment of dark under-eye circles.

Disorders of pigmentation are best treated using a combination of ingredients including tyrosinase inhibitors, PAR-2 blockers, and exfoliating agents. These should be combined with ingredients such as lignin peroxidase and laser or light devices, which attack or target melanin. Antioxidants can also be used to prevent hyperpigmentation by hindering inflammation. Polyphenol antioxidants have been found to be strong chelators of metal ions, such as Fe^{2+}, Fe^{3+}, Cu^{2+}, Zn^{2+}, and Mn^{2+}, and can interfere with the function of tyrosinase.[4,5] Sun protection as well as heat and sun avoidance are also vital for the successful treatment of dyschromia.

REFERENCES

1. Jimbow K, Quevedo WC Jr, Fitzpatrick TB, et al. Some aspects of melanin biology: 1950–1975. *J Invest Dermatol*. 1976;67:72.
2. Bolognia JL, Pawelek JM. Biology of hypopigmentation. *J Am Acad Dermatol*. 1988;19(2 Pt 1):217.
3. Matsumoto M, Kobayashi N, Hoshina O, et al. Study of causal factors of dark circles around the eyes. *IFCC Magazine*. 2001;4:281.
4. Brown JE, Khodr H, Hider RC, et al. Structural dependence of flavonoid interactions with Cu2+ ions: Implications for their antioxidant properties. *Biochem J*. 1998;330(Pt 3):1173.
5. Afanas'ev IB, Dorozhko AI, Brodskii AV, et al. Chelating and free radical scavenging mechanisms of inhibitory action of rutin and quercetin in lipid peroxidation. *Biochem Pharmacol*. 1989;38:1763.

CHAPTER 33

Overview of Melanin Production

Melanin production occurs inside the melanosomes located in the melanocytes. The process of melanin synthesis begins with the hydroxylation of tyrosine to 3,4-dihydroxyphenylalanine (DOPA) using the enzyme tyrosinase (Figure 33-1).[1] Two types of melanin are produced: eumelanin and pheomelanin. The relative amounts of these two forms of melanin determine hair

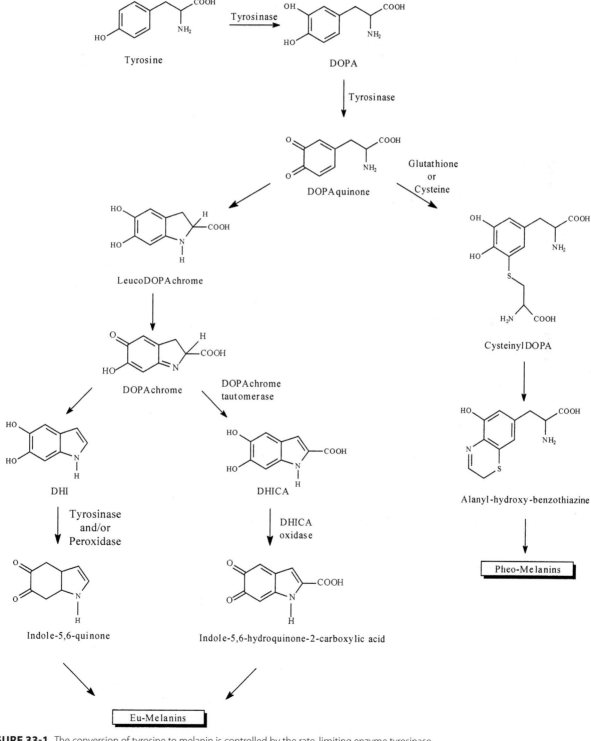

▲ **FIGURE 33-1** The conversion of tyrosine to melanin is controlled by the rate-limiting enzyme tyrosinase.

color and skin tone. Individuals with darker skin tones have mostly eumelanin and a lower level of pheomelanin, while the opposite is true in people with a light skin color.

Tyrosinase is the rate-limiting enzyme for melanin production. Tyrosinase is stimulated by ultraviolet (UV) radiation, DNA fragments such as thymidine dinucleotides that emerge as a result of UV exposure,[2] melanocyte-stimulating hormone (MSH), and growth factors such as bFGF and endothelin. Protein kinase C [3,4] and the cyclic adenosine monophosphate (cAMP)±protein kinase A pathway[2] play a role in increasing melanin production as do prostaglandins (D_2, E_2, and F_2), tumor necrosis factor-α (TNF-α), and interleukins (IL-α, IL-1β, and IL-6).[2–5] Vitamin D_3 may play a role in stimulating melanogenesis as well.[6] For more information, please see Chapter 13 of *Cosmetic Dermatology: Principles and Practice*, 2nd edition (McGraw-Hill 2009).

The most popular way to treat unwanted skin pigmentation is through the use of tyrosinase inhibitors. These do not eliminate melanin that is already present but help prevent future melanin production in the treated area. It is usually necessary to wait 8 to 16 weeks to see improvement in pigmentation. Tyrosinase inhibitors covered in this section include: aloesin, arbutin, hydroquinone, kojic acid, mulberry extract, vitamin C (ascorbic acid), and cucumber.

REFERENCES

1. Park HY, Yaar M. Disorders of melanocytes. In: Goldsmith LA, Katz SI, Gilchrest BA, et al. eds. *Fitzpatrick's Dermatology in General Medicine*. 8th ed. New York: McGraw-Hill; 2012:773–774.
2. Khlgatian MK, Hadshiew IM, Asawanonda P, et al. Tyrosinase gene expression is regulated by p53. *J Invest Dermatol*. 2002;118:126.
3. Chang MW. Disorders of hyperpigmentation. In: Bolognia JL, Jorizzo JL, Schaffer JV, eds. *Dermatology*. 3rd ed. London: Saunders; 2012:1051.
4. Park HY, Russakovsky V, Ohno S, et al. The beta isoform of protein kinase C stimulates human melanogenesis by activating tyrosinase in pigment cells. *J Biol Chem*. 1993;268:11742.
5. Lee JH, Park JG, Lim SH, et al. Localized intradermal microinjection of tranexamic acid for treatment of melasma in Asian patients: A preliminary clinical trial. *Dermatol Surg*. 2006;32:626.
6. Tomita Y, Torinuki W, Tagami H. Stimulation of human melanocytes by vitamin D_3 possibly mediates skin pigmentation after sun exposure. *J Invest Dermatol*. 1988;90:882.

CHAPTER 34

Aloesin

Activities:

Tyrosinase inhibition, antioxidant, anti-inflammatory

Important Chemical Components:

Aloesin (2-acetyonyl-8-glucopyranosyl-7-hydroxy-5-methylchromone)

Origin Classification:

This ingredient is natural, and a key constituent of *Aloe*. Organic forms exist.

Personal Care Category:

Depigmenting, sun protective (UVB)

Recommended for the following Baumann Skin Types:

DRPT, DRPW, DSPT, DSPW, ORPT, ORPW, OSPT, and OSPW

SOURCE

A moderately-high-molecular-weight hydroxymethyl C-glycosylated chromone derivative isolated from fresh *Aloe vera* leaves (as well as those from other *Aloe* species), aloesin is a natural compound that has been found to exert appreciable depigmenting activity. It is among the top choices for cosmetic and therapeutic applications to lighten skin.[1–4] While aloesin appears to be an important component in the armamentarium against hyperpigmentation disorders, its hydrophilic nature renders it less able than hydroquinone to penetrate the skin.[5] Some argue that its slower penetration into the skin endows aloesin with greater potential as a skin-lightening agent for cosmetic purposes as compared to hydroquinone, however.[6]

HISTORY

In traditional folk medicine, topical *A. vera* is used to treat inflammation, cicatrization, and dyspigmentation. Its constituent aloesin has been demonstrated to inhibit tyrosinase activity from human, murine, and mushroom sources.[7]

CHEMISTRY

Aloesin dose-dependently inhibits tyrosinase by blocking the hydroxylation of tyrosine to 3,4-dihydroxyphenylalanine (DOPA) as well as the oxidation of DOPA to dopaquinone; it has also been found to suppress melanin production in cultured normal melanocytes.[7] Aloesin and a few chemically related chromones, particularly the 5-methyl-7-methoxy-2(2'-benzyl-3'-oxobutyl)-chromone, have been demonstrated to exhibit stronger inhibitory activity on tyrosinase than arbutin and kojic acid.[6,8,9] This

is especially noteworthy because tyrosinase is the rate-limiting enzyme in melanin production and, thus, directly influences the development of skin pigment.

ORAL USES

Interestingly, aloesin has been suggested as having a potential role as a functional food. Lynch et al. have recently shown in experiments with Sprague-Dawley rats that aloesin appears to confer benefits pertaining to prediabetic states, including metabolic syndrome.[10] Aloesin is available in oral supplements and in aloe juice.

TOPICAL USES

Although less effective than hydroquinone when used as single therapy (Table 34-1), aloesin is safer, and has been most successfully used in hypopigmenting regimens for its synergistic activity in combination therapies with two or more agents acting on various mechanisms.[6]

SAFETY ISSUES

The Ames test has demonstrated no genotoxicity or mutagenicity linked to aloesin and cell-based assays have revealed no cytotoxicity.[8] More recent *in vitro* and *in vivo* genotoxicity assays conducted by Lynch et al., including the Ames test (bacterial mutation assay), *in vitro* mammalian cell cytogenetics assay, and mouse micronucleus test, have shown a lack of genotoxic potential in aloesin.[4]

ENVIRONMENTAL IMPACT

The effects of aloesin culling and processing depend directly on the impact of *Aloe* plant cultivation (see Chapter 65, Aloe Vera).

FORMULATION CONSIDERATIONS

Aloesin is difficult to synthesize.

TABLE 34-1
Pros and Cons of Aloesin

Pros	Cons
Effective as a depigmenting ingredient, particularly when used in combination	Less effective than hydroquinone
Good for type 2 (rosacea) sensitive skin	More research is necessary to determine what other ingredients are most effective in combination
Natural	
Organic forms exist	

USAGE CONSIDERATIONS

Aloesin is a good choice for Baumann Skin Type sensitive skin type 2 (rosacea) and should be combined with niacinamide and antioxidants for these types. For individuals with other skin types, aloesin can be combined with retinoids and another tyrosinase inhibitor and α-hydroxy acids.

SIGNIFICANT BACKGROUND

For many years, hydroquinone was the standard skin-whitening agent throughout the world, but its reputed cytotoxicity prompted a ban in 2000 in Europe and strict regulation in Asia. Several active constituents extracted from plants, including aloesin, arbutin, flavonoids, gentisic acid, hesperidin, licorice, niacinamide, yeast derivatives, and polyphenols, which inhibit melanogenesis through varying mechanisms without inducing melanocytotoxicity, have emerged as alternatives to hydroquinone used alone or in combination.[11] In 1999, aloesin and arbutin were shown to act synergistically in suppressing tyrosinase activity, and thus melanin production, in a combined treatment, but through different mechanisms, with aloesin noncompetitively inhibiting tyrosinase activity while arbutin acted competitively.[1]

In 2002, Jones et al. demonstrated that aloesin modulates melanogenesis by competitively inhibiting tyrosinase at the dihydroxyphenylalanine oxidation site, suppressing melanin synthesis in vitro, and that it is a tyrosinase inhibitor from mushroom, human, and murine sources. They also found that aloesin dose-dependently inhibited tyrosine hydroxylase and DOPA oxidase activities of tyrosinase from normal human melanocyte cell lysates. The researchers concluded that aloesin indeed demonstrated potential as a cosmetic or therapeutic agent for altering skin pigmentation.[7]

Also in that year, Choi et al. studied the inhibitory effects of aloesin and arbutin against UV-induced hyperpigmentation in humans. Subjects were exposed to UV radiation on the inner forearm and the treated areas were assigned to four daily treatments for 15 days with vehicle control, aloesin, arbutin, or a combination of the two botanical ingredients. Aloesin blocked pigmentation by 34 percent, arbutin, by 43.5 percent, and the combination treatment, 63.3 percent, as compared to the control. In addition, investigators noted that aloesin dose-dependently inhibited UV-induced pigmentation and concluded that the compound may be a suitable agent for blocking UV-induced melanin formation.[2]

In 2004, Yang et al. also investigated the synergistic effects of aloesin and arbutin. They treated normal cultured human melanocytes in vitro with an aloesin and arbutin mixture, which was found to have suppressed tyrosinase activity and resulted in a significant decline in melanin content in the cultured melanocytes. The mixture had little effect on melanocyte viability.[12] In 2008, many of the same researchers, led this time by Wang, explored the effects of aloesin on melanogenesis in an in vitro pigmented skin equivalent, based on recent success in the study of skin metabolism and depigmenting agents in such models, which have been shown to evince similar morphological and growth qualities to human skin. The investigators found that aloesin exhibited direct inhibitory effects on melanogenesis and dose-dependently initiated a reduction in tyrosinase activity and melanin content. Arbutin also exhibited dose-dependent inhibitory activity, but was less effective than aloesin. Tea polyphenols demonstrated greater inhibitory activity than aloesin but also greater toxicity. Consequently, the authors concluded that aloesin displayed the most potential of the ingredients tested as an agent intended to affect pigmentation for cosmetic or therapeutic purposes.[3]

Antioxidant and Anti-inflammatory Activity

In a wide-ranging study of the anti-inflammatory and antioxidant properties of various Aloe isolates, including cinnamoyl, p-coumaroyl, feruloyl, caffeoyl aloesin, and related compounds, Yagi et al. found that the involvement of the caffeoyl, feruloyl, and coumaroyl groups bound to aloesin was well established, and the contact hypersensitivity response suggested that aloesin prevented UVB-induced immune suppression. In addition, they noted that aloesin inhibited the tyrosine hydroxylase and DOPA oxidase activities of tyrosinase in normal human melanocyte cell lysates. The investigators concluded that the potent antioxidant and anti-inflammatory effects imparted by aloesin derivatives helped explain, in part, the anti-inflammatory and wound-healing properties of Aloe vera.[13,14]

CONCLUSION

Aloesin is a less effective but safe alternative to using hydroquinone to treat unwanted hyperpigmentation. It is an ideal choice in rosacea patients with hyperpigmented skin areas such as those seen in photoaging. Used with other skin-lightening agents, aloesin is a key ingredient in depigmenting regimens. Much more research is needed to ascertain whether aloesin can play a more independent role as a cosmetic and therapeutic depigmenting agent. Currently, aloesin is considered a useful adjuvant among skin-lightening options.

REFERENCES

1. Jin YH, Lee SJ, Chung MH, et al. Aloesin and arbutin inhibit tyrosinase activity in a synergistic manner via a different action mechanism. Arch Pharm Res. 1999;22:232.
2. Choi S, Lee SK, Kim JE, et al. Aloesin inhibits hyperpigmentation induced by UV radiation. Clin Exp Dermatol. 2002;27:513.
3. Wang Z, Li X, Yang Z, et al. Effects of aloesin on melanogenesis in pigmented skin equivalents. Int J Cosmet Sci. 2008;30:121.
4. Lynch B, Simon R, Roberts A. In vitro and in vivo assessment of the genotoxic activity of aloesin. Regul Toxicol Pharmacol. 2011;61:215.
5. Draelos ZD. Skin lightening preparations and the hydroquinone controversy. Dermatol Ther. 2007;20:308.
6. Solano F, Briganti S, Picardo M, et al. Hypopigmenting agents: An updated review on biological, chemical and clinical aspects. Pigment Cell Res. 2006;19:550.
7. Jones K, Hughes J, Hong M, et al. Modulation of melanogenesis by aloesin: A competitive inhibitor of tyrosinase. Pigment Cell Res. 2002;15:335.
8. Picardo M, Carrera M. New and experimental treatments of cloasma and other hypermelanoses. Dermatol Clin. 2007;25:353.
9. Piao LZ, Park HR, Park YK, et al. Mushroom tyrosinase inhibition activity of some chromones. Chem Pharm Bull. 2002;50:309.
10. Lynch B, Simon R, Roberts A. Subchronic toxicity evaluation of aloesin. Regul Toxicol Pharmacol. 2011;61:161.
11. Zhu W, Gao J. The use of botanical extracts as topical skin-lightening agents for the improvement of skin pigmentation disorders. J Investig Dermatol Symp Proc. 2008;13:20.
12. Yang ZQ, Wang ZH, Tu JB, et al. The effects of aloesin and arbutin on cultured melanocytes in a synergetic method. Zhonghua Zheng Xing Wai Ke Za Zhi. 2004;20:369.
13. Yagi A, Takeo S. Anti-inflammatory constituents, aloesin and aloemannan in Aloe species and effects of tanshinon VI in Salvia miltiorrhiza on heart. Yakugaku Zasshi. 2003;123:517.
14. Yagi A, Kabash A, Okamura N, et al. Antioxidant, free radical scavenging and anti-inflammatory effects of aloesin derivatives in Aloe vera. Planta Med. 2002;68:957.

CHAPTER 35

Arbutin

Activities:

Tyrosinase inhibition, antioxidant, anti-inflammatory

Important Chemical Components:

The molecular formula for arbutin is $C_{12}H_{16}O_7$.

Origin Classification:

β-arbutins are natural; deoxyarbutin and α-arbutins are synthetic.

Personal Care Category:

Depigmenting, sun protective

Recommended for the following Baumann Skin Types:

DRPT, DRPW, DSPT, DSPW, ORPT, ORPW, OSPT, and OSPW

SOURCE

Arbutin is a natural β-D-glucopyranoside derivative of hydroquinone (HQ) found in the dry leaves of bearberry, cranberry, blueberry, wheat, and other plants.[1,2] Arbutin is the primary active constituent in bearberry (*Arctostaphylos uva-ursi*).

HISTORY

Bearberry has been used for medicinal purposes at least since the 13th century, when it was thought to have been used in Wales.[3] It is official in most pharmacopoeias.[3] Arbutin, specifically, has been used in traditional medicine in Japan as a skin-lightening agent and has become an alternative to HQ for such purposes in the West (Table 35-1). Cosmetic products used for the purposes of skin whitening may include α- or β-arbutins. Of these glycosylated HQs, β-arbutin is naturally found in various plants, but α-arbutin and other arbutin derivatives, such as deoxyarbutin, are synthesized by chemical and enzymatic methods.[4] Approximately 50 years ago, scientists in Japan were the first to synthesize α-arbutin from the chemical reaction of penta-O-acetyl-β-D-glucopyranose and HQ.[4]

TABLE 35-1
Pros and Cons of Arbutin

Pros	Cons
May be allowed in countries that do not allow hydroquinone	Typically found to be less potent than hydroquinone
May confer antioxidant effects	Must be formulated properly to enhance skin penetration

CHEMISTRY

This β-D-glucopyranoside is composed of a molecule of HQ bound to glucose. Similar in structure to HQ, arbutin inhibits tyrosinase and 5,6-dihydroxyindole-2-carboxylic acid (DHICA) polymerase activities at noncytotoxic concentrations, with the hydrolyzation of the glycosidic bond resulting in a significant reduction in melanin synthesis.[5,6] In particular, arbutin seems to act as a reversible competitive inhibitor of tyrosinase (post-translational level).[5] That is, the depigmenting mechanism of arbutin involves a reversible inhibition of melanosomal tyrosinase activity rather than suppressing the expression and production of tyrosinase.[5] Tyrosinase is the rate-limiting enzyme that regulates melanin production and is a unique product of melanocytes. Therefore, agents that block tyrosinase activity, a crucial step in melanogenesis, prevent the production of the pigment melanin and are considered key cosmetic skin-whitening ingredients. In essence, arbutin is thought to inhibit tyrosinase activity and melanosome maturation.[7]

ORAL USES

Arbutin is available in oral supplements for bladder health. As the main active constituent of bearberry, which has been used in traditional medicine as a diuretic, arbutin is thought to play a role in treating urinary tract infections. Arbutin taken in oral form has not been shown to impact pigment in any way.

TOPICAL USES

Arbutin is included as an ingredient in several cosmetic products, typically for depigmenting purposes. But the synthetic arbutin derivative deoxyarbutin (4-[(tetrahydro-2H-pyran-2-yl)oxy]phenol) has displayed promising *in vitro* and *in vivo* results with a greater inhibition of tyrosinase than its plant-derived precursor,[8] and, similarly, evidence suggests that α-arbutin (4-hydroxyphenyl α-glucopyranoside) exhibits more potent inhibitory activity against human tyrosinase than arbutin.[9] This was previously demonstrated in studies of the effects of α- and β-arbutin on the tyrosinases from mushroom and murine melanoma.[10] The synthetic α-arbutin has also been found to be a safe and effective skin-lightening agent.[11]

SAFETY ISSUES

Although arbutin has been considered safe in a handful of studies, the European Union Scientists Committee on Consumer Products deemed, due to the release of HQ from the molecule, that the use of arbutin in cosmetic formulations is unsafe.[12,13] No such rulings have been issued in the United States, where arbutin is thought to be a safe alternative to HQ.

ENVIRONMENTAL IMPACT

It is not well established what impact the cultivation of arbutin sources has on the environment. Similarly, it is not yet known how the culling of plants containing arbutin for the processing of synthetic forms of the ingredient affects the environment.

FORMULATION CONSIDERATIONS

Skin penetration is an issue with many ingredients including arbutin. Various methods have been used to enhance skin penetration.[14]

USAGE CONSIDERATIONS

No interactions with other ingredients are known by the author.

SIGNIFICANT BACKGROUND

HQ, the gold standard cosmetic skin-lightening agent for many years, is more potent than arbutin but due to reports of cytotoxicity, nephrotoxicity, and genotoxicity was banned in Europe in 2000 and is strictly regulated in Asia.[15] Several skin-whitening formulations containing arbutin are available on the market; however, there are only a few small clinical studies in peer-reviewed journals on the depigmenting activity of this compound and its clinical efficacy is not firmly established. An open-label study on 10 melasma patients found that a gel formulation containing arbutin significantly decreased pigmentation in all of the patients, as assessed by Mexameter.[16]

Although the use of arbutin has been reported to be successful for cosmetic and therapeutic purposes, its suitability as an alternative depigmenting agent to HQ continues to be debated and much more study in humans is necessary. Fifteen years ago, tyrosinase activity was found to decrease in normal human melanocytes treated with arbutin, but an increase of pigmentation was also reported.[17] Indeed, Maeda and Fukuda had previously reported that while higher concentrations of arbutin displayed greater efficacy than lower concentrations, a paradoxical discoloration emerged as a result of postinflammatory hyperpigmentation.[2,5,18]

In a 2002 study examining the inhibitory effects of arbutin and/or aloesin on pigmentation in human skin after UV radiation, the administration of either or both compounds four times daily for 15 days revealed pigmentation suppression of 43.5 percent by arbutin, 34 percent by aloesin, and 63.3 percent by the co-treatment of the skin-lightening agents compared with the control.[19]

In January 2008, Yang et al. constructed a pigmented skin equivalent model *in vitro* and then studied the effects on melanocyte cell shape, tyrosinase activity, and melanin formation exerted by aloesin, tea polyphenols, and arbutin. A concentration-dependent inhibitory effect on melanocyte tyrosinase activity and melanin content was achieved by tea polyphenols, aloesin, and arbutin, in descending order, but significantly lower toxicity was associated with aloesin and arbutin.[20] Arbutin was also found to be less toxic than HQ in an *in vitro* study using a melanocyte-keratinocyte co-culture model in which four melanogenic-inhibiting compounds (i.e., arbutin, HQ, kojic acid, and niacinamide) were compared.[21]

Early in 2009, Lim et al. determined that arbutin both inhibited melanin production in B_{16} cells induced with α-melanocyte stimulating hormone (α-MSH) and reduced tyrosinase activity in a cell-free system. The addition of arbutin to brownish guinea pig and human skin tissues also resulted in neutralizing the hyperpigmentary impact of α-MSH. The authors concluded that arbutin is a useful skin-whitening agent.[22] Direct proof of its clinical efficacy as a depigmenting agent remains lacking, however.[23]

Antioxidant Activity

Antioxidant activity has also been attributed to arbutin and is thought to play a role in its potential therapeutic effectiveness. In September 2008, Bang et al. measured the hydrolytic activity of the primary skin microflora, *Staphylococcus epidermidis* and *Staphylococcus aureus*, in order to determine if skin microflora can hydrolyze arbutin to HQ. They found that arbutin was hydrolyzed by all strains, with the hydrolyzed HQ exhibiting greater 1,1-diphenyl-2-picrylhydrazyl radical-scavenging activity and tyrosinase inhibition than arbutin. The investigators concluded that the antioxidant activity of HQ allows the main skin microflora to enhance the skin-lightening properties of arbutin.[15]

In 2010, Takebayashi et al. used five assay systems to evaluate the antioxidant activity of arbutin and noted, in particular, that in two cell-based antioxidant assays using erythrocytes and skin fibroblasts, arbutin displayed potent antioxidant activity comparable to or greater than HQ.[24]

Synthetic Arbutin

While naturally-occurring arbutin has garnered attention in the cosmetic and therapeutic realm as an alternative to HQ use, recent evidence suggests that a synthetic version of the botanical is even more effective. In 2006, Hamed et al. evaluated the effects of deoxyarbutin in cultured human melanocytes, on xenographs, and in a clinical trial, finding it to be a safe, effective, and reversible tyrosinase inhibitor.[25]

In 2005, Boissy et al., using a hairless pigmented guinea pig model, observed that topically applied deoxyarbutin exhibited a more sustained effect than HQ, with the effect found to be completely reversible. Kojic acid and arbutin failed to induce skin lightening. The investigators also evaluated deoxyarbutin in a 12-week human clinical trial. Topical treatment with 3 percent deoxyarbutin induced a significant or slight decrease in overall skin lightness and amelioration of solar lentigines in light skin or dark skin patients, respectively.[8]

Building on previous work in which they showed that deoxyarbutin is a more effective and less toxic skin lightener than HQ, Chawla et al. used standard assays to evaluate the efficacy and reversibility of deoxyarbutin and its derivatives on inhibiting tyrosine hydroxylase and dihydroxyphenylalanine (DOPA)-oxidase. They found that the agents, when used in concentrations keeping 95 percent cell viability in culture, dose-dependently inhibited tyrosine hydroxylase and DOPA-oxidase activities, thus suppressing melanin synthesis by healthy melanocytes. Removal of the agents resulted in complete reversal of the depigmenting effect. An *in vitro* test using human and purified mushroom tyrosinase also revealed tyrosinase inhibition, which the authors cited as additional support for the notion that these agents directly inhibit the tyrosinase enzyme. They concluded that deoxyarbutin and its second-generation derivatives impede melanogenesis at safe concentrations by suppressing tyrosinase, and deserve consideration as effective agents to lighten the skin.[26]

In 2009, Hu et al. studied the impact of HQ, arbutin, and deoxyarbutin on melanogenesis and antioxidation using cultured melan-a melanocytes exposed or not exposed to UVA-induced oxidative stress and also sought to ascertain whether deoxyarbutin has the potential to serve as an alternative skin-whitening agent to HQ and arbutin. The notable differences among the treatments were seen when the melanocytes were exposed to a nontoxic dose of UVA; increases in the cytotoxicity of HQ and arbutin emerged. In addition, the production of reactive oxygen species was inhibited in association with the treatment of deoxyarbutin in comparison to arbutin and HQ and the investigators identified decreased protein expression of tyrosinase only in deoxyarbutin-treated melanocytes. The three whitening agents exhibited similar dose-dependent tyrosinase-inhibiting activity, with two- to threefold reductions in comparison to the untreated control cells. The researchers concluded that deoxyarbutin indeed is a safe and effective alternative to HQ, as it displays strong tyrosinase suppression, clear antioxidant potential, and reduced cytotoxicity in comparison to the long-time standard skin-whitening compound.[27]

Overall, the data appear to indicate that α-arbutin is somewhat more effective than β-arbutin, but as some have noted, both are HQ prodrugs and their antityrosinase activity is influenced by HQ release from the molecule.[12,28] Notably, synthetic α-arbutin (7 percent solution) has been successfully used in combination with the MedLite C_6 Q-switched Nd:YAG laser to treat refractory melasma, as shown in a prospective 10-week study of 35 patients. Treatments were well tolerated and at six months after initial therapy, 30 percent of the participants had excellent clearance (greater than 81 percent melasma reduction) and 36.7 percent experienced good clearance (51–80 percent reduction).[29]

It is also worth noting that recent *in vitro* and *in vivo* data suggest that 4-n-butylresorcinol is a more potent tyrosinase inhibitor than HQ, arbutin, and kojic acid.[12]

■ CONCLUSION

Arbutin has been traditionally used in Japan and recently in the West as a skin-lightening agent in cosmetic products. It is less effective but safer than HQ. Synthetic versions of arbutin appear to rival HQ in effectiveness while achieving a safety profile comparable to arbutin. The clinical efficacy of arbutin as a depigmenting agent has yet to be firmly established.

REFERENCES

1. Sheth VM, Pandya AG. Melasma: A comprehensive update Part II. *J Am Acad Dermatol.* 2011;65:699.
2. Draelos ZD. Skin lightening preparations and the hydroquinone controversy. *Dermatol Ther.* 2007;20:308.
3. Grieve M. *A Modern Herbal.* Vol 1. New York: Dover Publications; 1971:90.
4. Seo DH, Jung JH, Lee JE, et al. Biotechnological production of arbutins (α- and β-arbutins), skin-lightening agents, and their derivatives. *Appl Microbiol Biotechnol.* 2012;95:1417.
5. Maeda K, Fukuda M. Arbutin: mechanism of its depigmenting action in human melanocyte culture. *J Pharmacol Exp Ther.* 1996;276:765.
6. Chakraborty AK, Funasaka Y, Komoto M, et al. Effect of arbutin on melanogenic proteins in human melanocytes. *Pigment Cell Res.* 1998;11:206.
7. Davis EC, Callender VD. Postinflammatory hyperpigmentation: A review of the epidemiology, clinical features, and treatment options in skin of color. *J Clin Aesthet Dermatol.* 2010;3:20.
8. Boissy RE, Visscher M, DeLong MA. DeoxyArbutin: A novel reversible tyrosinase inhibitor with effective in vivo skin lightening potency. *Exp Dermatol.* 2005;14:601.
9. Zhu W, Gao J. The use of botanical extracts as topical skin-lightening agents for the improvement of skin pigmentation disorders. *J Investig Dermatol Symp Proc.* 2008;13:20.
10. Funayama M, Arakawa H, Yamamoto R, et al. Effects of alpha- and beta-arbutin on activity of tyrosinases from mushroom and mouse melanoma. *Biosci Biotechnol Biochem.* 1995;59:143.
11. Sugimoto K, Nishimura T, Nomura K, et al. Inhibitory effects of alpha-arbutin on melanin synthesis in cultured human melanoma cells and a three-dimensional human skin model. *Biol Pharm Bull.* 2004;27:510.
12. Kolbe L, Mann T, Gerwat W, et al. 4-n-butylresorcinol, a highly effective tyrosinase inhibitor for the topical treatment of hyperpigmentation. *J Eur Acad Dermatol Venereol.* 2013;27(Suppl 1):19.
13. Scientific Committee on Consumer Products (SCCP). Opinion on β-arbutin. April 15, 2008. http://ec.europa.eu/health/ph_risk/committees/04_sccp/docs/sccp_o_134.pdf. Accessed January 24, 2013.
14. Wiechers JW, Kelly CL, Blease TG, et al. Formulating for efficacy. *Int J Cosmet Sci.* 2004;26:173.
15. Bang SH, Han SJ, Kim DH. Hydrolysis of arbutin to hydroquinone by human skin bacteria and its effect on antioxidant activity. *J Cosmet Dermatol.* 2008;7:189.
16. Ertam I, Mutlu B, Unal I, et al. Efficiency of ellagic acid and arbutin in melasma: A randomized, prospective, open-label study. *J Dermatol.* 2008;35:570.
17. Nakajima M, Shinoda I, Fukuwatari Y, et al. Arbutin increases the pigmentation of cultured human melanocytes through mechanisms other than the induction of tyrosinase activity. *Pigment Cell Res.* 1998;11:12.
18. Halder RM, Richards GM. Topical agents used in the management of hyperpigmentation. *Skin Therapy Lett.* 2004;9:1.
19. Choi S, Lee SK, Kim JE, et al. Aloesin inhibits hyperpigmentation induced by UV radiation. *Clin Exp Dermatol.* 2002;27:513.
20. Yang ZQ, Wang ZH, Zhang TL, et al. The effect of aloesin on melanocytes in the pigmented skin equivalent model. *Zhonghua Zheng Xing Wai Ke Za Zhi.* 2008;24:50.
21. Lei TC, Virador VM, Vieira WD, et al. A melanocyte-keratinocyte coculture model to assess regulators of pigmentation in vitro. *Anal Biochem.* 2002;305:260.
22. Lim YJ, Lee EH, Kang TH, et al. Inhibitory effects of arbutin on melanin biosynthesis of alpha melanocyte stimulating hormone-induced hyperpigmentation in cultured brownish guinea pig skin tissues. *Arch Pharm Res.* 2009;32:367.
23. Leyden JJ, Shergill B, Micali G, et al. Natural options for the management of hyperpigmentation. *J Eur Acad Dermatol Venereol.* 2011;25:1140.
24. Takebayashi J, Ishii R, Chen J, et al. Reassessment of antioxidant activity of arbutin: Multifaceted evaluation using five antioxidant assay systems. *Free Radic Res.* 2010;44:473.
25. Hamed SH, Sriwiriyanont P, deLong MA, et al. Comparative efficacy and safety of deoxyarbutin, a new tyrosinase-inhibiting agent. *J Cosmet Sci.* 2006;57:291.
26. Chawla S, deLong MA, Visscher MO, et al. Mechanism of tyrosinase inhibition by deoxyArbutin and its second-generation derivatives. *Br J Dermatol.* 2008;159:1267.
27. Hu ZM, Zhou Q, Lei TC, et al. Effects of hydroquinone and its glucoside derivatives on melanogenesis and antioxidation: Biosafety as skin whitening agents. *J Dermatol Sci.* 2009;55:179.
28. Briganti S, Camera E, Picardo M. Chemical and instrumental approaches to treat hyperpigmentation. *Pigment Cell Res.* 2003;16:101.
29. Polnikorn N. Treatment of refractory melasma with the MedLite C6 Q-switched Nd:YAG laser and alpha arbutin: A prospective study. *J Cosmet Laser Ther.* 2010;12:126.

CHAPTER 36

Hydroquinone

Activities:

Tyrosinase inhibition

Important Chemical Components:

Chemical formula: 1,4 dihydroxybenzene

Origin Classification:

Derived from natural sources, but synthetic in topically applied form

Personal Care Category:

Depigmenting, brightening, lightening

Recommended for the following Baumann Skin Types:

DRPT, DRPW, DSPT, DSPW, ORPT, ORPW, OSPT, and OSPW. Hydroquinone (HQ) should be used with caution in sensitive skin types 2 and 4 because it may cause skin redness and irritation.

SOURCE

Hydroquinone (HQ), a hydroxyphenolic derivative of benzene, occurs naturally as an ingredient in various plant-derived foods and beverages, such as vegetables (e.g., onions), fruits (particularly cranberries, blueberries, and pears), grains (especially wheat, wheat germ, and rice), coffee, tea, beer, and red wine.[1–3] It is known to cause reversible inhibition of cellular metabolism by affecting both DNA and RNA synthesis. For many years, HQ has been the first-line therapy for postinflammatory hyperpigmentation and melasma. It is known to act as one of the most effective inhibitors of melanogenesis *in vitro* and *in vivo* (Table 36-1).[4]

HISTORY

In 1936, Oettel was the first to report that HQ exhibited a lightening effect on the coat of black-hair cats that was reversible after drug withdrawal.[2,5] Martin and Ansbacher were able to duplicate these results in 1941 in mice.[2,6] The use of HQ to lighten the skin finally

emerged in the 1950s after anecdotal reports from the southern United States of depigmentation resulting from the use of sunscreens containing HQ.[1,7] Dermatologists first started using HQ as a depigmenting agent in 1961, after Spencer's report that 45 percent of 98 subjects treated with 1.5 and 2 percent HQ showed improvement in hyperpigmentation without adverse side effects.[2,7] HQ has been used safely and effectively since that time for hypermelanosis, senile lentigos, vitiligo, and melasma, and has long been considered the most effective skin-lightening product for hyperpigmented skin disorders and the gold standard of treatment.[1,2,8–10]

Concerns about its safety and potential to cause cancer, however, led to its ban for general cosmetic purposes in Europe at the beginning of the millennium. In Asia, HQ is legal, but highly regulated. In the United States, the Food and Drug Administration (FDA) has long been considering the status of HQ but not yet decided whether to ban it in over-the-counter (OTC) products. HQ has never been etiologically linked with human cancer and has been safely used by dermatologists in the United States for decades. Consensus among dermatologists is that it is safe.[2] Pigmentation of the eye and permanent corneal damage are the most serious adverse health effects seen in workers exposed to HQ.[1] Exogenous ochronosis (darkening of the skin) is also associated with topically applied HQ, although only 30 cases of ochronosis have been ascribed to HQ use in North America.[2,11,12] Skin rashes and nail discoloration have also been linked to HQ use. The safety debate about HQ within the FDA has provided the impetus for manufacturers to research and develop newer skin-lightening agents. However, many of them are chemical derivatives of HQ, can cause the same types of complications, and are not as effective as HQ.

CHEMISTRY

HQ depletes glutathione and results in oxidative damage to membrane lipids and proteins, including tyrosinase.[13] It is a strong oxidant and is quickly converted to p-benzoquinone and hydroxybenzoquinone.[14] Its primary cutaneous use is in OTC products (2 percent concentration or less), prescription drugs (4 percent), and custom pharmacy formulations (2 to ≥10 percent) as an ingredient to inhibit melanin synthesis to achieve skin lightening. Cosmetic products containing HQ are often labeled as "skin brighteners." HQ imparts its depigmenting effect by efficiently inhibiting tyrosinase, lowering its activity by 90 percent,[15] and by virtue of its hampering of melanosome formation and cytotoxicity to melanocytes.[16,17] Further, HQ suppresses the enzymatic oxidation of tyrosine and phenol oxidases as well as melanin production by blocking sulfhydryl groups, in the latter case.[17] Although it is useful as a sole agent, HQ is often combined with other agents such as tretinoin, glycolic acid, kojic acid, and azelaic acid.[18]

ORAL USES

HQ is found in various foods and beverages as well as in the general environment and thus can be orally ingested or inhaled (it is also found in cigarette smoke).[2] However, oral use of HQ

TABLE 36-1
Pros and Cons of Hydroquinone

Pros	Cons
Most effective depigmenting agent	Questions about safety that scare patients
Suitable component in various combination products	Banned in Europe in OTC products
Preferred by dermatologists in the United States	Easily oxidized
	Difficult to formulate
	Reacts with other ingredients
	Allergic contact dermatitis can occur

does not confer any known or studied effects on skin pigmentation.

TOPICAL USES

For over half a century, HQ has been the standard-bearing topical treatment for disorders of pigmentation. Safety concerns about this benzene derivative have led to the introduction of various alternative treatments for skin lightening. Nevertheless, HQ remains in wide use and is well regarded by dermatologists. Although there are reports in the media about safety concerns pertaining to HQ and many consumers are afraid of it, most dermatologists consider it very safe and effective as it remains the gold standard of depigmentation products used in dermatology.

SAFETY ISSUES

Despite a lengthy record of medical usage, concerns have been raised about HQ because it is derived from benzene, which is known to engender aplastic anemia and leukemia in humans.[2,19] Therefore, fears that HQ may exhibit mutagenic properties have been expressed. In addition, there have been some side effects associated with the long-term use of cosmetic products with high HQ concentrations.[2] Consequently, since January 2001, HQ has been banned as an OTC cosmetic skin-bleaching agent in Europe, where it is available only by prescription,[20] and it is highly regulated in Asia.

Exogenous ochronosis is the most prevalent among the actual adverse events associated with HQ usage. By far, the highest number of cases have occurred among Bantu females in sub-Saharan Africa, particularly in South Africa, where other ingredients besides HQ, including quinine injection, resorcinol, and antimalarials, may be implicated.[17,21] It is also widely held that unsupervised and protracted use of adulterated HQ has played an important role in the incidence of HQ-induced exogenous ochronosis in Africa.[17]

Concerns about the effects of intermediate and particularly long-term use of HQ, such as leukomelanoderma en confetti and exogenous ochronosis, contributed to the European ban.[20,22] Ironically, exogenous ochronosis presents as yellow-brown or blue-black hyperpigmentary macules that can result from the treatment of other hyperpigmentary conditions with skin-bleaching formulations containing HQ.[21] Exogenous ochronosis occurs in the area of HQ application, usually after extended use of even low concentrations (2 percent) of HQ, and more often in patients with darker skin types. This adverse response is thought to be caused by the inhibition of the enzyme homogentisic acid oxidase in the skin, resulting in the local accumulation of homogentisic acid that then polymerizes to form ochronotic pigment.[23] Despite widespread use of HQ in North America, the number of reported cases of exogenous ochronosis due to HQ use has been limited to 30.[9] To reduce the likelihood of adverse effects seen with HQ, it is best to use it in four-month cycles, alternating it with kojic acid, azelaic acid, and other alternative lightening agents.[24]

Some studies have shown that large doses of HQ delivered systemically – not by topical application – resulted in some evidence of cancer in rats. However, rats metabolize HQ very differently than humans, who detoxify it in the liver.[2,25] In humans, HQ is probably metabolized to detoxified derivatives, such as glucuronide and sulfate conjugates of HQ.[26]

Recently, investigators conducted a literature search focusing on the biochemistry and toxicology of HQ, benzene, and related molecules, with an eye toward the potential long-term side effects of HQ use in cosmetics. After surveying the large body of literature, particularly since 1996, on the carcinogenicity of these compounds, the researchers concluded that the long-term use of topically applied HQ does pose an increased risk for cancer, and recommended that this benzene derivative no longer be used as a skin-lightening agent.[22] Nevertheless, there are no reports in the medical literature of any human cutaneous or internal malignancies linked to HQ.[2] In animal experiments, HQ use has been demonstrated to induce renal adenomas and leukemia. As absorption of HQ is more rapid than its elimination through urine, daily use is now known to accumulate in the body.[20] In workers exposed to HQ, the most serious health effects have been pigmentation of the eye and, in a very small number of cases, permanent corneal damage.[1]

At the time that this chapter was written, debate was ongoing in the United States as to whether the FDA will ban HQ in OTC formulations. Several companies have removed HQ from their products in anticipation of such a policy change. In addition, many companies with pharmaceutical products containing HQ that have not undergone the FDA approval process fear that the product will soon be banned by the FDA.

Irritant and allergic contact dermatitis as well as nail discoloration have also been associated with HQ use, with postinflammatory hyperpigmentation also resulting from contact dermatitis. In addition, hypopigmentation has been known to arise around the sites treated with HQ. Discontinuing HQ therapy resolves these side effects.[9,27] Despite the European ban and tight regulation in Asia, the American Academy of Dermatology and others have not found justification for restricting use of HQ and the FDA has not yet established new rules governing its use in the United States.[24]

Contact dermatitis to HQ can occur. The author had a patient that experienced an immediate hypersensitivity to HQ that occurred three minutes after application and had to be managed with Benadryl and topical steroids (Figure 36-1).

ENVIRONMENTAL IMPACT

In addition to the presence of HQ, or its β-D-glucopyranoside derivative arbutin, in various herbal formulations and foods, HQ is manufactured annually for use as a skin-lightening agent as well as industrial purposes, including use as a photographic developer for black and white film and a stabilizing component

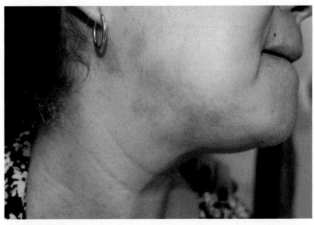

▲ **FIGURE 36-1** Contact dermatitis in response to hydroquinone use.

for paints, varnishes, motor fuels, and oils.[2] It is not clear how the environment is impacted by these processes, but exposure of workers to HQ has been studied extensively and not found to have significant long-range health implications.

FORMULATION CONSIDERATIONS

HQ is very difficult to formulate because it is a highly reactive oxidant that rapidly combines with oxygen. This renders it unstable, which, in turn, affects the stability of other ingredients combined in the same formulation or applied at the same time on the skin. HQ changes color when oxidized to a darker yellow or brown hue indicating that it has lost its effectiveness. For this reason, many preparations are kept refrigerated. Microsponge delivery systems have been developed with the intention of stabilizing HQ.[28]

USAGE CONSIDERATIONS

Although the 4 percent concentration is more effective than the more conventional 2 percent concentration, it is more irritating and may be more likely to lead to side effects such as skin redness. Prolonged application of HQ, often eight weeks or more, is necessary before any improvement becomes noticeable. A prescription is required in the United States for 4 percent HQ.

Most dermatologists recommend an HQ holiday after three months of use because patients can develop tachyphylaxis (a sudden or acute decrease in response or tolerance) to it. Stopping HQ for four weeks after three months of use seems to increase the effectiveness when it is restarted at month 4. In the author's practice, patients are advised to use a treatment regimen consisting of HQ. Once the spots clear, patients are switched to a maintenance regimen consisting of soy or niacinamide and a retinoid. The author also includes an antioxidant, which can chelate copper, hampering tyrosinase.[29]

SIGNIFICANT BACKGROUND

In a study of 16 women with idiopathic melasma, patients nightly applied 5 percent ascorbic acid cream on one side of the face and 4 percent HQ cream on the other side for 16 weeks, and applied sunscreen daily. The best subjective results were seen on the HQ side (93 percent vs. 62.5 percent), though no statistical differences were identified through colorimetric analysis. The side effect profile strongly favored the ascorbic acid side, with adverse reactions seen in 11 of 16 HQ sides as opposed to only 1 of 16 ascorbic acid sides.[30] The safety debate about HQ within the FDA has spurred companies to research newer, less controversial skin lighteners as well as combination therapies.

Tri-Luma

Because of escalating concerns regarding HQ monotherapy, numerous studies have been conducted that include HQ in combination topical therapy. HQ, along with tretinoin and topical corticosteroids, are well established as effective single agents for treating melasma and hyperpigmentation. In 1975, Kligman described combining HQ, tretinoin, and a topical steroid to treat skin pigmentations – a formula that to this day is referred to as the "Kligman formula."[31] Athough the Kligman formula is often compounded by independent pharmacists, the once-daily triple combination cream containing 0.05 percent

tretinoin, 4.0 percent HQ, and 0.01 percent fluocinolone acetonide (Tri-Luma) is the only commercially available combination of all three agents. In fact, this product is the only HQ-containing product that has been approved by the FDA to treat facial melasma.[32] Extensive studies have indicated an efficacious and safe profile for this triple combination cream in treating melasma.[32]

In a multicenter, open-label, 12-month study of once-daily application of Tri-Luma Cream for the treatment of facial melasma, which 173 out of 228 patients completed, the formulation was deemed to be safe and effective. Patient and physician assessment revealed complete or nearly complete clearing in over 90 percent of cases; 129 patients experienced at least one adverse event related to treatment, with most categorized as mild and transient.[33] More evidence to support the triple combination approach comes from an eight-week, multicenter, open-label, community-based study evaluating the hydrophilic cream formulation Tri-Luma used on 1,290 patients of diverse races/ethnicities and the full gamut of Fitzpatrick skin types. Global evaluations at the end of the study period revealed that 75 percent of patients exhibited "moderate or marked improvement" or were judged to be "almost clear" or "clear."[34] A 12-month extension of a randomized, investigator-blinded, multicenter, eight-week trial evaluating Tri-Luma Cream for facial melasma netted 389 patients completing six months of treatment and 327 patients completing 12 months, with 80 percent of patients exhibiting complete or nearly complete clearance of lesions. This study reinforced a previous smaller study indicating that once-daily application is effective, safe, and tolerable over a lengthy period for the treatment of moderate-to-severe melasma.[35]

If a ban on HQ is implemented, the one product that would remain unaffected is Tri-Luma™. When the FDA solicited safety data on HQ several years ago, only the manufacturers of Tri-Luma complied and it has now been approved for the short-term and intermittent long-term treatment of moderate-to-severe melasma.

Other Combination Therapies

In 2004, a 12-week open-label study with 28 patients (25 of whom completed the study) evaluated the safety and efficacy of a then-novel formulation of 4 percent HQ with 0.15 percent retinol entrapped in microsponge reservoirs, which were used for the gradual release of HQ to extend treatment exposure and limit skin irritation. With patients applying the study cream twice daily to the full face in the morning and evening and a broad-spectrum sunscreen 15 minutes after the morning application of the study product, patients were assessed at 4, 8, and 12 weeks. Improvement was seen in all study end points (including melasma or postinflammatory hyperpigmentation disease severity and intensity, as well as lesion area). The HQ/retinol combination was found to be safe and effective, with only one patient dropping out due to an adverse reaction not judged to be serious.[8]

Other studies of dual-combination formulations have yielded encouraging results. A 16-week comparison study revealed that an emollient cream containing 4 percent HQ and 0.3 percent retinol more effectively eliminated the signs of photodamage (i.e., dyspigmentation, fine wrinkles, and tactile roughness) than a 0.05 percent tretinoin emollient cream and, according to researchers, may represent a viable therapy for hyperpigmentation associated with photoaging.[36] Further, in a 24-week study in 2006, topical application of tazarotene plus HQ was found to be more effective in ameliorating the dyspigmentation associated with photodamage than tazarotene alone.[37] In addition to the various combination formulations containing HQ, various additives, such as antioxidants (e.g., vitamin C in addition to the more standard retinoids) and α-hydroxy acids, can be used to enhance efficacy and penetration.[9]

Alternatives

As the gold standard depigmenting agent, HQ is really the focus of this section of the book. The other chapters are a reaction to it, in a sense. Alternatives such as azelaic, thioctic (α-lipoic), kojic, and glycolic acids, as well as deoxyarbutin,[38] have been proposed as safer alternatives to the topical application of HQ.[20] Small proteins found in soy as well as niacinamide, a vitamin B_3 derivative, also appear to have potential as alternatives. The soy proteins, such as soybean trypsin inhibitor (STI) and Bowman-Birk Inhibitor (BBI), may inhibit skin pigmentation. These soy proteins have been found not only to exhibit depigmenting activity, but also to prevent UV-induced pigmentation both *in vitro* and *in vivo*.[39] Niacinamide has also been demonstrated to inhibit melanosome movement from melanocytes to keratinocytes.[40]

■ CONCLUSION

HQ has a long record of successful and safe use in medicine, particularly as a skin-lightening agent for dermatologic use. Recently, this agent has come under greater scrutiny due to its putative potential for inducing adverse effects. In 2006, the FDA published a monograph proposing a ban of all HQ products not approved through the New Drug Application process and asking companies that market HQ products to provide product safety data. Since then, we have been facing the prolonged possibility of a loss of a superlative cosmetic ingredient as the FDA mulls over the unpopular prospect of enacting its proposed ban (although the longer the FDA remains quiet on the issue, the less likely a ban appears to be, it might be argued). If a ban of HQ occurs, many dermatologists may choose to continue to have products containing HQ formulated for their patients in a pharmacy, which is becoming a very common practice in the United States. Unfortunately, it is difficult to stabilize a steroid, HQ, and tretinoin in a formulation, so this option may not be ideal for patients. The overwhelming opinion among dermatologists is that HQ warrants continued use in the prescription depigmenting armamentarium. The most challenging problem with HQ is that it is reactive with other ingredients and oxidizes rapidly. For that reason, the formulation of HQ, the order in which it is applied, and the other products with which it is used is very important in order to achieve maximum efficacy. HQ should only be used for three months and when the patient is experiencing pigmentation issues. Stopping HQ use for four weeks every three months may improve its efficacy. Combining HQ with skin lighteners that block protease-activated receptor-2 and exhibit sun protection factor is critical for success.

REFERENCES

1. DeCaprio AP. The toxicology of hydroquinone – Relevance to occupational and environmental exposure. *Crit Rev Toxicol.* 1999;29:283.
2. Nordlund JJ, Grimes PE, Ortonne JP. The safety of hydroquinone. *J Eur Acad Dermatol Venereol.* 2006;20:781.
3. Deisinger PJ, Hill TS, English JC. Human exposure to naturally occurring hydroquinone. *J Toxicol Environ Health.* 1996;47:31.
4. Parvez S, Kang M, Chung HS, et al. Survey and mechanism of skin depigmenting and lightening agents. *Phytother Res.* 2006;20:921.
5. Oettel H. Hydroquinone poisoning. *Arch Exp Pathol Pharmacol.* 1956;183:319.
6. Martin GJ, Ansbacher S. Confirmatory evidence of the chromotrichal activity of p-aminobenzoic acid. *J Biol Chem.* 1941;13:441.
7. Fitzpatrick TB, Arndt KA, el-Mofty AM, et al. Hydroquinone and psoralens in the therapy of hypermelansosis and vitiligo. *Arch Dermatol.* 1966;93:589.
8. Grimes PE. A microsponge formulation of hydroquinone 4% and retinol 0.15% in the treatment of melasma and postinflammatory hyperpigmentation. *Cutis.* 2004;74:362.
9. Halder RM, Richards GM. Topical agents used in the management of hyperpigmentation. *Skin Therapy Lett.* 2004;9:1.
10. Engasser PG, Maibach HI. Cosmetics and dermatology: Bleaching creams. *J Am Acad Dermatol.* 1981;5:143.
11. Lawrence N, Bligard CA, Reed R, et al. Exogenous ochronosis in the United States. *J Am Acad Dermatol.* 1988;18:1207.
12. Levin CY, Maibach H. Exogenous ochronosis: An update on clinical features, causative agents and treatment options. *Am J Clin Dermatol.* 2001;2:213.
13. Kim H, Choi HR, Kim DS, et al. Topical hypopigmenting agents for pigmentary disorders and their mechanisms of action. *Ann Dermatol.* 2012;24:1.
14. Dadzie OE, Petit A. Skin bleaching: Highlighting the misuse of cutaneous depigmenting agents. *J Eur Acad Dermatol Venereol.* 2009;23:741050.
15. Nordlund JJ. Postinflammatory hyperpigmentation. *Dermatol Clin.* 1988;6:185.
16. Penney KB, Smith CJ, Aleen JC. Depigmenting action of hydroquinone depends on disruption of fundamental cell processes. *J Invest Dermatol.* 1984;82:308.
17. Tse TW. Hydroquinone for skin lightening: Safety profile, duration of use and when should we stop? *J Dermatolog Treat.* 2010;21:272.
18. Guevara IL, Pandya AG. Melasma treated with hydroquinone, tretinoin and a fluorinated steroid. *Int J Dermatol.* 2001;40:212.
19. Rinsky RA, Smith AB, Hornung R, et al. Benzene and leukemia. An epidemiologic risk assessment. *N Engl J Med.* 1987;316:1044.
20. Kooyers TJ, Westerhof W. Toxicological aspects and health risks associated with hydroquinone in skin bleaching formula. *Ned Tijdschr Geneeskd.* 2004;148:768.
21. Bongiorno MR, Aricò M. Exogenous ochronosis and striae atrophicae following the use of bleaching creams. *Int J Dermatol.* 2005;44:112.
22. Kooyers TJ, Westerhof W. Toxicology and health risks of hydroquinone in skin lightening formulations. *J Eur Acad Dermatol Venereol.* 2006;20:777.
23. Kramer KE, Lopez A, Stefanato CM, et al. Exogenous ochronosis. *J Am Acad Dermatol.* 2000;42:869.
24. Burkhart CN, Katz KN. Chapter 222: Other topical medications. In: Goldsmith LA, Katz SI, Gilchrest BA, Paller AS, Leffell DJ, Wolff K, eds. *Fitzpatrick's Dermatology in General Medicine.* 8th ed. Vol. 2. New York: McGraw-Hill; 2012:2704.
25. Bates B. Derms react to possible FDA ban of hydroquinone: Cite poor scientific reasoning, ethnic bias. *Skin and Allergy News.* 2007;38:1.
26. Picardo M, Carrera M. New and experimental treatments of cloasma and other hypermelanoses. *Dermatol Clin.* 2007;25:353.
27. Grimes PE. Melasma. Etiologic and therapeutic considerations. *Arch Dermatol.* 1995;131:1453.
28. Mandava SS, Thavva V. Novel approach: Microsponge drug delivery system. *IJPSR.* 2012;3:967.
29. Kim YJ, Uyama H. Tyrosinase inhibitors from natural and synthetic sources: Structure, inhibition mechanism and perspective for the future. *Cell Mol Life Sci.* 2005;62:1707.
30. Espinal-Perez LE, Moncada B, Castanedo-Cazares JP. A double-blind randomized trial of 5% ascorbic acid vs. 4% hydroquinone in melasma. *Int J Dermatol.* 2004;43:604.
31. Kligman AM, Willis I. A new formula for depigmenting human skin. *Arch Dermatol.* 1975;111:40.
32. Torok HM. A comprehensive review of the long-term and short-term treatment of melasma with a triple combination cream. *Am J Clin Dermatol.* 2006;7:223.
33. Torok HM, Jones T, Rich P, et al. Hydroquinone 4%, tretinoin 0.05%, fluocinolone acetonide 0.01%: A safe and efficacious 12-month treatment for melasma. *Cutis.* 2005;75:57.

34. Grimes P, Kelly AP, Torok H, et al. Community-based trial of a triple-combination agent for the treatment of facial melasma. *Cutis*. 2006;77:177.

35. Torok H, Taylor S, Baumann L, et al. A large 12-month extension study of an 8-week trial to evaluate the safety and efficacy of triple combination (TC) cream in melasma patients previously treated with TC cream or one of its dyads. *J Drugs Dermatol*. 2005;4:592.

36. Draelos ZD. Novel approach to the treatment of hyperpigmented photodamaged skin: 4% hydroquinone/0.3% retinol versus tretinoin 0.05% emollient cream. *Dermatol Surg*. 2005;31:799.

37. Lowe N, Horwitz S, Tanghetti E, et al. Tazarotene versus tazarotene plus hydroquinone in the treatment of photodamaged facial skin: A multicenter, double-blind, randomized study. *J Cosmet Laser Ther*. 2006;8:121.

38. Hamed SH, Sriwiriyanont P, deLong MA, et al. Comparative efficacy and safety of deoxyarbutin, a new tyrosinase-inhibiting agent. *J Cosmet Sci*. 2006;57:291.

39. Paine C, Sharlow E, Liebel F, et al. An alternative approach to depigmentation by soybean extracts via inhibition of the PAR-2 pathway. *J Invest Dermatol*. 2001;116:587.

40. Hakozaki T, Minwalla L, Zhuang J, et al. The effect of niacinamide on reducing cutaneous pigmentation and suppression of melanosome transfer. *Br J Dermatol*. 2002;147:20.

CHAPTER 37

Kojic Acid

Activities:

Anti-inflammatory, antibiotic, anodyne, skin lightening[1]

Important Chemical Components:

Molecular formula: $C_6H_6O_4$

Origin Classification:

This agent is a natural metabolite of various bacterial species.

Personal Care Category:

Skin lightener

Recommended for the following Baumann Skin Types:

DRPT, DRPW, DSPT, DSPW, ORPT, ORPW, OSPT, and OSPW

SOURCE

Kojic acid (5-hydroxy-2-hydroxymethyl-γ-pyrone or 5-hydroxy-2-(hydroxymethyl)-4H-pyran-4-one) is a fungal metabolite of several species of bacteria, including *Acetobacter*, *Penicillium*, and *Aspergillus*, particularly *Aspergillus oryzae*, a fungus used for centuries in Asia in the production of soy sauce, miso, and sake.[2] Derivatives of kojic acid have been reported to display enhanced efficiency via greater skin penetration.[3]

HISTORY

Kojic acid was discovered as a fungal natural product in 1907.[4] It was used widely in cosmetic agents, particularly in Japan from 1988 to 2003, for its capacity to reduce pigmentation.[5–7] Kojic acid was deemed a "quasi-drug" and banned from the market in Japan by the Ministry of Health, Labor and Welfare in 2003 and subsequently in Korea and Switzerland due to safety concerns stemming from animal test results suggesting mutagenicity. Some countries have reportedly since reintroduced it as a skin-lightening agent, but it remains excluded in others.[8]

CHEMISTRY

Kojic acid inhibits tyrosinase activity, mainly by chelating copper, leading to a cutaneous whitening effect.[9] It is also believed to act by inhibiting the tautomerization of dopachrome to 5,6-dihydroxyindole-2-carboxylic acid.[5,10] In addition, the preservative and antibiotic activities of this agent contribute to extending product shelf life.[11] Such stability is one of the advantages of kojic acid in comparison to hydroquinone (HQ) as well as other skin-lightening ingredients (Table 37-1).[12] The efficacy of kojic acid in achieving such an effect is similar to that of HQ, the gold standard but controversial depigmenting

TABLE 37-1
Pros and Cons of Kojic Acid

PROS	CONS
More stable than hydroquinone	High sensitizing potential
Found to be effective in combination therapy	Lack of peer-reviewed data of monotherapy achieving depigmenting effect

agent.[13,14] However, while kojic acid yields greater stability than HQ, the fungal derivative does have labile oxidative properties, which are enhanced by light and heat exposure. Therefore, kojic acid is included in cosmetic formulations through its dipalmitic ester (as kojic dipalmitate).[15]

ORAL USES

Kojic acid is widely used as a food additive for preventing enzymatic browning, and to promote reddening of unripe strawberries.[16] It is used in Asia as a dietary antioxidant.[17,18]

TOPICAL USES

Kojic acid is second only to HQ in effectiveness as a skin-lightening agent in topical over-the-counter products, and is the most popular agent for treating melasma in East Asia.[8,18] Given the regulatory status of HQ, which has been banned in Europe and is tightly regulated in Asia, while remaining under scrutiny in the United States, this makes sense.

However, kojic acid is not a first-line therapy for melasma because it may cause skin irritation.[1,19,20] However, it can be effective in patients that do not tolerate the first-line products, particularly HQ.[20] Further, combining a topical corticosteroid with kojic acid can reduce the irritant qualities of the fungal derivative.[17,21] In the experimental setting, kojic acid is regularly used as a reference or positive control to test the skin-whitening potential of new agents.

Kojic acid products are typically used twice daily for one to two months or until the patient achieves the desired results.

SAFETY ISSUES

Despite the success of kojic acid at 1 percent concentrations, particularly in Japan, some studies have indicated that longer-term use of the agent may engender contact dermatitis and erythema.[14,22,23] In addition, an association between hepatic tumors in heterozygous p53-deficient mice and the topical application of kojic acid has been identified.[24,25] In 2003, Japan's health ministry ordered the removal of kojic acid from the market over fears, based on animal studies, that the fungal metabolite might cause cancer.[7]

In response to such findings and concerns, specifically the link between potential tumor promotion in mouse and rat livers due to kojic acid, Higa et al. examined the presence of initiation activity in rat liver and the potential of photogenotoxicity and carcinogenicity in mouse skin in relation to kojic acid. In one of the team's multiple experiments, a cream containing 1.0 or 3.0 percent kojic acid was applied twice to the backs of mice in a 24-hour period, with researchers noting that kojic acid failed to induce epidermal cell micronuclei. In addition, a skin carcinogenesis bioassay for initiation-promotion potential revealed the emergence of no skin nodules due to the topical application of 3.0 percent kojic acid cream to the backs of mice daily for seven days or five times a week for 19 weeks administered during either cancer stage. Overall, the investigators concluded that kojic acid poses a minimal risk of photocarcinogenesis in the skin and does not exhibit skin carcinogenesis initiation or promotion activity. They also supported the contention that kojic acid is a safe ingredient in cosmeceuticals.[26] In addition, in 2006, Lee et al. reported on derivatives of kojic acid displaying greater efficiency through increased penetration into the skin.[27]

Given its extensive use in foods, it may not be surprising to learn that there have been many reports on its oral safety. Toxicity resulting from an oral dose has been reported in a recent Japanese study, recording the occurrence of hepatocellular tumors in p53-deficient mice.[24] Furthermore, convulsions may occur if kojic acid is injected.[11,12]

ENVIRONMENTAL IMPACT

There is no known significant environmental impact associated with kojic acid preparation for medicinal purposes.

FORMULATION CONSIDERATIONS

Kojic acid has reportedly provoked contact allergies and is considered to display a high sensitizing potential.[23] Because preparations containing a 2.5 percent concentration of kojic acid have been associated with facial dermatitis,[28] a concentration of 1 percent has become more common. However, there have also been some reports of sensitization linked to 1 percent creams.[23] Mild facial erythema is the primary adverse effect reported in association with the typically well-tolerated fungal metabolite.[25]

USAGE CONSIDERATIONS

Kojic acid (1 percent) products are usually suggested for twice-daily use for one to two months or until the desired cosmetic result is achieved, though sensitization to 1 percent creams has been reported.[23] Concentrations of 2.5 percent have been associated with facial dermatitis, and it is considered to have a high sensitizing potential.[23,28]

SIGNIFICANT BACKGROUND

In 2003, Kim et al. studied the effects of a stable kojic acid derivative, 5-[(3-aminopropyl)phosphinooxy]-2-(hydroxymethyl)-4H-pyran-4-one (Kojyl-APPA), on tyrosinase activity and melanin production. They found that Kojyl-APPA is not a direct inhibitor of tyrosinase, but is enzymatically converted to kojic acid in cells. The derivative suppressed tyrosinase activity significantly 24 hours after treatment in normal human melanocytes and demonstrated a 30 percent inhibition of tyrosinase *in situ* (though not *in vitro*). The kojic acid derivative also lowered melanin content to 75 percent of control in melanoma cells and neomelanin

production to 43 percent of control in normal human melanocytes. Kojyl-APPA was also eightfold as capable of permeating the skin as kojic acid.[29] A kojic acid derivative identified as eight times more potent than kojic acid as a tyrosinase inhibitor was also synthesized in 2006. In addition, the compound produced by Lee et al. exhibited strong inhibitory activity toward melanin production.[27] This work suggests a fruitful area of research for the development of synthetic kojic acid agents for skin lightening.

Combination Therapy

In two separate studies in the mid-1990s, kojic acid combined with glycolic acid was found to be more effective than 10 percent glycolic acid and 4 percent HQ for the treatment of hyperpigmentation.[30,31] In one case, Garcia and Fulton evaluated and compared the effects on melasma and other pigmentary conditions of a glycolic acid/HQ formulation as well as a glycolic acid/kojic acid formulation. Wood's light and ultraviolet (UV) light photography were used to evaluate the effects of the different compounds, one on each side of the face, on 39 patients. No statistically significant differences were found between the reactions: 28 percent of the patients experienced marked improvements on the kojic acid side, 21 percent on the HQ side. The responses to each formulation were equal in 51 percent of the participants. While the kojic acid formulation was considered more irritating, the researchers found that both formulations effectively treated melasma.[31]

In 1999, Lim conducted a 12-week study of the effects on melasma of 2 percent kojic acid in a gel containing 10 percent glycolic acid and 2 percent HQ in 40 Chinese women with epidermal melasma. Subjects were randomized to receive the test formulation on one side of the face and the same formulation minus kojic acid on the other side. Self-assessment questionnaires every four weeks, photographs, and clinical evaluations were used to rate the efficacy of the treatment. Lim found that the addition of kojic acid to the glycolic acid/HQ gel reduced the signs of melasma. Specifically, more than half of the melasma cleared in 24 of 40 patients who received the kojic acid formulation as compared to 19 of 40 who received the kojic acid-free gel. Two patients experienced complete clearance, in both cases on the side of the face on which the kojic acid gel was used.[18] Two years later, Ferioli et al. found that combining HQ and kojic acid imparted a synergistic effect, with an equimolecular distribution leading to the optimal result.[32]

Further, in a recent three-month, paired, double-blind study comparing a combination of kojic acid, emblica extract, and glycolic acid to 4 percent HQ in 80 multiethnic patients with mild-to-moderate facial dyschromia, the two formulations were found to yield similar skin-lightening effects, suggesting that the combination therapy is a worthy alternative to HQ.[33] However, no peer-reviewed clinical studies have yet been reported that show a depigmenting effect from kojic acid monotherapy.[34]

Antiwrinkling Indication?

In 2001, Mitani et al. assessed the potential of kojic acid to deliver antiwrinkling effects given the iron-chelating properties of the acid and the known association between chronic photodamage and cutaneous iron. Over 20 weeks, the investigators topically applied kojic acid before exposing hairless mice to UV radiation. They found that the agent successfully suppressed wrinkle formation, epidermal hyperplasia, lower dermis fibrosis, as well as increases in upper dermis extracellular matrix components.[35]

CONCLUSION

A mainstay among skin-lightening agents over the last quarter century, the fungal derivative kojic acid is best used in combination with other depigmenting ingredients. This enhances the overall effect of the formulation and mitigates the irritating effects of the acid. Recent evidence has allayed fears regarding long-term carcinogenic effects, but, as always, research is ongoing to develop newer, safer derivatives.

REFERENCES

1. Prignano F, Ortonne JP, Buggiani G, et al. Therapeutical approaches in melasma. *Dermatol Clin*. 2007;25:337.
2. Bhat R, Hadi SM. Photoinactivation of bacteriophage lambda by kojic acid and Fe(III): role of oxygen radical intermediates in the reaction. *Biochem Mol Biol Int*. 1994;32:731.
3. Lee YS, Park JH, Kim MH, et al. Synthesis of tyrosinase inhibitory kojic acid derivative. *Arch Pharm Chem Life Sci*. 2006;339:11.
4. Bentley R. From miso, saké and shoyu to cosmetics: A century of science for kojic acid. *Nat Prod Rep*. 2006;23:1046.
5. Cabanes J, Chazarra S, Garcia-Carmona F. Kojic acid, a cosmetic skin whitening agent, is a slow-binding inhibitor of catecholase activity of tyrosinase. *J Pharm Pharmacol*. 1994;46:982.
6. Grimes PE. Management of hyperpigmentation in darker racial ethnic groups. *Semin Cutan Med Surg*. 2009;28:77.
7. Fuyuno I. Spotlight turns on cosmetics for Asian skin. *Nature*. 2004;432:938.
8. Draelos ZD. Skin lightening preparations and the hydroquinone controversy. *Dermatol Ther*. 2007;20:308.
9. Hira Y, Hatae S, Inoue T, et al. Inhibitory effects of kojic acid on melanin formation. In vitro and in vivo studies in black goldfish. *J Jpn Cosmet Sci Soc*. 1982;6:193.
10. Gillbro JM, Olsson MJ. The melanogenesis and mechanisms of skin-lightening agents – Existing and new approaches. *Int J Cosmet Sci*. 2011;33:210.
11. Uher M, Brtko J, Rajniakova O, et al. Kojic acid and its derivatives in cosmetics and health protection. *Parfuem Kosmet*. 1993;74:554.
12. Burdock GA, Soni MG, Carrabin IG. Evaluation of health aspects of kojic acid in food. *Regul Toxicol Pharmacol*. 2001;33:80.
13. Halder RM, Richards GM. Management of dyschromias in ethnic skin. *Dermatol Ther*. 2004;17:151.
14. Halder RM, Richards GM. Topical agents used in the management of hyperpigmentation. *Skin Therapy Lett*. 2004;9:1.
15. Balaguer A, Salvador A, Chisvert A. A rapid and reliable size-exclusion chromatographic method for determination of kojic dipalmitate in skin-whitening cosmetic products. *Talanta*. 2008;75:407.
16. Curtis PJ. Chemical induction of local reddening in strawberry fruits. *J Sci Food Agr*. 1977;28:243.
17. Parvez S, Kang M, Chung H-S, et al. Survey and mechanism of skin depigmenting and lightening agents. *Phytother Res*. 2006;20:921.
18. Lim JT. Treatment of melasma using kojic acid in a gel containing hydroquinone and glycolic acid. *Dermatol Surg*. 1999;25:282.
19. Lynde CB, Kraft JN, Lynde CW. Topical treatments for melasma and postinflammatory hyperpigmentation. *Skin Therapy Lett*. 2006;11:1.
20. Cayce KA, McMichael AJ, Feldman SR. Hyperpigmentation: an overview of the common afflictions. *Dermatol Nurs*. 2004;16:401.
21. Piamphongsant T. Treatment of melasma: a review with personal experience. *Int J Dermatol*. 1998;37:897.
22. Serra-Baldrich E, Tribo MJ, Camarasa JG. Allergic contact dermatitis from kojic acid. *Contact Dermatitis*. 1998;39:86.
23. Nakagawa M, Kawai K, Kawai K. Contact allergy to kojic acid in skin care products. *Contact Dermatitis*. 1995;32:9.
24. Takizawa T, Mitsumori K, Tamura T, et al. Hepatocellular tumor induction in heterozygous p53-deficient CBA mice by a 26-week dietary administration of kojic acid. *Toxicol Sci*. 2003;73:287.
25. Picardo M, Carrera M. New and experimental treatments of cloasma and other hypermelanoses. *Dermatol Clin*. 2007;25:353.
26. Higa Y, Kawabe M, Nabae K, et al. Kojic acid – Absence of tumor-initiating activity in rat liver, and of carcinogenic and photogenotoxic potential in mouse skin. *J Toxicol Sci*. 2007;32:143.
27. Lee YS, Park JH, Kim MH, et al. Synthesis of tyrosinase inhibitory kojic acid derivative. *Arch Pharm*. 2006;339:111.
28. Nakayama G, Watanabe N, Nishioka K, et al. Treatment of chloasma with kojic acid cream. *Jpn J Clin Dermatol*. 1982;36:715.
29. Kim DH, Hwang JS, Baek HS, et al. Development of 5-[(3-aminopropyl)phosphinooxy]-2-(hydroxymethyl)-4H-pyran-4-one as a novel whitening agent. *Chem Pharm Bull*. 2003;51:113.
30. Ellis DA, Tan AK, Ellis CS. Superficial micropeels: Glycolic acid and alpha-hydroxy acid with kojic acid. *Facial Plast Surg*. 1995;11:15.
31. Garcia A, Fulton JE Fr. The combination of glycolic acid and hydroquinone or kojic acid for the treatment of melasma and related conditions. *Dermatol Surg*. 1996;22:443.
32. Ferioli V, Rustichelli C, Pavesi G, et al. New combined treatment of hypermelanosis: Analytical studies on efficacy and stability improvement. *Int J Cosmet Sci*. 2001;23:333.
33. Draelos ZD, Yatskayer M, Bhushan P, et al. Evaluation of a kojic acid, emblica extract, and glycolic acid formulation compared with hydroquinone 4% for skin lightening. *Cutis*. 2010;86:153.
34. Leyden JJ, Shergill B, Micali G, et al. Natural options for the management of hyperpigmentation. *J Eur Acad Dermatol Venereol*. 2011;25:1140.
35. Mitani H, Koshiishi I, Sumita T, et al. Prevention of the photodamage in the hairless mouse dorsal skin by kojic acid as an iron chelator. *Eur J Pharmacol*. 2001;411:169.

CHAPTER 38

Emblica Extract

Activities:

Antioxidant, anti-inflammatory, antipyretic, antitumor, chemopreventive, hepatoprotective, analgesic, antibacterial[1,2]

Important Chemical Components:

Tannins (emblicanin A and B, corilagin, puningluconin, pedunclagin), ascorbic acid, amino acids, flavonoids, gallic acid, ellagic acid, rutin, curcuminoids, kaempferol, phyllembelic acid, linoleic acid, norsesquiterpenoids, pyrogallol[1,3–6]

Origin Classification:

Natural components isolated from various parts of *Emblica officinalis*. A standardized extract of *E. officinalis* (trade name Emblica) is 100 percent natural.

Personal Care Category:

Depigmenting, antiaging, sunscreen

Recommended for the following Baumann Skin Types:

DRPT, DRPW, DSPT, DSPW, ORPT, ORPW, OSPT, and OSPW

SOURCE

Emblica officinalis (also referred to taxonomically as *Phyllanthus emblica*, and popularly known as Indian gooseberry, *amla* in Hindi, *amaliki* in Sanskrit, as well as various other names in multiple languages) is a deciduous tree of the Euphorbiaceae family indigenous to India (and is variably classified in the Phyllanaceae family). Its fruit is a rich dietary source of ascorbic acid (vitamin C), various minerals, amino acids, as well as phenolic compounds and is the most important of the many parts of the plant used for food and medicinal purposes.[7] Amla has long been used in Ayurveda and Unani medicine, and is highly regarded for its unique array of tannins (particularly emblicanin A and emblicanin B) and flavonoids, which display potent antioxidant properties.[4,8,9] Indeed, it is actually one of the most important plants in Ayurveda.[10] The amla fruit is known to confer strong antioxidant activity and to protect human dermal fibroblasts against oxidative stress. For this reason, it is considered a useful and intriguing component in natural skin care.[11] In fact, *E. officinalis* is the foremost agent in the Ayurvedic arsenal for combating cutaneous aging and is considered a *rasayana* or restorative and adaptogenic agent.[9,12] Besides India, the plant is also found extensively throughout Asia, including Sri Lanka, Uzbekistan, Pakistan, Bangladesh, China, Thailand, Malaysia, and Indonesia, and has been used in other longstanding medical practices such as Siddha, Unani Tibetan, and Sri Lankan as well as traditional Chinese medicine and traditional Thai medicine.[1,7]

SOME TRADITIONAL MEDICAL SYSTEMS THAT USE EMBLICA

Ayurveda: derived from the Sanskrit *ayu* (life) and *veda* (knowledge), it is a 5,000-year-old traditional medical system in India.

Unani: Graeco-Arabic traditional medicine based on Arab and Persian adaptations of the teachings of the Greek physician Hippocrates and Roman physician Galen that has been broadly practiced by Muslims in the Middle East and South Asia.

Siddha: one of the oldest known traditional medical systems, traced back 10,000 years in India.

HISTORY

Emblica has been a staple in traditional medical practices throughout Asia for hundreds of years and is considered one of the most important plants in Ayurvedic medical practice (Table 38-1).[7] Traditional indications in Ayurveda include diarrhea, jaundice, and inflammation.[4] Amla has been used in folk medicine on the Indian subcontinent to treat inflammatory disease, liver disease, stomach and metabolic disorders, skin conditions, and geriatric issues as well as for beauty/cosmetic purposes including use as a hair tonic.[7,13] In addition, it is known to have been used for medicinal purposes during the Indian famine of 1939 to 1940 and to treat scurvy in what is now Rajasthan in 1837.[10] *P. emblica* has also been used in traditional medicine in Pakistan as a diuretic and to treat anemia and excessive bile.[14] Of note, the earlier taxonomic name *Phyllanthus emblica*, based on the Greek words *phyllom* (leaf) and *anthòs* (flower), was attributed to Carl Linnaeus based on observations about the branches of the tree, which appeared to be flat like leaves. It is thought that "emblica" comes from the bastardization of the Sanskrit *amlika* or Arabic *embelgi*.[10]

CHEMISTRY

Emblicanin A (2,3-di-O-galloyl-4,6-(S)-hexahydroxydiphenoyl-2-keto-glucono-δ-lactone) and emblicanin B (2,3,4,6-bis-(S)-hexahydroxydiphenoyl-2-keto-glucono-δ-lactone) are considered to be among the most important of the various active constituents of Indian gooseberry. However, the presence of emblicanins

TABLE 38-1

Pros and Cons of Emblica Extract

Pros	Cons
Can be used in countries that do not allow the use of hydroquinone or kojic acid	Not as effective as the standard-bearing depigmenting agents
Safer than hydroquinone or kojic acid	Limited clinical evidence of depigmenting efficacy
Long history of traditional medical use	
Potential for broad-spectrum applications	
Very affordable as part of the ayurvedic formula *triphala*	

A and B in the extract has been questioned by Majeed et al.[15] Nevertheless, the wide array of beneficial effects imparted by the fruit of *E. officinalis* are attributed to the complex interactions of these components along with ascorbic acid, gallic acid, ellagic acid, and key flavonoids. Majeed et al. have also investigated the role of vitamin C in amla, which is reputed to display greater antioxidant activity than vitamin C itself. Majeed et al. found that previous attempts to estimate ascorbic acid levels in amla failed to account for coeluting mucic acid gallates. They concluded that the potent antioxidant activity of amla should be ascribed to gallic acid esters.[15] Scartezzini et al. earlier claimed that the fruit contains vitamin C but in smaller amounts previously estimated, and that the constituent emblicanins recycle vitamin C, thus amplifying the overall antioxidant capacity exhibited by amla.[10]

A dynamic botanical source of several traditional medical practices, antidiabetic, hypolipidemic, antibacterial, antioxidant, antiulcerogenic, hepatoprotective, gastroprotective, and chemopreventive activity have all been associated with various parts of *E. officinalis*.[4] Regardless of what emerges regarding the source of the antioxidant strength of emblica or its relative richness as a source for vitamin C and tannins, its activity in suppressing tyrosinase activity has come to the fore in more recent research.[16,17]

ORAL USES

For centuries, the Indian gooseberry fruit has been consumed raw, cooked, or pickled alone and as a part of other food products, and is also used now in supplement form. It is considered an important dietary source of vitamin C as well as various minerals, amino acids, and tannins.[6,18]

It is worth noting the results of Banu et al. in assessing the capacity of orally administered *P. emblica* extract to protect against 7,12-dimethylbenz(a)anthracene (DMBA) in Swiss albino mice. Emblica was found to dose-dependently protect against the genotoxin, with the fruit-treated animals demonstrating significant elevation in liver antioxidants (e.g., glutathione, glutathione peroxidase, glutathione reductase, and detoxifying enzyme glutathione-S-transferase).[19]

TOPICAL USES

Among over-the-counter products, amla is contained in various hair care, skin care, color cosmetics, and soaps.[12] In particular, it is included in products intended to deliver antiaging and depigmenting activity.[16]

In a 2012 study of 17 Thai plants used traditionally to treat hair, particularly hair loss, Kumar et al. found *P. emblica* to be the second strongest inhibitor of 5α-reductase, behind *Carthamus tinctorius*, with a close relationship noted between inhibition of 5α-reductase and hair promotion.[20]

Skin Whitening

A standardized extract of *P. emblica* (trade name Emblica®) was found to exert long-lasting and broad-spectrum antioxidant activity. Due to its iron and chelating ability, the product does not provide pro-oxidation activity induced by iron and/or copper. Emblica helps to protect the skin from the deleterious effects of free radicals, non-radicals, and transition metal-induced oxidative stress. It contains emblicanins A and B and is photochemically and hydrolytically stable. Therefore, it is considered appropriate for incorporation into skin care formulations. The product is intended for use in antiaging, sunscreen, and general purpose skin care products.[17] Because

Emblica also acts at various sites in the melanogenesis pathway, as an inhibitor of tyrosinase and/or tyrosinase-related proteins (TRP-1 and 2) and peroxidase/H_2O_2,[17] as well as a broad-spectrum cascading antioxidant, it is conducive to use as a skin-whitening agent. It is thought to be as effective as hydroquinone (HQ) and kojic acid, without reports of provoking adverse side effects.

In 2010, Costa et al. assessed the efficacy and safety of a cream combining emblica, belides, and licorice 7 percent in comparison to HQ 2 percent for melasma treatment. Fifty-six women between 18 and 60 years of age (phototypes I to IV), with epidermal or mixed melasma, were instructed to use SPF 35 sunscreen for 60 days. At that point, they were assigned in a mono-blind clinical study to twice daily application of the botanical formulation or nightly use of HQ for a 60-day period. Follow-up occurred every 15 days, with the investigators observing no statistical differences between the groups in the successful improvement of melasma in most patients. Fewer side effects were noted in the group that received the botanical formulation, supporting the notion that it is a suitable alternative to HQ to treat melasma.[16]

Also that year, Draelos et al. conducted a double-blind skin-lightening activity comparison between HQ and a kojic acid, emblica extract, and glycolic acid topical formulation in 80 multiethnic subjects with mild-to-moderate facial dyschromia. Individuals were randomly assigned to use the study product or HQ 4 percent twice daily for 12 weeks, with results showing parity between the products. The researchers concluded that the new combination preparation including emblica is an effective alternative to HQ 4 percent for individuals with mild-to-moderate facial dyschromia.[21]

SAFETY ISSUES

The use of emblica is considered safe and effective with no adverse side effects reported.

ENVIRONMENTAL IMPACT

E. officinalis is found extensively throughout Asia. No significant environmental risks related to its cultivation have been established.

FORMULATION CONSIDERATIONS

There is a wide variety of commercial preparations of Indian gooseberry available, with varying levels of key ingredients. Thus, standardization is necessary across the broad range of products.[22] Scartezzini et al. have noted that processed emblica fruit contains more ascorbic acid and polyphenols than the dried fruit.[10]

USAGE CONSIDERATIONS

No interactions with other ingredients are known by the author.

SIGNIFICANT BACKGROUND

Antioxidant and Antiaging Activity

In 2002, a standardized extract of *P. emblica* (trade name, Emblica) was noted for delivering long-lasting and broad-spectrum antioxidant activity, appropriate for use in antiaging, sunscreen, and general purpose skin formulations, given its demonstrated capacity to protect the skin from damage engendered by free radicals, non-radicals, and transition metal-induced oxidative stress.[17]

The protective effects of emblica have also been found to extend to activity against arsenic. Specifically, Sharma et al. showed that adult Swiss albino mice treated with emblica fruits before and after exposure to arsenic evinced significantly less oxidative stress in the liver as compared to the rats treated only with arsenic.[6]

In 2009, Poltanov et al. studied the chemistry and antioxidant properties of four commercial *E. officinalis* fruit extracts and found different levels of antioxidative efficacy, with each nonetheless demonstrating free radical-scavenging capacity, primarily attributed to total phenolic and tannin content.[22]

In addition, Yokozawa et al., studying the effects of an ethyl acetate extract of amla on lipid metabolism and protein expression pertaining to the aging process in young and aged rats, determined that the administration of the botanical extract prevented dyslipidemia and oxidative stress.[18]

Chemopreventive Activity

In 2005, Sancheti et al. performed a two-stage skin carcinogenesis study in Swiss albino mice to ascertain the chemopreventive action of *E. officinalis* fruit extract. A single application of DMBA was used to induce skin cancer, followed two weeks later by thrice weekly applications of croton oil (through the end of the 16-week experiment) to promote tumors. A statistically significant difference in tumor incidence, yield, and burden as well as cumulative number of papillomas favored the mice treated with *E. officinalis* as opposed to the control group. The investigators concluded that *E. officinalis* fruit extract exhibited chemopreventive potential against DMBA-induced skin cancer in Swiss albino mice.[8]

In 2010, Ngamkitidechakul et al. investigated the reputed anticancer activity of an aqueous extract of *P. emblica* against cancer cell lines, and in terms of mouse skin tumorigenesis, *in vitro* invasiveness, and *in vitro* apoptosis. They found that cell growth was suppressed in six human cancer cell lines [A549 (lung), HepG2 (liver), HeLa (cervical), MDA-MB-231 (breast), SK-OV3 (ovarian), and SW620 (colorectal)] with an extract of 50 to 100 µg/mL. In addition, *P. emblica* extract treatment of mouse skin yielded a 50 percent decrease in tumor numbers and volumes in the two-stage skin carcinogenesis model initiated by DMBA and promoted by 12-O-tetradecanoylphorbol-13-acetate (TPA). The investigators also noted apoptosis in HeLa cells spurred by the extract and inhibited invasiveness of MDA-MB-231 cells in the *in vitro* Matrigel invasion assay. They concluded that *P. emblica* displays anticancer activity and merits additional investigation as a potential chemopreventive agent.[1]

Photoprotection

In 2002, Morganti et al. assessed the *in vitro* and *in vivo* activity of various topical antioxidants and nutritional supplements in a randomized, double-blind, placebo-controlled study conducted over eight weeks on 30 female volunteers (aged 48–59 years) with moderate dry skin and photodamage. All subjects twice daily applied a nanocolloidal gel (α-lipoic acid 05. mg, melatonin/emblica 15 mg) and/or daily took two capsules of an oral diet supplement (ascorbic acid 45 mg, tocopherol 5 mg, lutein 3 mg, α-lipoic acid 2.5 mg). Oral and topical administration of the antioxidant-rich compounds resulted in significant reduction in oxidative stress and lipid peroxidation. Free radicals recovered

in blood serum and on skin, *in vivo*, and reactive oxygen species (ROS) induced by *in vitro* irradiation of leukocytes with ultraviolet B (UVB) were also decreased in antioxidant-treated patients. The investigators concluded that all of the compounds showed therapeutic potential, in topical or systemic form, as photoprotectants and agents intended to lower the oxidative stress of photoaging-affected individuals, with the α-lipoic and melatonin/emblica combination showing promise as a topical preparation.[23]

In 2010, Adil et al. investigated the efficacy of amla to suppress UVB-induced photoaging in human skin fibroblasts. They found that the botanical agent had broad effects, protecting procollagen 1 against UVB damage by suppressing UVB-induced matrix metalloproteinase-1 (MMP-1) proliferation in fibroblasts, inhibiting hyaluronidase activity, and preventing UVB from disrupting the normal cell cycle. They observed that amla concentration-dependently promoted fibroblast proliferation and provided a potent photoprotective effect against UVB-induced cytotoxicity.[13] In 2011, Majeed et al. showed that *P. emblica* fruit extract effec-tively protected against UVB-induced ROS and collagen damage in normal human dermal fibroblasts and demonstrates potential as a topical component of the dermatologic armamentarium against photoaging.[24]

Previously, Fujii et al. conducted an *in vitro* investigation of the effects of amla extract on human skin fibroblasts, particularly in relation to the synthesis of procollagen and MMPs. They noted that amla concentration-dependently stimulated fibroblast production and concentration- and time-dependently spurred procollagen synthesis. In addition, the extract markedly reduced MMP-1 production while significantly elevating tissue inhibitors of MMP-1 (TIMP-1). The researchers concluded that amla can play an important role in controlling collagen metabolism and thus shows therapeutic and cosmetic potential.[11] Chanvorachote et al. also reported on their findings that *P. emblica* extract exhibited procollagen type I-promoting and collagenase-inhibiting effects in murine fibroblasts, which the investigators suggested was an indication of its potential as an antiaging agent.[25]

Combination Therapy: Triphala

Based on evidence that *triphala* (an antioxidant-rich herbal formulation that combines dried fruits of *Terminalia chebula*, *Terminalia bellirica*, and *E. officinalis*; the word is derived from the Sanskrit *tri*, three, and *phala*, fruits), long used in Ayurveda, has demonstrated *in vitro* antimicrobial activity against wound pathogens, including *Staphylococcus aureus*, *Pseudomonas aeruginosa*, and *Streptococcus pyogenes*, Kumar et al. recently prepared a triphala ointment and evaluated its effects for *in vivo* wound healing on infected rats. The investigators identified significantly improved wound closure and bacterial count decreases in the treated group, along with significant hexosamine, uronic acid, and superoxide dismutase levels and diminished MMP expression. They concluded that triphala ointment exhibited antioxidant, antibacterial, and wound-healing activities suitable for treating infected wounds and that the active constituents of the ointment warrant further consideration for wound therapy.[26] Subsequently, the same team successfully demonstrated the healing effects of triphala incorporated into a collagen sponge to treat the infected dermal wounds in albino rats.[27] Triphala, also used as a colon cleanser, digestive aid, diuretic, and laxative, is useful in the prevention of cancer and exhibits antineoplastic, radioprotective, and chemoprotective effects, according to recent studies.[5]

In 2005, Naik et al. studied the aqueous extract of the fruits of *E. officinalis*, *Terminalia chebula*, and *Terminalia belerica* as well as their equiproportional mixture triphala to compare their *in vitro* antioxidant activity. The investigators found that the individual triphala constituents displayed somewhat different activities under various conditions, with emblica exhibiting the greatest efficiency in lipid peroxidation and the plasmid DNA assay, while *Terminalia chebula* was the most effective at scavenging free radicals. They concluded that the combination formulation triphala appears to show the greatest efficiency by virtue of combining the strengths of each of its constituents.[28]

In a 2009 study by Nariya et al. comparing an equiproportional formulation of triphala with an unequal one (1:2:4 proportion of *T. chebula*, *T. belerica*, and *E. officinalis*, respectively), the one favoring a much larger percentage of emblica was found to confer much greater intestinal protection against methotrexate-induced damage in rats. The investigators attributed their results to the greater proportion of antioxidants, particularly the ellagic and gallic acids and flavonoids found in *E. officinalis*.[29]

In 2010, Hazra et al. studied the 70 percent methanol extracts of *Terminalia chebula*, *Terminalia belerica*, and *E. officinalis* fruit to assess their *in vitro* antioxidant and ROS-scavenging properties against 2,2-diphenyl-1-picrylhydrazyl (DPPH), hydroxyl, superoxide, nitric oxide, H_2O_2, peroxynitrite, singlet oxygen, and hypochlorous acid. The investigators identified varying orders of potency of the extracts in the manifestation of antioxidative properties, scavenging of particular ROS, as well as flavonoid and phenolic content but each of these components of the Ayurvedic staple triphala demonstrated significant antioxidative capacity, and the researchers concluded that these compounds represent strong natural antioxidant sources.[2]

In a 2012 review, Baliga et al. noted that scientific studies over the previous two decades have confirmed numerous ethnomedical claims and investigators have found that triphala exhibits a broad array of beneficial activities, including free radical scavenging, antioxidant, anti-inflammatory, analgesic, antibacterial, antimutagenic, wound healing, antistress, adaptogenic, hypoglycemic, anticancer, chemoprotective, radioprotective, and chemopreventive among others.[30] Baliga and Dsouza had previously reported that preclinical studies have shown that antipyretic, analgesic, antitussive, antiatherogenic, adaptogenic, cardioprotective, gastroprotective, antianemia, antihypercholesterolemia, wound-healing, antidiarrheal, antiatherosclerotic, hepatoprotective, nephroprotective, and neuroprotective properties have been ascribed to amla alone.[7] In addition, they noted that amla reportedly exerts radiomodulatory, chemomodulatory, chemopreventive, free radical-scavenging, antioxidant, anti-inflammatory, antimutagenic, immunomodulatory, and wound-healing activities.[7]

Extracts of *E. officinalis* have also been combined with those of *Terminalia chebula*, *Terminalia bellerica*, *Albizia lebbeck*, *Piper nigrum*, *Zingiber officinale*, and *Piper longum* in a polyherbal formulation (Aller-7/NR-A2) that has been found safe for the treatment of allergic rhinitis.[31]

In Vitro Studies with Dermatologic Implications

In 2008, Fujii et al. studied the effects of amla extract on human skin fibroblasts, with a focus on *in vitro* production of procollagen and MMPs. They employed the WST-8 assay to assess human skin fibroblast mitochondrial activity and an immunoassay to measure procollagen, MMPs, and TIMP-1 released from the fibroblasts. The researchers found that amla extract controls collagen metabolism in therapeutic and cosmetic applications. Specifically, they found that in a concentration-dependent fashion, amla promoted fibroblast proliferation and in a concentration- and time-dependent manner stimulated procollagen synthesis. They also noted that amla significantly lowered MMP-1 production, with significant increases in TIMP-1, but had no effect on MMP-2. The authors concluded that their findings suggest the potential of amla to confer mollifying and therapeutic as well as cosmetic benefits.[11]

CONCLUSION

The fruit and most other parts of *E. officinalis* have long been used in various traditional medical practices in Asia, especially India, for a wide range of indications. Recent evidence suggests broad potential for the extract of the amla fruit in modern Western medical treatment and, in particular, as an ingredient in general purpose dermatologic topical formulations as well as antiaging, hypopigmenting, and sunscreen agents. Much more research is necessary to establish the effectiveness of such products, but current findings are encouraging.

REFERENCES

1. Ngamkitidechakul C, Jaijoy K, Hansakul P, et al. Antitumor effects of Phyllanthus emblica L.: Induction of cancer cell apoptosis and inhibition of in vivo tumour promotion and in vitro invasion of human cancer cells. *Phytother Res.* 2010;24:1405.
2. Hazra B, Sarkar R, Biswas S, et al. Comparative study of the antioxidant and reactive oxygen species scavenging properties in the extracts of the fruits of Terminalia chebula, Terminalia belerica and Emblica officinalis. *BMC Complement Altern Med.* 2010;10:20.
3. Pozharitskaya ON, Ivanova SA, Shikov AN, et al. Separation and evaluation of free radical-scavenging activity of phenol components of Emblica officinalis extract by using an HPTLC-DPPH* method. *J Sep Sci.* 2007;30:1250.
4. Krishnaveni M, Mirunalini S. Therapeutic potential of Phyllanthus emblica (amla): The ayurvedic wonder. *J Basic Clin Physiol Pharmacol.* 2010;21:93.
5. Baliga MS. Triphala, Ayurvedic formulation for treating and preventing cancer: A review. *J Altern Complement Med.* 2010;16:1301.
6. Sharma A, Sharma MK, Kumar M. Modulatory role of Emblica officinalis fruit extract against arsenic induced oxidative stress in Swiss albino mice. *Chem Biol Interact.* 2009;180:20.
7. Baliga MS, Dsouza JJ. Amla (Emblica officinalis Gaertn), a wonder berry in the treatment and prevention of cancer. *Eur J Cancer Prev.* 2011;20:225.
8. Sancheti G, Jindal A, Kumari R, et al. Chemopreventive action of emblica officinalis on skin carcinogenesis in mice. *Asian Pac J Cancer Prev.* 2005;6:197.
9. Datta HS, Mitra SK, Patwardhan B. Wound healing activity of topical application forms based on Ayurveda. *Evid Based Complement Alternat Med.* 2011;134378.
10. Scartezzini P, Antognoni F, Raggi MA, et al. Vitamin C content and antioxidant activity of the fruit and of the Ayurvedic preparation of Emblica officinalis Gaertn. *J Ethnopharmacol.* 2006;104:113.
11. Fujii T, Wakaizumi M, Ikami T, et al. Amla (Emblica officinalis Gaertn.) extract promotes procollagen production and inhibits matrix metalloproteinase-1 in human skin fibroblasts. *J Ethnopharmacol.* 2008;119:53.
12. Datta HS, Paramesh R. Trends in aging and skin care: Ayurvedic concepts. *J Ayurveda Integr Med.* 2010;1:110.
13. Adil MD, Kaiser P, Satti NK, et al. Effect of Emblica officinalis (fruit) against UVB-induced photo-aging in human skin fibroblasts. *J Ethnopharmacol.* 2010;132:109.
14. Ishtiaq M, Hanif W, Khan MA, et al. An ethnomedicinal survey and documentation of important medicinal folklore food phytonims of flora of Samahni valley, (Azad Kashmir) Pakistan. *Pak J Biol Sci.* 2007;10:2241.

15. Majeed M, Bhat B, Jadhav AN, et al. Ascorbic acid and tannins from Emblica officinalis Gaertn. Fruits–A revisit. *J Agric Food Chem*. 2009;57:220.

16. Costa A, Moisés TA, Cordero T, et al. Association of emblica, licorice and belides as an alternative to hydroquinone in the clinical treatment of melasma. *An Bras Dermatol*. 2010;85:613.

17. Chaudhuri RK. Emblica cascading antioxidant: A novel natural skin care ingredient. *Skin Pharmacol Appl Skin Physiol*. 2002;15:374.

18. Yokozawa T, Kim HY, Kim HJ, et al. Amla (Emblica officinalis Gaertn.) prevents dyslipidaemia and oxidative stress in the ageing process. *Br J Nutr*. 2007;97:1187.

19. Banu SM, Selvendiran K, Singh JP, et al. Protective effect of Emblica officinalis ethanolic extract against 7,12-dimethylbenz(a) anthracene (DMBA) induced genotoxicity in Swiss albino mice. *Hum Exp Toxicol*. 2004;23:527.

20. Kumar N, Rungseevijitprapa W, Narkkhong NA, et al. 5α-reductase inhibition and hair growth promotion of some Thai plants traditionally used for hair treatment. *J Ethnopharmacol*. 2012;139:765.

21. Draelos ZD, Yatskayer M, Bhushan P, et al. Evaluation of a kojic acid, emblica extract, and glycolic acid formulation compared with hydroquinone 4% for skin lightening. *Cutis*. 2010;86:153.

22. Poltanov EA, Shikov AN, Dorman HJ, et al. Chemical and antioxidant evaluation of Indian gooseberry (Emblica officinalis Gaertn., syn. Phyllanthus emblica L.) supplements. *Phytother Res*. 2009;23:1309.

23. Morganti P, Bruno C, Guarneri F, et al. Role of topical and nutritional supplement to modify the oxidative stress. *Int J Cosmet Sci*. 2002;24:331.

24. Majeed M, Bhat B, Anand S, et al. Inhibition of UV-induced ROS and collagen damage by Phyllanthus emblica extract in normal human dermal fibroblasts. *J Cosmet Sci*. 2011;62:49.

25. Chanvorachote P, Pongrakhananon V, Luanpitpong S, et al. Type I pro-collagen promoting and anti-collagenase activities of Phyllanthus emblica extract in mouse fibroblasts. *J Cosmet Sci*. 2009;60:395.

26. Kumar MS, Kirubanandan S, Sripriya R, et al. Triphala promotes healing of infected full-thickness dermal wound. *J Surg Res*. 2008;144:94.

27. Kumar MS, Kirubanandan S, Sripriya R, et al. Triphala incorporated collagen sponge–a smart biomaterial for infected dermal wound healing. *J Surg Res*. 2010;158:162.

28. Naik GH, Priyadarsini KI, Bhagirathi RG, et al. In vitro antioxidant studies and free radical reactions of triphala, an ayurvedic formulation and its constituents. *Phytother Res*. 2005;19:582.

29. Nariya M, Shukla V, Jain S, et al. Comparison of enteroprotective efficacy of triphala formulations (Indian Herbal Drug) on methotrexate-induced small intestinal damage in rats. *Phytother Res*. 2009;23:1092.

30. Baliga MS, Meera S, Mathai B, et al. Scientific validation of the ethnomedicinal properties of the Ayurvedic drug Triphala: a review. *Chin J Integr Med*. 2012;18:946.

31. Amit A, Joshua AJ, Bagchi M, et al. Safety of a novel botanical extract formula for ameliorating allergic rhinitis. Part II. *Toxicol Mech Methods*. 2005;15:193.

CHAPTER 39

Mulberry Extract

Activities:

Antityrosinase, antihyperglycemic,[1,2] antitumorigenic,[3] anti-inflammatory,[3] antiypyretic,[3] antioxidant,[3,4] antiatherogenic,[4] antimicrobial,[5] chemopreventive,[5] neuroprotective[5]

Important Chemical Components:

Morus alba: Mulberroside F (the phytoalexin moracin M-6, 3'-di-O-beta-D-glucopyranoside), mulberroside A, various polyphenols, including moracetin, rutin, isoquercitrin, gallic acid, quercetin 3-(6-malonylglucoside), and astragalin,[1,4] oxyresveratrol (the aglycone of mulberroside A),[6] and fatty acids (e.g., linoleic and palmitic)[7]

Morus australis: Oxyresveratrol, multiple chalcones, austraone A, moracenin D, sanggenon T, and kuwanon O[8]

Morus nigra: Mulberroside A, 5'-geranyl-5,7,2',4'-tetrahydroxyflavone, steppogenin-7-O-beta-D-glucoside, morachalcone A, 2,4,2',4'-tetrahydroxychalcone, moracin N, kuwanon H, mulberrofuran G, morachalcone A, oxyresveratrol-3'-O-beta-D-glucopyranoside, and oxyresveratrol-2-O-beta-D-glucopyranoside[9]

Morus notabilis: Moracin O, moracin P[10]

Morus papyrifera (or *Broussonetia papyrifera*): Prenylated, polyhyrdroxylated mono- and bis-phenyl derivatives, flavonoids (quercetin, luteolin), linoleic acid, methyl palmitate, oleic acid, linoleic acid ester, and diterpenes (three different broussonetones)[11,12]

Origin Classification:

Natural components isolated from various Moraceae species

Personal Care Category:

Depigmenting

Recommended for the following Baumann Skin Types:

DRPT, DRPW, DSPT, DSPW, ORPT, ORPW, OSPT, and OSPW

SOURCE

The family Moraceae, which is native to eastern Asia, is the source of multiple species of deciduous trees associated with skin-lightening activity, including *Morus alba*, *Morus australis*, *Morus Nigra*, *Morus notabilis*, and *Morus papyrifera*. Moraceae are fast-growing perennial trees that now are cultivated in tropical, subtropical, and temperate climates.[5] The fruits of these trees are consumed throughout the world and various parts of the plants have been and continue to be used in traditional medicine.

The genus Broussonetia, a member of the Moraceae family and closely related to the genus Morus, is found throughout Asia and the Pacific Islands.[11] *Broussonetia papyrifera* (also known as *Morus papyrifera* and, commonly, as paper mulberry) is a deciduous tree native to eastern Asia. Its bark is used for making high-quality paper, but other parts of the tree have been used in traditional medicine and such uses continue today.

HISTORY

The leaves of *Morus alba* are an important source of nutrition for the silkworm (*Bombyx mori*).[1,3,5,13] Therapeutic uses of the leaves, bark, and branches for human beings have long been found in traditional Chinese medicine (TCM).[4,11,14] *M. alba* has been deployed in TCM as a wind-heat-effusing agent.[15] In addition, various parts of several Moraceae species have been used in TCM to treat tinea, dysentery, hernia, and edema.[11] Ayurvedic medicine has also employed this herb to treat diarrhea, intestinal ulcers, small pox, back pain, vocal cord inflammation, and cutaneous cracks on the soles of the feet.[3] From a global finance perspective, mulberry is one of the most important plants in the economy of India.[5] The roots, barks, and stems of *Morus australis* have also been long used in traditional Japanese medicine (known as Kampo) to treat diabetes and arthritis.[16] In China, the leaves, stem, leaf juice, roots, fruits, and bark of *B. papyrifera* have all been utilized for various health benefits, with the stem and leaf juice used to treat skin disorders and insect bites.[11]

CHEMISTRY

Tyrosinase is the rate-limiting enzyme for melanogenesis. In the early stages of melanin production, it catalyzes the hydroxylation of L-tyrosine to 3,4-dihydroxyphenylalanine (DOPA) and the oxidation of DOPA to dopaquinone.[16] Several Moraceae species represent a new frontier of natural tyrosinase inhibitors, which are thought to be less expensive to process than synthetic agents such as hydroquinone and, importantly, less likely to induce adverse side effects (Table 39-1).

Tyrosinase activity has been demonstrated to be suppressed by dried white mulberry (*M. alba*) leaves (85 percent ethanol extract).[7] The primary active component of white mulberry, mulberroside F (moracin M-6, 3'-di-O-β-D-glucopyranoside), which is extracted from the dried leaves of the tree, has also been shown to inhibit tyrosinase activity as well as melanin formation in melan-a cells.[7,17] Other potent constituents found in *M. alba* leaves include phenolic flavonoids, such as gallic acid and quercetin, and fatty acids, such as linoleic and palmitic acids.

TABLE 39-1
Pros and Cons of Mulberry Extract

PROS	CON
Potent inhibitors of tyrosinase	Dearth of clinical studies of each species
Indications that mulberry is more effective than kojic acid and arbutin	
Safer than hydroquinone	

Mulberroside A is the main active constituent of black mulberry (*M. nigra*), but it has weak tyrosinase-inhibitory properties.[9] Nevertheless, it has been utilized in Korea as a raw material in cosmetic products intended for skin whitening.[18] Black mulberry also contains morachalcone A, among several other compounds, with reported inhibitory activity against mushroom tyrosinase and melanin biosynthesis.[9,19] *M. nigra* and *M. alba* are believed to have especially potent antioxidant potential, and mulberroside F has displayed superoxide-scavenging activity in particlar.[1,20]

The methanol extract of *Morus australis* (known as Chinese mulberry or, in Japan, as *shimaguwa*), found in China, Japan, Korea, and parts of Southeast Asia, is also known to confer a skin-whitening effect due to tyrosinase inhibition.[16]

Extracts of paper mulberry have been demonstrated to inhibit L-DOPA oxidation, more potently than arbutin, and to scavenge free radicals such as 2,2-diphenyl-1-picrylhydrazyl (DPPH) and hydrogen peroxide among others.[11]

ORAL USES

White mulberry is consumed regularly in Korea, Japan, India, and Chile. It is sometimes used in preserves or syrup.[4] The fruits of black and red mulberry (*Morus rubra*, which is native to North America), in particular, are used in baked goods and alcoholic beverages. Mulberry is also available in oral supplement form.

It is also worth noting that the dietary consumption of mulberry leaf powder derived from *M. alba* or especially quercetin 3-(6-malonylglucoside), its quantitatively primary active flavonol glycoside, has been shown to ameliorate hyperglycemia in obese mice and lowered oxidative stress in the liver.[21]

Animal Study: Antioxidant Effects

In a 2010 study of the effects of daily administration of mulberry leaves (*M. alba*) in rats fed a high-fat diet, Kobayashi et al. found that the botanical lowered plasma triglyceride reactive oxygen species synthesis and limited oxidative stress by upregulating the expression of genes involved in responding to oxidative stress.[14]

TOPICAL USES

Extracts of *M. alba* are currently in use as additives in cosmetic products for the purposes of skin lightening.[15]

In 2013, Singh et al. evaluated the effects of mulberry, kiwi, and Sophora extracts on melanogenesis and melanin transfer in human melanocytes and in co-cultures with phototype-matched normal adult epidermal keratinocytes. They assessed these botanicals against isobutylmethylxanthine, hydroquinone, vitamin C, and niacinamide, finding that compared with unstimulated control, the extracts significantly lowered melanogenesis in normal adult epidermal melanocytes as well as human melanoma cells. Melanin transfer was also decreased as was filopodia expression on melanocytes. The investigators concluded that their results, comparable to standard-bearing depigmenting agents, suggest the effectiveness of the tested extracts as topical agents for reducing hyperpigmentation.[22]

Morus alba (White Mulberry)

Lee et al. studied the *in vitro* effects of an 85 percent methanol extract of dried *M. alba* leaves on melanin biosynthesis in 2002 and found that one of the primary bioactive constituents, mulberroside F (moracin M-6, 3'-di-O-β-D-glucopyranoside), suppressed the tyrosinase activity that converts dopa to dopachrome in the melanin synthesis process and also inhibited the melanin formation of melan-a cells. This study was one of the earlier indications that mulberry, specifically the component mulberroside F, which also displayed some superoxide-scavenging capacity, may be a viable skin-whitening agent. Further, the mulberry extracted more potently inhibited tyrosinase activity than kojic acid.[1] In 2003, a different team of investigators observed that the young twigs of *M. alba* also displayed the ability to inhibit tyrosinase activity as well as melanin production in B16 melanoma cells. *In vivo*, the extracts reduced melanin synthesis in a guinea pig model without exhibiting toxicity.[23]

In 2006, Wang et al. investigated 25 traditional Chinese herbal medicines potentially useful in dermatology, particularly for skin whitening. *M. alba* was one of four species of extracts that displayed strong inhibitory activity against tyrosinase, more potent, in fact, than arbutin.[15] Extracts of *M. alba* were also found to be one of the seven species among 52 crude Nepalese drugs tested by Adhikari et al. for mushroom tyrosinase inhibitory activity in 2008 to concentration-dependently exhibit potent properties in this realm.[6]

A 2008 study by Nattapong and Omboon showed *in vitro* that the extracts from Thai mulberry, a hybrid of *M. alba* and *M. rotundiloba*, were effective as a whitening agent, partly owing to the presence of the pentacyclic triterpenoid betulinic acid.[24]

In 2011, Park et al. found that topically applied mulberroside A isolated from the roots of *M. alba* as well as its derivatives oxyresveratrol and oxyresveratrol-3-*O*-glucoside inhibited melanogenesis in UV-induced hyperpigmented guinea pig skin. Specifically, they showed that the mulberry ingredients caused depigmentation and lowered melanin content, with oxyresveratrol more strongly suppressing melanogenesis than mulberroside A.[25] The investigators concluded that these ingredients warrant attention as potential cosmetic skin-whitening agents.[26]

Morus australis (Chinese Mulberry/Shimaguwa)

In 2012, Takahashi et al. isolated the components of a 95 percent methanol extract of the dried stems of shimaguwa to study the mechanism of the plant's skin-whitening activity. They identified four chalcones, all of which were found to inhibit mushroom tyrosinase activity more effectively than arbutin. Three of the four chalcones were actually measured as exhibiting 100-fold greater tyrosinase inhibitory activity than arbutin, with minimal or no cytotoxicity, as assessed in assays to evaluate the effects of the chalcones on melanin production, without altering cell growth, in melanin-producing B16 murine melanoma cells. The investigators concluded that these three chalcones may account for the depigmenting activity of shimaguwa. Further, they noted that the skin-whitening activity of *M. australis* is not limited to the inhibition of tyrosinase.[16]

Also that year, Zheng et al. isolated constituents from the roots of *M. australis* and conducted tyrosinase inhibitory testing. They found that several ingredients, including oxyresveratrol, moracenin D, sanggenon T, and kuwanon O, displayed more potent tyrosinase suppression than that of kojic acid. The investigators concluded that *M. australis*, widespread in Asia, is a good natural source of tyrosinase inhibitors potentially useful in cosmetic skin-lightening products as well as in foods as antibrowning agents.[8]

Morus nigra (Black Mulberry)

In 2010, Zheng et al. compared the phytochemical profiles of *M. nigra* roots and twigs with old and young *M. alba* twigs. In the process, the researchers discovered one previously unknown compound (5'-geranyl-5,7,2',4'-tetrahydroxyflavone) as well as eight others, among 28 known phenolic compounds in *M. nigra*, which exhibited better tyrosinase inhibition than kojic acid. The other compounds include steppogenin-7-O-β-D-glucoside, 2,4,2',4'-tetrahydroxychalcone, moracin N, kuwanon H, mulberrofuran G, morachalcone A, oxyresveratrol-3'-O-β-D-glucopyranoside and oxyresveratrol-2-O-β-D-glucopyranoside, with 2,4,2',4'-tetrahydroxychalcone and morachalcone A associated with significantly lower $IC_{(50)}$ (half maximal inhibitory concentration) values than kojic acid, suggesting their viability as effective natural suppressors of tyrosinase.[9]

Morus notabilis

In 2012, Hu et al. conducted a phytochemical evaluation of the stem of *M. notabilis*, isolating and characterizing several compounds in the process, including moracins O and P. These Moraceae family constituents demonstrated stronger mushroom tyrosinase-inhibiting effects as compared to kojic acid.[10]

Morus papyrifera (Paper Mulberry)

In a 2007 study of 101 plant extracts screened for their inhibitory activities against tyrosinase, L-DOPA oxidation, and melanin biosynthesis in B_{16} mouse melanoma cells, Hwang and Lee noted that extracts of *Broussonetia papyrifera* (also known as *Morus papyrifera*), one of the 31 extracts to exhibit greater than 50 percent inhibition of mushroom tyrosinase, concentration-dependently suppressed tyrosinase activity and L-DOPA oxidation. Further, extracts of *Morus bombycis* (also known as *Morus australis* or Chinese mulberry), one of the 17 groups of tyrosinase-inhibiting extracts tested on melanogenesis, significantly inhibited melanin production. These two species of mulberry were deemed by the authors to be among a group of botanicals to represent potential sources of skin-whitening agents for skin particularly sensitive to ultraviolet radiation.[27]

In 2008, Ko et al. isolated three previously unknown constituents of *B. papyrifera* leaves along with seven known compounds. The newly discovered diterpenes (broussonetones) were found to marginally block tyrosinase but to significantly inhibit xanthine oxidase. In their preliminary screening, the investigators found that the parent flavonoids of the isolated diterpenes from methanolic extracts of the ground leaves of the plant exhibited greater mushroom tyrosinase inhibition than kojic acid as well as significant DPPH free radical-scavenging activity. The authors concluded that their results suggest the utility of the active constituents of paper mulberry as ingredients in skin-protecting cosmetics.[12] Also in 2008, Zheng et al. isolated one new compound and 10 known ones from *B. papyrifera* twigs and found greater tyrosinase-inhibitory activity as compared to arbutin.[11,28]

The bark of paper mulberry is composed of extremely strong fibers used to produce high-quality paper and cloth. The roots of the tree have been found to display potent tyrosinase-inhibiting properties. In one study, a 0.4 percent concentration of paper mulberry extract was demonstrated to suppress tyrosinase activity by 50 percent compared to 5.5 percent hydroquinone and 10 percent kojic acid. Notably, paper mulberry is not considered a significant irritant even at 1 percent concentration.[29,30]

■ SAFETY ISSUES

Pollen from the *M. alba* tree has been associated with respiratory allergies as well as contact urticaria.[13,31] There are no known adverse side effects from topical use.

■ ENVIRONMENTAL IMPACT

The availability of mulberry leaves, particularly white mulberry, for the silkworm and the silk industry are important factors related to the environmental impact of mulberry cultivation. Several varieties of mulberry species are cultivated in China, Japan, Korea, and India for the sericulture, or silk farming, industry.[32] For economic reasons, efforts to develop higher yield mulberry varieties are ongoing.[32] High water demands are associated with high-yielding mulberry cultivars.[5]

■ FORMULATION CONSIDERATIONS

Optimal solvents have been found to extract the active ingredients from the plant.[33]

■ USAGE CONSIDERATIONS

No interactions with other ingredients are known by the author.

■ SIGNIFICANT BACKGROUND

Cancer

In 2004, Prasad et al. showed that *Morus indica* (very similar to or another designation for *M. alba*) exhibited *in vitro* and *in vivo* activity against tumorigenesis in mice. Investigators studied the inhibitory activity and level of aryl hydrocarbon hydroxylase, cytochrome P450, DNA sugar damage in calf thymus DNA, and Fe(++)/ascorbate-induced lipid peroxidation in microsomes of mice, finding significant elevation in the activity of antioxidant enzymes and reduction in cutaneous malondialdehyde levels at three doses of the extract *in vitro*. Using the two-stage 12-O-tetradecanoyl-phorbol-13-acetate (TPA)-induced oxidative stress initiation and 7,12-dimethylbenz(a)anthracene (DMBA)-induced and croton oil-promoted skin tumorigenesis model in Swiss albino mice, the researchers also found that applying the mulberry extract one hour before croton oil application extended the tumor latency period and also led to the reduction in the number of tumors per mouse and percentage of mice developing tumors. Pretreatment with *M. indica* also dose-dependently suppressed TPA-induced stimulation of mouse epidermal ornithine decarboxylase activity. The authors concluded that white mulberry extract appears to have potential as a therapeutic agent for cancer control.[3]

Melasma

In 2011, Alvin et al. conducted a randomized, single-blind, placebo-controlled trial of 50 Filipino patients (49 women, 1 man) to assess the safety and efficacy of 75 percent white mulberry extract oil in a comparison with placebo for melasma treatment. Patients were followed up at weeks 4 and 8. The mulberry extract group performed significantly better than the placebo group in each measurement [i.e., the melasma area and severity score (MASI), Mexameter reading, and melasma quality of life score (MelasQOL)]. The 25 patients treated with mulberry extract improved from a baseline MASI reading of 4.076 (±0.24) to 2.884 (±0.25) at week 8 with a mean difference of 1.19; the placebo group mean difference of improvement was 0.06. The mean Mexameter reading showed a significant difference, with a slight increase for the mulberry group (indicating lighter pigmentation) and the placebo group scoring a slightly higher value. Further, the MelasQOL score for the mulberry group markedly increased from baseline to week 8 [58.84 (SD: ± 3.18) to 44.16 (SD: ± 4.29)], whereas the placebo group improved slightly from 57.44 (SD: ± 4.66) at baseline to 54.28 (SD: ± 4.79) at week 8. The only adverse events reported were mild itching in four patients from the mulberry group; 12 cases of either itching or erythema were reported by the placebo group. The researchers concluded that 75 percent mulberry extract oil objectively ameliorates melasma in Fitzpatrick skin types III to V, though they recommend further research with a larger sample size and longer treatment duration and follow-up.[34]

CONCLUSION

The Moraceae family of deciduous trees includes several species that have been used as food and in traditional medical practices throughout Asia. Such uses have expanded in recent years as evidence has emerged that multiple constituents of these trees exert potent antityrosinase activity, in some cases more than kojic acid and arbutin. As such, mulberry has joined the ranks of naturally sourced dermatologic skin-whitening agents.

REFERENCES

1. Lee SH, Choi SY, Kim H, et al. Mulberroside F isolated from the leaves of *Morus alba* inhibits melanin biosynthesis. *Biol Pharm Bull*. 2002;25:1045.
2. Hoffmann D. The endocrine system. In: *Medical Herbalism: The Science and Practice of Herbal Medicine*. Rochester, VT: Healing Arts Press; 2003:464.
3. Prasad L, Khan TH, Sehrawat A, et al. Modulatory effect of *Morus indica* against two-stage skin carcinogenesis in Swiss albino mice: Possible mechanism by inhibiting aryl hydrocarbon hydroxylase. *J Pharm Pharmacol*. 2004;56:1291.
4. Enkhmaa B, Shiwaku K, Katsube T, et al. Mulberry (*Morus alba L.*) leaves and their major flavonol quercetin 3-(6-malonylglucoside) attenuate atherosclerotic lesion development in LDL receptor-deficient mice. *J Nutr*. 2005;135:729.
5. Khurana P, Checker VG. The advent of genomics in Mulberry and perspectives for productivity enhancement. *Plant Cell Rep*. 2011;30:825.
6. Adhikari A, Devkota HP, Takano A, et al. Screening of Nepalese crude drugs traditionally used to treat hyperpigmentation: In vitro tyrosinase inhibition. *Int J Cosmet Sci*. 2008;30:353.
7. Zhu W, Gao J. The use of botanical extract as topical skin-lightening agents for the improvement of skin pigmentation disorders. *J Investig Dermatol Symp Proc*. 2008;13:20.
8. Zheng ZP, Tan HY, Wang M. Tyrosinase inhibition constituents from the roots of *Morus australis*. *Fitoterapia*. 2012;83:1008.
9. Zheng ZP, Cheng KW, Zhu Q, et al. Tyrosinase inhibitory constituents from the roots of *Morus nigra*: A structure-activity relationship study. *J Agric Food Chem*. 2010;58:5368.
10. Hu X, Wang M, Yan GR, et al. 2-Arylbenzofuran and tyrosinase inhibitory constituents of Morus notabilis. *J Asian Nat Prod Res*. 2012;14:1103.
11. Wang GW, Huang BK, Qin LP. The genus *Broussonetia*: A review of its phytochemistry and pharmacology. *Phytother Res*. 2012;26:1.
12. Ko HH, Chang WL, Lu TM. Antityrosinase and antioxidant effects of ent-kaurane diterpenes from leaves of *Broussonetia papyrifera*. *J Nat Prod*. 2008;71:1930.
13. Navarro AM, Orta JC, Sánchez MC, et al. Primary sensitization to *Morus alba*. *Allergy*. 1997;52:1144.
14. Kobayashi Y, Miyazawa M, Kamei A, et al. Ameliorative effects of mulberry (*Morus alba L.*) leaves on hyperlipidemia in rats fed a high-fat diet: Induction of fatty acid oxidation, inhibition of lipogenesis, and suppression of oxidative stress. *Biosci Biotechnol Biochem*. 2010;74:2385.
15. Wang KH, Lin RD, Hsu FL, et al. Cosmetic applications of selected traditional Chinese herbal medicines. *J Ethnopharmacol*. 2006;106:353.
16. Takahashi M, Takara K, Toyozato T, et al. A novel bioactive chalcone of *Morus australis* inhibits tyrosinase activity and melanin biosynthesis in B$_{16}$ melanoma cells. *J Oleo Sci*. 2012;61:585.
17. Konda S, Geria AN, Halder RM. New horizons in treating disorders of hyperpigmentation in skin of color. *Semin Cutan Med Surg*. 2012;31:133.
18. Kim JK, Kim M, Cho SG, et al. Biotransformation of mulberroside A from Morus alba results in enhancement of tyrosinase inhibition. *J Ind Microbiol Biotechnol*. 2010;37:631.
19. Zhang X, Hu X, Hou A, et al. Inhibitory effect of 2,4,2',4'-tetrahydroxy-3-(3-methyl-2-butenyl)-chalcone on tyrosinase activity and melanin biosynthesis. *Biol Pharm Bull*. 2009;32:86.
20. Arfan M, Khan R, Rybarczyk A, et al. Antioxidant activity of mulberry fruit extracts. *Int J Mol Sci*. 2012;13:2472.
21. Katsube T, Yamasaki M, Shiwaku K, et al. Effect of flavonol glycoside in mulberry (*Morus alba L.*) leaf on glucose metabolism and oxidative stress in liver in diet-induced obese mice. *J Sci Food Agric*. 2010;90:2386.
22. Singh SK, Baker R, Wibawa JI, et al. The effects of Sophora angustifolia and other natural plant extracts on melanogenesis and melanin transfer in human skin cells. *Exp Dermatol*. 2013;22:67.
23. Lee KT, Lee KS, Jeong JH, et al. Inhibitory effects of Ramulus mori extracts on melanogenesis. *J Cosmet Sci*. 2003;54:133.
24. Nattapong S, Omboon L. A new source of whitening agent from a Thai Mulberry plant and its betulinic acid quantitation. *Nat Prod Res*. 2008;22:727.
25. Kim YM, Yun J, Lee CK, et al. Oxyresveratrol and hydroxystilbene compounds. Inhibitory effect on tyrosinase and mechanism of action. *J Biol Chem*. 2002;277:16340.
26. Park KT, Kim JK, Hwang D, et al. Inhibitory effect of mulberroside A and its derivatives on melanogenesis induced by ultraviolet B irradiation. *Food Chem Toxicol*. 2011;49:3038.
27. Hwang JH, Lee BM. Inhibitory effects of plant extracts on tyrosinase, L-DOPA oxidation, and melanin synthesis. *J Toxicol Environ Health A*. 2007;70:393.
28. Zheng ZP, Cheng KW, Chao J, et al. Tyrosinase inhibitors from paper mulberry (*Broussonetia papyrifera*). *Food Chem*. 2008;106:529.
29. Baumann L, Woolery-Lloyd H, Friedman A. "Natural" ingredients in cosmetic dermatology. *J Drugs Dermatol*. 2009;8:s5.
30. Dong-Il Jang. Melanogenesis inhibitor from paper Mulberry. *Cosm Toiletr*. 1997;112:59.
31. Muñoz FJ, Delgado J, Palma JL, et al. Airborne contact urticaria due to mulberry (*Morus alba*) pollen. *Contact Dermatitis*. 1995;32:61.
32. Umate P. Mulberry improvements via plastid transformation and tissue culture engineering. *Plant Signal Behav*. 2010;5:785.
33. Kim J-M, Chang S-M, Kim I-H, et al. Design of optimcal solvent for extraction of bio-active ingredients from mulberry leaves. *Biochem Eng J*. 2007;37:271.
34. Alvin G, Catambay N, Vergara A, et al. A comparative study of the safety and efficacy of 75% mulberry (*Morus alba*) extract oil versus placebo as a topical treatment for melasma: a randomized, single-blind, placebo-controlled trial. *J Drugs Dermatol*. 2011;10:1025.

CHAPTER 40

Vitamin C (Ascorbic Acid)

Activities:

Anti-inflammatory, antioxidant, photoprotectant, depigmenting

Important Chemical Components:

Esterified forms of L-ascorbic acid, such as ascorbyl-6-palmitate and magnesium ascorbyl phosphate. Its molecular formula is $C_6H_8O_6$.

Origin Classification:

Ascorbic acid is natural and found throughout the plant kingdom. Organic forms are available. Numerous synthetic topical formulations contain ascorbic acid.

Personal Care Category:

Depigmenting

Recommended for the following Baumann Skin Types:

DRNW, DRPT, DRPW, ORNW, ORPT, and ORPW

SOURCE

Vitamin C (ascorbic acid) can be found in citrus fruits and green leafy vegetables. Although this essential nutrient cannot be synthesized by the human body, dietary consumption renders it the most abundant antioxidant in human skin and vitamin C plays an important role in endogenous collagen production.[1,2] This chapter will discuss the use of vitamin C in skin pigmentation. Its antiaging and antioxidant properties are discussed in Chapter 55, Ascorbic Acid (Vitamin C).

HISTORY

Ascorbic acid, also known as vitamin C, is an essential nutrient. It is necessary for the formation of bone and connective tissue. Scurvy, a disease caused by the lack of vitamin C, was first described in the 13th century. In the 18th century, it was discovered that citrus fruits cured scurvy. Vitamin C was first isolated by Dr. Albert Szent-Györgyi, who won the Nobel Prize in Physiology or Medicine in 1937 for this work. *Ascorbic* is derived from the Latin *a-*(without) and *scorbuticus* (scurvy). Nobel Laureate Linus Pauling championed the use of oral vitamin C in 1971 in his book *Vitamin C and the Common Cold*. The capacity of vitamin C to inhibit melanin formation was known as early as 1950.[3,4] In the late 1980s, Dr. Sheldon Pinnell from Duke University began looking at vitamin C as a photoprotectant. In 1987, he published a paper in the *Archives of Dermatology* demonstrating that collagen synthesis could be induced by ascorbic acid.[5] He filed a patent in 1989 on a way to stabilize vitamin C in a topical formulation that later became the basis for the company Skinceuticals. His diligence and adherence to evidence-based science made a great impact and now vitamin C is one of the ingredients most recognized by consumers in the antiaging skin care market. Vitamin C is less known as an ingredient to decrease skin pigmentation because the form of ascorbic acid (magnesium ascorbyl phosphate) that is the best inhibitor of tyrosinase does not easily penetrate into the skin.[6]

CHEMISTRY

Ascorbic acid is necessary for the hydroxylation of lysine and proline in procollagen to form the structural protein known as collagen. It is the loss of this process that leads to scurvy in vitamin C deficiency because the loss of collagen results in blood vessel fragility and other symptoms of scurvy.

Ascorbic acid is very unstable and upon exposure to light and air reversibly oxidizes to dehydroascorbic acid, ascorbate-2-sulfate, and oxalic acid. These metabolites are excreted in the urine.[7]

Ascorbic acid suppresses melanin formation and diminishes oxidized melanin through its capacity to reduce *o*-quinones, specifically *o*-dopaquinone, back to dopa, thus preventing melanin formation. Ascorbic acid also inhibits pigmentation by interacting with copper ions that are needed by tyrosinase to function.[8–10]

ORAL USES

Of course, vitamin C is readily available in a wide range of fruits and vegetables. It is also widely available in oral supplement form. Notably, most data buttressing the beneficial effects of vitamin C have arisen from investigations of oral vitamin C or vitamin C applied to tissue cultures. Although oral vitamin C is easily absorbed into the circulation because low stomach pH provides the optimal environment, studies suggest that oral ingestion alone is not sufficient for skin protection. No studies have examined the effects of oral vitamin C on skin pigmentation.

TOPICAL USES

Among cosmetic indications, vitamin C has been shown to be effective in treating skin aging, melasma, postlaser erythema, and stretch marks. This chapter will focus on the effects of ascorbic acid on skin pigmentation.

Melasma

In 1996, Kameyama et al. showed *in vitro* that magnesium-L-ascorbyl-2-phosphate inhibited melanin formation on purified tyrosinase or cultured cells and suppressed such formation without hindering cell growth on cultured human melanoma cells.[4] In addition, the twice-daily topical application of 10 percent magnesium-L-ascorbyl-2-phosphate was effective or fairly effective in lightening ephelides, melasma, or senile lentigos in 19 of 34 subjects.[4]

In 2004, Espinal-Perez et al. conducted a double-blind randomized trial of 5 percent ascorbic acid as compared to 4 percent hydroquinone (HQ) water–oil emulsion in 16 female patients, aged 23 to 43 years (mean, 36 years) with melasma. Of those treated with vitamin C, 62.5 percent exhibited good or excellent subjectively evaluated skin lightening. There was no statistically significant difference in depigmenting activity in the HQ group, but 68.7 percent of patients experienced irritation whereas vitamin C was well tolerated.[11]

In a randomized, double-blind, placebo-controlled study, investigators used iontophoresis to enhance the penetration of vitamin C into the skin and significantly decrease pigmentation compared to placebo.[12]

Ascorbic acid is largely viewed as ineffective as a depigmenting agent alone but effective, particularly in 5 to 10 percent concentrations, when used in combination with other ingredients, such as HQ.[13] In the magnesium-L-ascorbyl-2-phosphate esterified form, however, vitamin C is among the most popular prescribed depigmenting agents around the world, especially in countries where HQ and its derivatives are banned.[14]

PIPA

Vitamin C can be used to prevent postinflammatory pigment alteration (PIPA) after procedures because it inhibits tyrosinase, decreases inflammation and quenches free radicals. In one study, the application of topical vitamin C two or more weeks after surgery reduced the duration and degree of erythema in a study of 10 patients receiving skin resurfacing with a carbon dioxide laser.[15]

Stretch Marks

Stretch marks can be red, white, or brown in color. Ascorbic acid can improve the texture of stretch marks by increasing collagen synthesis. The depigmenting effects can lighten the pigmentation associated with stretch marks. The anti-inflammatory capabilities of ascorbic acid may also help diminish the redness associated with these lesions. This unique combination of properties renders ascorbic acid an ideal ingredient to treat all types of stretch marks. In a comparison of topical vitamin C and glycolic acid to tretinoin and glycolic acid for the treatment of striae alba, both preparations resulted in an objective improvement, though only the tretinoin/glycolic acid combination increased elastin content of the striae.[16]

SAFETY ISSUES

Vitamin C is an essential nutrient and is safe for oral consumption. After a thorough review by the Cosmetic Ingredient Review Expert Panel, L-ascorbic acid and various esters, including calcium ascorbate, magnesium ascorbate, magnesium ascorbyl phosphate, sodium, ascorbate, and sodium ascorbyl phosphate, were deemed safe in topical cosmetic formulations.[17]

ENVIRONMENTAL IMPACT

Vitamin C is not the specific target in the cultivation of the numerous fruits and vegetables that contain it but its collection is implicit and essential for human health. It is unlikely that its use has any deleterious effects on the environment. Organic forms of vitamin C are available.

FORMULATION CONSIDERATIONS

Ascorbic acid is hydrophilic and very unstable due to its ability to rapidly oxidize. Multiple topical preparations contain vitamin C; however, many of these products have problems with stability and their utility is questionable (Table 40-1). The companies IS

TABLE 40-1
Pros and Cons of Vitamin C

Pros	Cons
Potent anti-inflammatory and antioxidant activity	Difficult to formulate
Strong safety profile	Topical forms are expensive
Tyrosinase inhibitor	Does not readily penetrate the skin
Oral ingestion results in increased skin levels	Not very effective when used as monotherapy
Oral forms are inexpensive	
Readily found in diet	

Clinical, Skinceuticals, and La Roche-Posay have developed stabilized vitamin C preparations that are packaged in a manner intended to minimize inactivation of this easily degraded product. Specifically, the packaging of these products limits ultraviolet (UV) and air exposure from rapidly oxidizing vitamin C. However, these formulations do not contain magnesium-L-ascorbyl-2-phosphate, the form of ascorbic acid that is the strongest tyrosinase inhibitor.

Magnesium-L-ascorbyl-2-phosphate is a stable derivative of ascorbic acid, an ascorbate ester developed specifically to improve stability, absorption, and hypopigmenting activity.[18] One study examining the effects of daily topical application of magnesium-L-ascorbyl-2-phosphate on patients with melasma or senile lentigos demonstrated a significant lightening effect in 19 of 34 patients.[4] However, percutaneous absorption of magnesium ascorbyl phosphate is marginal because it is a charged molecule, making it difficult to traverse the stratum corneum.

USAGE CONSIDERATIONS

Ascorbic acid penetrates best in a pH of 2-2.5; therefore, an acidic environment is necessary. For this reason, it is optimal to use ascorbic acid after a low-pH cleanser such as a glycolic acid or a salicylic acid product. Combining with other acidic agents such as azelaic acid may be useful. However, ascorbic acid is unstable and can be so easily oxidized that it is crucial to apply it in the correct order in a regimen to ensure its stability and maximize the chance of penetration. Combining ascorbic acid with ferulic acid has been shown to enhance its stability (see Chapter 54, Ferulic Acid). Combinations with phloretin may enhance its depigmentation ability as well (see Chapter 52, Phloretin), but more studies are needed to determine its usefulness in the treatment and prevention of pigmentation disorders when combined with other ingredients.

SIGNIFICANT BACKGROUND

In addition to its utility as a depigmenting agent, vitamin C has antioxidant properties and has been shown to stimulate collagen synthesis [see Chapter 55, Ascorbic Acid (Vitamin C)].

CONCLUSION

Vitamin C preparations are safe and effective in ameliorating hyperpigmentation, striae, and postlaser erythema, as well as preventing or mitigating the harmful effects of UV radiation. While a versatile agent in dermatology, vitamin C is more commonly used to treat pigmentation disorders in countries that do not allow hydroquinone and its derivatives. It is most effective when used in combination with another agent.

REFERENCES

1. Shindo Y, Witt E, Han D, et al. Enzymic and non-enzymic antioxidants in epidermis and dermis of human skin. *J Invest Dermatol.* 1994;102:122.
2. Farris PK. Topical vitamin C: A useful agent for treating photoaging and other dermatologic conditions. *Dermatol Surg.* 2005;31:814.
3. Lerner AB, Fitzpatrick TB. Biochemistry of melanin formation. *Physiol Rev.* 1950;30:91.
4. Kameyama K, Sakai C, Kondoh S, et al. Inhibitory effect of magnesium l-ascorbyl-2-phosphate (VC-PMG) on melanogenesis in vitro and in vivo. *J Am Acad Dermatol.* 1996;34:29.
5. Pinnell SR, Murad S, Darr D. Induction of collagen synthesis by ascorbic acid: A possible mechanism. *Arch Dermatol.* 1987;123:1684.
6. Wang PC, Huang YL, Hou SS, et al. Lauroyl/palmitoyl glycol chitosan gels enhance skin delivery of magnesium ascorbyl phosphate. *J Cosmet Sci.* 2013;64:273.
7. National Library of Medicine Hazardous Substances Database. Ascorbic Acid – Compound Summary: Biomedical Effects and Toxicity – Absorption, Distribution and Excretion. http://pubchem.ncbi.nlm.nih.gov/summary/summary.cgi?cid=54670067. Accessed October 22, 2013.
8. Ros JR, Rodríguez-López JN, García-Cánovas F. Effect of l-ascorbic acid on the monophenolase activity of tyrosinase. *Biochem J.* 1993;295:309.
9. Gukasyan GS. Study of the kinetics of oxidation of monophenols by tyrosinase: The effect of reducers. *Biochemistry (Mosc).* 2002;67:277.
10. Kim H, Choi HR, Kim DS, et al. Topical hypopigmenting agents for pigmentary disorders and their mechanisms of action. *Ann Dermatol.* 2012;24:1.
11. Espinal-Perez LE, Moncada B, Castanedo-Cazares JP. A double-blind randomized trial of 5% ascorbic acid vs. 4% hydroquinone in melasma. *Int J Dermatol.* 2004;43:604.
12. Huh CH, Seo KI, Park JY, et al. A randomized, double-blind, placebo-controlled trial of vitamin C iontophoresis in melasma. *Dermatology.* 2003;206:316.
13. Callender VD, St Surin-Lord S, Davis EC, et al. Postinflammatory hyperpigmentation: Etiologic and therapeutic considerations. *Am J Clin Dermatol.* 2011;12:87.
14. Parvez S, Kang M, Chung HS, et al. Survey and mechanism of skin depigmenting and lightening agents. *Phytother Res.* 2006;20:921.
15. Alster TS, West TB. Effect of topical vitamin C on postoperative carbon dioxide laser resurfacing erythema. *Dermatol Surg.* 1998;24:331.
16. Ash K, Lord J, Zukowski M, et al. Comparison of topical therapy for striae alba (20% glycolic acid/0.05% tretinoin versus 20% glycolic acid/10% L-ascorbic acid). *Dermatol Surg.* 1998;24:849.
17. Elmore AR. Final report of the safety assessment of l-ascorbic acid, calcium ascorbate, magnesium ascorbate, magnesium ascorbyl phosphate, sodium ascorbate, and sodium ascorbyl phosphate as used in cosmetics. *Int J Toxicol.* 2005;24(Suppl 2):51.
18. Solano F, Briganti S, Picardo M, et al. Hypopigmenting agents: An updated review on biological, chemical and clinical aspects. *Pigment Cell Res.* 2006;19:550.

CHAPTER 41

Cucumber

Activities:

Antityrosinase, antioxidant, anti-inflammatory, anti-hyaluronidase, anti-elastase

Important Chemical Components:

Extracts: glycosides, steroids, flavonoids, lutein, carbohydrates, tannins, and terpenoids.[1,2] A group of triterpenoids known as cucurbitacins (particularly cucurbitacin D and 23, 24-dihydrocucurbitacin D),[3] cucumegastigmanes I and II, cucumerin A and B, vitexin, orientin, isoscoparin 2"-O-(6"-(E)-p-coumaroyl) glucoside, apigenin 7-O-(6"-O-p-coumaroylglucoside)[4]

Pulp: Water, ascorbic acid (vitamin C), caffeic acid, lactic acid[4]

Seeds: α- and β-amyrin, sitosterols, cucurbitasides[2]

Origin Classification:

This ingredient is considered natural. Organic forms are available.

Personal Care Category:

Depigmenting, anti-inflammatory, occlusive, emollient, sun protective, antioxidant, antiwrinkle, scar treatment, and first aid for burns

Recommended for the following Baumann Skin Types:

DRPT, DRPW, DSPT, DSPW, ORPT, ORPW, OSPT, and OSPW

SOURCE

Cucumis sativus, an annual creeping vine, is a member of the Cucurbitaceae family, which also includes pumpkin, zucchini, watermelon, and squash. Found wildly in the Himalayan region and commonly referred to as cucumber in English, *khira* in Hindi, *sakusa* as well as *trapusah* in Sanskrit, *sasa* in Bengali, and *vellarikkay* in Tamil, the plant is cultivated throughout India and China, in particular, as well as Europe and the United States.[2,5] It is grown as a food crop, with its fruit, the cucumber, found in many cuisines as well as a component in traditional medicine and folk cosmetics.[6]

HISTORY

C. sativus has been cultivated in Asia for 3,000 years as a food source (Table 41-1).[7] It has also long been used for cosmetic purposes as the cucumber is known to impart a healing, soothing, and cooling effect to irritated skin.[7] Its use for treating hyperpigmentation dates back centuries.[5] The leaves, fruits, and seeds of *C. sativus* have been used in traditional Indian medicine, especially Ayurveda, to treat numerous skin

TABLE 41-1
Pros and Cons of Cucumber

Pros	Cons
Uses for skin care date back to antiquity	Paucity of research and clinical data to buttress traditional claims
Broad spectrum of reported activity	No studies on use in rosacea
Anti-inflammatory activity makes cucumber a good choice for treating sensitive skin	

conditions, including sunburn and under-eye swelling, and it has been noted for its soothing, antipruritic, emollient effects.[5] Other medical indications for cucumber arose during its early use, and included headaches and acne (for which the fruit juice was used as a demulcent in lotions); the seeds were also used as a diuretic.[2] In traditional Chinese medicine, the leaves, roots, and stems of the plant have been used to detoxify as well as to treat diarrhea and gonorrhea.[6] In addition, the application of cucumber slices to ameliorate swelling or dark circles under the eyes has long been accepted throughout the world as an effective treatment.

CHEMISTRY

The activity that cucumber exhibits in suppressing tyrosinase and melanin production is attributed to its primary bioactive components cucurbitacin D and 23, 24-dihydrocucurbitacin D.[3,8] These bitter compounds are also thought to be characteristic of the species and have displayed anti-inflammatory, purgative, and antifertility activity *in vitro* and *in vivo*.[4] Other important constituents of cucumber include lutein and ascorbic acid.

ORAL USES

By far, its primary use is in the culinary realm. Cucumber, considered a fruit botanically but a vegetable gastronomically, is cultivated throughout the world as a seasonal vegetable and is particularly popular in India and the Middle East.

TOPICAL USES

Cucumber extracts can be found in a wide range of over-the-counter skin care creams, lotions, and eye gels for various indications, primarily to soothe and soften skin and to treat wrinkles and sunburn. Skin whitening, though, is also one of the indications increasingly seen for this botanical.

Early in 2011, Akhtar et al. reported on their efforts to formulate a topical water in oil (w/o) emulsion of 3 percent cucumber extracts and evaluate it according to multiple parameters versus its base as a control (lacking cucumber ingredients) in 21 healthy volunteers over four weeks. The use of the cucumber formulation yielded statistically significant reductions in sebum and a decline in melanin content that was not statistically significant. Transepidermal water loss and erythema were elevated by the test formulation, but these changes were also not statistically significant. There were also statistically nonsignificant differences found between the base and formulation in altering melanin content through four weeks, gradually reducing melanin content over the final three weeks after an initial mild increase in the case of the formulation. The authors concluded that their findings point to the potential for cucumber extracts to be effective ingredients in skin care agents for medical and cosmetic purposes, particularly skin whitening, though more research is necessary.[3]

SAFETY ISSUES

Though rare, there have been a few reports of contact dermatitis and urticaria in reaction to cucumber.[9,10] Of course, this edible plant is considered safe and its fruit is consumed throughout the world.

ENVIRONMENTAL IMPACT

Despite a long history of traditional use and anecdotal evidence, there is no scientific basis for the use of *C. sativus* in folk cosmetics.[6] Not surprisingly, then, the harvesting of cucumber fruits typically results in the remaining plant parts being left as waste. No significant environmental damage from the industry has been reported.

FORMULATION CONSIDERATIONS

None known by author.

USAGE CONSIDERATIONS

No interactions with other ingredients are known by the author.

SIGNIFICANT BACKGROUND

Analgesic, Antioxidant, Anticancer, Antiwrinkle Activity

In 2002, Villaseñor et al. assessed the comparative effectiveness of sugar beet roots, cucumber fruits, New Zealand spinach leaves, and turmeric rhizomes against dimethylbenz[a]anthracene (DMBA)-initiated and croton oil-promoted skin tumors in a Swiss Webster albino mouse model using three different protocols. The four species were selected based on prior findings of antioxidant activity and effectiveness in preventing skin tumors induced in laboratory settings. All four displayed antioxidant activity and all were found to be effective in lowering skin tumor incidence and the number of skin tumors as well as delaying the onset of skin tumor formation in comparison to the control, with turmeric exhibiting the greatest potency.[11]

In 2010, Kumar et al. evaluated the aqueous fruit extract of *C. sativus* for free radical-scavenging and analgesic activities using *in vitro* and *in vivo* models. Preliminary phytochemical screening indicated that cucumber contains various classes of compounds known to exert antioxidant as well as analgesic activity, including flavonoids and tannins. The investigators found that the fruit extract showed maximum antioxidant and analgesic effect at 500 µg/mL and 500 mg/kg, respectively, though the exact constituents of *C. sativus* fruits responsible for the promising effects were not elucidated by the study.[2]

In 2011, Nema et al. subjected the lyophilized juice of *C. sativus* fruit to 1,1-diphenyl-2-picrylhydrazyl (DPPH) and

superoxide radical-scavenging assays, in reference to butylated hydroxytoluene, as well as hyaluronidase and elastase inhibitory assays, in reference to oleanolic acid. The cucumber juice, rich in ascorbic acid, was found to display significant free radical scavenging activity as well as potent anti-hyaluronidase and anti-elastase activity. The researchers concluded that *C. sativus* warrants consideration for its potential use as an antiwrinkle ingredient in cosmetic formulations.[5]

Skin Whitening

In 2008, Kai et al. assessed six plant parts of *C. sativus* to compare inhibitory effects on melanogenesis. They found that methanol extracts of the leaves and stems suppressed melanin production in cultured B_{16} mouse melanoma cells. Although they did not alter mushroom tyrosinase activity or crude enzyme lysate activity in these cells, the methanol extracts did reduce tyrosinase expression at the protein level. The researchers suggested that these findings indicate that the depigmenting activity of *C. sativus* extracts is associated with the downregulation rather than inhibition of tyrosinase. They also found that lutein, of eight compounds isolated from the leaves, inhibited melanogenesis, significantly lowering tyrosinase expression. The investigators concluded that *C. sativus* leaves and, especially, lutein effectively suppress tyrosinase expression and deserve consideration for skin-whitening indications.[6]

The roots of Chinese cucumber (*Trichosanthes kirilowii*), a member of the Cucurbitaceae family, have been used in traditional Chinese medicine as an anti-inflammatory agent and also as an abortifacient. Significantly, *T. kirilowii* and *C. sativus* share some of the same primary active constituents. In 2002, Oh et al. isolated cucurbitacin D and 23,24-dihydrocucurbitacin D from the root of *T. kirilowii* via tyrosinase inhibitory activity-guided fractionation. The investigators found that the compounds effectively inhibited tyrosinase activity as well as melanin synthesis in B_{16}/F_{10} melanoma cells.[12]

CONCLUSION

The use of cucumber as an effective agent for the temporary relief of swollen eyes, or dark circles under the eyes, has been established. Also, cucumber has an anecdotal reputation as a diuretic systemically and topically acting against water retention, thus ameliorating burns, dermatitis, and swollen eyes. This folk medicine success or popularity has, perhaps, spurred the inclusion of *C. sativa* in various skin care products. There is a dearth of research on the dermatologic benefits of the plant, however. Its anti-inflammatory activity nevertheless makes it a good choice as a lightening ingredient for individuals with sensitive skin types. In the author's experience, the anti-inflammatory activities are mild and have not proven to be of much benefit in the treatment of rosacea. Much more research is necessary to determine the appropriate role of cucumber in dermatology but its potential is intriguing.

REFERENCES

1. Gandía-Herrero F, Jiménez M, Cabanes J, et al. Tyrosinase inhibitory activity of cucumber compounds: Enzymes responsible for browning in cucumber. *J Agric Food Chem*. 2003;51:7764.
2. Kumar D, Kumar S, Singh J, et al. Free radical scavenging and analgesic activities of Cucumis sativus L. fruit extract. *J Young Pharm*. 2010;2:365.
3. Akhtar N, Mehmood A, Khan BA, et al. Exploring cucumber extract for skin rejuvenation. *African J Biotechnol*. 2011;10:1206.

4. Mukherjee PK, Nema NK, Maity N, et al. Phytochemical and therapeutic potential of cucumber. *Fitoterapia*. 2013;84:227.

5. Nema NK, Maity N, Sarkar B, et al. Cucumis sativus fruit-potential antioxidant, anti-hyaluronidase, and anti-elastase agent. *Arch Dermatol Res*. 2011;303:247.

6. Kai H, Baba M, Okuyama T. Inhibitory effect of Cucumis sativus on melanin production in melanoma B_{16} cells by downregulation of tyrosinase expression. *Planta Med*. 2008;74:1785.

7. Grieve M. *A Modern Herbal*. Vol. 1. New York: Dover Publications; 1971:239–240.

8. Chen JC, Chiu MH, Nie RL, et al. Cucurbitacins and cucurbitane glycosides: structures and biological activities. *Nat Prod Rep*. 2005;22:386.

9. Zachariae CO. Cucumber contact dermatitis. *Contact Dermatitis*. 2000;43:240.

10. Weltfriend S, Kwangsukstith C, Maibach HI. Contact urticaria from cucumber pickle and strawberry. *Contact Dermatitis*. 1995;32:173.

11. Villaseñor IM, Simon MK, Villanueva AM. Comparative potencies of nutraceuticals in chemically induced skin tumor prevention. *Nutr Cancer*. 2002;44:66.

12. Oh H, Mun YJ, IM SJ, et al. Cucurbitacins from Trichosanthes kirilowii as the inhibitory components on tyrosinase activity and melanin synthesis of B_{16}/F_{10} melanoma cells. *Planta Med*. 2002;68:832.

CHAPTER 42

Lignin Peroxidase

Activities:

Skin lightening

Important Chemical Components:

Also known as diarylpropane oxygenase, diarylpropane peroxidase, ligninase I, and LiP, lignin peroxidase catalyzes the following reaction: 1,2-bis(3,4-dimethoxyphenyl) propane-1,3-diol+H_2O_2 ⇌ 3,4-dimethoxybenzaldehyde + 1-(3,4-dimethoxyphenyl)ethane-1,2-diol + H_2O. The molecular formulae for lignin are $C_9H_{10}O_2$, $C_{10}H_{12}O_3$, $C_{11}H_{14}O_4$.

Origin Classification:

This a naturally occurring enzyme derived from one of the most abundant organic polymers that is highly processed for commercial use.

Personal Care Category:

Depigmenting, toning

Recommended for the following Baumann Skin Types:

DRPT, DRPW, DSPT, DSPW, ORPT, ORPW, OSPT, and OSPW

SOURCE

Derived from the white-rot tree fungus *Phanerochaete chrysosporium*, lignin peroxidase is a naturally occurring enzyme identified as the enzyme responsible for breaking down lignin in decaying trees, resulting in rapid decolorization.[1] Lignin peroxidase emerges extracellularly during submerged fermentation of the *P. chrysosporium* fungus and is then purified from the fermented liquid medium.[2,3]

HISTORY

The enzyme lignin peroxidase was first identified in 1984, and has been studied for many years as a potential agent to break down lignin in order to whiten wood pulp in paper production.[4] It was subsequently found to break down eumelanin, which has a similar chemical structure to lignin. The development of lignin peroxidase as a skin-lightening agent resulted from these discoveries.[3,5] In 2004, Woo et al. published the first report indicating that lignin peroxidase/hydrogen peroxide (H_2O_2) had the capacity to eliminate the pigment in synthetic melanin.[1,3]

CHEMISTRY

Lignin, an organic polymer found in the cell walls of plants, is similar in molecular structure to melanin as well as coal. In 1994, *P. chrysosporium* was found to cause decolorization and depolymerization of low-grade coal in culture conditions conducive to mineralization of lignin.[3,6] Recent research has verified that lignin peroxidase has the potential to break down or depolymerize melanin.[3]

ORAL USES

This agent is for topical use only.

TOPICAL USES

A trademarked (by Syneron of Israel) lignin peroxidase formulation, Melanozyme is a glycoprotein active at pH 2 to 4.5, above which it is inactive (5.5 is the normal pH of skin, with some variation between 5.0 and 6.5), that identifies epidermal eumelanin and breaks it down without suppressing tyrosinase or affecting melanin biosynthesis. Melanozyme, produced in liquid form by Lonza of Switzerland in a proprietary, high-yield production process that produces a commercially concentrated formulation, is available only in the new skin-lightening product known as Elure.

The two-sided product includes Melanozyme on one side and an activator containing H_2O_2 0.12 percent that oxidizes, thereby activating the lignin peroxidase to lighten the skin and even skin tone.[7] Melanozyme could not lighten the skin without the activating role of H_2O_2, which is applied to the skin surface after Melanozyme. After the enzyme is oxidized, it is reduced by a substrate molecule, such as veratryl alcohol, before the melanin is oxidized. After application of the formulation (lotion or cream), the individual's cutaneous pH temporarily declines to 3.5 before rebounding to the normal level, as the enzyme is inactivated. At that stage, it becomes a simple glycoprotein hydrolyzed in the skin into amino acids by naturally occurring proteases and other glycosidases. At the time this book was published, Melanozyme was the only lignin peroxidase established as an effective skin-lightening agent.

SAFETY ISSUES

The safety of lignin peroxidase as a skin-lightening active ingredient has been demonstrated in preclinical studies with doses that are 17,000 times the recommended dose without prompting any side effects.[8] Lignin peroxidase is nonmutagenic and nonirritating to eyes. The potential for skin irritation is very low and in studies of 50 subjects each, there were no reports of skin irritation during acute sensitivity, cumulative sensitivity, or when used in sensitized skin (Table 42-1).

ENVIRONMENTAL IMPACT

Global production of lignin is approximately 1.1 million metric tons annually.[9] Lignin peroxidase represents a very small fraction of this output. The culling and processing of lignin is a highly industrialized process and likely exacts some toll, but this is a renewable resource.

TABLE 42-1
Pros and Cons of Lignin Peroxidase

Pro	Cons
Strong safety profile	Paucity of research to establish effectiveness
	H_2O_2 is required to potentiate its activity in current formulations
	No activity on pheomelanin

FORMULATION CONSIDERATIONS

New formulations that do not contain H_2O_2 are currently being researched.[7]

USAGE CONSIDERATIONS

The Melanozyme ingredient is active at pH 2 to 4.5 so it needs to be in an acidic environment. It can be used in combination with acidic agents such as hydroxy acids.

SIGNIFICANT BACKGROUND

In 2004, Woo et al. isolated and identified the melanin decolorization fungus and depigmented the melanin biopolymer with lignin peroxidase and H_2O_2, and further showed that crude lignin peroxidase prepared from culture broth could also decolorize human skin pigment.[3]

In 2011, Mauricio et al. conducted a randomized, double-blind, placebo-controlled, split-face, single-center study of 51 women of East Asian (Chinese and Korean) and Southeast Asian (Filipino, Thai, and Vietnamese) ethnicity (ranging in age from 20 to 60 years and Fitzpatrick skin types 3 to 5) to assess the skin-lightening safety and efficacy of lignin peroxidase creams compared with 2 percent hydroquinone (HQ) cream and placebo. Participants were randomized to receive lignin peroxidase day and night creams for one side of the face and HQ cream or placebo for the other. Whereas no statistically significant lightening effect was seen with either HQ or placebo, the researchers noted a statistically significant mean reduction in the melanin index of 7.6 percent from baseline associated with the lignin peroxidase side. In addition, patients preferred the lignin peroxidase products. Overall, a more rapid and observable skin-lightening effect was observed with the lignin peroxidase creams.[7]

CONCLUSION

Lignin peroxidase shows potential to enter the ever-expanding list of viable skin-lightening agents. While the few extant results suggest such efficacy, much more research is necessary to establish this ingredient as a suitable alternative in the depigmenting armamentarium. In the author's experience, this ingredient works well in skin types with an Asian ancestry and less well in other demographic groups, likely due to the ratio of eumelanin to pheomelanin in various ethnicities. Those with a preponderance of eumelanin will have better efficacy with this ingredient.

REFERENCES

1. Nagasaki K, Kumazawa M, Murakami S, et al. Purification, characterization, and gene cloning of Ceriporiopsis sp. Strain MD-1 peroxidases that decolorize human hair melanin. *Appl Environ Microbiol.* 2008;74:5106.
2. Spruit D. The interference of some substances with the water vapour loss of human skin. *Dermatologica.* 1971;142(2):89–92.
3. Woo S, Cho J, Lee B, et al. Decolorization of melanin by lignin peroxidase from Phanerochaete chrysosporium. *Biotechnol Bioprocess Eng.* 2004;9:256.
4. Gold MH, Kuwahara M, Chiu AA, et al. Purification and characterization of an extracellular H_2O_2-requiring diarylpropane oxygenase from the white rot basidiomycete, Phanerochaete chrysosporium. *Arch Biochem Biophys.* 1984;234:353.
5. USPTO Patent Applicatioin 20060051305. Methods of producing lignin peroxidase and its use in skin and hair lightening.
6. Ralph JP, Catchesidex DEA. Decolourisation and depolymerisation of solubilised low lank coal by the white rot basidiomycete Phanerochaete chrysosporium. *Appl Microbiol Biotechnol.* 1994;42:536.
7. Mauricio T, Karmon Y, Khaiat A. A randomized and placebo-controlled study to compare the skin-lightening efficacy and safety of lignin peroxidase cream vs. 2% hydroquinone cream. *J Cosmet Dermatol.* 2011;10:253.
8. Data on file. Rakuto Bio Technologies, 5 Carmel Street, P.O. Box 528, New Industrial Park, Yokneam, 20692.
9. Higson A, Smith C. The National Non-Food Crops Centre (NNFCC) Renewable Chemicals Factsheet: Lignin. http://www.nnfcc.co.uk/publications/nnfcc-renewable-chemicals-factsheet-lignin. Accessed June 17, 2013.

CHAPTER 43

Overview of the PAR-2 Receptor

Protease-activated receptor-2 (PAR-2) is a G-protein-coupled receptor that is able to enhance the capacity of keratinocytes to ingest melanosomes from the neighboring melanocyte. Each melanocyte is in contact with an average of 36 keratinocytes forming an "epidermal melanin unit" (Figure 43-1).[1,2] Once melanin is created within melanosomes, it migrates into the dendrite tips of the melanocyte and is then incorporated into other keratinocytes of the epidermal melanin unit. Although the exact process of melanin transfer is not completely understood, PAR-2 has been shown to play an important role.[3] The PAR-2 can be up- or downregulated, and is upregulated by ultraviolet radiation.[4] It is thought to be important in hyperpigmentation disorders because it has been found that serine protease inhibitors that interfere with PAR-2 activation induce depigmentation by reducing melanosome transfer and distribution.[5] Soybeans, which contain the serine protease inhibitors soybean trypsin inhibitor (STI) and Bowman–Birk protease inhibitor (BBI),

have been demonstrated to inhibit melanosome transfer, resulting in an improvement of mottled facial pigmentation.[6] In addition, activation of PAR-2 with trypsin and other synthetic peptides has been shown to result in visible skin darkening.[5]

Other systems play a role in melanosome transfer as well. For example, β-amyloid precursor protein (APP) is a newly detected epidermal growth factor that has been demonstrated to increase the release of melanin as well as enhance the movements of the melanocyte dendritic tips.[7] Keratinocyte growth factor also promotes melanosome transfer by stimulating the phagocytic process.[8] Many different factors affect melanosome transfer and play a role in the complex pigmentation process. At this time, only PAR-2 blockers have been added in cosmeceutical skin care products to block the transfer of melanosomes, so this section will focus on these agents. PAR-2 blockers do not break down melanin that is already in keratinocytes; therefore, results will not be seen for 8 to 16 weeks of using such skin care products.

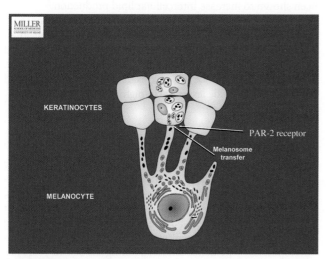

▲ **FIGURE 43-1** Epidermal melanin unit. One melanocyte can intercalate with many keratinocytes.

REFERENCES

1. Jimbow K, Quevedo WC Jr, Fitzpatrick TB, et al. Some aspects of melanin biology: 1950–1975. *J Invest Dermatol.* 1976;67:72.
2. Nordlund JJ. The melanocyte and the epidermal melanin unit: An expanded concept. *Dermatol Clin.* 2007;25:271.
3. Seiberg M, Paine C, Sharlow E, et al. Inhibition of melanosome transfer results in skin lightening. *J Invest Dermatol.* 2000;115:162.
4. Seiberg M. Keratinocyte-melanocyte interactions during melanosome transfer. *Pigment Cell Res.* 2001;14:236.
5. Seiberg M, Paine C, Sharlow E, et al. The protease-activated receptor 2 regulates pigmentation via keratinocyte-melanocyte interactions. *Exp Cell Res.* 2000;254:25.
6. Wallo W, Nebus J, Leyden JJ. Efficacy of a soy moisturizer in photoaging: a double-blind, vehicle-controlled, 12-week study. *J Drugs Dermatol.* 2007;6:917.
7. Quast T, Wehner S, Kirfel G, et al. sAPP as a regulator of dendrite motility and melanin release in epidermal melanocytes and melanoma cells. *FASEB J.* 2003;17:1739.
8. Cardinali G, Bolasco G, Aspite N, et al. Melanosome transfer promoted by keratinocyte growth factor in light and dark skin-derived keratinocytes. *J Invest Dermatol.* 2008;128:558.

CHAPTER 44

Niacinamide

Activities:

PAR-2 inhibition, anti-inflammatory, antioxidant, antiaging, photoprotective

Important Chemical Components:

Also known as nicotinamide (and 3-pyridinecarboxamide), molecular formula is $C_6H_6N_2O$

Origin Classification:

Natural vitamin constituent of various foods but the cosmetic ingredient is laboratory made

Personal Care Category:

Depigmenting, exfoliant

Recommended for the following Baumann Skin Types:

Is a superior choice for dry, sensitive and wrinkle-prone skin types. Best for DRNT, DRNW, DRPT, DRPW, DSNT, DSNW, DSPT, DSPW, ORPT, ORPW, OSPT, OSPW, OSNT, and OSNW.

SOURCE

Niacinamide, also known as nicotinamide, is the biologically active amide of niacin (vitamin B_3). This form of the vitamin is found naturally in a wide variety of foods, particularly root vegetables, mushrooms, yeasts, some fruits, peanuts, and seeds.[1,2] Significantly, the effects of niacinamide on pigmentation have been shown to be reversible (Table 44-1).[3]

HISTORY

Research on and the use of oral niacinamide dates back to the 1930s, but the data on the use of topical niacinamide are relatively new. The first use of topical niacinamide to ameliorate skin barrier function in individuals with pellagra, which is characterized by pronounced cutaneous sensitivity to sunlight, was reported in 1976.[4–6] For over 40 years, niacinamide has been used in dermatology for a broad array of disorders including acne, atopic dermatitis, autoimmune bullous dermatoses, excess sebum, as well as rosacea,

TABLE 44-1
Pros and Cons of Niacinamide

Pros	Cons
PAR-2 blocking agent	Not well known by consumers
Water soluble	Not as potent as hydroquinone
Easily tolerated	No organic or natural forms are available on the market
Anti-inflammatory	
Can be formulated in SPF	
No interactions with other ingredients	

and more recently to treat hyperpigmentation and to prevent photoaging and photoimmunosuppression.[7,8]

CHEMISTRY

Niacinamide is an important part of the niacin coenzymes nicotinamide adenine dinucleotide (NAD+) and nicotinamide adenine dinucleotide phosphate (NADP+), and their respective reduced forms the antioxidants NADH and NADPH. These compounds contribute to cellular oxidation and reduction reactions as well as DNA synthesis and repair, are involved in over 200 enzymatic reactions, and may play a role in providing cosmetic benefits.[2,9–11] Surjana and Damian suggest that niacinamide is able to confer clinical effects because of its role as a cellular energy precursor, a modulator of inflammatory cytokines, and a suppressor of the nuclear enzyme poly(adenosine diphosphate-ribose) polymerase-1.[7] It has also been shown to increase intercellular lipid production.[3,12]

Niacinamide has been demonstrated to suppress melanosome transfer to epidermal keratinocytes, by up to 68 percent in an *in vitro* model, and to render improvement in undesired facial pigmentation.[9] This inhibition of melanosome transfer from melanocytes to keratinocytes is considered the primary method by which niacinamide lessens skin pigmentation.

ORAL USES

The nutritional value of niacin or niacinamide has been long understood. Niacinamide is found in various vegetables (particularly asparagus and root vegetables), mushrooms, yeasts, some fruits, peanuts, and seeds. Oral niacinamide is best known for curing pellagra, but it has also been linked to playing a role in preventing insulin-dependent diabetes mellitus development.[9,13] Evidence amassed during the last 15 years has also shown that oral niacinamide has prevented photocarcinogenesis in mice, as well as protected against photoimmunosuppression in humans and mice.[14–16] In addition, recent results of phase II double-blinded randomized controlled trials led by Surjana et al. indicate that oral niacinamide (500 mg) effectively diminishes actinic keratoses and shows potential for chemopreventive activity against skin cancer.[17]

TOPICAL USES

Niacinamide has been used for various indications in dermatology, including acne and rosacea.[18–20] This water-soluble vitamin is known to be a significant active ingredient in moisturizers intended to improve xerosis and stratum corneum (SC) barrier function.[4] In addition, it has recently been shown in topical form to protect against UVA and UVB radiation and is thought to be a promising agent to prevent against skin cancer.[21]

In a 2005 study, twice daily application of a 5 percent niacinamide preparation for 8 weeks yielded significant improvement in hyperpigmentation as did the use of 3.5 percent niacinamide combined with retinyl palmitate.[22]

In 2013, Mohammed et al. studied the effects of twice-daily application of a niacinamide-containing formulation for 28 days on the left and right mid-volar forearms of 20 healthy volunteers in terms of transepidermal water loss (TEWL), corneocyte surface area and maturity, SC thickness, and selected protease activities. Overall, areas treated with niacinamide-containing formulations exhibited larger and more mature corneocytes, less inflammatory activity and TEWL, and greater SC thickness as compared to pre-treatment baseline and areas left untreated or treated with vehicle control. The investigators concluded that niacinamide displays unique SC barrier-bolstering qualities and merits consideration as a topical formulation adjunct.[4] During the last decade, though, its greatest application in dermatology has been thought to be in relation to its activity as a depigmenting agent.

Combination Therapy

In 2006, Hakozaki et al. studied the effects of combining high-frequency ultrasound with topical skin-lightening agents (ascorbyl glucoside and niacinamide) on facial hyperpigmentation in 60 Japanese women. They found in their four-week clinical trial that the use of ultrasound radiation along with skin-lightening gel significantly diminished facial hyperpigmentation spots as compared with no treatment and skin-lightening gel alone, which they attributed to the facilitating effect of ultrasound on the transepidermal transport of the topical agents.[23]

In 2009, Bissett et al. performed two double-blind, 10-week, left-right randomized, split-face clinical studies to ascertain if the combination of N-undecyl-10-enoyl-L-phenylalanine, which has reportedly lowered melanin production in cultured melanocytes, and niacinamide is more effective than niacinamide alone in diminishing facial hyperpigmentation. In one study, 80 Japanese women (76 of whom completed the study) randomized into two groups each applied one of two formulation pairs to the randomly assigned side of the face, a vehicle control and a 5 percent niacinamide formulation, or a 5 percent niacinamide and a 5 percent niacinamide plus 1 percent N-undecylenoyl phenylalanine formulation. In the other study, 152 Caucasian women (of whom 147 completed the study) applied either vehicle control, a 5 percent niacinamide formulation, or a 5 percent niacinamide and 1 percent N-undecylenoyl-phenylalanine combination formulation to the randomly assigned side of the face. The investigators found that the combination formulation was more effective than the vehicle or niacinamide alone in improving the appearance of hyperpigmentation in both studies. They concluded that this combination formulation is an effective antiaging agent for facial skin.[24]

Early in the next year, Jerajani et al. measured the effects in 246 Indian women (aged 30–60 years) with epidermal hyperpigmentation of the daily use of a lotion containing niacinamide, panthenol, and tocopherol acetate for 10 weeks. In this randomized, double-blind trial, which 207 women completed, those who used the well-tolerated test formulation experienced significant improvements in the appearance of hyperpigmentation, skin tone, and texture as compared to controls.[25]

Also in 2010, Kimball et al. conducted a 10-week, double-blind, vehicle-controlled, full-face, parallel-group clinical study in 202 women (aged 40–60 years) to evaluate the effects of a combination of niacinamide and N-acetyl glucosamine in a topical moisturizing formulation on irregular facial pigmentation. The evenly divided groups daily applied either a morning sun protection factor (SPF) 15 sunscreen moisturizing lotion and evening moisturizing cream each containing 4 percent niacinamide and 2 percent N-acetyl glucosamine or the SPF 15 lotion and cream vehicles. All measurement parameters revealed that the test formulation was significantly more effective in alleviating detectable hyperpigmentation than the control product and yielded results superior to using an SPF sunscreen alone.[26]

Niacinamide was also a key active ingredient in an SPF 30 moisturizing lotion used in a recent randomized, controlled comparative study on wrinkle reduction. In this eight-week parallel-group study of 196 women with moderate to moderately severe periorbital wrinkles, 99 women used the SPF moisturizer containing 5 percent niacinamide, peptides, and antioxidants; a moisturizing cream containing niacinamide and peptides; and a targeted wrinkle product containing niacinamide, peptides, and 0.3 percent retinyl propionate. The remaining cohort of 97 women used 0.02 percent tretinoin plus moisturizing SPF 30 sunscreen. The niacinamide regimen was significantly better tolerated and provided significantly improved wrinkle appearance compared to the tretinoin group.[27]

SAFETY ISSUES

Niacinamide is very well tolerated by the skin and has an excellent safety profile.

ENVIRONMENTAL IMPACT

Given the widespread availability of plants containing niacinamide, no discrete environmental toll is exacted in the culling of niacinamide specifically.

FORMULATION CONSIDERATIONS

Niacinamide is chemically stable, easily formulated, and compatible with various other potential cosmetic formulation ingredients.[28]

USAGE CONSIDERATIONS

Niacinamide can be used in conjunction with retinoids, sunscreens, hydroxy acids, and other ingredients without concern for cross-reactivity.

SIGNIFICANT BACKGROUND

In 2002, Hakozaki et al. examined the *in vitro* effects of niacinamide on melanogenesis and *in vivo* effects on 18 Japanese women with hyperpigmentation. In cultured melanocytes, niacinamide exerted no effect on mushroom tyrosinase catalytic activity or melanogenesis but significantly inhibited melanosome transfer in a keratinocyte/melanocyte coculture model and decreased cutaneous pigmentation in a pigmented reconstructed epidermis model. In the clinical trial over four weeks, the 18 participants with hyperpigmentation used 5 percent niacinamide moisturizer and a vehicle moisturizer in a paired design, and 120 subjects with facial tanning were assigned to two of three treatments (vehicle, sunscreen, and 2 percent niacinamide plus sunscreen). The investigators found that niacinamide significantly reduced hyperpigmentation and enhanced skin lightness in comparison to vehicle alone. They concluded that niacinamide effectively lightens skin by suppressing melanosome transfer from melanocytes to keratinocytes.[9]

In 2004, Bissett et al. conducted a 12-week, double-blind, placebo-controlled, split-face, left-right randomized clinical study with 50 Causcasian women (aged 40–60 years) to compare a moisturizer containing 5 percent niacinamide and a control moisturizer. The investigators found that the well-tolerated niacinamide formulation imparted significant improvements in fine lines/wrinkles, hyperpigmentation, skin texture, red blotchiness, and sallowness compared to the control product.[28]

The next year, Bissett et al. sought to clinically determine the antiaging effects of topical niacinamide in addition to the well-established improvement on hyperpigmentation. In this 12-week, double-blind, left-right randomized study, 50 white females with clinical signs of facial photoaging twice daily applied 5 percent niacinamide to half of the face and its vehicle control to the other half. The researchers observed that the niacinamide-treated areas demonstrated marked improvement in elasticity as well as in reducing fine lines and wrinkles, hyperpigmented spots, red blotchiness, and skin sallowness.[29]

Also in 2005, Greatens et al. used an *in vitro* melanocyte-keratinocyte coculture to find that both agents are reversible inhibitors of melanosome transfer at concentrations not affecting cell viability. In a related study, the investigators observed that topically applied niacinamide dose-dependently and reversibly diminished hyperpigmented lesions.[3]

CONCLUSION

Niacinamide, the biologically active amide of niacin (vitamin B$_3$), the dearth of which leads to pellagra, has long been known to play an important role in cutaneous health. This versatile vitamin exhibits its most dynamic dermatologic activity as a depigmenting agent. It is a safe and effective alternative to hydroquinone, though not as potent or effective as the standard-bearing depigmenting agent. However, niacinamide has a well-established role in dermatology and its range of indications appears to be broadening. Niacinamide is one of the author's favorite ingredients because of its utility in treating inflammation and pigmentation, and preventing of skin aging and skin cancer, as well as its tolerability.

REFERENCES

1. Leydenx JJ, Shergillx B, Micalix G, et al. Natural options for the management of hyperpigmentation. *J Eur Acad Dermatol Venereol.* 2011;25:1140.
2. Zhu W, Gao J. The use of botanical extracts as topical skin-lightening agents for the improvement of skin pigmentation disorders. *J Investig Dermatol Symp Proc.* 2008;13:20.
3. Greatens A, Hakozaki T, Koshoffer A, et al. Effective inhibition of melanosome transfer to keratinocytes by lectins and niacinamide is reversible. *Exp Dermatol.* 2005;14:498.
4. Mohammed D, Crowther JM, Matts PJ, et al. Influence of niacinamide containing formulations on the molecular and biophysical properties of the stratum corneum. *Int J Pharm.* 2013;441:192.
5. Comaish JS, Felix RH, McGrath H. Topically applied niacinamide in isoniazid-induced pellagra. *Arch Dermatol.* 1976;112:70.
6. Benavente CA, Schnell SA, Jacobson EL. Effects of niacin restriction on sirtuin and PARP responses to photodamage in human skin. *PLoS One.* 2012;7:e42276.
7. Surjana D, Damian DL. Nicotinamide in dermatology and photoprotection. *Skinmed.* 2011;9:360.
8. Namazi MR. Nicotinamide in dermatology: A capsule summary. *Int J Dermatol.* 2007;46:1229.
9. Hakozaki T, Minwalla L, Zhuang J, et al. The effect of niacinamide on reducing cutaneous pigmentation and suppression of melanosome transfer. *Br J Dermatol.* 2002;147:20.
10. Konda S, Geria AN, Halder RM. New horizons in treating disorders of hyperpigmentation in skin color. *Semin Cutan Med Surg.* 2012;31:133.
11. Gillbro JM, Olsson MJ. The melanogenesis and mechanisms of skin-lightening agents – Existing and new approaches. *Int J Cosmet Sci.* 2011;33:210.
12. Sharlow ER, Paine CS, Babiarz L, et al. The protease-activated receptor-2 upregulates keratinocyte phagocytosis. *J Cell Sci.* 2000;113:3093.
13. Elliott RB, Pilcher CC, Fergusson DM, et al. A population based strategy to prevent insulin-dependent diabetes using nicotinamide. *J Pediatr Endocrinol Metab.* 1996;9:501.
14. Gensler HL, Williams T, Huang AC, et al. Oral niacin prevents photocarcinogenesis and photoimmunosuppression in mice. *Nutr Cancer.* 1999;34:36.
15. Damian DL. Photoprotective effects of nicotinamide. *Photochem Photobiol Sci.* 2010;9:578.
16. Yiasemides E, Sivapirabu G, Halliday GM, et al. Oral nicotinamide protects against ultraviolet radiation-induced immunosuppression in humans. *Carcinogenesis.* 2009;30:101.
17. Surjana D, Halliday GM, Martin AJ, et al. Oral nicotinamide reduces actinic keratoses in phase II double-blinded randomized controlled trials. *J Invest Dermatol.* 2012;132:1497.
18. Callender VD, St Surin-Lord S, Davis EC, et al. Postinflammatory hyperpigmentation: Etiologic and therapeutic considerations. *Am J Clin Dermatol.* 2011;12:87.
19. Niren NM, Torok HM. The Nicomide Improvement in Clinical Outcomes Study (NICOS): results of an 8-week trial. *Cutis.* 2006;77(1 Suppl):17.
20. Fowler JF Jr, Woolery-Lloyd H, Waldorf H, et al. Innovations in natural ingredients and their use in skin care. *J Drugs Dermatol.* 2010;9(6 Suppl):S72.
21. Sivapirabu G, Yiasemides E, Halliday GM, et al. Topical nicotinamide modulates cellular energy metabolism and provides broad-spectrum protection against ultraviolet radiation-induced immunosuppression in humans. *Br J Dermatol.* 2009;161:1357.
22. Otte N, Borelli C, Korting HC. Nicotinamide – Biologic actions of an emerging cosmetic ingredient. *Int J Cosmet Sci.* 2005;27:255.
23. Hakozaki T, Takiwaki H, Miyamoto K, et al. Ultrasound enhanced skin-lightening effect of vitamin C and niacinamide. *Skin Res Technol.* 2006;12:105.
24. Bissett DL, Robinson LR, Raleigh PS, et al. Reduction in the appearance of facial hyperpigmentation by topical N-undecyl-10-enoyl-L-phenylalanine and its combination with niacinamide. *J Cosmet Dermatol.* 2009;8:260.
25. Jerajani HR, Mizoguchi H, Li J, et al. The effects of a daily facial lotion containing vitamins B$_3$ and E and provitamin B$_5$ on the facial skin of Indian women: a randomized, double-blind trial. *Indian J Dermatol Venereol Leprol.* 2010;76:20.
26. Kimball AB, Kaczvinsky JR, Li J, et al. Reduction in the appearance of facial hyperpigmentation after use of moisturizers with a combination of topical niacinamide and N-acetyl glucosamine: Results of a randomized, double-blind, vehicle-controlled trial. *Br J Dermatol.* 2010;162:435.
27. Fu JJ, Hillebrand GG, Raleigh P, et al. A randomized, controlled comparative study of the wrinkle reduction benefits of a cosmetic niacinamide/peptide/retinyl propionate product regimen vs. a prescription 0.02% tretinoin product regimen. *Br J Dermatol.* 2010;162:647.
28. Bissett DL, Miyamoto K, Sun P, et al. Topical niacinamide reduces yellowing, wrinkling, red blotchiness, and hyperpigmented spots in aging facial skin. *Int J Cosmet Sci.* 2004;26:231.
29. Bissett DL, Oblong JE, Berge CA. Niacinamide: A B vitamin that improves aging facial skin appearance. *Dermatol Surg.* 2005;31:860.

CHAPTER 45

Soy

Activities:

PAR-2 inhibition, anti-inflammatory, antioxidant, photoprotectant, moisturizing

Important Chemical Components:

Isoflavones (e.g., genistein and daidzein), phytoestrogens, vitamin E, and serine protease inhibitors, including the proteins soybean trypsin inhibitor (STI) and the Bowman-Birk inhibitor (BBI)

Origin Classification:

Soybean is a natural ingredient. Organic forms are available. Forms that have been altered in the lab to remove the estrogenic components are referred to as "active naturals."

Personal Care Category:

Depigmenting, brightening, lightening, moisturizing, antiaging

BST Treatable with this Ingredient:

DRPT, DRPW, DSPT, DSPW, ORPT, ORPW, OSPT, and OSPW

SOURCE

The soybean plant belongs to the pea family, Leguminosae. It contains a higher amount of oil than other legumes. Soy is usually divided into two categories: nonfermented and fermented. Nonfermented soy foods include whole dry soy beans, soy nuts, fresh green soybeans (edamame), soymilk, tofu, okara and yuba. Soymilk, also known as soy juice, soy drink or soya milk, is produced by soaking dry soybeans and grinding them with water. Soy ice cream, soy yogurt, and soy-based cheeses are derived from soymilk. Soybean cake is a by-product obtained during the processing of soybean oil. Tofu is made by coagulating soymilk with a curdling agent and then pressing the curds into blocks.

Fermented soy products include tempeh, miso, soy sauce, natto, and fermented tofu and soymilk products. Miso is produced from fermented soybeans and used as a soup base and flavoring ingredient. Soy sauce is made in a process similar to that of miso except that the paste is pressed to yield a liquid.[1] The fermentation process breaks down many of the soy components, including the proteins soybean trypsin inhibitor (STI) and the Bowman-Birk inhibitor (BBI) as well as saponins, but some studies suggest that the isoflavones are spared and one found that lactic fermentation increased levels of aglycone, an important bioactive form of isoflavone.[2] The important point is that there are various forms of soy and fractions of soy used in cosmeceuticals. Therefore, "soy" on the label does not provide enough information. It is necessary to look at the clinical trials using the final formulation of a soy product before making any assumptions about efficacy.

HISTORY

Soy is considered one of the earliest crops cultivated by humans, dating back to the 11th century BCE in Northern China. In North America, the first soybean plants emerged in the 1700s.[3] In the United States, the earliest terminology for soy oil was "Chinese bean oil" by Roelofsen in 1894.[4] The expression "soy oil" was first used by Jordan in 1918, but it was not widely adopted until the 1940s.[4] In the early 1940s, the protein proteinase inhibitors STI and BBI were isolated from soybeans.[5] Today, soy is one of the most commonly used ingredients in cosmeceutical moisturizers as well as extremely popular worldwide in foods, beverages, food additives, and livestock feed.[6]

CHEMISTRY

Soy contains many components that render it useful as a cosmeceutical ingredient. Important soy constituents include linoleic acid, phospholipids, polysaccharides, B vitamins, tocopherol, phytosterols, isoflavones, and saponins.[7] Flavonoids are polyphenolic components of plants with active properties. Isoflavones are a subtype of flavonoids (see Chapter 46, Antioxidants) found in soy (Table 45-1). The most potent isoflavones in soy are genistein and daidzein.[8] Isoflavones are present in leguminous plants but are particularly abundant in soy. Isoflavones have 2-phenylnaphthalene-type chemical structures similar to those of estrogens and have been found to bind to estrogen receptors and engender estrogen-like activity.[9] For this reason they are classified as phytoestrogens (Figure 45-1). There are 12 different isoforms among soy isoflavones that can

TABLE 45-1
Pros and Cons of Soy

Pros	Cons
Good source of isoflavone antioxidants	Serine protease inhibitors are inactivated by heat in the processing of soybeans and soymilk
Strong safety profile	Confusing labeling
Crops are good for the environment	Many companies add "soy" to their products without using the right formulation of soy and without testing efficacy
Organic forms are available	Insufficient trials looking at efficacy of the various formulations
"Total soy" imparts proven benefits	Estrogenic activity
Dietary soy may have antiaging and anti-inflammatory properties	Safety concerns about unfermented soy
Moisturizing	Dietary soy does not affect pigmentation disorders
Good option for sensitive skin, including rosacea types	

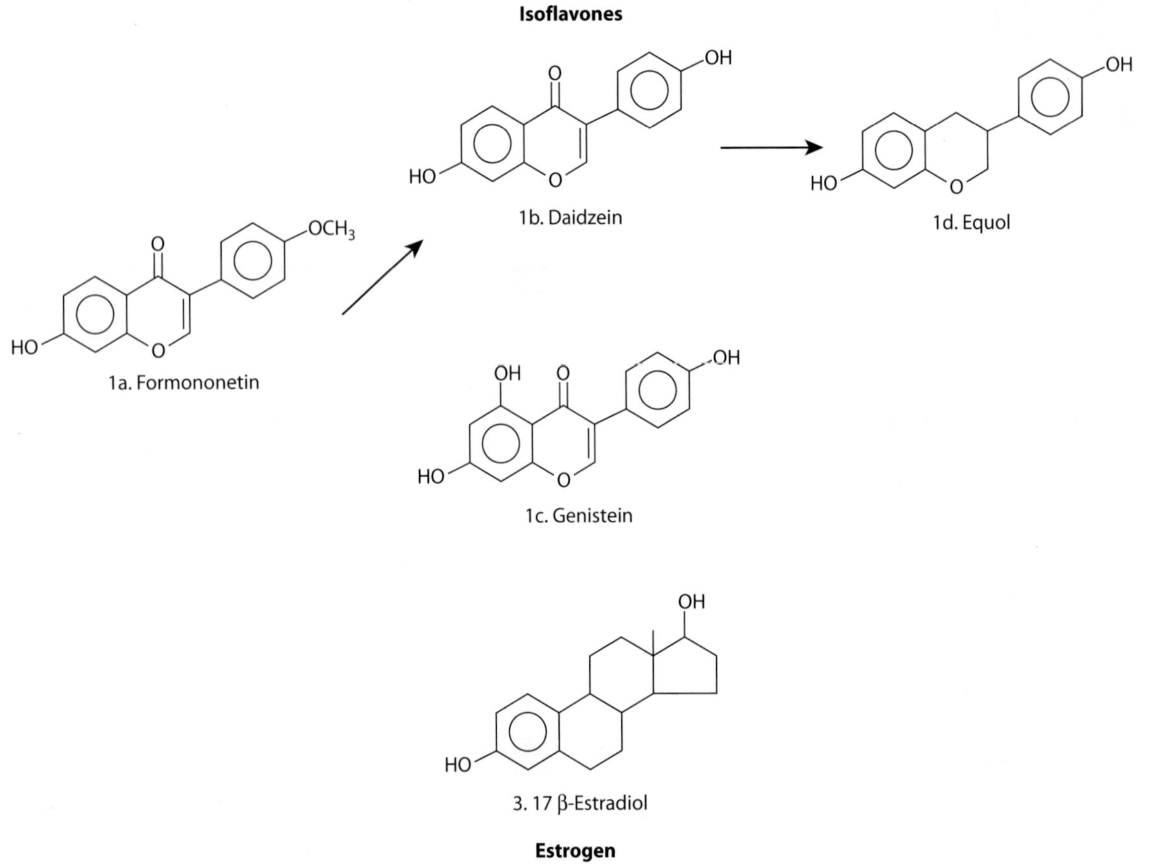

▲ FIGURE 45-1 The family of isoflavones have a chemical structure similar to that of estradiol (estrogen).

be divided into four chemical forms: aglycone (daidzein, genistein, and glycitein), glucoside (daidzin, genistin, and glycitin),acetylglucoside (acetyldaidzin, acetylgenistin, and acetylglycitin), and malonylglucoside (malonyldaidzin, malonylgenistin, and malonylglycitin).[10] The aglycone and acetylglucoside groups possess stronger antioxidant properties than the other isoforms.[11]

ORAL USES

Soybean has been a staple of the Asian diet for thousands of years and some credit this botanical for the greater longevity seen in subsets of the Japanese population. Soy is thought to yield the following unproven health benefits: lowering cholesterol, decreasing cardiovascular disease, decreasing breast and other cancers,[12] preventing osteoporosis, slowing skin aging,[13] and improving menopausal symptoms.[9] These benefits are partially explained by the estrogenic effects of soy.

The health impact of plant-derived estrogens depends on several factors, including concentration, the concentrations of endogenous estrogens, and individual characteristics, such as gender and menopausal status.[9,14] The beneficial effects of these compounds may be due to their influence on estrogen receptors but they are also known to affect enzymes, protein synthesis, cell proliferation, angiogenesis, calcium transport, Na+/K+ adenosine triphosphatase, growth factor action, vascular smooth muscle cells, lipid oxidation, and cell differentiation.[9]

Oral soy may help protect skin through its antioxidant activities, especially the genistein component.[15] After oral administration, soy isoflavones have been shown to protect

against ultraviolet B (UVB)-induced oxidative stress and keratinocyte death.[10,11,13,16,17]

Dietary soy does not play a role in treating skin pigmentation because fermentation of the soy seeds is required for dietary consumption. This fermentation process eliminates the STI and BBI proteins. Stomach acids would also break down the STI and BBI proteins, preventing them from being absorbed when taken orally.[5] However, dietary soy may play a role in skin moisturization and antiaging. Phosphatidylserine synthesized from soy lecithin was shown to increase skin moisturization and decrease wrinkles in human subjects when taken orally.[18] Another double-blind study demonstrated that a supplemental drink containing soy isoflavones, lycopene, vitamins C and E, and fish oil resulted in increased deposition of collagen fibers in the dermis; however, these effects could be due to the presence of vitamin C in the supplement, which is well known to increase collagen synthesis[19] [(see Chapter 55, Ascorbic Acid (Vitamin C)].

TOPICAL USES

In addition to systemic activity, many key soy constituents (i.e., isoflavones, vitamin E, and serine protease inhibitors) have demonstrated cutaneous benefits. The soy isoflavones genistein and daidzein are classified as phytoestrogens with weak estrogenic activity and have reportedly displayed anticarcinogenic, antiphotocarcinogenic, photoprotective, and antiphotodamage activity.[10,13,20–22] In addition, they have been shown, *in vitro*, to increase collagen content and to act as antioxidants by scavenging free radicals.[10,11,13,16,17]

Depigmenting Activity

Soy is an interesting treatment for skin pigmentation when used properly and when the proper forms of it are used. Soy can exacerbate melasma because natural soy contains estrogenic phytoestrogens and melasma is known to be an estrogen-responsive disorder. Soybean seeds, but not other parts of the plant, contain the soymilk-derived proteins STI and BBI that inhibit the activation of protease-activated receptor 2 (PAR-2). PAR-2 allows phagocytosis of melanosomes by keratinocytes during keratinocyte–melanocyte interaction and is upregulated by UV exposure, leading to increased skin pigmentation.[23,24] PAR-2 is a seven transmembrane G-protein-coupled receptor on the surface of keratinocytes that is necessary for the keratinocyte to engulf and phagocytize melanosomes. The soy small protein components known as STI and BBI block PAR-2,[5] thereby preventing skin pigmentation by diminishing the transfer of melanin-containing melanosomes to keratinocytes[5,25–27] (see Chapter 43, Overview of the PAR-2 Receptor). STI and BBI have been shown to reversibly reduce pigmentation or prevent UVB-induced photodamage in preclinical studies, suggesting that UVB-induced skin pigmentation may be regulated by PAR-2 activation.[5,25,28,29]

The depigmenting activity of soy-derived STI and BBI and their capacity to prevent UV-induced pigmentation has been shown both *in vitro* and *in vivo*. Unfortunately, BBI and STI become denatured during heat processing, fermentation, and when exposed to stomach acids. A patented technology was created to preserve the proteins in their active nondenatured state so that they can be applied topically in skin care formulations. In this process the estrogenic components of soy are removed but the BBI and STI proteins are retained. This ingredient is found on cosmetic labels as "active soy" or "total soy." The topical application of total soy formulations has been convincingly shown in human trials to lighten various dyschromias including melasma.[30,31] For that reason, total soy (which contains STI and BBI) has been incorporated into several cosmetic formulations to impart skin-lightening activity and many studies show improvement of skin hyperpigmentation.[27,32] In addition, whole soy extract has demonstrated some efficacy when combined with salicylic acid and retinol in treating postinflammatory hyperpigmentation resulting from acne.[27,33]

Anti-inflammatory Activity

There are several mechanisms by which soy can reduce inflammation. Flavonoids are known to inhibit eicosanoid-generating enzymes (see Chapter 64, Anti-Inflammatory Agents) and modulate proinflammatory gene expression.[34] The flavonoids genistein and daidzein have been shown to inhibit the activation of nuclear factor-κB (NF-κB).[35] Soy isoflavones are known to decrease the secretions of interleukin-1 (IL-1), IL-6, nitric oxide (NO) and prostaglandin E_2 (PGE_2) in the cell supernatant and fluid of mouse peritoneal exudate.[36,37] Soy contains large amounts of isoflavones that are known to affect the inflammatory process at multiple levels.[38]

Anticarcinogenic Activity

Nondenatured soymilk has been demonstrated to prevent or decrease the formation of UVB-induced thymine dimers and apoptotic cells in the epidermis, to enhance UVB-induced checkpoint kinase-1 activation (yielding more time for DNA repair), and to lower the incidence or progression of UVB-induced skin tumors.[39,40] Soy also appears to hinder UVB-induced inflammation, as suggested by a decrease in UVB-induced cyclooxygenase-2 (COX-2) expression and PGE_2 secretion.[40]

Antiaging Activity

Skin aging manifests from the loss of collagen, elastin, and hyaluronic acid (see Chapter 5, Epidermis and Dermis). Nondenatured "total soy" soybean extracts have also been shown to promote collagen synthesis and bolster the elastic fiber framework.[41,42] Because total soy has had the estrogenic components removed, an increase in collagen production cannot be attributed to estrogenic effects. Liu et al. found that the elastic tissue in total soy-treated skin displayed augmented fine and highly branched elastin fibers in the upper dermis similar to the "repair zone" seen after retinoid treatment.[41] These changes are thought to be due to elevated elastin promoter activity, suppression of elastase activity, and protection of elastic fibers from exogenous elastases.[42]

Chiu et al. demonstrated that an isoflavone extracted from soy decreased expression of c-Jun N-terminal kinases (JNK) and extracellular signal-regulated kinase (ERK) genes and p38 signaling pathways known to play a role in the destruction of collagen that occurs after sun exposure.[8,43] Soy fractions containing daidzein, genistein, and glycitein were shown to inhibit UVB-induced apoptosis of human keratinocytes and reduce the level of desquamation, transepidermal water loss, erythema, and epidermal thickness in mouse skin.[10] The UVB-protective effects of soy isoflavones might be related to their antioxidant activities.[11,44]

A recent study examined the activity of a soy fraction on the retinoic acid receptor (RAR), which is known to be responsible for many of the antiaging properties demonstrated by retinoids such as tretinoin [see Chapter 83, Retinoids (Retinol)]. This study showed that the daidzein fraction of soy directly binds to the RAR and increases expression of RAR mRNA.[45]

The effects of *Bifidobacterium*-fermented and nonfermented soymilk extracts were compared in cultures of human keratinocytes, human fibroblasts, and in hairless mouse skin following topical application for two weeks. The fermented soymilk, but not the nonfermented one, enhanced the production of hyaluronic acid (HA) in all of these models. Genistein and daidzein were detected in the fermented soymilk at a concentration of 0.18 and 0.07 mM, respectively, but not in the nonfermented product. The researchers concluded that genistein released from its glycoside during fermentation with *Bifidobacterium* has the potential to enhance HA production in the epidermis and dermis.[46]

Moisturizing Activity

Soybeans are composed of 19 percent oil (high for a legume), characterized by triglycerides and polyunsaturated fatty acids such as linoleic and α-linoleic acids. Linoleic acid helps the skin produce ceramides. Recall that ceramides and fatty acids help form the skin barrier that prevents water from evaporating off of the skin (see Chapter 7, Moisturizing Agents). Oligosaccharides in soy can function as humectants, attracting water to the skin's surface while the oil component functions as an occlusive, preventing water from evaporating from the skin's surface. The fact that soy has been shown to increase levels of HA in skin might help explain why skin appears more hydrated when exposed to soy.

SAFETY ISSUES

The safety of fermented versus unfermented soy in the diet has been debated for several years.[47] A 2003 review of the literature concluded that soy in the diet is generally safe even though it has estrogenic activity; however, long-term studies are needed.[47]

ENVIRONMENTAL IMPACT

Soy is one of the primary commodity crops in the United States. It is often used as a cover crop to improve soil for future crops because it increases levels of organic matter, improves the water-holding capacity of soil, enhances drainage in clay soils, and provides a range of macro- and micronutrients that optimize plant health.[48] Soybeans form a symbiotic relationship between various strains of *Rhizobium* bacteria found in the soil. The bacteria infect the soy plant roots and extract nitrogen from the atmosphere and metabolize it into a form that the soy plants can use to make protein. In return, these "nitrogen-fixing bacteria" receive sugars from the plant for their own nutrition. That is why farmers rotate soybeans with corn, to take advantage of this legume's nitrogen-fixing ability to improve the soil.

FORMULATION CONSIDERATIONS

Formulation of soy depends on the type of soy or soy fractions used. The final formula must be studied in order to make statements about efficacy. For this reason, products labeled "*clinically proven*" to reduce skin pigmentation are preferred to products that do not say clinically proven. Generic "copied" products with soy are unreliable because of the many issues relating to formulating soy, including whether the estrogenic components have been removed, if the STI and BBI proteins are present, and whether the soy is fermented or nonfermented. A manufacturing process was developed in 2001 to incorporate a wide array of nondenatured soy proteins, essential fatty acids, carbohydrates, and vitamins in topical formulations, enhancing the capacity of products to harness soy potency.[3]

USAGE CONSIDERATIONS

The polyunsaturated fatty acids in soy leave products susceptible to going rancid, so they should be kept in a cold, dark place and discarded on their expiration date. Soy products can be used in conjunction with retinoids and glycolic acids and other ingredients without increasing the risk of irritation. In fact, the anti-inflammatory and hydrating properties of soy may help mitigate irritation due to retinoids.

SIGNIFICANT BACKGROUND

Animal Studies

In 2000, Seiberg et al. conducted *in vitro* and *in vivo* studies to demonstrate the interference with PAR-2 activation displayed by serine protease inhibitors that results in the suppression of melanosome transfer and distribution. They showed that *in vitro* treatment with a serine protease inhibitor resulted in reduced pigmentation in swine skin samples. They also reported from their *in vivo* experiments that twice-daily application of a serine protease inhibitor for eight or nine weeks visibly and dose-dependently lightened the skin of Yucatan swine.[25]

In 2001, Paine et al. performed *in vitro* and *in vivo* studies in which dark-skinned Yucatan microswine were treated with soybean extract serine protease inhibitor. Diminished skin color was observed visually and confirmed by F&M staining of histologic sections that displayed decreased melanin deposition in the skin biopsies of treated skin. The effect was associated only with fresh soymilk and not pasteurized soymilk preparations. This suggests that a heat-labile component of the soymilk, STI, is the active depigmenting agent. Soymilk treatment also prevented UVB-induced hyperpigmentation of the animals' skin.[5]

Clinical Studies

In 2000, Hermanns et al. conducted a clinical study of 44 Caucasian men with solar lentigines (ages 52–61 years) in which subjects applied either stabilized soy extract, 15 percent azelaic acid, or 12 percent glycolic acid formulation once daily to the face for three weeks. Analysis of videomicroscopic images showed that the soy formulation produced a significant decrease in pigmentation at the end of three weeks and performed better than the other two products.[30]

In a 12-week study in 2001, 16 Hispanic women with melasma applied stabilized soy extract once daily to one lesion, leaving a second lesion untreated. Fourteen of the subjects showed some depigmentation from using the soy formulation, with an average 12 percent reduction in clinical score at the end of the study.[49]

In 2002, Hermanns et al. conducted a two-month open randomized trial in Belgium in 30 women of Southeast Asian ancestry (between the ages of 42 and 57 years) who presented with hyperpigmentation on the dorsal forearms and backs of the hands. Twice daily, the volunteers applied a stabilized soy extract to the lesions and surrounding area, with the other arm/hand serving as a control. The investigators reported that a modest lightening effect was revealed using corneomelametry. In addition, they noted that the faintly mottled skin as indicated by UV light examination responded better to the soy formulation.[50]

In 2007, Wallo et al. examined the effects of a novel soy moisturizer containing nondenatured STI and BBI on pigmentation, skin tone amelioration, and other signs of photoaging in a double-blind, parallel, vehicle-controlled study. Sixty-three women, aged 30 to 61 with Fitzpatrick phototypes I to III, with moderately severe mottled hyperpigmentation, lentigines, blotchiness, tactile roughness, and dullness completed the study. The moisturizer and the vehicle respectively were administered twice daily for a period of 12 weeks. By clinical observation, self-assessment, colorimetry, and digital photography, the researchers noted a significant improvement of mottled pigmentation, blotchiness, dullness, fine lines, as well as overall texture, skin tone, and appearance in the soy moisturizer group as compared to the vehicle subjects. Improvement in the soy group was seen as early as the second week of treatment.[51]

CONCLUSION

There are many different forms of soy and soy extracts on the market; therefore, looking for "soy" on the label is not sufficient information on which to base a purchasing decision. Soy delivers antioxidant, anti-inflammatory, moisturizing, and depigmenting benefits to the skin. However, the nondenatured soy extracts, as opposed to the more processed ingredients, appear to be more effective as topical agents for pigmentation disorders. Dietary soy can play an important role in skin care, but does not influence skin pigmentation because stomach acids destroy the STI and BBI proteins.

REFERENCES

1. Golbitz P. Traditional soyfoods: Processing and products. *J Nutr.* 1995;125:570S.
2. Lai LR, Hsieh SC, Huang HY, et al. Effect of lactic fermentation on the total phenolic, saponin and phytic acid contents as well as anti-colon cancer cell proliferation activity of soymilk. *J Biosci Bioeng.* 2013;115:552.
3. Leyden JJ, Shergill B, Micali G, et al. Natural options for the management of hyperpigmentation. *J Eur Acad Dermatol Venereol.* 2011;25:1140.
4. Shurtleff W, Aoyagi A. A special report on the history of soy oil, soybean meal, and modern soy products. Soy Info Center. http://www.soyinfocenter.com/HSS/soybean_crushing1.php. Accessed September 7, 2013.
5. Paine C, Sharlow E, Liebel F, et al. An alternative approach to depigmentation by soybean extracts via inhibition of the PAR-2 pathway. *J Invest Dermatol.* 2001;116:587.
6. Draelos ZD. Skin lightening preparations and the hydroquinone controversy. *Dermatol Ther.* 2007;20:308.
7. Dixit AK, Antony JIX, Sharma NK, et al. Soybean constituents and their functional benefits. In: Tiwari VK, ed. *Opportunity, Challenge and Scope of Natural Products in Medicinal Chemistry.* Kerala, India: Research Signpost; 2011:367–383.
8. Chiu TM, Huang CC, Lin TJ, et al. In vitro and in vivo anti-photoaging effects of an isoflavone extract from soybean cake. *J Ethnopharmacol.* 2009;126:108.
9. Tham DM, Gardner CD, Haskell WL. Clinical review 97: Potential health benefits of dietary phytoestrogens: A review of the clinical, epidemiological, and mechanistic evidence. *J Clin Endocrinol Metab.* 1998;83:2223.
10. Huang CC, Hsu BY, Wu NL, et al. Anti-photoaging effects of soy isoflavone extract (aglycone and acetylglucoside form) from soybean cake. *Int J Mol Sci.* 2010;11:4782.
11. Kao TH, Chen BH. Functional components in soybean cake and their effects on antioxidant activity. *J Agric Food Chem.* 2006;54:7544.
12. Ingram D, Sanders K, Kolybaba M, et al. Case-control study of phyto-oestrogens and breast cancer. *Lancet.* 1997;350:990.
13. Kim SY, Kim SJ, Lee JY, et al. Protective effects of dietary soy isoflavones against UV-induced skin-aging in hairless mouse model. *J Am Coll Nutr.* 2004;23:157.
14. Knight DC, Eden JA. A review of the clinical effects of phytoestrogens. *Obstet Gynecol.* 1996;87:897.
15. Wei H, Bowen R, Cai Q, et al. Antioxidant and antipromotional effects of the soybean isoflavone genistein. *Proc Soc Exp Biol Med.* 1995;208:124.
16. Südel KM, Venzke K, Mielke H, et al. Novel aspects of intrinsic and extrinsic aging of human skin: Beneficial effects of soy extract. *Photochem Photobiol.* 2005;81:581.
17. Accorsi-Neto A, Haidar M, Simões R, et al. Effects of isoflavones on the skin of postmenopausal women: A pilot study. *Clinics (Sau Paulo).* 2009;64:505.
18. Choi HD, Han JJ, Yang JH, et al. Effect of soy phosphatidylserine supplemented diet on skin wrinkle and moisture in vivo and clinical trial. *J Kor Soc Appl Biol Chem.* 2013;56:227.
19. Jenkins G, Wainwright LJ, Holland R, et al. Wrinkle reduction in post-menopausal women consuming a novel oral supplement: a double-blind placebo-controlled randomised study. *Int J Cosmet Sci.* 2013 August 8. [Epub ahead of print]
20. Barnes S. Effect of genistein on in vitro and in vivo models of cancer. *J Nutr.* 1995;125:777S.
21. Moore JO, Wang Y, Stebbins WG, et al. Photoprotective effect of isoflavone genistein on ultraviolet B-induced pyrimidine dimer formation and PCNA expression in human reconstituted skin and its implications in dermatology and prevention of cutaneous carcinogenesis. *Carcinogenesis.* 2006;27:1627.
22. Cassidy A, Albertazzi P, Lise Nielsen I, et al. Critical review of health effects of soyabean phyto-oestrogens in post-menopausal women. *Proc Nutr Soc.* 2006;65:76.
23. Seiberg M. Keratinocyte-melanocyte interactions during melanosome transfer. *Pigment Cell Res.* 2001;14:236.
24. Scott G, Deng A, Rodriguez-Burford C, et al. Protease-activated receptor 2, a receptor involved in melanosome transfer, is upregulated in human skin by ultraviolet irradiation. *J Invest Dermatol.* 2001;117:1412.
25. Seiberg M, Paine C, Sharlow E, et al. Inhibition of melanosome transfer results in skin lightening. *J Invest Dermatol.* 2000;115:162.
26. Parvez S, Kang M, Chung HS, et al. Survey and mechanism of skin depigmenting and lightening agents. *Phytother Res.* 2006;20:921.
27. Callender VD, St Surin-Lord S, Davis EC, et al. Postinflammatory hyperpigmentation: Etiologic and therapeutic considerations. *Am J Clin Dermatol.* 2011;12:87.
28. Seiberg M, Paine C, Sharlow E, et al. The protease-activated receptor 2 regulates pigmentation via keratinocyte-melanocyte interactions. *Exp Cell Res.* 2000;254:25.
29. Konda S, Geria AN, Halder RM. New horizons in treating disorders of hyperpigmentation in skin of color. *Semin Cutan Med Surg.* 2012;31:133.
30. Hermanns JF, Petit L, Martalo O, et al. Unraveling the patterns of subclinical pheomelanin-enriched facial hyperpigmentation: Effect of depigmenting agents. *Dermatology.* 2000;201:118.
31. Leyden J, Wallo W. The mechanism of action and clinical benefits of soy for the treatment of hyperpigmentation. *Int J Dermatol.* 2011;50:470.
32. Finkey MB, Herndon J, Stephens T, et al. Soy moisturizer SPF 15 improves dyschromia [poster]. *J Am Acad Dermatol.* 2005;52(Suppl):P170.
33. Sah A, Stephens TJ, Kurtz ES. Topical acne treatment improves postacne postinflammatory hyperpigmentation (PIH) in skin of color [poster]. *J Am Acad Dermatol.* 2005;52(Suppl):P25.
34. Kim HP, Son KH, Chang HW, et al. Anti-inflammatory plant flavonoids and cellular action mechanisms. *J Pharmacol Sci.* 2004;96:229.
35. Hämäläinen M, Nieminen R, Vuorela P, Heinonen M, Moilanen E. Anti-inflammatory effects of flavonoids: Genistein, kaempferol, quercetin, and daidzein inhibit STAT-1 and NF-kappaB activations, whereas flavones, isorhamnetin, naringenin, and pelargonidin inhibit only NF-kappaB activation along with their inhibitory effect on iNOS expression and NO production in activated macrophages. *Mediators Inflamm.* 2007;45673.
36. Kao TH, Wu WM, Hung CF, et al. Anti-inflammatory effects of isoflavone powder produced from soybean cake. *J Agric Food Chem.* 2007;55:11068.
37. Kao TH, Huang RF, Chen BH. Antiproliferation of hepatoma cell and progression of cell cycle as affected by isoflavone extracts from soybean cake. *Int J Mol Sci.* 2007;8:1095.
38. Stoner G, Wang LS. Natural products as anti-inflammatory agents. In: AJ Dannenberg, NA Berger, eds. *Energy Balance and Cancer Vol. 7: Obesity, Inflammation and Cancer.* New York: Springer; 2013:341–361.
39. Huang MT, Xie JG, Lin CB, et al. Inhibitory effect of topical applications of nondenatured soymilk on the formation and growth of UVB-induced skin tumors. *Oncol Res.* 2004;14:387.
40. Chen N, Scarpa R, Zhang L, et al. Nondenatured soy extracts reduce UVB-induced skin damage via multiple mechanisms. *Photochem Photobiol.* 2008;84:1551.
41. Liu JC, Seiberg M, Chen T, et al. Pre-clinical and clinical evaluation of total soy preparations in improving skin physical tone parameters. Poster presented at the 60th American Academy of Dermatology meeting, New Orleans, LA, 2002.
42. Zhao R, Bruning E, Rossetti D, et al. Extracts from Glycine max (soybean) induce elastin synthesis and inhibit elastase activity. *Exp Dermatol.* 2009;18:883.
43. Peus D, Vasa RA, Beyerle A, et al. UVB activates ERK1/2 and p38 signaling pathways via reactive oxygen species in cultured keratinocytes. *J Invest Dermatol.* 1999;112:751.
44. Chiang HS, Wu WB, Fang JY, et al. UVB-protective effects of isoflavone extracts from soybean cake in human keratinocytes. *Int J Mol Sci.* 2007;8:651.
45. Oh HJ, Kang YG, Na TY, et al. Identification of daidzein as a ligand of retinoic acid receptor that suppresses expression of matrix metalloproteinase-9 in HaCaT cells. *Mol Cell Endocrinol.* 2013;376:107.

46. Miyazaki K, Hanamizu T, Iizuka R, et al. Bifidobacterium-fermented soy milk extract stimulates hyaluronic acid production in human skin cells and hairless mouse skin. *Skin Pharmacol Appl Skin Physiol*. 2003;16:108.

47. Munro IC, Harwood M, Hlywka JJ, et al. Soy isoflavones: A safety review. *Nutr Rev*. 2003;61:1.

48. Reed BH. The Texas Gardener. http://www.texasgardener.com/pastissues/mayjun05/Soybean.html. Accessed September 7, 2013.

49. Piérard G, Graf J, Gonzalez R, et al. Effects of soy on hyperpigmentation in Caucasian and Hispanic populations. Poster presented at the 59th American Academy of Dermatology meeting. Washington, DC, 2001.

50. Hermanns JF, Petit L, Piérard-Franchimont C, et al. Assessment of topical hypopigmenting agents on solar lentigines of Asian women. *Dermatology*. 2002;204:281.

51. Wallo W, Nebus J, Leyden JJ. Efficacy of a soy moisturizer in photoaging: A double-blind, vehicle-controlled, 12-week study. *J Drugs Dermatol*. 2007;6:917.

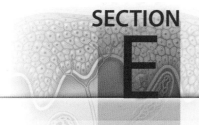

SECTION E
Antioxidants

CHAPTER 46

Antioxidants

The skin has naturally occurring antioxidants that protect against the ravages of free radicals by reducing and neutralizing them (see Chapter 2, Basic Cosmetic Chemistry, for an explanation of free radicals). Antioxidative enzymes that naturally occur in the skin include superoxide dismutase, catalase, and glutathione peroxidase; nonenzymatic endogenous antioxidative molecules are α-tocopherol (vitamin E), ascorbic acid (vitamin C), glutathione, and ubiquinone (better known as coenzyme Q_{10} or CoQ_{10}).[1] However, as part of the natural aging process our defense mechanisms decrease. This leads to an imbalance and increased number of unchecked free radicals, which engender damage to DNA, cytoskeletal elements, cellular proteins, and cellular membranes. Moreover, many of these antioxidant defense mechanisms are inhibited by ultraviolet (UV) and visible light.[2,3] Topical antioxidants are currently marketed for the prevention of aging and UV-mediated skin damage. The free radical theory of aging explains why antioxidants are thought to prevent wrinkles, but this theory does not justify the use of antioxidants to treat wrinkles that are already present. Several companies claim that their antioxidant-containing products "treat" wrinkles; however, this is an exaggeration. The only antioxidant that can improve wrinkles that have already been formed is ascorbic acid, through its effects on collagen synthesis.[4]

In addition to the effects associated with their antioxidative activity, many antioxidants exhibit anti-inflammatory properties or depigmenting activities, which are described in more detail in other sections. There are several important factors to consider when evaluating the efficacy of antioxidants. In order to be considered biologically active, orally administered products must be absorbed and shown to raise antioxidant levels in the skin. Topically administered products must be absorbed into the skin and delivered to the target tissue in the active form and remain there long enough to exert the desired effects. Antioxidants can

be activated or inactivated by enzymes in the skin. Some antioxidants are very unstable; therefore, some ingredients such as vitamin C become oxidized and rendered inactive before reaching the target. Stabilizing them in formulation and packaging them to minimize air and light exposure are challenging tasks. Absorption is also important and depends on several factors such as the molecular form of the compound, its pH, whether it is water soluble or fat soluble, and the vehicle that contains the product. This section will discuss the most popular types of antioxidants found in topical cosmetic products.

Fat-soluble antioxidants function in the lipophilic portion of the cell membrane and include vitamin E, idebenone, lycopene, curcumin, and CoQ_{10}.[5] Other antioxidants are water soluble and found in hydrophilic areas of the cell. These include ascorbic acid, green tea, silymarin, coffeeberry, and resveratrol.

POLYPHENOLS AND THE CLASSIFICATION OF ANTIOXIDANTS

Polyphenols are widely distributed in nature and in the plant kingdom in particular. They are synthesized by plants in response to environmental hazards that induce enhanced free-radical production.[6] Polyphenol biosynthesis begins when phenylalanine ammonia-lyase is induced by exposure to UV light, γ-irradiation, ozone, low temperatures, organic toxins, and/or heavy metals. Phenylalanine is catalytically deaminated to cinnamic acid and then cinnamic acid is converted to various polyphenols, which share a definitive structural component: a phenol or an aromatic ring with at least one hydroxyl group. Polyphenols are an exceedingly important source of antioxidants and are found in a vast spectrum of vegetables, fruits, herbs, grains, tea, coffee beans, honey, and red wine (Table 46-1).

TABLE 46-1
Subclasses of the Most Abundant Polyphenols, Flavonoids, and Food Sources of Each Class[7-9]

FLAVONES	FLAVONOLS	FLAVANONES	ISOFLAVONES	FLAVANOLS (CATECHINS)	ANTHOCYANINS	PROANTHOCYANIDINS
Celery	Apples	Oranges	Soy	Apples	Blackberries	Apples
Fresh parsley	Broccoli	Grapefruit		Cocoa	Cherries	Dark chocolate
Sweet red pepper	Olives			Dark chocolate	Currants (black and red)	Grapes
	Onions			Tea (black and green)	Grapes	Pears
	Tea (black and green)				Plums	Red wine
					Raspberries	Tea (black and green)
					Strawberries	

TABLE 46-2
Categories of Polyphenols Currently Pertinent to Skin Care

A. Flavonoids

FLAVONES	FLAVONOLS	FLAVANONES	ISOFLAVONES	FLAVANALS (CATECHINS)	ANTHOCYANINS	PROANTHOCYANIDINS	DIHYDROCHALCONE[10]
Apigenin	Quercetin		Genistein	Green tea		Pycnogenol	Phloretin[11]
Luteolin							

B. Nonflavonoids

TANNINS	STILBENES OR PHYTOALEXINS	LIGNANS	HYDROXYCINNAMIC ACIDS
Ellagic acid	Resveratrol	Flaxseed	Caffeic acid
		Sesame seed	Ferulic acid

Note: Some categories have been excluded.

When the "parent polyphenol" known as cinnamic acid is further catalytically transformed, myriad polyphenolic compounds result that are divided into classes: glycosylated phenylpropanoids, flavonoids, isoflavonoids, stilbenoids, coumarins, curcuminoids, phenolic polymers such as tannins, proanthocyanidins, suberin, lignins, and lignans. Flavonoids are the most abundant polyphenols in the human diet as well as the most studied polyphenols, and can be further divided into several categories (Table 46-2). An ingredient does not have to be a polyphenol to have antioxidant abilities. Vitamins, minerals, substances that confer pigments to plants, and other ingredients may exhibit antioxidant activity as well. This section will discuss various antioxidants used in skin care. The particular characteristics that these ingredients display are derived from the subcategories they fall into based on their chemical structure.

REFERENCES

1. Shindo Y, Witt E, Han D, et al. Enzymic and non-enzymic antioxidants in epidermis and dermis of human skin. *J Invest Dermatol.* 1994;102:122.
2. Fuchs J, Huflejt ME, Rothfuss LM, et al. Acute effects of near ultraviolet and visible light on the cutaneous antioxidant defense system. *Photochem Photobiol.* 1989;50:739.
3. Fuchs J, Huflejt ME, Rothfuss LM, et al. Impairment of enzymic and nonenzymic antioxidants in skin by UVB irradiation. *J Invest Dermatol.* 1989;93:769.
4. Pinnell SR, Murad S, Darr D. Induction of collagen synthesis by ascorbic acid: A possible mechanism. *Arch Dermatol.* 1987;123:1684.
5. Baumann S, Bogdan Allemann I. Antioxidants. In: Baumann L, Saghari S, Weisberg E, eds. *Cosmetic Dermatology: Principles and Practice.* 2nd ed. New York: McGraw-Hill Medical; 2009:294–296.
6. Korkina L, De Luca C, Pastore S. Plant polyphenols and human skin: Friends or foes. *Ann N Y Acad Sci.* 2012;1259:77.
7. Scalbert A, Williamson G. Dietary intake and bioavailability of polyphenols. *J Nutr.* 2000;130:2073S.
8. Ross JA, Kasum CM. Dietary flavonoids: Bioavailability, metabolic effects, and safety. *Annu Rev Nutr.* 2002;22:19.
9. Grove K. Catechins are the major source of flavonoids in a group of Australian women. *Asia Pac J Clin Nutr.* 2004;13(Suppl):S72.
10. Nakamura Y, Watanabe S, Miyake N, et al. Dihydrochalcones: Evaluation as novel radical scavenging antioxidants. *J Agric Food Chem.* 2003;51:3309.
11. Rezk BM, Haenen GR, van der Vijgh WJ, et al. The antioxidant activity of phloretin: The disclosure of a new antioxidant pharmacophore in flavonoids. *Biochem Biophys Res Commun.* 2002;295:9.

CHAPTER 47

Green Tea

Activities:

Antioxidant, antiaging,[1] antiacne, antiangiogenic, anticarcinogenic, anticariogenic, anti-inflammatory, antimicrobial, chemopreventive, immunomodulatory,[2] photoprotective

Important Chemical Components:

ECG [(-)EpiCatechin-3-*O*-Gallate]
GCG [(-)GalloCatechin-3-*O*-Gallate]
EGC [(-)EpiGalloCatechin]
EGCG [(-)EpiGalloCatechin-3-*O*-Gallate]

Origin Classification:

This ingredient is considered natural. Organic forms are available.

Personal Care Category:

Antiaging, moisturizing, antiacne, anogenital wart treatment

Recommended for the following Baumann Skin Types:

DRNW, DRPW, DSNT, DSPT, DSNW, DSPW, ORNW, ORPW, OSNT, OSPT, OSNW, and OSPW

TABLE 47-1
Pros and Cons of Green Tea

PROS	CONS
More evidence than other antioxidants	Clinical efficacy has not yet been clearly established[73,86]
Wide range of health benefits conferred	Insufficient number of clinical studies[9,73]
Found in many topical products	Products often contain an insufficient amount
Tolerated by sensitive skin types	Does not treat wrinkles that are already present
Minimal reaction with other ingredients	May turn the cream brown when included in large concentrations

SOURCE

Derived from *Camellia sinensis*, an evergreen tree belonging to the Theaceae family (Figure 47-1), green tea has long been a popular beverage worldwide, particularly in Asian countries. Its use by human beings is thought to date back 4,000 years.[3] During the last 15 years, it has also gained notable attention because of its purported antioxidant and anticarcinogenic properties. In fact, green tea is one of the most heavily researched of the antioxidants and myriad studies on the cutaneous effects of green tea appear in the literature.[4] Green tea, rife with plant polyphenols, displays significant antioxidant, chemopreventive, immunomodulatory, and anti-inflammatory activity and affects the biochemical pathways important in cell proliferation, when administered either topically or orally.[2,5,6] For this reason, and because of its widespread popularity as a beverage, green tea polyphenols are among the most frequently studied herbal agents used in medicine.

Polyphenols, many of which are potent antioxidants, are a large, diverse family of thousands of chemical substances found in plants (Table 47-1). The four major polyphenolic catechins found in green tea include: ECG [(-)EpiCatechin-3-*O*-Gallate], GCG [(-)GalloCatechin-3-*O*-Gallate], EGC [(-)EpiGalloCatechin], and EGCG [(-)EpiGalloCatechin-3-*O*-Gallate], the most abundant and biologically active green tea constituent. Like green tea, white tea is derived from *C. sinensis*, but it is more expensive because it is harder to obtain. White tea actually comes from the tips of the green tea leaves or leaves not yet fully opened, with buds still covered by fine white hair. Of the four primary "true teas," green and white are unfermented; black tea is fermented; and oolong tea is semi-fermented.[2,7]

In a wide-ranging evidence-based review of the use of botanicals in dermatology, Reuter et al. concluded in 2010 that the oral administration and topical application of antioxidant plant extracts of green and black tea, among other botanicals, can protect skin against the deleterious effects of ultraviolet (UV) exposure, including erythema, premature aging, and cancer.[8]

HISTORY

Tea has been consumed as a beverage for thousands of years, becoming popular on a wide scale about 700 years ago; currently, it is second in global popularity only to water.[3,9–11] Chinese records trace the use of tea as a beverage to the time of Emperor Shen Nung circa 2700 BCE,[3] though it is thought that its use for medicinal purposes may date back 300 years earlier.[10] Traditional Chinese medicine (TCM) began emphasizing the consumption of tea circa 1100 BCE.[10] It was introduced in Japan in the 500s CE, and its pharmacological properties, among others, were described in text by a Japanese Zen priest, Yeisai, in 1211.[12] It was also cultivated in India and

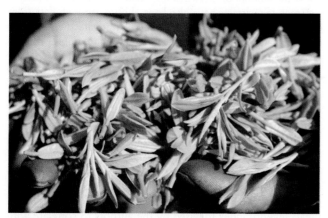

▲ **FIGURE 47-1** Leaves of *Camellia sinensis*. Reprinted with permission from Meltzer SM, Mon BJ, Tewari KS. Green tea catechins for treatment of external genital warts. *Am J Obstet Gynecol* 2009;200:233.e2 with permission from Elsevier.

Indonesia, through which the respective imperial powers of the English and Dutch imported and, in the case of the English, popularized the beverage on a large scale.[3]

Research into the health benefits of tea, particularly green tea, is a relatively recent phenomenon, as is the research into and topical application of green tea. In the late 1980s and early 1990s, several early studies with mice demonstrated, using a two-stage skin tumorigenesis model, that green tea polyphenols (GTPs), administered orally or applied topically, exhibit broad activity against skin tumor initiation and promotion involving multiple tumor-inducing agents.[13–25]

CHEMISTRY

In particular, studies in mouse skin tumor bioassay systems in the 1990s showed that topically applied GTPs protected skin against skin cancer induced, initiated, or promoted by 3-methylcholanthrene, initiated by 7,12-dimethylbenz(a) anthracene (DMBA), promoted by 12-O-tetradecanoylphorbol-13-acetate (TPA), or enhanced by benzoyl peroxide- and 4-nitroquinoline N-oxide, and other agents.[15] GTPs are also known to have the capacity to scavenge a vast range of free radicals, including 1,1-diphenyl-2-picryl-hydrazyl (DPPH), hydroxyl radicals, and lipid-derived radicals.[26]

Ras and activator protein (AP)-1, both of which are involved in the mitogen-activated protein kinase (MAPK) pathway, are among the molecular targets of GTPs.[27] The antiapoptotic effects exhibited by EGCG on UVB-irradiated keratinocytes appear to be brought about by increased expression of the antiapoptotic molecule Bcl-2 and a decline in the proapoptotic protein Bax.[28] EGCG reduces UV-induced immunosuppression by limiting interleukin (IL)-10 synthesis and increasing IL-12 production; both are major cytokines that mediate UV-induced immunosuppression.[29] Further, the EGCG-induced IL-12 increase enhances the production of enzymes that repair UV-induced DNA damage.[30] EGCG also appears to lower UVB-induced immunosuppression by decreasing CD11b, a cell surface marker for activated macrophages and neutrophils in animals treated with UVB.[31]

In mice, EGCG has been demonstrated to downregulate UV-induced expression of AP-1 and NF-κB while inhibiting matrix metalloproteinases (MMPs), which are known to degrade collagen, thus leading to photodamage. In one study, GTPs were administered in drinking water to SKH-1 hairless mice, which were then exposed to multiple doses of UVB. The result was suppression of UVB-induced protein oxidation *in vivo* in mouse skin; these findings were also observed *in vitro* in human skin fibroblast HS68 cells. Oral administration of GTPs was also demonstrated to inhibit UVB-induced expression of matrix-degrading MMPs in the hairless mouse skin, suggesting the antiphotoaging activity of GTPs.[32]

ORAL USES

Green tea is one of the most popular beverages worldwide. Many of the salutary effects associated with green tea are based on oral administration. Recent evidence also suggests that green tea exerts an anticariogenic effect when used as an oral rinse, as it has been shown to reduce the acidity of saliva and plaque.[33] In addition to its popularity in liquid form, green tea extracts are also available as dietary pill supplements.

A 2007 review article by Katiyar et al. on the photoprotective efficacy of GTPs against UV-induced carcinogenesis concluded that the oral administration of GTPs or topical application of EGCG prevents the development of UVB-induced skin tumors in mice. The investigators suggested that this chemopreventive activity is mediated via several mechanisms involving IL-12, angiogenesis suppression, and the stimulation of cytotoxic T cells in a tumor microenvironment.[34]

TOPICAL USES

Green tea is found in several over-the-counter (OTC) skin care products. The formulations vary by the type of green tea polyphenol component (e.g., EGCG), and the amount of polyphenol, both of which are important to know when evaluating product efficacy. Green tea seems to decrease skin inflammation and neutralize free radicals, which explains its popularity as an additive in rosacea and antiaging skin care products. The antiaging effects of green tea are difficult to measure because it functions as an antioxidant that prevents aging and does not have the capacity to increase collagen synthesis or ameliorate extant wrinkles. However, there is relatively good evidence (compared to other antioxidants) to suggest that topically applied green tea can help protect skin from UV radiation.

In 2012, Pazyar performed a thorough literature search of all *in vitro*, *in vivo*, and controlled clinical trials involving green tea formulations and their dermatologic applications. They evaluated 20 studies, with evidence suggesting that orally administered green tea displays a broad range of healthy activity, including quenching free radicals, cancer prevention, treating hair loss, slowing cutaneous aging, and protecting against the side effects of psoralen-UVA therapy. Further, they found supportive data for the use of topically applied green tea extract to treat several cutaneous conditions, including acne, rosacea, atopic dermatitis, androgenetic alopecia, hirsutism, candidiasis, keloids, leishmaniasis, and genital warts.[35]

Also, a green tea topical formulation, green tea sinecatechin polyphenon E (Veregen®) ointment, has recently been shown to exert antioxidant, antiviral, and antitumor activity, and has demonstrated efficacy in treating condylomata acuminata (external anogenital warts).[36] In addition, topically applying GTPs in the morning in combination with traditional sunscreens is believed to have the potential to protect the skin from UV-induced damage. Topical green tea may improve rosacea, prevent retinoid dermatitis, and play a role in managing pigmentation disorders. Few of the many OTC products that contain GTPs have been tested in controlled clinical trials and the concentration of polyphenols in these products is too low to demonstrate efficacy. It is necessary to know the amount of GTPs in a formulation to judge its efficacy.

Green tea extracts have also been shown, through data from 60 patients analyzed retrospectively, to mitigate the effects of acute radiation-induced skin toxicity, through complex mechanisms that do not rely only on the effects of EGCG.[37]

Acne

In 2009, Elsaie et al. enrolled 20 patients in a six-week study to investigate the efficacy of 2 percent green tea lotion for the treatment of mild-to-moderate acne vulgaris. Participants applied lotion twice daily and were evaluated every two weeks. The researchers reported a statistically significant reduction in mean total lesion count from 24 to 10 after the treatment period (a decrease of 58.33 percent). A statistically significant decline in mean severity index (devised by the authors to correlate with total lesion count in increasing intensity, scaled from 1 to 3) from 2.05 to 1.25 (39.02 percent decrease) was also noted. The investigators concluded that 2 percent green tea lotion is both an effective and cost-effective approach for ameliorating mild-to-moderate acne lesions.[38]

A 2012 study revealed that ethanol extracts of several herbs, including green tea, exhibited the potential for inhibiting acne when incorporated into a topical moisturizer, specifically acting against acne-causing bacteria without provoking irritation.[39] Earlier that year, Jung et al. conducted *in vitro* and *in vivo* experiments to evaluate the effects against acne of polyphenon-60, which contains various green tea catechins (now referred to as sinecatechins in the United States).[40] In their clinical study, patients exhibited improvement in acne symptoms, including a reduction in the number of pustules and comedones. *In vitro* work revealed that *Propionibacterium acnes*-enhanced toll-like receptor 2 (TLR2) and IL-8 levels in THP-1 cells were diminished by polyphenon-60. Human monocyte cell lines and human primary monocytes were also decreased. The investigators concluded that polyphenon-60 inhibits inflammation through the downregulation of the extracellular signal-regulated kinases 1/2 (ERK1/2) pathway and AP-1 pathway, thus suppressing TLR2 expression and IL-8 secretion.[41]

In 2013, Mahmood et al. conducted a single-blind, placebo-controlled, split-face comparative study in 22 individuals to evaluate the efficacy of green tea as well as green tea plus lotus as compared to placebo for controlling casual sebum secretions in healthy adults. Over a 60-day period, volunteers in Group 1 applied a multiple emulsion formulation containing green tea extract; Group 2 applied a multiple emulsion with green tea and lotus extract. Compared to placebo, consistent and statistically significant decreases in sebum secretions were observed in both treatment groups. The combination of green tea and lotus extracts also achieved statistically sounder results than green tea alone. The investigators concluded that a synergistic interaction between green tea and lotus extract constituents appears to hold promise for the treatment of skin conditions in which elevated sebum levels are involved.[42]

Anogenital Warts

Gross et al. reported in 2007 on a randomized, double-blind, placebo-controlled Phase II/III 12-week clinical efficacy and safety study of polyphenon E, consisting of more than 85 percent catechins,[43] in 242 outpatients with external genital warts at 28 hospitals in Germany and Russia. Polyphenon E 15 percent ointment was found efficacious and safe for men and women in clearing external genital warts, with statistically significant differences seen compared to placebo and higher clearance and lower recurrence compared to the 10 percent ointment.[44]

In 2006, the United States Food and Drug Administration (USFDA) approved of the use of a green tea extract formulation (Veregen) for the topical treatment of genital and perianal warts, typically caused by the human papillomavirus (HPV)-6 or HPV-11.[40,45,46] In 2008, Tatti et al. conducted a randomized, double-blind, vehicle-controlled trial to evaluate the efficacy of topical sinecatechins, a defined green tea extract, in 502 male and female patients (aged 18 years and older) for the treatment of anogenital warts. For 16 weeks or until complete clearance, subjects applied sinecatechins ointment 15 or 10 percent or vehicle (placebo) three times daily. A 12-week follow-up to gauge recurrence ensued. Complete clearance was achieved in 57.2 percent of patients treated with 15 percent ointment, 56.3 percent using 10 percent ointment, and 33.7 percent who used only the vehicle. Respective recurrence rates were 6.5 percent, 8.3 percent, and 8.8 percent. The investigators concluded that topical sinecatechins in 15 and 10 percent concentrations represent effective and well-tolerated options for anogenital wart treatment.[47] Similarly favorable results

regarding polyphenon E 15 percent were reported by Gross that year in reference to three placebo-controlled clinical studies in 1,400 patients with genital warts from Europe, North and South America, and South Africa.[48]

In 2010, Tatti et al. conducted randomized, double-blind, vehicle-controlled safety and efficacy trials in nearly 1,000 patients with external genital warts who were treated with polyphenon E ointment 10 percent, polyphenon E ointment 15 percent, or vehicle. They concluded that the sinecatechin formulation was effective and well tolerated, with complete clearance observed in 54.9 percent of subjects taking the 15 percent ointment, 53.6 percent of those taking the 10 percent ointment, and 35.4 percent using only the vehicle.[40]

Hoy et al. reported in 2012 on the evaluation of polyphenon E 10 percent ointment in two double-blind, multinational studies in adults with external genital and perianal warts. Polyphenon E 10 percent was found to be significantly more effective than vehicle in completely or partially clearing all warts (baseline and those emerging during treatment) in both studies. During 12-week follow-up periods in both studies, rates of recurrence or new warts appearing were less than 9 percent in both treatment arms. Polyphenon E 10 percent was well tolerated, with most adverse effects involving minor skin irritation at the treatment site.[49]

Earlier that year, Stockfleth and Meyer reviewed the use of sinecatechins (polyphenon E) ointment for the treatment of external anogenital warts. They noted that while clearance rates are similar among sinecatechins and other indicated topical medications such as imiquimod and podophyllotoxin, recurrence rates are lower for patients treated with sinecatechins. The authors concluded that the use of sinecatechins for condylomata acuminata is safe and effective and its various molecular activities suggest broader applications to other viral and tumor lesions.[50] Previously, Stockfleth et al., in 2008, had found, in a randomized controlled trial of 503 patients, that polyphenon E (15 and 10 percent) was safe and efficacious for the treatment of external genital and perianal warts.[51] Ahn et al. showed earlier, in a study with 51 patients, that polyphenon E and EGCG delivered topically or in capsule form were also effective in treating HPV-infected cervical lesions.[52]

Sinecatechins, derived from green tea catechins and other constituents of *C. sinensis*, in a topical 15 percent ointment (Veregen®), is the first botanical drug formulation to be approved by the FDA for the treatment of external genital and perianal warts.[40,53,54] Sinecatechins have been shown *in vitro* to suppress HPV-infected tumor cell lines, and to manifest antiproliferative activity that Tyring speculates may be involved in the overall anticancer and antiviral properties associated with these GTPs that also lead to the clearance of external genital and perianal warts.[55] Interestingly, sinecatechins have been recently shown to hinder, often dose-dependently, several kinases and enzymes, including MMPs (MMP-1, MMP-2, MMP-7, and MMP-9), lipoxygenases, cyclooxygenases, and proteases, which are involved in inflammatory mediator generation.[53,54]

Other Antimicrobial Uses

In 2013, De Oliveira et al. showed that modified EGCG (palmitoyl-EGCG) has potential as a topical antiviral agent for herpes simplex virus (HSV-1) infection.[56]

Indeed, EGCG has been demonstrated to exhibit significant activity against HSV, inactivating several clinical isolates of HSV-1 as well as HSV-2, and, given its stability in pH ranges characteristic in the vagina, is emerging as a viable microbicidal agent for lowering HSV transmission, according to Isaacs et al.[57]

In addition, EGCG has been found in one study to suppress the human immunodeficiency virus-1 (HIV-1) infectivity-enhancing activity of human semen, though with significant variability. The investigators speculate that topically applied EGCG may emerge as an additional tactic to reduce the likelihood of sexual transmission of HIV, but note that more information regarding the differences in efficacy is necessary before therapeutic human trials can commence.[58] EGCG has also been demonstrated to lower the number of plaques in HIV-infected cultured cells.[56]

Further, Shin et al. recently developed and used an experimental skin contact model for influenza virus to assess a green tea handwash disinfectant, finding that viral infectivity was eliminated on skin cell layers washed with the green tea solution.[59]

Other Indications

Hsu et al. showed in 2007 that the topical application of 0.5 percent GTPs attenuated the symptoms of psoriasis in a flaky skin mouse model, suggesting that GTP-induced caspase 14 may serve as a potential target of novel formulations aimed at alleviating psoriasis.[60] Green tea extracts have also protected against the phototoxic effects engendered by the psoriasis treatment psoralen plus UVA, by inhibiting DNA damage and attenuating the inflammatory effects of the treatment.[11,61]

Kwon et al. observed *in vitro* the growth stimulation of dermal papilla cells by EGCG as well as on human scalps *in vivo* in a 2007 study. The investigators suggested that EGCG exerts dual proliferative and antiapoptotic effects on dermal papilla cells and has potential to thwart androgenetic alopecia.[62]

In a small randomized, double-blind, six-week split-face trial in 2010, Domingo et al. found that the topical application of a cream containing 2.5 percent EGCG may have potential in preventing telangiectasias.[63]

A small pilot study of four atopic dermatitis patients conducted by Kim et al. in 2012 revealed that all four patients using bath therapy with green tea extracts three times each week over four weeks improved markedly. The investigators concluded that the green tea-infused bath therapy is a safe and effective alternative to corticosteroid treatment for patients with atopic dermatitis associated with *Malassezia sympodialis*.[64]

In addition, the use of green tea catechins in a local delivery system was shown in a clinical pilot study in 2002 to be effective in ameliorating periodontal status.[65] Green tea had previously been shown in human and laboratory studies to impart protection against dental caries.[10,66,67]

Combination Therapy

Green tea has been shown to work in combination with red light to exert a rejuvenating effect on the skin, as Sommer and Zhu reported in 2009 that green tea-filled cotton pads applied once daily for 20 minutes prior to treatment with light-emitting diodes (central wavelength 670 nm, dermal dose 4 J/cm^2) diminished wrinkles in one month comparably to 10 months of light treatment alone.[68]

In a small 2013 study with 16 subjects with facial redness, a topical formulation combining GTPs, resveratrol, and caffeine was found to reduce erythema after six weeks of treatment, with no adverse effects seen.[69]

SAFETY ISSUES

Green tea and green tea extracts are generally recognized as safe (GRAS). After extensive safety testing of oral and topical preparations of EGCG in rats, guinea pigs, rabbits, and dogs,

Isbrucker et al. established a no-observed adverse effect level of 500 mg EGCG preparation/kg/day.[70] Previously, Stratton et al. found no toxicity associated with daily topical EGCG use in studies with female SKH-1 hairless mice, but noted that use of topical depilatories could activate dermal toxicity from EGCG use.[61]

ENVIRONMENTAL IMPACT

It is improbable that the cultivation of *C. sinensis* adversely effects the environment. Rather, it is more likely that the sustainability of tea plantations may be challenged or threatened by global climate change. In a recent study by Wijeratne et al., the investigators concluded that tea yields are likely to decrease in lower and moderate elevations and increase in higher elevations.[71]

FORMULATION CONSIDERATIONS

Green tea is thought to be challenging to formulate because of the inherent hydrophilicity of EGCG, which limits penetration into human skin.[72,73]

Dvorakova et al. ascertained, in a 1999 study of the pharmacokinetics of EGCG applied topically in mouse and human skin, that the stability of the green tea constituent in hydrophilic ointment depends on time, temperature, and degree of oxidation. Stability was enhanced by the supplementation of butylated hydroxytoluene.[74]

A 2011 study by Bianchi et al. showed that use of the water-soluble UVB filter benzophenone-4 rendered EGCG more photostable in topical formulations designed to protect the skin from photodamage.[75]

In 2013, Silva et al. evaluated the efficacy of five commercial green tea extracts in cosmetic formulations in protecting against UV-induced damage to human and mouse fibroblasts and compared the results to the effects of a fluid preparation meeting Brazilian Pharmacopoeia standards. As comparative parameters, they used individual EGCG content, catalase and superoxide dismutase status, and MMP-1, MMP-9, and MMP-13 levels. The researchers found substantial variability in EGCG content, unlike the fluid product, which was also the only formulation capable of markedly lowering MMP degradation while increasing superoxide dismutase and catalase levels. The investigators stated that their findings represent the first report indicating that the methods of preparing herbal mixtures can substantially interfere with constituents with inherent photoprotective properties, and, specifically, the efficacy of *C. sinensis* extracts can be compromised in such products.[76]

USAGE CONSIDERATIONS

EGCG is the component in green and white tea responsible for antioxidant activity.[26,77] Therefore, one must know which polyphenols are present in a skin care formulation to assess product usefulness. Learning the percentage of polyphenols in the product is also important. Some products turn brown due to the inclusion of a large amount of green tea components. Green tea does not easily react with other ingredients and seems to facilitate or support their stability; therefore, it is relatively easy to combine with other ingredients.

SIGNIFICANT BACKGROUND

In a 2010 systematic database review (MEDLINE, Embase, CINAHL®, CENTRAL, and AMED databases) of randomized clinical trials or controlled clinical trials showing evidence for the effectiveness or efficacy of botanical treatments in reducing skin aging and wrinkling, Hunt et al. reported that of the 11 trials of botanical extracts that met all the inclusion criteria, no significant reduction in skin wrinkling was associated with green tea or Vitaphenol® (a combination of green and white teas, mangosteen, and pomegranate extract). They noted, though, that all trials were of poor methodological quality and more rigorous studies are necessary to explain or validate their finding.[78] Elbling et al. also cautioned against the excessive consumption of green tea or topical use of green tea products before the performance of extensive *in vivo* investigations given their *in vitro* findings that EGCG increased hydrogen peroxide-induced oxidative stress and DNA damage.[79]

Nonetheless, GTPs are believed to impart broad photoprotective effects against UV-induced carcinogenic activity as well as sunburn response, immunosuppression, and photoaging. Therefore, green tea is thought to be a potentially significant agent to be combined with traditional sunscreens to buttress photoprotection.[80]

Photoprotection

Early studies of GTPs demonstrated inhibition of chemical- and UV-induced carcinogenesis in hairless or Sencar mice receiving orally administered or topically applied test drug.[81–83] Such evidence has been confirmed in subsequent work, with EGCG emerging as a potent suppressor of photocarcinogenesis.[84] The photoprotective effects of topically applied GTPs have also been noted in human skin, with a dose-dependent decline of UV-induced erythema, diminished sunburn cell formation, protection of epidermal Langerhans cells, and limitation of DNA damage.[85]

As Mnich et al. noted in 2009, the limited studies conducted in humans of the effects of topical green tea extracts have typically included high concentrations of extracts over short test periods. In their five-week study with 21 volunteers, however, stabilized low-dose green tea extracts incorporated into a cosmetic product (OM24) were found to be effective, at cosmetically usable concentrations, in conferring photochemopreventive activity, lowering UVB-mediated epithelial damage without tachyphylaxis.[86]

Also that year, Camouse et al. analyzed skin samples from volunteers or skin explants and showed that topically applied green or white tea extracts provided protection to human skin from solar-simulated UV light, concluding that both agents are potential photoprotective agents.[87]

In 2011, a study by Katiyar elucidated aspects of the mechanisms of action of GTPs, topically applied or orally administered in the drinking water of mice, which have been shown to prevent UVB-induced nonmelanoma skin cancer development. The process appears to be at least partly mediated through DNA repair.[88] Another recent study with Katiyar at the helm showed that GTPs prevent UV-induced immunosuppression through a similar mechanism, rapid DNA damage repair and amelioration of nucleotide excision repair genes. The authors suggest that this process may explain the chemopreventive effects of GTPs in warding off photocarcinogenesis.[89]

In Vitro Studies

A study comparing the effects of EGCG and retinoic acid on alterations in the extracellular matrix induced by UVA exposure revealed, using artificial skin and cultured keratinocytes and fibroblasts, that topically applied EGCG can reverse UV-induced changes. EGCG was also found by Lee et al., in this 2005 study, to be slightly more effective than retinoic acid.[90]

In 2009, Osterburg et al. demonstrated *in vitro* that EGCG acts as an effective bactericidal against antibiotic-resistant *Acinetobacter baumannii*, an increasingly common source of infections in intensive care units worldwide.[91]

Additional antibacterial activity exhibited by green tea has been recently supported. In 2012, Sharma et al. found that selected bacterial strains, including *Staphylococcus epidermidis*, *Micrococcus luteus*, *Brevibacterium linens*, *Pseudomonas fluorescens*, and *Bacillus subtilis*, were sensitive to green tea extract via disc diffusion assay.[1]

Using A375 (BRAF-mutated) and Hs294t (Non-BRAF-mutated) melanoma cell lines in 2011, Singh and Katiyar ascertained the effect of green tea catechins on the invasive potential of human melanoma cells in an *in vitro* model. They determined that EGCG exhibited the capacity to suppress melanoma cell invasion/migration by targeting the endogenous expression of cyclooxygenase-2, and prostaglandin E_2 receptors, as well as the cellular epithelial-to-mesenchymal transition or transformation.[92]

Recent *in vitro* evidence also suggests that green tea extracts have the potential for efficacy against leishmaniasis.[93]

Additional Animal Studies

The preponderance of studies supporting anticarcinogenic, anti-inflammatory, antioxidant, and photoprotective activity associated with green tea has been performed in animals.[9,15,34,94,95]

In 2003, Vayalil et al. demonstrated in an *in vivo* mouse model that the topical application of GTPs or EGCG in hydrophilic ointment prior to single or multiple UVB exposures led to a significant prevention of UVB-induced antioxidant enzyme depletion, particularly glutathione peroxidase and catalase. Treatment with EGCG also substantially inhibited, in a time-dependent manner, the phosphorylation of the ERK1/2, JNK, and p38 proteins of the MAPK family after one or multiple UVB exposures.[96]

In 2006, Meeran et al. demonstrated that EGCG can prevent photocarcinogenesis in mice by inducing an IL-12 DNA repair mechanism.[30]

The next year, Sevin et al. determined that 2 percent EGCG topically applied to the skin of Wistar albino rats rendered a photoprotective effect against UVA when applied before but not after UV exposure.[97]

EGCG, through injection or topical application, has also been shown to enhance neovascularization and regional perfusion leading to the amelioration of skin flap survival in a rat dorsal skin flap model.[98]

Human Studies

The broad effects of GTPs in human beings have been examined in a spate of studies during the last 15 years.

Katiyar et al., in 1999, demonstrated that the topical application of EGCG to human skin displays the potential to hinder the UVB-generated infiltration of inflammatory leukocytes and the ensuing development of reactive oxygen species.[99] The next year, Katiyar et al. extended a mouse model to an *in vivo* demonstration in humans that topically applied GTPs prevent the formation of UVB-induced DNA damage as manifested by the inhibition of cutaneous cyclobutane pyrimidine dimers, at least partially accounting for the suppression of photocarcinogenesis associated with green tea.[100] In 2001, Katiyar et al.

showed that pretreatment of human skin with EGCG prior to UV irradiation prevents the cascade of oxidative stress, including the protection of the antioxidant enzyme glutathione peroxidase. It also suppresses UV-induced infiltration of inflammatory leukocytes and significantly reduces the UV-induced synthesis of hydrogen peroxide and nitric oxide.[101]

Chiu et al. conducted, in 2005, a double-blind, placebo-controlled, eight-week trial with 40 women with moderate photoaging who were randomized for treatment with either a 10 percent green tea cream and 300 mg twice-daily green tea oral supplement or a placebo regimen. The investigators found significant histologic (elastic content of treated specimens) but no clinical signs of improvement in photoaged skin. They concluded that a longer treatment period might be necessary to achieve clinical improvement.[102]

In 2013, Hong et al. conducted an eight-week study in 42 healthy Korean females (aged 30–59 years) to examine the antiwrinkle effects of topically applied green tea extract displaying high antioxidant activity after tannase treatment, with increased levels of gallic acid, EGC, and EC. Subjects were randomly divided into two groups, one of which applied tannase-converted green tea extract on their crow's feet and the other, normal green tea extract. Reductions in the average roughness of skin values were much greater in the tannase group as were the scavenging abilities against free radicals. In addition, marked or moderate improvements in wrinkles were reported in the tannase group (63.6 percent) compared to the normal green tea group (36.3 percent). The researchers concluded that tannase treatment enhanced the antioxidant activity of green tea extract, rendering it better able to combat wrinkles, adding that the tannase green tea formulation warrants attention as an antiwrinkle agent.[103]

At around the same time, Gianeti conducted clinical studies in 24 volunteers to assess the effects of a cosmetic formulation containing 6 percent *C. sinensis* glycolic leaf extracts. The experimental formulation was compared to vehicle alone in the treatment of forearm skin, which was evaluated before and after two hours of application as well as after 15 and 30 days of use. Skin moisture was enhanced after 30 days of topical application as was the viscoelastic-to-elastic ratio as compared with vehicle and control (a forearm area left untreated). Skin roughness was significantly diminished after 30 days. The investigators concluded that the use of green tea in a topical cosmetic formulation yielded salient moisturizing and cutaneous microrelief benefits.[104]

Also in 2013, Rhodes et al. found that the oral intake of green tea catechins in 16 healthy human subjects (with 14 completing the study) appeared to result in the integration of catechin metabolites into human skin linked to the negation of UV-induced 12-hydroxyeicosatetraenoic acid (12-HETE). They speculated that this incorporation of catechins may render protection against sunburn inflammation and even cumulative UV-induced harm.[105]

In addition, in a small study of 10 healthy male volunteers conducted over a 60-day period, Mahmood et al. found that a green tea extract cream had a significant impact on the viscoelastic properties of the skin.[106]

After earlier showing the efficacy of green tea and lotus extracts in skin disorders involving excess sebum, Mahmood and Akhtar conducted a 60-day, placebo-controlled, and comparative, split-face study in 33 healthy Asian men to evaluate the efficacy of two cosmetic formulations (green tea and lotus extract) in treating facial wrinkles. The participants were divided into three groups, with one applying multiple emulsions with green tea, one applying multiple emulsions with lotus extract, and one applying a combination of both botanicals. Applications were once daily, with each of the active formulations applied to one side of the face and placebo on the other side. All of the formulations yielded improvements in skin roughness, scaliness, smoothness, and wrinkling, with the greatest reduction in wrinkling conferred by the combination formulation. The investigators concluded that the synergistic activity of green tea and lotus extracts exerted significant improvement along several skin parameters, suggesting the potential for these ingredients in antiaging products.[105]

CONCLUSION

Investigations into the health benefits of green tea and its constituent polyphenols represents one of the most fertile areas of antioxidant research. While broad-spectrum clinical efficacy of topically applied green tea polyphenols (particularly EGCG) has not been established, evidence is amassing that these constituents due indeed deliver cutaneous benefits. Green tea polyphenols are in use for a growing number of indications, especially acne and genital warts, and there is reason for optimism that topically applied green tea will gain favor as an adjuvant therapy option in several cases. More clinical studies are necessary to further elucidate the versatile role of green tea in the dermatologic armamentarium. This popular herbal agent holds particular promise in relation to photoprotection against UV-induced skin cancer and aging.

REFERENCES

1. Sharma A, Gupta S, Sarethy IP, et al. Green tea extract: Possible mechanism and antibacterial activity on skin pathogens. *Food Chem.* 2012;135:672.
2. Oyetakin White P, Tribout H, Baron E. Protective mechanisms of green tea polyphenols in skin. *Oxid Med Cell Longev.* 2012;2012:560682.
3. Weisburger JH. Tea and health: A historical perspective. *Cancer Lett.* 1997;114:315.
4. Hsu S. Green tea and the skin. *J Am Acad Dermatol.* 2005;52:1049.
5. Katiyar SK, Ahmad N, Mukhtar H. Green tea and skin. *Arch Dermatol.* 2000;136:989.
6. Katiyar SK, Elmets CA, Agarwal R, et al. Protection against UVB radiation-induced local and systemic suppression of contact hypersensitivity and edema responses in C3H/HeN mice by green tea polyphenols. *Photochem Photobiol.* 1995;62:855.
7. Thornfeldt C. Cosmeceuticals containing herbs: fact, fiction, and future. *Dermatol Surg.* 2005;31:873.
8. Reuter J, Merfort I, Schempp CM. Botanicals in dermatology: An evidence-based review. *Am J Clin Dermatol.* 2010;11:247.
9. Wright TI, Spencer JM, Flowers FP. Chemoprevention of nonmelanoma skin cancer. *J Am Acad Dermatol.* 2006;54:933.
10. Cooper R, Morré DJ, Morré DM. Medicinal benefits of green tea: Part I – Review of noncancer health benefits. *J Altern Complement Med.* 2005;11:521.
11. Bickers DR, Athar M. Novel approaches to chemoprevention of skin cancer. *J Dermatol.* 2000;27:691.
12. Suzuki Y, Miyoshi N, Isemura M. Health-promoting effects of green tea. *Proc Jpn Acad Ser B Phys Biol Sci.* 2012;88:88.
13. Katiyar SK, Mohan RR, Agarwal R, et al. Protection against induction of mouse skin papillomas with low and high risk of conversion to malignancy by green tea polyphenols. *Carcinogenesis.* 1997;18:497.
14. Katiyar SK, Rupp CO, Korman NJ, et al. Inhibition of 12-O-tetradecanoylphorbol-13-acetate and other skin tumor-promoter-caused induction of epidermal interleukin-1 alpha mRNA and protein expression in SENCAR mice by green tea polyphenols. *J Invest Dermatol.* 1995;105:394.
15. Mukhtar H, Katiyar SK, Agarwal R. Green tea and skin – Anticarcinogenic effects. *J Invest Dermatol.* 1994;102:3.
16. Katiyar SK, Agarwal R, Mukhtar H. Inhibition of both stage I and stage II skin tumor promotion in SENCAR mice by a polyphenolic fraction isolated from green tea: Inhibition depends on the duration of polyphenol treatment. *Carcinogenesis.* 1993;14:2641.

17. Katiyar SK, Agarwal R, Mukhtar H. Protection against malignant conversion of chemically induced benign skin papillomas to squamous cell carcinomas in SENCAR mice by a polyphenolic fraction isolated from green tea. *Cancer Res.* 1993;53:5409.

18. Katiyar SK, Agarwal R, Ekker S, et al. Protection against 12-O-tetradecanoylphorbol-13-acetate-caused inflammation in SENCAR mouse ear skin by polyphenolic fraction isolated from green tea. *Carcinogenesis.* 1993;14:361.

19. Katiyar SK, Agarwal R, Wood GS, et al. Inhibition of 12-O-tetradecanoylphorbol-13-acetate-caused tumor promotion in 7,12-dimethylbenz[a]anthracene-initiated SENCAR mouse skin by a polyphenolic fraction isolated from green tea. *Cancer Res.* 1992;52:6890.

20. Agarwal R, Katiyar SK, Zaidi SI, et al. Inhibition of skin tumor promoter-caused induction of epidermal ornithine decarboxylase in SENCAR mice by polyphenolic fraction isolated from green tea and its individual epicatechin derivatives. *Cancer Res.* 1992;52:3582.

21. Wang ZY, Khan WA, Bickers DR, et al. Protection against polycyclic aromatic hydrocarbon-induced skin tumor initiation in mice by green tea polyphenols. *Carcinogenesis.* 1989;10:411.

22. Conney AH, Wang ZY, Huang MT, et al. Inhibitory effect of green tea on tumorigenesis by chemicals and ultraviolet light. *Prev Med.* 1992;21:361.

23. Katiyar SK, Agarwal R, Wang ZY, et al. (-)-Epigallocatechin-3-gallate in Camellia sinensis leaves from Himalayan region of Sikkim: Inhibitory effects against biochemical events and tumor initiation in Sencar mouse skin. *Nutr Cancer.* 1992;18:73.

24. Huang MT, Ho CT, Wang ZY, et al. Inhibitory effect of topical application of a green tea polyphenol fraction on tumor initiation and promotion in mouse skin. *Carcinogenesis.* 1992;13:947.

25. Wang ZY, Huang MT, Ferraro T, et al. Inhibitory effect of green tea in the drinking water on tumorigenesis by ultraviolet light and 12-O-tetradecanoylphorbol-13-acetate in the skin of SKH-1 mice. *Cancer Res.* 1992;52:1162.

26. Shi X, Ye J, Leonard SS, et al. Antioxidant properties of (-)-epicatechin-3-gallate and its inhibition of Cr(VI)-induced DNA damage and Cr(IV)- or TPA-stimulated NF-kappaB activation. *Mol Cell Biochem.* 2000;206:125.

27. Stratton SP, Dorr RT, Alberts DS. The state-of-the-art in chemoprevention of skin cancer. *Eur J Cancer.* 2000;36:1292.

28. Chung JH, Han JH, Hwang EJ, et al. Dual mechanisms of green tea extract (EGCG)-induced cell survival in human epidermal keratinocytes. *FASEB J.* 2003;17:1913.

29. Katiyar SK, Challa A, McCormick TS, et al. Prevention of UVB-induced immunosuppression in mice by the green tea polyphenol (-)-epigallocatechin-3-gallate may be associated with alterations in IL-10 and IL-12 production. *Carcinogenesis.* 1999;20:2117.

30. Meeran SM, Mantena SK, Elmets CA, et al. (-)-Epigallocatechin-3-gallate prevents photocarcinogenesis in mice through interleukin-12-dependent DNA repair. *Cancer Res.* 2006;66:5512.

31. Katiyar SK, Bergamo BM, Vayalil PK, et al. Green tea polyphenols: DNA photodamage and photoimmunology. *J Photochem Photobiol B.* 2001;65:109.

32. Vayalil PK, Mittal A, Hara Y, et al. Green tea polyphenols prevent ultraviolet light-induced oxidative damage and matrix metalloproteinases expression in mouse skin. *J Invest Dermatol.* 2004;122:1480.

33. Awadalla HI, Ragab MH, Bassuoni MW, et al. A pilot study of the role of green tea use on oral health. *Int J Dent Hyg.* 2011;9:110.

34. Katiyar S, Elmets CA, Katiyar SK. Green tea and skin cancer: photoimmunology, angiogenesis and DNA repair. *J Nutr Biochem.* 2007;18:287.

35. Pazyar N, Feily A, Kazerouni A. Green tea in dermatology. *Skinmed.* 2012;10:352.

36. Tzellos TG, Sardeli C, Lallas A, et al. Efficacy, safety and tolerability of green tea catechins in the treatment of external anogenital warts: A systematic review and meta-analysis. *J Eur Acad Dermatol Venereol.* 2011;25:345.

37. Pajonk F, Riedisser A, Henke M, et al. The effects of tea extracts on proinflammatory signaling. *BMC Med.* 2006;4:28.

38. Elsaie ML, Abdelhamid MF, Elsaaiee LT, et al. The efficacy of topical 2% green tea lotion in mild-to-moderate acne vulgaris. *J Drugs Dermatol.* 2009;8:358.

39. Rasheed A, Shama SN, Joy JM, et al. Formulation and evaluation of herbal anti-acne moisturizer. *Pak J Pharm Sci.* 2012;25:867.

40. Tatti S, Stockfleth E, Beutner KR, et al. Polyphenon E: A new treatment for external anogenital warts. *Br J Dermatol.* 2010;162:176.

41. Jung MK, Ha S, Son JA, et al. Polyphenon-60 displays a therapeutic effect on acne by suppression of TLR2 and IL-8 expression via down-regulating the ERK1/2 pathway. *Arch Dermatol Res.* 2012;304:655.

42. Mahmood T, Akhtar N, Moldovan C. A comparison of the effects of topical green tea and lotus on facial sebum control in healthy humans. *Hippokratia.* 2013;17:64.

43. Meltzer SM, Monk BJ, Tewari KS. Green tea catechins for treatment of external genital warts. *Am J Obstet Gynecol.* 2009;200:233.e1.

44. Gross G, Meyer KG, Pres H, et al. A randomized, double-blind, four-arm parallel-group, placebo-controlled Phase II/III study to investigate the clinical efficacy of two galenic formulations of Polyphenon E in the treatment of external genital warts. *J Eur Acad Dermatol Venereol.* 2007;21:1404.

45. Wu KM, Ghantous H, Birnkrant DB. Current regulatory toxicology perspectives on the development of herbal medicines to prescription drug products in the United States. *Food Chem Toxicol.* 2008;46:2606.

46. Chen ST, Dou J, Temple R, et al. New therapies from old medicines. *Nat Biotechnol.* 2008;26:1077.

47. Tatti S, Swinehart JM, Thielert C, et al. Sinecatechins, a defined green tea extract, in the treatment of external anogenital warts: a randomized controlled trial. *Obstet Gynecol.* 2008;111:1371.

48. Gross G. Polyphenon E. A new topical therapy for condylomata acuminate. *Hautarzt.* 2008;59:31.

49. Hoy SM. Polyphenon E 10% ointment: In immunocompetent adults with external genital and perianal warts. *Am J Clin Dermatol.* 2012;13:275.

50. Stockfleth E, Meyer T. The use of sinecatechins (polyphenon E) ointment for treatment of external genital warts. *Expert Opin Biol Ther.* 2012;12:783.

51. Stockfleth E, Beti H, Orasan R, et al. Topical Polyphenon E in the treatment of external genital and perianal warts: a randomized controlled trial. *Br J Dermatol.* 2008;158:1329.

52. Ahn WS, Yoo J, Huh SW, et al. Protective effects of green tea extracts (polyphenon E and EGCG) on human cervical lesions. *Eur J Cancer Prev.* 2003;12:383.

53. Berman B, Wolf J. The role of imiquimod 3.75% cream in the treatment of external genital warts. *Skin Therapy Lett.* 2012;17:5.

54. Tyring SK. Sinecatechins: Effects on HPV-induced enzymes involved in inflammatory mediator generation. *J Clin Aesthet Dermatol.* 2012;5:19.

55. Tyring SK. Effect of sinecatechins on HPV-activated cell growth and induction of apoptosis. *J Clin Aesthet Dermatol.* 2012;5:34.

56. De Oliveira A, Adams SD, Lee LH, et al. Inhibition of herpes simplex virus type 1 with the modified green tea polyphenol palmitoyl-epigallocatechin gallate. *Food Chem Toxicol.* 2013;52:207.

57. Isaacs CE, Wen GY, Xu W, et al. Epigallocatechin gallate inactivates clinical isolates of herpes simplex virus. *Antimicrob Agents Chemother.* 2008;52:962.

58. Hartjen P, Frerk S, Hauber I, et al. Assessment of the range of the HIV-1 infectivity enhancing effect of individual human semen specimen and the range of inhibition of EGCG. *AIDS Res Ther.* 2012;9:2.

59. Shin WJ, Kim YK, Lee KH, et al. Evaluation of the antiviral activity of a green tea solution as a hand-wash disinfectant. *Biosci Biotechnol Biochem.* 2012;76:581.

60. Hsu S, Dickinson D, Borke J, et al. Green tea polyphenol induces caspase 14 in epidermal keratinocytes via MAPK pathways and reduces psoriasiform lesions in the flaky skin mouse model. *Exp Dermatol.* 2007;16:678.

61. Zhao JF, Zhang YJ, Jin XH, et al. Green tea protects against psoralen plus ultraviolet A-induced photochemical damage to skin. *J Invest Dermatol.* 1999;113:1070.

62. Kwon OS, Han JH, Yoo HG, et al. Human hair growth enhancement in vitro by green tea epigallocatechin-3-gallate (EGCG). *Phytomedicine.* 2007;14:551.

63. Domingo DS, Camouse MM, Hsia AH, et al. Anti-angiogenic effects of epigallocatechin-3-gallate in human skin. *Int J Clin Exp Pathol.* 2010;3:705.

64. Kim HK, Chang HK, Baek SY, et al. Treatment of atopic dermatitis associated with Malassezia sympodialis by green tea extracts bath therapy: A pilot study. *Mycobiology.* 2012;40:124.

65. Hirasawa M, Takada K, Makumura M, et al. Improvement of periodontal status by green tea catechin using a local delivery system: A clinical pilot study. *J Periodontal Res.* 2002;37:433.

66. Otake S, Makimura M, Kuroki T, et al. Anticaries effects of polyphenolic compounds from Japanese green tea. *Caries Res.* 1991;25:438.

67. Horiba N, Maekawa Y, Ito M, et al. A pilot study of Japanese green tea as a medicament: antibacterial and bactericidal effects. *J Endod.* 1991;17:122.

68. Sommer AP, Zhu D. Green tea and red light – A powerful duo in skin rejuvenation. *Photomed Laser Surg.* 2009;27:969.

69. Ferzil G, Patel M, Phrsai N, et al. Reduction of facial redness with resveratrol added to topical product containing green tea polyphenols and caffeine. *J Drugs Dermatol.* 2013;12:770.

70. Isbrucker RA, Edwards JA, Wolz E, et al. Safety studies on epigallocatechin gallate (EGCG) preparations – Part 2: dermal, acute and short-term toxicity studies. *Food Chem Toxicol.* 2006;44:636.

71. Wijeratne MA, Anandacoomaraswamy A, Amarathunga MSKLD, et al. Assessment of impact of climate change on productivity of tea (Camellia sinensis L.) plantations in Sri Lanka. *J Natn Sci Foundation Sri Lanka.* 2007;35:119.

72. Farris P. Idebenone, green tea, and Coffeeberry extract: New and innovative antioxidants. *Dermatol Ther.* 2007;20:322.

73. Levin J, Momin SB. How much do we really know about our favorite cosmeceutical ingredients? *J Clin Aesthet Dermatol.* 2010;3:22.

74. Dvorakova K, Dorr RT, Valcic S, et al. Pharmacokinetics of the green tea derivative, EGCG, by the topical route of administration in mouse and human skin. *Cancer Chemother Pharmacol.* 1999;43:331.

75. Bianchi A, Marchetti N, Scalia S. Photodegradation of (-)-epigallocatechin-3-gallate in topical cream formulations and its photostabilization. *J Pharm Biomed Anal.* 2011;56:692.

76. Silva AR, Seidl C, Furusho AS, et al. In vitro evaluation of the efficacy of commercial green tea extracts in UV protection. *Int J Cosmet Sci.* 2013;35:69.

77. Wei H, Zhang X, Zhao JF, et al. Scavenging of hydrogen peroxide and inhibition of ultraviolet light-induced oxidative DNA damage by aqueous extracts from green and black teas. *Free Radic Biol Med.* 1999;26:1427.

78. Hunt KJ, Hung SK, Ernst E. Botanical extracts as anti-aging preparations for the skin: A systematic review. *Drugs Aging.* 2010;27:973.

79. Elbling L, Weiss RM, Teufelhofer O, et al. Green tea extract and (-)-epigallocatechin-3-gallate, the major tea catechin, exert oxidant but lack antioxidant activities. *FASEB J.* 2005;19:807.

80. Yusuf N, Irby C, Katiyar SK, et al. Photoprotective effects of green tea polyphenols. *Photodermatol Photoimmunol Photomed.* 2007;23:48.

81. Wang ZY, Agarwal R, Bickers DR, et al. Protection against ultraviolet B radiation-induced photocarcinogenesis in hairless mice by green tea polyphenols. *Carcinogenesis.* 1991;12:1527.

82. Gensler HL, Timmermann BN, Valcic S, et al. Prevention of photocarcinogenesis by topical administration of pure epigallocatechin gallate isolated from green tea. *Nutr Cancer.* 1996;26:325.

83. Khan WA, Wang ZY, Athar M, et al. Inhibition of the skin tumorigenicity of (+/-)-7 beta,8 alpha-dihydroxy-9 alpha,10 alpha-epoxy-7,8,9,10-tetrahydrobenzo[a]pyrene by tannic acid, green tea polyphenols and quercetin in Sencar mice. *Cancer Lett.* 1988;42:7.

84. Mittal A, Piyathilake C, Hara Y, et al. Exceptionally high protection of photocarcinogenesis by topical application of (-)- epigallocatechin-3-gallate in hydrophilic cream in SKH-1 hairless mouse model: relationship to inhibition of UVB-induced global DNA hypomethylation. *Neoplasia.* 2003;5:555.

85. Elmets CA, Singh D, Tubesing K, et al. Cutaneous photoprotection from ultraviolet injury by green tea polyphenols. *J Am Acad Dermatol.* 2001;44:425.

86. Mnich CD, Hoek KS, Virkki LV, et al. Green tea extract reduces induction of p53 and apoptosis in UVB-irradiated human skin independent of transcriptional controls. *Exp Dermatol.* 2009;18:69.

87. Camouse MM, Domingo DS, Swain FR, et al. Topical application of green and white tea extracts provides protection from solar-simulated ultraviolet light in human skin. *Exp Dermatol.* 2009;18:522.

88. Katiyar SK. Green tea prevents non-melanoma skin cancer by enhancing DNA repair. *Arch Biochem Biophys.* 2011;508:152.

89. Katiyar SK, Vaid M, van Steeg H, et al. Green tea polyphenols prevent UV-induced immunosuppression by rapid repair of DNA damage and enhancement of nucleotide excision repair genes. *Cancer Prev Res (Phila).* 2010;3:179.

90. Lee JH, Chung JH, Cho KH. The effects of epigallocatechin-3-gallate on extracellular matrix metabolism. *J Dermatol Sci.* 2005;40:195.

91. Osterburg A, Gardner J, Hyon SH, et al. Highly antibiotic-resistant Acinetobacter baumannii clinical isolates are killed by the green tea polyphenol (-)-epigallocatechin-3-gallate (EGCG). *Clin Microbiol Infect.* 2009;15:341.

92. Singh T, Katiyar SK. Green tea catechins reduce invasive potential of human melanoma cells by targeting COX-2, PGE2 receptors and epithelial-to-mesenchymal transition. *PLoS One.* 2011;6:e25224.

93. Feily A, Saki J, Maraghi S, et al. In vitro activity of green tea extract Leishmania major promastigotes. *Int J Clin Pharmacol Ther.* 2012;50:233.

94. Katiyar SK. Skin photoprotection by green tea: Antioxidant and immunomodulatory effects. *Curr Drug Targets Immune Endocr Metabol Disord.* 2003;3:234.

95. Katiyar SK, Elmets CA. Green tea polyphenolic antioxidants and skin photoprotection (Review). *Int J Oncol.* 2001;18:1307.

96. Vayalil PK, Elmets CA, Katiyar SK. Treatment of green tea polyphenols in hydrophilic cream prevents UVB-induced oxidation of lipids and proteins, depletion of antioxidant enzymes and phosphorylation of MAPK proteins in SKH-1 hairless mouse skin. *Carcinogenesis.* 2003;24:927.

97. Sevin A, Ozta ş P, Senen D, et al. Effects of polyphenols on skin damage due to ultraviolet A rays: An experimental study on rats. *J Eur Acad Dermatol Venereol.* 2007;21:650.

98. Cheon YW, Tark KC, Kim YW. Better survival of random pattern skin flaps through the use of epigallocatechin gallate. *Dermatol Surg.* 2012;38:1835.

99. Katiyar SK, Matsui MS, Elmets CA, et al. Polyphenolic antioxidant (-)-epigallocatechin-3-gallate from green tea reduces UVB-induced inflammatory responses and infiltration of leukocytes in human skin. *Photochem Photobiol.* 1999;69:148.

100. Katiyar SK, Perez A, Mukhtar H. Green tea polyphenol treatment to human skin prevents formation of ultraviolet light B-induced pyrimidine dimers in DNA. *Clin Cancer Res.* 2000;6:3864.

101. Katiyar SK, Afaq F, Perez A, et al. Green tea polyphenol (-)-epigallocatechin-3-gallate treatment of human skin inhibits ultraviolet radiation-induced oxidative stress. *Carcinogenesis.* 2001;22:287.

102. Chiu AE, Chan JL, Kern DG, et al. Double-blinded, placebo-controlled trial of green tea extracts in the clinical and histologic appearance of photoaging skin. *Dermatol Surg.* 2005;31:855.

103. Hong YH, Jung EY, Shin KS, et al. Tannase-converted green tea catechins and their anti-wrinkle activity in humans. *J Cosmet Dermatol.* 2013;12:137.

104. Gianeti MD, Mercurio DG, Campos PM. The use of green tea extract in cosmetic formulations: Not only an antioxidant active ingredient. *Dermatol Ther.* 2013;26:267.

105. Mahmood T, Akhtar N. Combined topical application of lotus and green tea improves facial skin surface parameters. *Rejuvenation Res.* 2013;16:91.

106. Mahmood T, Akhtar N, Khan BA, et al. Changes in skin mechanical properties after long-term application of cream containing green tea extract. *Aging Clin Exp Res.* 2011;23:333.

CHAPTER 48

Rosa Damascena

Activities:

Antioxidant, antibacterial, antimicrobial, anti-inflammatory, antiseptic, and anxiolytic

Important Chemical Components:

Geraniol, which exhibits potent antiseptic activity (seven times that of phenol), and citronellol are the main constituents[1,2].
Phenyl ethyl alcohol, nerol, linalool, eugenol, quercetin, kaempferol, myricetin, β-carotene, tocopherol, γ-tocopherol, ascorbic acid, farnesol, stearpoten, and phenolic acids are also key active ingredients.

Origin Classification:

This ingredient is considered natural. As an ingredient used for dermatologic purposes, it is laboratory made.

Personal Care Category:

Antioxidant

Recommended for the following Baumann Skin Types:

DRNW, DRPW, DSNW, DSPW, ORNW, ORPW, OSNW, and OSPW

SOURCE

Known as the Damask Rose and Rose of Castile (and Gole Mohammadi in Iran), *Rosa damascena*, a member of the Rosaceae family, is a rose hybrid the flowers of which have been used for rose oil in perfume and for rosewater.[3] The petals are rich sources of vitamin C and flavonoids and water extracts of the flower are important components of the ancient herbal remedy "Safi" (cleansing agent), used safely for centuries in Unani medicine (practiced in South Asia and founded on traditional Graeco-Arabic medicine) in Pakistan.[4] Indeed, various medicinal properties have been associated with this species. *R. damascena* is an important ingredient in the food and cosmetics industries in addition to traditional medicine.

HISTORY

Originally found in the Middle East (the name "Damask Rose" is based on Damascus, Syria), *R. damascena* was introduced to Europe during the Crusades.[5] It is no longer found in the wild, but is cultivated for rose oil in several countries, primarily Bulgaria, Turkey, France, Morocco, Iran, and India.[6] Rosewater has been used for centuries in religious rites and for physical, emotional, and spiritual purposes or healing. Thriving rosewater industries are found in Bulgaria, France, and Iran.[3,7] The first use of rosewater has been attributed to the Persian doctor Avicenna (an anglicized version of Ibn Sina) in the early 11th century.[8] The use of *R. damascena* in Unani medicine,

particularly as an anti-inflammatory agent, has a long history and includes gastrointestinal and cardiovascular indications.[3,9] *R. damascena* is also used for culinary purposes in several global cuisines. The climatic conditions of the northern Indian state of Uttarakhand have been found to be especially conducive to the production of rose oil meeting international standards.[10]

Recent History

Some of the earliest work to indicate the potential health and dermatologic benefits of *R. damascena* dates to the late 1970s. Murphy and Hamilton isolated a strain of cultured cells of the plant that displayed strong resistance to ultraviolet (UV) radiation (254 nm) and generated a greater amount of polyphenols (primarily flavonoids) during the latter stages of culture growth. They found that this UV resistance was associated with increased polyphenolic production.[11] Flavonoids are the most prevalent and frequently studied polyphenols, which are the most abundant source of antioxidants in the human diet, often linked to a preventive role in cancer and heart disease as well as cutaneous signs of aging.[12-17] These phenolics, found throughout the *R. damascena* plant (i.e., fruits, seeds, leaves, roots, bark) are thought to be the main constituents responsible for the strong antioxidant activity exhibited by extracts of the plant (Table 48-1).[3]

CHEMISTRY

The rosewater and rose oil produced in mountainous northern India contains phenyl ethyl alcohol as a major constituent, with geraniol and citronellol appearing in many cultivars, as well as nerol nonadecane, heneicosane, and linalool.[10] Other chemical components include farnesol and stearpoten.

Ulusoy et al. examined the phenolic content as well as the antioxidant and antibacterial activities of *R. damascena* flower extracts absolute, essential oil, and hydrosol. The major constituents of rose essential oil and hydrosol (>55 percent) were found to be citronellol and geraniol, with phenylethyl alcohol (78.83 percent) identified as the primary component of rose absolute. The levels of key antioxidants (i.e., β-carotene, tocopherol, and γ-tocopherol) were found to be higher in rose absolute as compared to hydrosol and rose oil. High levels of phenolics were noted in rose absolute and the essential oil, which exhibited potent antibacterial activity against *Escherichia coli*, *Pseudomonas aeruginosa*, *Bacillus subtilis*, *Staphylococcus aureus*, *Chromobacterium violaceum*, and *Erwinia carotovora*.[2] Hydrosols, also referred to as floral waters, flower waters, hydroflorates, or distillates, are derived from steam distilling plant materials.

TABLE 48-1
Pros and Cons of Rosa Damascena

PROS	CON
Promising data to support antibacterial, antioxidant reputation	Insufficient research to establish potential in the dermatologic armamentarium
Wide range of medical benefits reported	

ORAL USES

R. damascena is edible and is found as a spice in the cuisine of Morocco, Turkey, and Iran.

TOPICAL USES

In 2003, Tabrizi et al. assessed various extracts of *R. damascena* for its capacity as an antisolar agent in absorbing UV. The presence of flavonoids as the primary constituents of the extracts was verified before investigators identified the UV absorption spectra, with all three extracts found to be effective in absorbing UV in the 200 to 400 nm range. The team then incorporated the extracts into oil-in-water creams at 5 and 8 percent concentrations. The hydroalcoholic extract provided the highest SPF, but the cream containing 5 percent ether extract yielded the most satisfactory appearance and stability. The investigators ascribed the UV absorption ability of the extracts to the flavonoid constituents and suggested that other synthetic antisolar compounds might be added to *R. damascena* extracts to enhance overall product efficacy. In addition, they concluded that the presence of *R. damascena* in the tested formulation would confer cooling, soothing, and anti-inflammatory properties suitable for a general skin care product as well as a photoprotective agent.[7]

SAFETY ISSUES

R. damascena has a long history of safe use in traditional medicine and cuisine. Although the sample size is small, there are no significant reports of adverse effects from products with *R. damascena* as a main active ingredient.

ENVIRONMENTAL IMPACT

Like any botanical crop cultivated for industrial uses, the industry itself exacts an environmental toll, but *R. damascena* is considered a friendly-to-the environment rural crop.[6]

FORMULATION CONSIDERATIONS

R. damascena has been formulated into various food products, including teas, in Korea.[18] Rosewater, rose oil, and rose hips are the main products extracted and processed from this plant. Due to the low oil content in *R. damascena* and the dearth of natural and synthetic alternatives, the essential oil is one of the most expensive in the world, earning the epithet "fluid gold."[3,6]

USAGE CONSIDERATIONS

The author knows of no interactions with other ingredients.

SIGNIFICANT BACKGROUND

Antioxidant Activity

In 2005, Schiber et al. extracted and characterized flavonol glycosides from *R. damascena* petals following industrial distillation for essential oil recovery. After analyzing 22 constituents, kaempferol and quercetin were the only flavonoids (specifically, flavonols) detected, with kaempferol compounds accounting for 80 percent of the compounds measured. In noting the high flavonol content (approximately 16 g/kg in dry weight), the researchers concluded that *R. damascena* represents a promising source of natural antioxidants.[19]

In a late 2010 study using a reversed-phase high-performance liquid chromatographic (RP-HPLC) method to simultaneously measure the flavonols, flavones, and phenolic acids as important compounds in various fruits, vegetables, and medicinal plants, *R. damascena* was identified as one of the species, along with *Solidago virgaurea, Ginkgo biloba,* and *Camellia sinensis* (the source of green tea), as having the highest flavonoid content.[17]

Also in late 2010, Kalim et al. assessed the antioxidant activity of plants typically used in Unani medicine, of which the 10 displaying the most promising effects, including *R. damascena,* an astringent used for cardiac health and as an anti-inflammatory and astringent in Unani, were identified for additional analysis. The total phenolic, flavonoid, and ascorbic acid contents were ascertained from methanol (50 percent) extract preparations of all 10 species and researchers also evaluated the *in vitro* scavenging of reactive oxygen and nitrogen species and the ability of the plant extracts to prevent oxidative DNA harm. *R. damascena* was among seven of the extracts to display moderate antioxidant activity and one of three species found to potentially have significant preventive activity against oxidative DNA damage as well as antioxidant activity. The investigators concluded that *R. damascena, Cleome icosandra,* and *Cyperus scariosus,* all of which are commonly used in Unani medicine and reportedly deliver substantial benefits in the treatment of various human disorders, are potentially useful as natural antioxidants in pharmaceutical products.[20] In 2012, Moein et al. investigated plants growing in Iran that are used for medicinal purposes and confirmed the antioxidant potency of *R. damascena.*[21]

Antibacterial Activity

In 2002, *R. damascena* was among eight essential oils studied for composition and antimicrobial characteristics. The antibacterial activities of the aromatic extracts were ascertained by disk diffusion testing. Among the standard test bacterial strains *Escherichia coli, Staphylococcus aureus,* and *Pseudomonas aeruginosa, R. damascena* demonstrated antimicrobial activity against *S. aureus.*[22] Recent work has provided additional evidence of its antibacterial activity. In 2010, Zu et al. tested 10 essential oils for antibacterial activity against *Propionibacterium acnes* as well as *in vitro* toxicology against three human cancer cell lines. Among the essential oils tested, which included mint, ginger, lemon, grapefruit, jasmine, lavender, chamomile, thyme, rose (*R. damascena*), and cinnamon, thyme, cinnamon, and rose exhibited the greatest antibacterial potency against *P. acnes.*[23]

The antimicrobial activity of *R. damascena* extract has been further established in recent tests. In a study published in the dental literature, the antimicrobial effects of 2 percent *R. damascena* extract were compared to those of a 5.25 percent sodium hypochlorite (NaOCl) and 2 percent chlorhexidine (CHX) on endodontic pathogens, including *Enterococcus faecalis, Actinomyces naeslundii, Porphyromonas gingivalis, Fusobacerium nucleatum,* and *Candida albicans.* The minimum inhibitory concentrations (MIC) for *R. damascena* were lower than those for CHX except in the case of *F. nucelatum*; the MIC for *R. damascena* was lower than that for NaOCl for *C. albicans* and otherwise equal. In each case, test microorganisms were destroyed within one minute. The researchers concluded that the botanical exhibited strong activity against gram-positive (*E. faecalis, A. naeslundii,* and *C. albicans*) as well as gram-negative (*P. gingivalis* and *F. nucleatum*) strains.[24]

Also, in a 2010 investigation of the antimicrobial activity and cytotoxicity of 51 ethanol, methanol, aqueous, butanol, and n-hexane extracts of different parts of 14 plants all used in traditional medicine in Jordan, the highest activity (100 percent inhibition) reported was for the butanol extract of *R. damascena* against *Salmonella typhimurium* and *Bacillus cereus*. The aqueous extract of *R. damascena* was also active against *C. albicans*. In addition, the butanol and aqueous extracts of *R. damascena* suppressed methicillin-resistant *Staphylococcus aureus*.[25]

Anxiolytic Activity

In a recent study on the relaxing effects of rose oil administered by transdermal absorption, 40 healthy volunteers were assessed based on autonomic parameters (i.e., blood pressure, breathing rate, blood oxygen saturation, pulse rate, and skin temperature) as well as self-report after receiving rose oil or placebo. Olfactory stimulation was prevented through the use of breathing masks. Significant reductions in systolic blood pressure, breathing rate, and blood saturation were observed as compared to placebo. The rose oil group also self-reported as calmer, more relaxed, and less alert. The author suggested that this small study lends support for the use of rose oil in aromatherapy for the relief of stress and depression.[26]

In 2011, Hoseinpour et al. conducted a randomized, double-blind, placebo-controlled two-week study in 50 patients of a *R. damascena* mouthwash to treat aphthous stomatitis (canker sores) based on the reputed anti-inflammatory and antinociceptive activity of the plant. The investigators found that by days 4 and 7, there were statistically significant differences between the placebo and test groups according to all parameters (i.e., pain, size, and number of ulcers), with the *R. damascena* mouthwash showing greater effectiveness than the placebo.[27] Rose oil is one of several popular anxiolytic essential oils used in aromatherapy.[28]

Other Activities

In 1996, water and methanol extracts of *R. damascena* were found to display moderate anti-HIV activity, with the pure compounds quercetin and kaempferol playing an important role.[29]

More recently, in 2010, flavonoids isolated from *R. damascena* buds were demonstrated to hinder the activity of 3-hydroxy-3-methylglutaryl-coenzyme A (HMG-CoA) reductase as well as angiotensin I-converting enzyme (ACE), suggesting the potential for the herb to impart beneficial effects on the cardiovascular system.[18]

■ CONCLUSION

The data that exist on *R. damascena* are interesting and suggest a wide range of medical benefits but do not yet establish its use in the dermatologic realm. Much more research is necessary to determine the potential efficacy of this botanical, particularly for its antioxidant and antimicrobial activities, in topical products.

REFERENCES

1. Hoffmann D. *Medical Herbalism: The Science and Practice of Herbal Medicine*. Rochester, VT: Healing Arts Press; 2003:64.
2. Ulusoy S, Bosgelmez-Tinaz G, Seçilmiş-Canbay H. Tocopherol, carotene, phenolic contents and antibacterial properties of rose essential oil, hydrosol and absolute. *Curr Microbiol*. 2009;59:554.
3. Boskabady MH, Shafei MN, Saberi Z, et al. Pharmacological effects of rosa damascena. *Iran J Basic Med Sci*. 2011;14:295.
4. Mahmood N, Piacente S, Pizza C, et al. The anti-HIV activity and mechanisms of action of pure compounds isolated from Rosa damascena. *Biochem Biophys Res Commun*. 1996;229:73.
5. Grieve M. A *Modern Herbal*. Vol 2. New York: Dover Publications; 1971:684.
6. Tsanaktsidis CG, Tamoutsidis E, Kasapidis G, et al. Preliminary results on attributes of distillation products of the rose rosa damascena as a dynamic and friendly to the environment rural crop. *ICESD*. 2012;1:66.
7. Tabrizi H, Mortazavi SA, Kamalinejad M. An in vitro evaluation of various Rosa damascene flower extracts as a natural antisolar agent. *Int J Cosmet Sci*. 2003;25:259.
8. Ericksen M. *Healing with Aromatherapy*. New York: McGraw-Hill Professional; 2000:9.
9. Zaidi SF, Muhammad JS, Shahryar S, et al. Anti-inflammatory and cytoprotective effects of selected Pakistani medicinal plants in Helicobacter pylori-infected gastric epithelial cells. *J Ethnopharmacol*. 2012;141:403.
10. Verma RS, Padalia RC, Chauhan A, et al. Volatile constituents of essential oil and rose water of damask rose (Rosa damascena Mill.) cultivars from North Indian hills. *Nat Prod Res*. 2011;25:1577.
11. Murphy TM, Hamilton CM. A strain of Rosa damascene cultured cells resistant to ultraviolet light. *Plant Physiol*. 1979;64:936.
12. Svobodvá A, Psotová J, Walterová D. Natural phenolics in the prevention of UV-induced skin damage: A review. *Biomed Pap Med Fac Univ Palacky Olomouc Czech Repub*. 2003;147:137.
13. Scalbert A, Williamson G. Dietary intake and bioavailability of polyphenols. *J Nutr*. 2000;130:2073S.
14. Ross JA, Kasum CM. Dietary flavonoids: Bioavailability, metabolic effects, and safety. *Annu Rev Nutr*. 2002;22:19.
15. Birt DF, Hendrich S, Wang W. Dietary agents in cancer prevention: Flavonoids and isoflavonoids. *Pharmacol Ther*. 2001;90:157.
16. Rechner AR, Spencer JP, Kuhnle G, et al. Novel biomarkers of the metabolism of caffeic acid derivatives in vivo. *Free Radic Biol Med*. 2001;30:1213.
17. Haghi G, Hatami A. Simultaneous quantification of flavonoids and phenolic acids in plant materials by a newly developed isocratic high-performance liquid chromatography approach. *J Agric Food Chem*. 2010;58:10812.
18. Kwon EK, Lee DY, Lee H, et al. Flavonoids from the buds of Rosa damascena inhibit the activity of 3-hydroxy-3-methylglutaryl-coenzyme a reductase and angiotensin I-converting enzyme. *J Agric Food Chem*. 2010;58:882.
19. Schiber A, Mihalev K, Berradini N, et al. Flavonol glycosides from distilled petals of Rosa damascene Mill. *Z Naturforsch C*. 2005;60:379.
20. Kalim MD, Bhattacharyya D, Banerjee A, et al. Oxidative DNA damage preventive activity and antioxidant potential of plants used in Unani system of medicine. *BMC Complement Altern Med*. 2010;10:77.
21. Moein S, Moein M, Khoshnoud MJ, et al. In vitro antioxidant properties evaluation of 10 Iranian medicinal plants by different methods. *Iran Red Crescent Med J*. 2012;14:771.
22. Aridoğan BC, Baydar H, Kaya S, et al. Antimicrobial activity and chemical composition of some essential oils. *Arch Pharm Res*. 2002;25:860.
23. Zu Y, Yu H, Liang L, et al. Activities of ten essential oils towards Propionibacterium acnes and PC-3, A-549 and MCF-7 cancer cells. *Molecules*. 2010;15:3200.
24. Shokouhinejad N, Emaneini M, Aligholi M, et al. Antimicrobial effect of Rosa damascena extract on selected endodontic pathogens. *J Calif Dent Assoc*. 2010;38:123.
25. Talib WH, Mahasneh AM. Antimicrobial, cytotoxicity and phytochemical screening of Jordanian plants used in traditional medicine. *Molecules*. 2010;15:1811.
26. Hongratanaworakit T. Relaxing effect of rose oil on humans. *Nat Prod Commun*. 2009;4:291.
27. Hoseinpour H, Peel SA, Rakhshandeh H, et al. Evaluation of Rosa damascena mouthwash in the treatment of recurrent aphthous stomatitis: a randomized, double-blinded, placebo-controlled clinical trial. *Quintessence Int*. 2011;42:483.
28. Setzer WN. Essential oils and anxiolytic aromatherapy. *Nat Prod Commun*. 2009;4:1305.
29. Mahmood N, Piacente S, Pizza C, et al. The anti-HIV activity and mechanisms of action of pure compounds isolated from Rosa damascena. *Biochem Biophys Res Commun*. 1996;229:73.

CHAPTER 49

Pycnogenol

Activities:

Antioxidant, anti-inflammatory, anticarcinogenic, photoprotective, antimicrobial

Important Chemical Components:

Flavonoids, primarily procyanidins (which are biopolymers of catechin and epicatechin subunits),[1] taxifolin,[2] and phenolic acids (i.e., ferulic, caffeic, p-hydroxybenzoic, vanillic, gallic, and protocatechuic acids)[1,3–5]

Origin Classification:

Pycnogenol is a legal trademark for a process of extracting flavonoids and other compounds from French maritime pine bark.[6] Thus, its origin is natural but the marketed standardized pine bark extract product is synthesized and processed in the laboratory.

Personal Care Category:

Anti-inflammatory, hydrating

Recommended for the following Baumann Skin Types:

DRNT, DRNW, DRPW, DSNT, DSNW, DSPW, ORNT, ORNW, ORPW, OSNT, OSNW, and OSPW

SOURCE

Growing in the coastal areas of southwest France, *Pinus pinaster* (previously known as *Pinus maritima*) is the source of the procyanidin (also known as proanthocyanidin)-rich standardized extract Pycnogenol.[7,8] Twenty years ago, it was found that procyanidol oligomers (PCOs) bind to elastic skin fibers when intradermally injected into young rabbits. Research showed that PCOs and (+) catechin (catechins are the fundamental antioxidant elements in green tea) bound to insoluble elastin significantly decelerating the rate of degradation engendered by elastases, which is characteristic of inflammatory processes.[9] Since this time, a small but cogent body of research has evolved regarding PCOs (now referred to as oligomeric proanthocyanidins, or OPCs), particularly in grape seed extract and French maritime pine bark extract. OPCs, usually referred to simply as proantho-cyanidins, are the most potent antioxidant free-radical scavengers yet identified. Great varieties of fruits, vegetables, nuts, seeds, flowers, and bark, particularly, grape seed, grape skin, bilberry, cranberry, black currant, green tea, black tea, blueberry, blackberry, strawberry, black cherry, red wine, red cabbage, and red apple skins are the sources of widely available OPCs.[10] Grape seed and pine bark are the most commercially viable sources. *P. pinaster*, like the extract of grape seed, is emerging as a versatile component in the medical armamentarium against several diseases, and appears to offer potential dermatologic applications.

HISTORY

"Pycnogenols," based on the ancient Greek *puknos* ("condensed") and *genos* ("class, family"), is a term originally coined to describe a class of polyphenols (flavan-3-ol derivatives), but "Pycnogenol" has come to refer to the patented name for a proprietary mix of procyanidins extracted from French maritime pine bark, *Pinus pinaster*, standardized, and sold primarily as a nutritional supplement.[3,11] The use of pine bark itself dates back to the 4th century BCE and records showing that Hippocrates recommended it to treat inflammation.[3]

Native Americans are said to have been well aware of pine bark's medicinal benefits for centuries, as far back as the 1500s, and reportedly used pine bark (thought to be white pine) to treat scurvy during the winter in Canada in 1535.[12–14] It has been used as a health supplement since 1853.[15] Today, Pycnogenol continues to be used worldwide as a nutritional supplement and to treat various conditions including chronic inflammation, circulatory dysfunction, and several psychophysiological impairments.[7] It has also been shown to be effective treating mild-to-moderate asthma and inflammatory bowel disorders,[2,16] and is thought to be useful in various other conditions, including diabetes, attention deficit hyperactivity disorder, systemic lupus erythematosus (as a second-tier therapy for inflammation), and some cancers.[1,17] In addition, the extract has been shown to be effective in inhibiting the growth of several different prokaryotic (gram-positive and gram-negative) and eukaryotic (yeast and fungi) microorganisms.[18]

CHEMISTRY

Proanthocyanidins are polyphenolic bioflavonoids believed to confer a vast array of biological, pharmacological, chemopro-tective, and antioxidant activity.[19] Between 65 and 75 percent of Pycnogenol is made up of procyanidins composed of catechin and epicatechin subunits with varying chain lengths.[7] Polyphenolic monomers, phenolic or cinnamic acids, and their glycosides are additional constituents.[7] These compounds acting synergistically are thought to have the capacity to stabilize collagen and elastin, by neutralizing collagenase and elastase,[9,15] which would improve the elasticity, flexibility, and appearance of skin, and protect the skin from ultraviolet (UV) B damage. The constituents of Pycnogenol are considered to be highly bioavailable.[3,7]

ORAL USES

In 2004, Segger et al. conducted a double-blind, placebo-controlled trial in 62 women between the ages of 45 and 73 years to evaluate the efficacy of a proprietary oral supplement (Evelle) in treating skin roughness and elasticity. Pycnogenol is a key active ingredient of the formulation along with amino acids, blueberry extract, carotenoids, glycosaminoglycans, selenium, vitamins C and E, and zinc. The investigators used an optical cutometer to measure skin elasticity, which was found to be statistically significantly greater (by 9 percent) as compared to placebo after six weeks of treatment. After 12 weeks of treatment, skin roughness, assessed using three-dimensional microtopography imaging, was statistically significantly reduced by 6 percent compared with the control group. The authors concluded that the oral supplement Evelle displays the potential to reduce the signs of skin aging.[20]

Pycnogenol has also been proposed as one among several nutritional supplements as part of a new therapeutic approach to a collagen tissue disorder known as Ehlers–Danlos syndrome classic type, including cutaneous and vascular manifestations such as easy bruising, bleeding, varicose veins, and inadequate tissue healing.[21]

A daily supplement dosage of 100 mg of Pycnogenol® has also recently been found to ease early symptoms of menopause, as shown in an eight-week study of 38 women. Hot flashes, night sweats, mood swings, irregular periods, loss of libido, and vaginal dryness subsided in the treatment group, with no changes experienced by the control group. The investigators concluded that Pycnogenol significantly diminished major and minor symptoms of early menopause in the women studied due, in part, to the reduced oxidative stress imparted by the antioxidant.[22]

The efficacy of oral Pycnogenol for the treatment and management of chronic venous insufficiency (CVI) and venous microangiopathy has also been suggested by a series of prospective controlled trials by Cesarone et al., with the extract rapidly limiting edema, cramps, and the feeling of heavy legs.[2,23,24]

TOPICAL USES

Pycnogenol is known to have potent antioxidant, anti-inflammatory, and anticarcinogenic properties.[25–27] In fact, in a 2007 study comparing the total oxygen radical scavenging capacity of 11 different phytochemicals using the oxygen radical absorbance capacity (ORAC) assay and the total oxyradical scavenging capacity (TOSC) assay, quercetin, Pycnogenol, grape skin extract, and green tea polyphenols were found to exhibit the greatest antioxidant activity.[28] Significantly, Pycnogenol also reportedly confers cardiovascular benefits, exhibits strong free radical-scavenging against reactive oxygen and nitrogen species, and plays a role in the cellular antioxidant network, as supported by its demonstrated capacity to regenerate the ascorbyl radical and to protect endogenous vitamin E and glutathione from oxidative stress (Table 49-1).[3]

TABLE 49-1
Pros and Cons of Pycnogenol

Pros	Cons
Potent antioxidant	Brief history of investigation and use of topical formulations
Protects vitamin E from oxidation	"Pycnogenol" is a trademarked name for a particular formulation of French pine bark
Recycles oxidized vitamin C	More data on French pine bark are needed
Highly bioavailable	
Reportedly 50 times more potent than vitamin E and 30 times more potent than vitamin C[15]	
No reported cases of contact dermatitis	

Most research on Pycnogenol has been conducted *in vitro* using cell cultures or in animal models. Some small studies on the topical application of this potent antioxidant have been performed on humans, however. In a study evaluating the capacity of pine bark extract to protect human skin against erythema induced by solar radiation, 21 fair-skinned volunteers were given oral supplementation of Pycnogenol. During supplementation, the UV radiation (UVR) level necessary to reach one minimal erythema dose (MED) was significantly elevated, suggesting that oral pine bark extract supplementation mitigates the effects of UVR on the skin, lowering erythema. The investigators noted that the extract inhibited nuclear factor-κB-dependent gene expression, a marker of the UV-induced proinflammatory response in HaCaT cells.[4]

The efficacy of Pycnogenol in protecting against UVR prompted a 30-day clinical trial of 30 women with melasma in which patients were given one 25 mg tablet of Pycnogenol at each meal, three times daily. Investigators found that the average surface area of melasma significantly decreased, showing Pycnogenol to be an effective and safe treatment for this condition.[26] This dynamic OPC is also said to exhibit potential or actual efficacy in treating other dermatologic conditions. Pine bark extract has been found to downregulate calgranulin A and B genes, both of which are characteristically upregulated in psoriasis and various dermatoses.[13]

In a study of another application of pine bark extract, 40 patients with diagnosed CVI were treated daily in an open, controlled comparative study with either 600 mg Venostasin (horse chestnut seed extract) or 360 mg Pycnogenol over a four-week period (see Chapter 74, Horse Chestnut). Pycnogenol significantly reduced lower limb circumference, as well as cholesterol and low-density lipoprotein values though not high-density lipoproteins, and significantly improved subjective symptoms. Both treatments were tolerated equally well, but Venostasin had only marginal effects on the lower limbs and overall symptoms and no effect on lipid values. Investigators found that for the treatment of CVI, Pycnogenol showed greater efficacy than Venostasin, a well-regarded therapy for this indication.[29]

In 2012, Marini et al. conducted a 12-week investigation to ascertain whether nutritional supplementation with Pycnogenol® could improve the cosmetic appearance of 20 healthy postmenopausal women. The skin condition of the volunteers was evaluated before, during, and after supplementation using corneometry, cutometry, visioscan and ultrasound analyses as well as biopsies and subsequent polymerase chain reaction (PCR) analyses. The investigators found that the well-tolerated supplementation led to improved skin hydration and elasticity, a manifestation that was marked in the subjects who initially presented with dry skin. They also noted a significant increase in the mRNA expression of hyaluronic acid synthase-1 (HAS-1), a key enzyme involved in hyaluronic acid production, as well as salient increases in gene expression involved in collagen synthesis, to which the researchers attributed the clinical improvements. The investigators concluded that their results, including the first molecular evidence of the cutaneous benefits of improved hydration and elasticity, suggest the potential for Pycnogenol supplementation to mitigate the clinical signs of aging skin.[30]

SAFETY ISSUES

Oral Pycnogenol is generally recognized as safe (GRAS) for consumption at prescribed doses and is not associated with any adverse side effects.[24,26] It is included in many dietary supplements and multivitamins.[31]

ENVIRONMENTAL IMPACT

The wood industry considered pine bark an inconvenient residue with limited practical use until recent years; now it is used as a vegetal substrate and combustible.[7] *P. pinaster* is a fast-growing evergreen tree widely planted for timber (and cut after 30–50 years of cultivation) in its native Mediterranean climates and for use as a nutritional source.[1] It is an invasive species in South Africa, where it was introduced in the late 1600s. *P. pinaster* is cultivated in large monocultures, which environmentalists criticize for limiting biodiversity.

FORMULATION CONSIDERATIONS

The quality of aqueous pine bark extract is specified in the United States Pharmacopeia (USP 28).[7,31]

USAGE CONSIDERATIONS

Pycnogenol is thought to be unique in that it displays greater biologic effects as a whole compound or mixture than its purified constituents do individually, which suggests synergistic interaction among its components.[3,7]

SIGNIFICANT BACKGROUND

In Vitro Studies

In vitro studies of Pycnogenol have indicated a wide range of benefits imparted by this botanical extract. Research has demonstrated that Pycnogenol is significantly more potent than vitamins C and E and exhibits the capacity to recycle vitamin C, regenerate vitamin E (as does vitamin C), and facilitate the activity of endogenous antioxidant enzymes.[26] Protective effects against UV radiation have also been associated with Pycnogenol.[26]

The known antioxidant and anti-inflammatory characteristics of Pycnogenol spurred the study of the interaction, and related molecular mechanisms, of T cells with human keratinocytes after activation with interferon (IFN)-γ. Various pretreatment regimens of HaCaT cells with Pycnogenol significantly inhibited IFN-γ-induced adherence of T cells to HaCaT cells as well as IFN-γ-induced expression of ICAM-1 expression in such cells, suggesting Pycnogenol's potential as a treatment component for inflammatory skin disorders.[27]

In an *in vitro* study aimed at identifying natural compounds capable of stimulating human growth hormone (HGH) as a viable replacement for the successful but problematic recombinant human growth hormone (rHGH), equal amounts of L-arginine, L-lysine, aged garlic extract, S-allyl cysteine and Pycnogenol significantly raised the secretion of HGH.[32] This potential application has antiaging implications given the association of decreased levels of HGH and increased signs of aging, including the thinning of the skin.

Animal Studies

In 1997, Blazsó et al. showed that topically applied Pycnogenol on the shaved backs of rats delivered protection from UVB-induced erythema.[33] In 2004, Sime and Reeve exposed Skh:hr hairless mice to solar-simulated ultraviolet radiation (SSUVR) and after irradiation topically applied lotions containing Pycnogenol. Dose-dependent reductions in the inflammatory sunburn reaction and immunosuppression (as manifested by suppression of contact hypersensitivity reactions) were observed as a result of Pycnogenol treatment. Tumor formation, induced by chronic exposure to SSUVR five days/week for 10 weeks, was delayed in mice treated with Pycnogenol and tumor prevalence was significantly reduced (from 100 percent of control mice to 85 percent of 0.2 percent Pycnogenol-treated mice) as was tumor multiplicity. The investigators concluded that topical Pycnogenol exhibits potential as a photoprotective complement to sunscreens, clearly showing biologic activity when applied after exposure to UV radiation.[25]

In 2009, Ince et al. demonstrated the strong anti-inflammatory properties of Pycnogenol as well as *Pinus brutia* (Turkish pine) in a rat model of carageenan-induced inflammation, with intraperitoneal administration of each dose-dependently suppressing paw swelling.[14]

Earlier that year, in a study on the effects of tobacco smoke and UV light radiation on murine skin, Pavlou et al. also considered the potential protective effects conferred by Pycnogenol and found that the potent antioxidant appeared to protect male and female hairless SKH-2 mouse skin from squamous cell carcinoma induced by exposure to cigarette smoke and UV radiation.[34]

Pycnogenol was also a key constituent in an oral antioxidant mixture that has shown promising dermatologic results. In 2007, Cho et al. investigated the effects on UVB-induced wrinkle formation in female SKH-1 hairless mice of an orally administered antioxidant compound composed of vitamins C and E, Pycnogenol, and evening primrose oil. In addition, the researchers also examined the potential molecular mechanisms of photoprotection against UVB damage. After 10 weeks of oral administration of the antioxidant solution or a vehicle control and thrice weekly UVB irradiation, wrinkle formation was found to be significantly decreased in mice given the antioxidant cocktail. Further, significant declines in epidermal thickness, UVB-induced hyperplasia, acanthosis, and hyperkeratosis were observed. The investigators concluded that the significant inhibition of UVB-induced wrinkle formation rendered by the oral antioxidant mixture occurred by virtue of the antioxidants suppressing matrix metalloproteinase activity spurred by UVB exposure while bolstering collagen production.[35]

In addition, in 2012, Lee et al. showed that topical application of pine bark extract imparted protection against hexavalent chromium-induced dermatotoxicity in rats, significantly and dose-dependently reducing the incidence and severity of cutaneous irritation and histopathological lesions caused by the heavy metal found commonly in the environment. Treatment with the extract also lowered malondialdehyde concentrations and augmented catalase and glutathione-S-transferase activity in skin tissues. The investigators concluded that pine bark extract is a viable agent for the protection against the formation of oxidative stress-induced dermal lesions.[31]

In a 2013 *in vivo* comparison of Pycnogenol and *P. brutia* bark extract in an incision wound model in rats, both topical formulations were found to inhibit lipid peroxidation, increase vascularization, and reduce necrotic areas, though the wound-healing activity of the *P. brutia* extract was found to be more substantial, as it significantly accelerated wound healing.[36]

CONCLUSION

Though the body of research is not exhaustive, extant evidence suggests that pine bark extract confers significant beneficial biological effects. In particular, research indicates that pine bark extract possesses notable antioxidant, anti-inflammatory, photoprotective, and anticarcinogenic capacity. In addition, several authors suggest that OPCs inhibit enzymes involved in cutaneous breakdown, that is, collagenase, elastase, and hyaluronidase. Pine bark extract might not have the same media buzz as its fellow proanthocyanidin grape seed extract, but current research provides just as much reason for optimism. That said, the efficacy of oral pine bark extract is much more firmly established than that of topical formulations. Much more research is necessary to evaluate the current limited range of topical products and to determine the viability of translating promising laboratory findings into effective and safe topical clinical and over-the-counter products.

REFERENCES

1. Rohdewald P. A review of the French maritime pine bark extract (Pycnogenol), a herbal medication with a diverse clinical pharmacology. *Int J Clin Pharmacol Ther.* 2002;40:158.
2. Cesarone MR, Belcaro G, Rohdewald P, et al. Comparison of Pycnogenol and Daflon in treating chronic venous insufficiency: A prospective, controlled study. *Clin Appl Thromb Hemost.* 2006;12:205.
3. Packer L, Rimbach G, Virgili F. Antioxidant activity and biologic properties of a procyanidin-rich extract from pine (Pinus maritime) bark, pycnogenol. *Free Radic Biol Med.* 1999;27:704.
4. Saliou C, Rimbach G, Moini H, et al. Solar ultraviolet-induced erythema in human skin and nuclear factor-kappa-B-dependent gene expression in keratinocytes are modulated by a French maritime pine bark extract. *Free Radic Biol Med.* 2001;30:154.
5. Svobodová A, Psotová J, Walterová D. Natural phenolics in the prevention of UV-induced skin damage: A review. *Biomed Pap Med Fac Univ Palacky Olomouc Czech Repub.* 2003;147:137.
6. Hoffmann D. The endocrine system. In: *Medical Herbalism: The Science and Practice of Herbal Medicine.* Rochester, VT: Healing Arts Press; 2003:13.
7. D'Andrea G. Pycnogenol: A blend of procyanidins with multifaceted therapeutic applications? *Fitoterapia.* 2010;81:724.
8. Baumann L. How to prevent photoaging? *J Invest Dermatol.* 2005;125:xii.
9. Tixier JM, Godeau G, Robert AM, et al. Evidence by in vivo and in vitro studies that binding of pycnogenols to elastin affect its rate of degradation by elastases. *Biochem Pharmacol.* 1984;33:3933.
10. Bagchi D, Bagchi M, Stohs SJ, et al. Free radicals and grape seed proanthocyanidin extract: Importance in human health and disease prevention. *Toxicology.* 2000;148:187.
11. Masquelier J, Michaud J, Laparra J, et al. Flavonoids and pycnogenols. *Int J Vitam Nutr Res.* 1979;49:307.
12. Chandler RF, Freeman L, Hooper SN. Herbal remedies for the Maritime Indians. *J Ethnopharmacol.* 1979;1:49.
13. Rihn B, Saliou C, Bottin MC, et al. From ancient remedies to modern therapeutics: Pine bark uses in skin disorders revisited. *Phytother Res.* 2001;15:76.
14. Ince I, Yesil-Celiktas O, Karabay-Yavasoglu NU, et al. Effects of Pinus brutia bark extract and Pycnogenol in a rat model of carrageenan induced inflammation. *Phytomedicine.* 2009;16:1101.
15. Rona C, Vailati F, Berardesca E. The cosmetic treatment of wrinkles. *J Cosmet Dermatol.* 2004;3:26.
16. Lau BH, Riesen SK, Truong KP, et al. Pycnogenol as an adjunct in the management of childhood asthma. *J Asthma.* 2004;41:825.
17. Stefanescu M, Matache C, Onu A, et al. Pycnogenol efficacy in the treatment of systemic lupus erythematosus patients. *Phytother Res.* 2001;15:698.
18. Torras MA, Faura CA, Schönlau F, et al. Antimicrobial activity of pycnogenol. *Phytother Res.* 2005;19:647.
19. Bagchi D, Garg A, Krohn RL, et al. Oxygen free radical scavenging abilities of vitamins C and E, and a grape seed proanthocyanidin extract in vitro. *Res Commun Mol Pathol Pharmacol.* 1997;95:179.
20. Segger D, Schönlau F. Supplementation with Evelle improves skin smoothness and elasticity in a double-blind, placebo-controlled study with 62 women. *J Dermatolog Treat.* 2004;15:222.
21. Mantle D, Wilkins RM, Preedy V. A novel therapeutic strategy for Ehlers–Danlos syndrome based on nutritional supplements. *Med Hypotheses.* 2005;64:279.
22. Errichi S, Bottari A, Belcaro G, et al. Supplementation with Pycnogenol® improves signs and symptoms of menopausal transition. *Panminerva Med.* 2011;53:65.
23. Cesarone MR, Belcaro G, Rohdewald P, et al. Rapid relief of signs/symptoms in chronic venous microangiopathy with pycnogenol: A prospective, controlled study. *Angiology.* 2006;57:569.
24. Cesarone MR, Belcaro G, Rohdewald P, et al. Improvement of diabetic microangiopathy with pycnogenol: A prospective, controlled study. *Angiology.* 2006;57:431.
25. Sime S, Reeve VE. Protection from inflammation, immunosuppression and carcinogenesis induced by UV radiation in mice by topical Pycnogenol. *Photochem Photobiol.* 2004;79:193.
26. Ni Z, Mu Y, Gulati O. Treatment of melasma with pycnogenol. *Phytother Res.* 2002;16:567.
27. Bito T, Roy S, Sen CK, et al. Pine bark extract pycnogenol downregulates IFN-gamma-induced adhesion of T cells to human keratinocytes by inhibiting inducible ICAM-1 expression. *Free Radic Biol Med.* 2000;28:219.
28. Tomer DP, McLeman LD, Ohmine S, et al. Comparison of the total oxyradical scavenging capacity and oxygen radical absorbance capacity antioxidant assays. *J Med Food.* 2007;10:337.
29. Koch R. Comparative study of Venostasin and Pycnogenol in chronic venous insufficiency. *Phytother Res.* 2002;16(Suppl 1):S1.
30. Marini A, Grether-Beck S, Jaenicke T, et al. Pycnogenol® effects on skin elasticity and hydration coincide with increased gene expressions of collagen type I and hyaluronic acid synthase in women. *Skin Pharmacol Physiol.* 2012;25:86.
31. Lee IC, Kim SH, Shin IS, et al. Protective effects of pine bark extract on hexavalent chromium-induced dermatotoxicity in rats. *Phytother Res.* 2012;26:1534.
32. Buz'Zard AR, Peng Q, Lau BH. Kyolic and Pycnogenol increase human growth hormone secretion in genetically-engineered keratinocytes. *Growth Horm IGF Res.* 2002;12:34.
33. Blazsó G, Gábor M, Rohdewald P. Antiinflammatory activities of procyanidin-containing extracts from Pinus pinaster Ait. after oral and cutaneous application. *Pharmazie.* 1997;52:380.
34. Pavlou P, Rallis M, Deliconstantinos G, et al. In-vivo data on the influence of tobacco smoke and UV light on murine skin. *Toxicol Ind Health.* 2009;25:231.
35. Cho HS, Lee MH, Lee JW, et al. Anti-wrinkling effects of the mixture of vitamin C, vitamin E, pycnogenol and evening primrose oil, and molecular mechanisms on hairless mouse skin caused by chronic ultraviolet B irradiation. *Photodermatol Photoimmunol Photomed.* 2007;23:155.
36. Cetin EO, Yesil-Celiktas O, Cavusoglu T, et al. Incision wound healing activity of pine bark extract containing topical formulations: A study with histopathological and biochemical analyses in albino rats. *Pharmazie.* 2013;68:75.

CHAPTER 50

Resveratrol

Activities:

Antioxidant, antibacterial, anticancer, anti-inflammatory, antitumorigenic, antityrosinase, cardioprotective

Important Chemical Components:

Also known as *trans*-3,5,4′,-trihydroxystilbene, or 3, 4′, 5-stilbenetriol

Origin Classification:

Resveratrol is natural and found in approximately 70 plants, including many plant foods. It can also be synthesized chemically.

Personal Care Category:

Antiaging, anticancer

Recommended for the following Baumann Skin Types:

DRNW, DRPW, DSNW, DSPW, ORNW, ORPW, OSNW, and OSPW

SOURCE

Resveratrol (*trans*-3,5,4′-trihydroxystilbene), a polyphenolic phytoalexin synthesized in nearly 70 species and found notably in the skin and seeds of grapes, berries (e.g., blueberries, cranberries, mulberries, bilberries, lingberries, partridgeberries, sparkleberries, and deerberries), peanuts (in the nonedible as well as edible parts of the plant), red wine, purple grape juice, jackfruit, pomegranate, eucalyptus, the roots of *Polygonum cuspidatum* (Japanese knotweed, known as *Ko-jo-kon* in Japanese), scots pine, spruce, corn lily, gnetum, and butterfly orchid tree, displays a wide range of biological and pharmacological properties.[1–13] It is particularly abundant in the skin and seeds of *Vitis vinifera*, known as the grapevine, which is native to southern Europe and western Asia.[14] *P. cuspidatum* is used in traditional Chinese and Japanese medicine to treat dermatitis, among other conditions.[15]

Studies have shown that resveratrol possesses potent antioxidant, antiproliferative, and anti-inflammatory characteristics (Table 50-1).[15–18] Specifically, *in vitro* and *in vivo* studies have shown that resveratrol exerts chemopreventive and antiproliferative activity against various cancers, including skin cancer, by suppressing cellular events associated with tumor initiation, promotion, and progression and triggering apoptosis in such tumor cells.[10,19,20]

HISTORY

Vitis vinifera, the primary source of resveratrol (particularly in the form of red wine), has been used since antiquity. The use of grapevine or grapeseed as food is believed to predate recorded history and its use for wine has been traced back 4,500 years to ancient Egypt.[17] Resveratrol itself was first identified from the roots of *Veratrum grandiflorum* (white hellebore), though, in 1940.[21–24] The so-called "French paradox," the phenomenon identified in the early 1990s indicating that the low rate of heart disease seen in France despite a rich diet including regular consumption of red wine, has been partially attributed to the antioxidant properties of the resveratrol found in red wine and prompted great interest in the compound.[5,13,25–28] Indeed, resveratrol has been shown in several *in vitro* and *in vivo* models to have the capacity to mitigate damage in heart ischemia reperfusion as well as brain ischemia/reperfusion in rodent models.[29]

Research on resveratrol really exploded after a seminal report in the journal *Science* in 1997 suggesting chemopreventive properties. In that study, purified resveratrol was found to exhibit major inhibitory activity against cancer initiation, promotion, and progression. Specifically, its antioxidant and antimutagenic potency and induction of phase II drug-metabolizing enzymes were seen as counter to carcinogenic initiation. Resveratrol hindered cyclooxygenase (COX) and hydroperoxidase and initiated anti-inflammatory effects thereby demonstrating antipromotion activity. The induction of human promyelocytic leukemia cell differentiation by this newly-discovered botanical ingredient also thwarted the progress of carcinogenic activity. In addition, significant inhibitory effects were demonstrated by resveratrol *in vitro*, with carcinogen-induced preneoplastic lesions in mouse mammary glands, and *in vivo*, with tumorigenesis in the two-stage mouse skin cancer model.[1]

Since then, copious research has been performed on this botanical compound that has developed a strong reputation as a potent antioxidant, anti-inflammatory, and antiproliferative agent.[15,30,31] Most importantly, it is considered to act as a chemopreventive agent against skin cancer and to exert antiproliferative influence on oral squamous, breast, colon, and prostate cancer cells,[19] triggering apoptosis in such tumor cells.[20] Generally, it has been shown to inhibit tumor initiation, promotion, and progression in chemically- and ultraviolet B (UVB)-induced skin carcinogenesis in mice and multiple murine models of human cancers.[10,31,32]

The most recent data indicate that resveratrol protects against UVB-mediated skin damage in SKH-1 hairless mice, particularly by suppressing survivin, the overexpression of which is associated with various forms of cancer.[33,34] Significantly, this antioxidant has come to develop a reputation for having the capacity to prevent cardiovascular disease and cancer.[35] Not surprisingly then, resveratrol is one of the most often studied polyphenolic compounds.

TABLE 50-1
Pros and Cons of Resveratrol

Pros	Cons
Wide-ranging biological and pharmacological properties	Poor bioavailability[28]
Potent anticancer properties demonstrated in preclinical studies	More clinical evidence of topical efficacy is needed

CHEMISTRY

There are two isoforms of resveratrol: *trans*-resveratrol, the more stable form and the one to which most of its salutary effects are attributed, and *cis*-resveratrol.[36,37] Among its numerous antioxidant activities, resveratrol has been demonstrated to potently inhibit nitric oxide generation and inducible nitric oxide synthase protein expression.[38] Its chemopreventive activity was further supported in 2008 by a study in which resveratrol induced apoptosis through mitochondrial pathway modulation by stimulating p53 activity in mouse skin tumors.[39] In human skin, resveratrol has been found to sensitize keratinocytes to UVA-induced apoptosis.[3] In addition, resveratrol has also been shown to act as a sensitizer to enhance the therapeutic effects of ionizing radiation against cancer cells.[12]

Boyer et al. showed that oxidative stress to mitochondria engendered by UVA and resveratrol reduces the mitochondrial membrane potential resulting in the opening of mitochondrial pores and then apoptosis in human keratinocytes. They suggested that this understanding may lead to developing future chemotherapeutic approaches to cutaneous tumors.[3]

In 2013, Choi et al. analyzed whether resveratrol influences autophagy in human dermal fibroblasts grown in complete medium and found that resveratrol-induced autophagy can be mediated by death-associated protein kinase 1 (DAPK1). They concluded that some of the health benefits derived from resveratrol may be ascribed to its capacity to regulate DAPK1.[40]

In 2010, Bastianetto et al. found that resveratrol appears to act on specific polyphenol binding sites in the epidermis, knowledge that they suggest might be applied to the prevention of skin conditions linked to aging.[11]

Also, five new stilbenoids, vatalbinosides A-E, and 13 known compounds were isolated from the stem of *Vatica albiramis* by Abe et al. They examined the effects of these new compounds on interleukin (IL)-1β-induced production of matrix metalloproteinase (MMP)-1 in human dermal fibroblasts and identified three resveratrol tetramers [(-)-hopeaphenol, vaticanol C, and stenophyllol C] as potent inhibitors of MMP-1 production.[41]

ORAL USES

Resveratrol is consumed regularly as a key active ingredient in several foods, beverages, and dietary supplements. Its bioavailability is extremely limited, however.

In 2012, Buonocore et al. conducted a placebo-controlled, double-blind study for 60 days with 50 participants (25 taking supplements and 25 taking placebo) to assess the topical and systemic effects of a resveratrol- and procyanidin-containing dietary supplement on age-related changes in the skin. The investigators found that after 60 days of treatment, significant increases in systemic oxidative stress, plasmatic antioxidant capacity, and skin antioxidant power emerged. Further, skin moisturization and elasticity were enhanced and decreases were noted in skin roughness and wrinkle depth. Age spots also subsided. The researchers concluded that the use of a dietary supplement containing resveratrol and procyanidin exhibits potential for contributing to an antiaging regimen in support of wrinkle reduction and lowering systemic and cutaneous oxidative stress.[42]

TOPICAL USES

In 2013, Ikeda et al., studying the effect of resveratrol on the regulation of extracellular matrix expression, proliferation, and apoptosis of keloid fibroblasts, found that type I collagen,

α-smooth muscle actin, and heat shock protein 47 expression dose-dependently diminished in resveratrol-treated keloid fibroblasts but not in normal skin fibroblasts. Resveratrol also reduced transforming growth factor (TGF)-β1 synthesis by keloid fibroblasts, inhibited their proliferation, and induced apoptosis of the fibroblasts. The investigators concluded that resveratrol appears to confer an antifibrogenic effect on keloid fibroblasts without harming normal skin fibroblasts, indicating its potential use for treating keloids.[43]

Skin Lightening

Resveratrol was previously shown to work synergistically with 4-n-butylresorcinol (a derivative of resorcinol, one of the primary phenols found in argan oil; see Chapter 10, Argan Oil) to lower tyrosinase levels and significantly reduce melanin synthesis more effectively than either compound alone.[44] As Franco et al. also noted that year, resveratrol can inhibit tyrosinase but it does not sufficiently suppress melanin production to justify its use as a lone skin-whitening agent in pharmaceutical formulations, but warrants attention as a coadjuvant for treating hyperpigmentation.[45] The potential role of resveratrol in skin lightening was reinforced by a recent study in which 52 medicinal plants grown in Korea were tested for human tyrosinase activity and the dried stems of the grape tree *V. vinifera* were found to potently inhibit human tyrosinase, and more effectively than arbutin.[46] In addition, it is worth noting that resveratrol, through its antioxidant activity and potentially inhibitory impact on cytochrome P450 2E1 expression, has been shown to protect mouse primary hepatocytes from hydroquinone-induced cytotoxicity.[47] Also, Galgut and Ali, studying the effects of topical ethanolic extract of *Arachis hypogaea* (peanuts, which contain half the resveratrol of red wine) on the tail melanophores of tadpole *Bufo melanostictus*, observed discrete gathering of pigment cells and resultant skin lightening. They concluded that resveratrol, the main active ingredient in *A. hypogaea*, warrants attention for potential clinical use as a nontoxic melanolytic agent to treat hyperpigmentation.[7,48]

Acne

In a single-blind pilot study in 2011, Fabbrocini et al. investigated the potential therapeutic impact of resveratrol on 20 patients with acne. A resveratrol-containing hydrogel was applied daily on the right side of the face for 60 days, with the left side receiving the hydrogel vehicle as control. No adverse effects were reported and all patients were satisfied with the treatment. Investigators reported a 53.75 percent mean decrease in the Global Acne Grading System score on the resveratrol-treated sides and a 6.10 percent decline on the control sides. In addition, histologic analysis revealed a statistically significant reduction of lesions in areas treated with resveratrol (66.7 percent mean reduction in the average area of microcomedones on the resveratrol-treated sides vs. 9.7 percent reduction on the control sides).[37]

Erythema

In a small 2013 study by Ferzli et al., 16 subjects with erythema applied a formulation containing resveratrol, green tea polyphenols, and caffeine twice daily to the whole face. Clinical photographs and spectrally enhanced images taken before treatment and every two weeks through three months were evaluated. The researchers reported that improvement was seen in 16 of 16 clinical images and 13 of 16 spectrally enhanced images. Erythema reduction was observable by six weeks of treatment.[49]

SAFETY ISSUES

Resveratrol is associated with low toxicity and minimal side effects.[28] In higher doses, it has been shown to exhibit pro-apoptotic activity toward healthy cells as well as tumor cells.[13]

ENVIRONMENTAL IMPACT

Resveratrol is present in roughly 70 species of plants. Few if any of the plants are cultivated to harness resveratrol specifically, though. As such, the environmental impact of cultivating plants such as *V. vinifera*, in particular, might be extrapolated to understand the effects from the industrial harvesting of plants containing resveratrol. Interestingly, resveratrol itself is generated in plants as a reaction to infection with the fungus *Botrytis cinera* as well as other environmental conditions, such as injury, exposure to ozone, sunlight, and heavy metals, as well as water deprivation.[10,13,50]

FORMULATION CONSIDERATIONS

In 2009, Kobierski et al. identified two nonionic stabilizers to achieve a nanosuspension of resveratrol stable at room temperature and for 30 days. The nanosuspensions are thought to be capable of improving skin penetration and solubility.[28,51] The previous year, Gelo-Pujic et al. synthesized new resveratrol precursors, combining resveratrol and lipoic acid as well as resveratrol and vitamin E, to improve on photostability and lipophilicity of the antioxidants; both new molecules demonstrated good chemical stability under heat and photoaging conditions.[9]

In 2013, Pando et al. showed that novel niosomes formulated with Plurol oleique or Peceol were more effective than liposomes in cutaneous delivery of resveratrol.[52] Investigations of various nanoformulations of resveratrol in phospholipid vesicles by Caddeo et al. revealed that conventional phosphatidylcholine liposomes prepared with penetration enhancer-containing vesicles were able to include resveratrol in satisfactory yields (>74 percent). Researchers noted that the lamellarity of the vesicles relied on formulation composition and the antioxidant activity of resveratrol was not influenced by vesicular formulation. Estimated shelf life for the preparations ranged from three to six months.[53]

Significantly, Detoni et al. caution that preventing the photoisomerization of resveratrol from its *E*-isomeric form to its *Z*-configuration is integral in maintaining the biological and pharmacological activities of the polyphenol in topical skin formulations. In their study of various supramolecular structures infused with *E*-resveratrol, they found that *E*-resveratrol concentration was maintained for the longest time by liposomes but their size decreased after UVA exposure. Nanocarriers were most successful in achieving higher levels of *E*-resveratrol in the epidermis under UVA exposure. Skin penetration profiles of the different tested vehicles were similar in the dark.[54]

Interestingly, resveratrol has been incorporated into cosmeto-textile products (i.e., cotton and polyamide fabrics) and shown *in vitro* to be delivered into the stratum corneum (SC), epidermis, and dermis. The skin penetration efficacy of these resveratrol-containing products was also tested in volunteers, with an *in vitro* percutaneous absorption method detecting resveratrol in the SC, epidermis, and dermis and an *in vivo* method (i.e., stripping) detecting resveratrol in the SC. Less resveratrol penetrated the skin when incorporated in the cosmeto-textile preparations as compared to direct topical application.[55]

Ndiaye et al. point out that the many commercially available skin care products that contain resveratrol have not been rigorously tested. In addition, several deliver the polyphenol through microparticles, which ostensibly extend resveratrol release into the skin but actually lower the amount of the compound available to penetrate the skin.[28]

USAGE CONSIDERATIONS

Resveratrol is associated with poor bioavailability and the fact that it is rapidly metabolized limits its viability as a systemic therapy.[28] However, some topical delivery systems have recently been cited as effective in the laboratory and worthy of consideration for development, including a hydrogel patch successful in preventing resveratrol from escaping into the body as well as nonionic nanosuspensions.[51,56] That said, there are already a few topical products available that feature resveratrol as a key ingredient. Like many such preparations, their marketing claims have not been confirmed by stringent testing, such as randomized, double-blind clinical studies.

In a 2013 study by Pastore et al. of the molecular mechanisms of resveratrol activity in normal human epidermal keratinocytes, the phytoalexin was found to synergize with tumor necrosis factor (TNF)-α to engender delayed, enduring IL-8 expression via consistent activation of the epidermal growth factor receptor (EGFR)-extracellular signal regulated kinase (ERK) axis. They cautioned that patients with psoriasis who overexpress TNF-α, IL-8, and EGFR-ERK in the skin should be wary of topically applying resveratrol. In addition, the authors suggested that habitual topical application of resveratrol might pose risk given that high nuclear levels of EGFR correlate to elevated tumorigenesis risk. Finally, they expressed skepticism regarding the potential of resveratrol to accelerate wound healing because of its antiproliferative impact on normal keratinocytes.[57] Further, Mukherjee et al. note that at lower doses, resveratrol is effective in contributing to health maintenance, but at higher doses it displays proapoptotic activity toward healthy cells as well as tumor cells.[13]

SIGNIFICANT BACKGROUND

Resveratrol is known to exert a wide range of biologic activities as demonstrated in multiple preclinical studies.

In Vitro Studies

In 2001, human epidermoid carcinoma A432 cells treated with resveratrol were demonstrated to suppress cell growth, G_1 phase arrest of the cell cycle, apoptosis, and dose- and time-dependent induction of WAF1/p21 and multiple decreases in various protein expressions.[58,59] Also that year, Khanna et al. reported that grape seed proanthocyanidin extract (GSPE) containing 5,000 parts per million resveratrol was found to facilitate oxidant-induced vascular endothelial growth factor (VEGF) expression in cultured keratinocytes, with GSPE pretreatment of human keratinocyte (HaCaT) cells upregulating hydrogen peroxide (H_2O_2) and TNF-α-induced VEGF expression and release. The authors concluded that resveratrol-containing GSPE has potential to ameliorate dermal wounds and similar skin conditions.[60] The ensuing year, Khanna et al. reported on the *in vivo* success of topically applied GSPE on dermal wounds. Specifically, the compound increased the rate of wound contractions and closure as well as the expression of VEGF and tenascin in wound edge tissue. Greater cell density and definition in the hyperproliferative epithelial region along with augmented deposition of connective tissue were also observed as a result of grape seed extract topical application.[61] Many of the same investigators, reporting that year that grape seed extract and resveratrol were shown in combination to promote VEGF expression, suggested that such activity is an important step in wound-angiogenesis.[62] It is worth noting that the anti-inflammatory and wound-healing activity of polyphenols such as resveratrol have been found to be dependent on their interaction with EGFR-regulated cytoplasmic and nuclear pathways, not their redox characteristics.[63]

In 2008, Park et al. examined the effect of resveratrol pretreatment on UVB-treated HaCaT cells. They found that resveratrol increased cell survival and diminished caspase-3 and caspase-8 activation, suggesting the potential of the botanical ingredient as a photoprotective agent in sunscreen formulations.[64]

In a 2009 *in vitro* study of the potential cancer-preventive properties exhibited by several phytochemicals (i.e., ellagic acid, grape seed extract, lycopene, N-acetylcysteine, resveratrol, and ursolic acid) against murine skin carcinogenesis, Kowalczyk et al. observed that resveratrol, ellagic acid, and grape seed extract strongly scavenged peroxyl and superoxide radicals. All of the tested phytochemicals also protected cells from H_2O_2-induced DNA damage.[65]

Also that year, Roy et al. determined that resveratrol and UVB can work synergistically against skin cancer cells, with the polyphenol sensitizing A431 human epidermoid carcinoma cells to UVB-induced apoptosis.[66]

In 2010, Jagdeo et al. demonstrated that resveratrol dose-dependently imparted a significant reduction of intracellular H_2O_2-induced upregulation of reactive oxygen species in normal human skin fibroblasts *in vitro*.[67]

Liu et al. conducted an *in vitro* study the following year to examine the protective role of resveratrol in HaCaT cells against UVA-induced oxidative damage and found that resveratrol degrades Kelch-like-ECH-associated protein 1 (Keap 1) and expedites Nrf2 accretion in cell nuclei, thus shielding the HaCaT cells from oxidative harm.[68]

In 2012, Osmond et al. conducted *in vitro* and *in vivo* experiments to assess the potential of resveratrol as a chemotherapy adjunct for melanoma treatment. Resveratrol significantly reduced melanoma cell viability in both melanoma cell lines tested. The polyphenol was also found to selectively spare cells in the nonmalignant fibroblast lines as compared to its cytotoxic impact on melanoma cells. In addition, cytotoxicity to malignant cells was greatly amplified by 72 hours of treatment with resveratrol and temozolomide as compared to temozolomide treatment alone. No significant differences were seen *in vivo*. The authors concluded that the *in vitro* antitumor activity of resveratrol positions the botanical as a potential therapeutic agent in melanoma management.[69]

Animal Studies

In one of the early studies with resveratrol, pretreatment of mouse skin with this potent antioxidant significantly lowered the oxidative stress induced by 12-*O*-tetradecanoylphorbol-13-acetate (TPA) and restored glutathione levels and superoxide dismutase activity.[70] Resveratrol pretreatment also dose-dependently reversed or reduced several of the carcinogenic effects induced by TPA by disrupting the pathways of reactive oxidants.[71] TPA-mediated increases in the expression of COX-1, COX-2, c-myc, c-fos, c-jun, TGF-β1, and TNF-α were all inhibited by resveratrol pretreatment.[58,71]

In an investigation involving the two-stage mouse skin carcinogenesis model [7,12 dimethylbenz(a)anthracene (DMBA)-initiated, TPA-promoted], resveratrol was shown to exhibit significant inhibitory activity against Epstein-Barr virus early antigen induction. Resveratrol also conferred a 60 percent reduction in papillomas at 20 weeks in an *in vivo* assay at a 50-fold molar ratio to TPA.[72]

The molecular mechanisms of its antitumorigenic properties were suggested by the results of an investigation by Kundu et al. of the effects of resveratrol on TPA-induced COX-2 expression in mouse skin. Researchers observed dose-dependent inhibition of COX-2 expression following pretreatment of dorsal skin of female ICR mice with resveratrol. Decreases in the phosphorylation of ERK and the catalytic activity of ERK and p38 mitogen-activated protein kinases (MAPK) were also noted as was the DNA binding of activator protein-1 (AP-1) induced by TPA.[73]

In a 2005 study of the effects of resveratrol on UVB-mediated skin tumorigenesis in SKH-1 hairless mice, controls were chronically exposed to UVB, twice weekly for 28 weeks, while resveratrol was topically applied pretreatment (30 minutes before each UVB exposure) or posttreatment (5 minutes after). Pre- and posttreatment were found to confer equal benefit, both equally inhibiting tumor incidence and postponing tumorigenesis onset. Resveratrol treatment was also found to mitigate the deleterious effects of UVB on survivin as well as on apoptosis in UVB-mediated skin tumors. The authors concluded that their findings are the first results with direct implications regarding human skin cancers. Further, they speculated that resveratrol is suitable for inclusion in various product types (e.g., emollient, patch, sunscreens, and other skin care products) intended to prevent skin cancer and other conditions thought to be generated by the sun.[34]

Researchers assessing the effects of pretreatment with resveratrol on H_2O_2-induced oxidative stress and apoptosis in cultured rat pheochromocytoma (PC12) cells found several effects of the oxidizer, including cytotoxicity, DNA fragmentation, transient activation of nuclear factor (NF)-κB, and intracellular accumulation of reactive oxygen species, to be diminished.[26] Another potential application of resveratrol was suggested by a study in which resveratrol pretreatment suppressed the NF-κB activation in cultured rat PC12 cells transiently induced by β-amyloid. Resveratrol also thwarted other effects of the β-amyloid peptide, which is believed to account for the senile plaques characteristic of the brains of Alzheimer's patients. Specifically, the polyphenol was found to have attenuated the cytotoxicity, apoptosis, and intracellular reactive oxygen intermediate formation.[74] In 2005, resveratrol was found to increase cellular antioxidant defense capacity, specifically protecting the tested cultured PC12 cells from oxidative damage.[4]

In 2009, Roy et al. evaluated the chemopreventive potential of resveratrol in DMBA-induced mouse skin tumorigenesis over 28 weeks. Resveratrol was topically applied to the animals one hour before DMBA exposure. The results showed definite chemopreventive activity, specifically a delay in tumorigenesis onset as well as decreases in tumor volume and total number of tumors. Notably, resveratrol increased apoptotic protease-activating factor-1 as well as DMBA-inhibited p53 and Bax and suppressed skin tumorigenesis by regulating phosphatidylinositol-3-kinase (PI3K) and AKT proteins, which are thought to foster cancer by facilitating proliferation and inhibiting apoptosis. The investigators concluded that resveratrol warrants consideration as a chemopreventive agent.[75]

Later that year, Yusuf et al. examined whether Toll-like receptor 4 (TLR4), which like other Toll-like receptors plays an important role in immune responses, was necessary for the chemopreventive activity imparted by resveratrol against DMBA-induced cutaneous carcinogenesis. Investigators compared mice with normal and deficient TLR4 function when pretreated with resveratrol and then exposed to a DMBA-induced skin carcinogenesis protocol. Fewer tumors/group were observed in resveratrol-treated TLR4-competent mice as opposed to TLR4-deficient mice. Tumor size was also diminished *in vivo* and their survival suppressed *in vitro* by resveratrol much more so in the TLR4-competent mice. In addition, angiogenesis was more significantly inhibited in TLR4-competent mice. The researchers concluded that TLR4 plays a key mediating role in the chemoprevention of DMBA-induced skin carcinogenesis exerted by resveratrol.[76]

In 2011, Kim et al. demonstrated that orally administered resveratrol inhibits UV-induced skin tumorigenesis in highly tumor-susceptible p53(±)/SKH-1 mice and suppresses the invasiveness of human A432 squamous cell carcinoma partly by targeting and downregulating TGF-β2.[77]

Recently, resveratrol was also found by Hao et al. to suppress the growth of a human skin squamous cell carcinoma A431 xenograft in nude mice.[78] Several of the same investigators showed that the inhibition mechanism of resveratrol is the upregulation of the protein and mRNA expression of p53 and the downregulation of the protein and mRNA expression of survivin, leading to tumor cell apoptosis.[21]

Photoprotection

Resveratrol has been demonstrated to protect against UVB-mediated cutaneous damage in SKH-1 hairless mice. Specifically, a significant decline in UVB-mediated generation of H_2O_2 as well as infiltration of leukocytes and inhibition of skin edema has been associated with the topical application of resveratrol to SKH-1 hairless mice before UVB exposure. Topically applied resveratrol also significantly hinders UVB-mediated induction of COX-2 and ornithine decarboxylase (ODC) enzyme activities and protein expression of ODC, which are markers for tumor promotion. In addition, it inhibits the UVB-mediated rise in lipid peroxidation, a marker of oxidative stress.[33,34] Pretreatment of normal human epidermal keratinocytes with resveratrol was shown in one study to inhibit UVB-induced activation of the NF-κB pathway.[79] This protective effect delivered by resveratrol against the damage from multiple UVB exposures has been ascribed to the inhibition of the MAPK pathway and mediated via modulation in the expression and function of the cell cycle regulatory protein cki–cyclin–cdk network.[80] In short-term experiments, resveratrol topically applied to SKH-1 hairless mouse skin before UVB irradiation led to marked suppression of cell proliferation and phosphorylation of survivin.[81] Inhibition of UVB-induced tumor incidence and delay in the onset of skin tumorigenesis has been demonstrated in long-term studies entailing the topical application of resveratrol both pre- and postexposure.[82] The postexposure application of resveratrol yielded equal protection to the pre-exposure application, suggesting that resveratrol-mediated responses may not be sunscreen effects. Evidence pointing to the photoprotective effects of resveratrol continues to be collected.[12,83]

Other deleterious effects of UV exposure have been mitigated by resveratrol. Afaq et al. showed that UVB-induced skin edema was significantly inhibited by the topical application of resveratrol to SKH-1 hairless mice.[84] In another experiment by Afaq et al., topically applied resveratrol significantly inhibited

UVB-mediated increases in bifold skin thickness and edema and greatly diminished UVB-induced lipid peroxidation, COX and ODC activities, as well as protein expression of the ODC enzyme in SKH-1 hairless mice.[15] The authors concluded that topically applied resveratrol appears to impart significant photoprotective capacity against the damage wrought by UVB radiation. Additional research by this team buttresses their position, as they demonstrated that resveratrol dose- and time-dependently blocked UVB-mediated activation of NF-κB in normal human epidermal keratinocytes and that this pathway plays an important role in the photoprotective activity expressed by stilbene.[16] In an experiment by some of the same investigators, resveratrol was topically applied to SKH-1 hairless mice 30 minutes before exposure to UVB; 24 hours later, significant reductions were observed in bifold skin thickness, hyperplasia, and infiltration of leukocytes. Critical cell cycle regulatory proteins, the target of the investigation, were substantially downregulated as a result of the resveratrol treatment. The researchers concluded that this potent antioxidant may have the potential to play a significant role in preventing UVB-mediated photodamage and carcinogenesis.[80]

Antiaging Activity

In 2008, Baxter reported that in an oxygen radical absorbance capacity (ORAC) comparison, a new skin formulation with 1 percent resveratrol exhibited 17 times the antioxidant activity of a 1 percent idebenone formulation.[2] Idebenone has been reported to be the most potent topical antioxidant (see Chapter 61, Idebenone).[85]

In 2010, Giardina et al. conducted an *in vitro* study to assess the tonic-trophic characteristics of resveratrol as well as resveratrol plus N-acetylcysteine on cultured skin fibroblasts. They found that both formulations dose-dependently yielded an increase in cell proliferation and inhibition of collagenase activity.[86]

In 2012, Wu et al. studied the protective effects of resveratrate, a stable derivative of resveratrol, against damage to human skin caused by repetitive solar simulator UV radiation (SSUVR) in 15 healthy human volunteers. Six sites on nonexposed dorsal skin of each participant were studied, with four sites exposed to SSUVR and the remaining sites serving as positive control (SSUVR only) and baseline control (no treatment or exposure). The investigators observed minimal erythema on areas treated with resveratrate and the resveratrol derivative significantly suppressed sunburn cell formation. They concluded that resveratrate protects the skin against sunburn and suntan provoked by repetitive SSUVR.[6]

In a 2013 *in vitro* study of the skin permeation kinetics of polyphenols using diffusion cells via *ex vivo* pig skin and a cellulose membrane, Zillich et al. demonstrated that several polyphenols, including resveratrol, (-)epigallocatechin-3-O-gallate (EGCG), quercetin, rutin, and protocatechuic acid formulated in oil-in-water (o/w) emulsions could pass through the SC and were identified in the epidermis and dermis. The investigators concluded that their findings validate the use of polyphenols as active ingredients in antiaging products.[87]

Antimicrobial and Antiviral Activity

Resveratrol has also been evaluated as an antifungal or antimicrobial because this potent compound is synthesized in response to injury or fungal attack.[88,89] In one study, researchers assessed the antimicrobial activity of resveratrol against bacteria and dermatophytes known to be important causes of human skin infections, including the bacteria *Staphylococcus aureus*, *Enterococcus faecalis*, and *Pseudomonas aeruginosa*. Resveratrol was found to inhibit the growth of the tested bacteria as well as the growth of the fungal species *Trichophyton mentagrophytes*, *Trichophyton tonsurans*, *Trichophyton rubrum*, *Epidermophyton floccosum*, and *Microsporum gypseum*. Investigators concluded that the potential dermatologic applications of resveratrol, and its analogs, appear to be even wider than previously believed and may even come to include clinical applications for diabetic wounds.[30]

In another study with direct implications regarding new dermatologic applications, investigators evaluated the *in vivo* effects of resveratrol on herpes simplex virus (HSV) given prior success *in vitro*. Topical application of two concentrations of resveratrol (12.5 and 25 percent) cream to the abraded epidermis of SKH-1 mice infected with HSV-1 effectively suppressed lesion development when applied multiple times a day within one or six hours after infection, but not at after 12 hours of infection. In comparisons between resveratrol cream, 10 percent docosanol cream (Abreva) and 5 percent acyclovir ointment (Zovirax), resveratrol cream and acyclovir were comparably effective whereas mice treated with docosanol developed lesions at the same rate as cream-only control mice. In addition, the resveratrol creams successfully inhibited lesion formation when the experiment was repeated with an HSV-1 acyclovir-resistant virus.[90]

CONCLUSION

Grape skin and seeds, berries, peanuts, and some other foods that contain the potent antioxidant resveratrol are the main sources of what is emerging as a compound with the potential to deliver significant health benefits, particularly in the realm of cardioprotective, cancer-preventive, and photoprotective activity. While there has been intense research over the last two decades, more is necessary to establish resveratrol for consideration as a standard first-line therapy and to further elucidate its range of cutaneous applications. Data and preclinical evidence do appear to support the use of resveratrol in various product types (e.g., emollients, patches, sunscreens, and additional skin care products) intended to prevent skin cancer and other conditions caused or exacerbated by solar exposure, such as photoaging. More clinical evidence is needed, though, to establish the full potential of topically applied resveratrol.

REFERENCES

1. Jang M, Cai L, Udeani GO, et al. Cancer chemopreventive activity of resveratrol, a natural product derived from grapes. *Science*. 1997;275:218.
2. Baxter RA. Anti-aging properties of resveratrol: Review and report of a potent new antioxidant skin care formulation. *J Cosmet Dermatol*. 2008;7:2.
3. Boyer JZ, Jandova J, Janda J, et al. Resveratrol-sensitized UVA induced apoptosis in human keratinocytes through mitochondrial oxidative stress and pore opening. *J Photochem Photobiol B*. 2012;113:42.
4. Chen CY, Jang JH, Li MH, et al. Resveratrol upregulates heme oxygenase-1 expression via activation of NF-E2-related factor 2 in PC12 cells. *Biochem Biophys Res Commun*. 2005;331:993.
5. She QB, Bode AM, Ma WY, et al. Resveratrol-induced activation of p53 and apoptosis is mediated by extracellular-signal-regulated protein kinases and p38 kinase. *Cancer Res*. 2001;61:1604.
6. Wu Y, Jia LL, Zheng YN, et al. Resveratrate protects human skin from damage due to repetitive ultraviolet irradiation. *J Eur Acad Dermatol Venereol*. 2012 Jan 5. Venereol. 2013;27:345.
7. Konda S, Geria AN, Halder RM. New horizons in treating disorders of hyperpigmentation in skin of color. *Semin Cutan Med Surg*. 2012;31:133.
8. Saraf S, Kaur CD. Phytoconstituents as photoprotective novel cosmetic formulations. *Pharmacogn Rev*. 2010;4:1.
9. Gelo-Pujic M, Desmurs JR, Kassem T, et al. Synthesis of new antioxidant conjugates and their in vitro hydrolysis with stratum corneum enzymes. *Int J Cosmet Sci*. 2008;30:195.
10. Athar M, Back JH, Tang X, et al. Resveratrol: A review of preclinical studies for human cancer prevention. *Toxicol Appl Pharmacol*. 2007;224:274.
11. Bastianetto S, Dumont Y, Duranton A, et al. Protective action of resveratrol in human skin: Possible involvement of specific receptor binding sites. *PLoS One*. 2010;5:e12935.
12. Reagan-Shaw S, Mukhtar H, Ahmad N. Resveratrol imparts photoprotection of normal cells and enhances the efficacy of radiation therapy in cancer cells. *Photochem Photobiol*. 2008;84:415.
13. Mukherjee S, Dudley JI, Das DK. Dose-dependency of resveratrol in providing health benefits. *Dose Response*. 2010;8:478.
14. Nassiri-Asl M, Hosseinzadeh H. Review of the pharmacological effects of Vitis vinifera (Grape) and its bioactive compounds. *Phytother Res*. 2009;23:1197.
15. Afaq F, Adhami VM, Admad N. Prevention of short-term ultraviolet B radiation-mediated damages by resveratrol in SKH-1 hairless mice. *Toxicol Appl Pharmacol*. 2003;186:28.
16. Adhami VM, Afaq F, Ahmad N. Suppression of ultraviolet B exposure-mediated activation of NF-kappaB in normal human keratinocytes by resveratrol. *Neoplasia*. 2003;5:74.
17. Foster S. *101 Medicinal Herbs: An Illustrated Guide*. Loveland, CO: Interweave Press; 1998:108-9.
18. Hoffmann D. *Medical Herbalism: The Science and Practice of Herbal Medicine*. Rochester, VT: Healing Arts Press; 2003:99-100.
19. Ding XZ, Adrian TE. Resveratrol inhibits proliferation and induces apoptosis in human pancreatic cancer cells. *Pancreas*. 2002;25:e71.
20. Delmas D, Rébé C, Lacour S, et al. Resveratrol-induced apoptosis is associated with Fas redistribution in the rafts and the formation of a death-inducing signaling complex in colon cancer cells. *J Biol Chem*. 2003;278:41482.
21. Hao Y, Huang W, Liao M, et al. The inhibition of resveratrol to human skin squamous cell carcinoma A431 xenografts in nude mice. *Fitoterapia*. 2013;86:84.
22. Namasivayam N. Chemoprevention in experimental animals. *Ann N Y Acad Sci*. 2011;1215:60.
23. Das S, Das DK. Resveratrol: A therapeutic promise for cardiovascular diseases. *Recent Pat Cardiovasc Drug Discov*. 2007;2:133.
24. Aggarwal BB, Bhardwaj A, Aggarwal RS, et al. Role of resveratrol in prevention and therapy of cancer: Preclinical and clinical studies. *Anticancer Res*. 2004;24:2783.
25. Simini B. Serge Renaud: From French paradox to Cretan miracle. *Lancet*. 2000;355:48.
26. Jang JH, Surh YJ. Protective effects of resveratrol on hydrogen peroxide-induced apoptosis in rat pheochromocytoma (PC12) cells. *Mutat Res*. 2001;496:181.
27. Hoffmann D. *Medical Herbalism: The Science and Practice of Herbal Medicine*. Rochester, VT: Healing Arts Press; 2003:110.
28. Ndiaye M, Philippe C, Mukhtar H, et al. The grape antioxidant resveratrol for skin disorders: Promise, prospects, and challenges. *Arch Biochem Biophys*. 2011;508:164.
29. Zhuang H, Kim YS, Koehler RC, et al. Potential mechanism by which resveratrol, a red wine constituent, protects neurons. *Ann N Y Acad Sci*. 2003;993:276.
30. Chan MM. Antimicrobial effect of resveratrol on dermatophytes and bacterial pathogens of the skin. *Biochem Pharmacol*. 2002;63:99.
31. Svobodová A, Psotová J, Walterová D. Natural phenolics in the prevention of UV-induced skin damage. A review. *Biomed Pap Med Fac univ Palacky Olomouc Czech Repub*. 2003;147:137.
32. Afaq F, Mukhtar H. Photochemoprevention by botanical antioxidants. *Skin Pharmacol Appl Skin Physiol*. 2002;15:297.
33. Aziz MH, Afaq F, Ahmad N. Prevention of ultraviolet-B radiation damage by resveratrol in mouse skin is mediated via modulation in surviving. *Photochem Photobiol*. 2005;81:25.
34. Aziz MH, Reagan-Shaw S, Wu J, et al. Chemoprevention of skin cancer by grape constituent resveratrol: Relevance to human disease? *FASEB J*. 2005;19:1193.
35. Hebbar V, Shen G, Hu R, et al. Toxicogenomics of resveratrol in rat liver. *Life Sci*. 2005;76:2299.
36. Puizina-Ivić N, Mirić L, Carija A, et al. Modern approach to topical treatment of aging skin. *Coll Antropol*. 2010;34:1145.

37. Fabbrocini G, Staibano S, De Rosa G, et al. Resveratrol-containing gel for the treatment of acne vulgaris: A single-blind, vehicle-controlled, pilot study. *Am J Clin Dermatol.* 2011;12:133.

38. Bhat KP, Pezzuto JM. Cancer chemopreventive activity of resveratrol. *Ann N Y Acad Sci.* 2002;957:210.

39. Kalra N, Roy P, Prasad S, et al. Resveratrol induces apoptosis involving mitochondrial pathways in mouse skin tumorigenesis. *Life Sci.* 2008;82:348.

40. Choi MS, Kim Y, Jung JY, et al. Resveratrol induces autophagy through death-associated protein kinase 1 (DAPK1) in human dermal fibroblasts under normal culture conditions. *Exp Dermatol.* 2013;22:491.

41. Abe N, Ito T, Ohguchi K, et al. Resveratrol oligomers from Vatica albiramis. *J Nat Prod.* 2010;73:1499.

42. Buonocore D, Lazzeretti A, Tocabens P, et al. Resveratrol-procyanidin blend: Nutraceutical and antiaging efficacy evaluated in a placebocontrolled, double-blind study. *Clin Cosmet Investig Dermatol.* 2012;5:159.

43. Ikeda K, Torigoe T, Matsumoto Y, et al. Resveratrol inhibits fibrogenesis and induces apoptosis in keloid fibroblasts. *Wound Repair Regen.* 2013;21:616.

44. Kim SY, Park KC, Kwon SB, et al. Hypopigmentary effects of 4-n-butylresorcinol and resveratrol in combination. *Pharmazie.* 2012;67:542.

45. Franco DC, de Carvalho GS, Rocha PR, et al. Inhibitory effects of resveratrol analogs on mushroom tyrosinase activity. *Molecules.* 2012;17:11816.

46. Park J, Booy YC. Isolation of resveratrol from vitis viniferae caulis and its potent inhibition of human tyrosinase. *Evid Based Complement Alternat Med.* 2013;2013:645257.

47. Wang DH, Ootsuki Y, Fujita H, et al. Resveratrol inhibited hydroquinone-induced cytotoxicity in mouse primary hepatocytes. *Int J Environ Res Public Health.* 2012;9:3354.

48. Galgut JM, Ali SA. Effect and mechanism of action of resveratrol: A novel melanolytic compound from the peanut skin of Arachis hypogaea. *J Recept Signal Transduct Res.* 2011;31:374.

49. Ferzli G, Patel M, Phrsai N, et al. Reduction of facial redness with resveratrol added to topical product containing green tea polyphenols and caffeine. *J Drugs Dermatol.* 2013;12:770.

50. De Nisco M, Manfra M, Bolognese A, et al. Nutraceutical properties and polyphenolic profile of berry skin and wine of Vitis vinifera L. (cv. Aglianico). *Food Chem.* 2013;140:623.

51. Kobierski S, Ofori-Kwakye K, Müller RH, et al. Resveratrol nanosuspensions for dermal application—production, characterization, and physical stability. *Pharmazie.* 2009;64:741.

52. Pando D, Caddeo C, Manconi M, et al. Nanodesign of olein vesicles for the topical delivery of the antioxidant resveratrol. *J Pharm Pharmacol.* 2013;65:1158.

53. Caddeo C, Manconi M, Fadda AM, et al. Nanocarriers for antioxidant resveratrol: Formulation approach, vesicle self-assembly and stability evaluation. *Colloids Surf B Biointerfaces.* 2013;111C:327.

54. Detoni CB, Souto GD, da Silva AL, et al. Photostability and skin penetration of different E-resveratrol-loaded supramolecular structures. *Photochem Photobiol.* 2012;88:913.

55. Alonso C, Martí M, Martínez V, et al. Antioxidant cosmeto-textiles: Skin assessment. *Eur J Pharm Biopharm.* 2013;84:192.

56. Hung CF, Lin YK, Huang ZR, et al. Delivery of resveratrol, a red wine polyphenol, from solutions and hydrogels via the skin. *Biol Pharm Bull.* 2008;31:955.

57. Pastore S, Lulli D, Maurelli R, et al. Resveratrol induces long-lasting IL-8 expression and peculiar EGFR activation/distribution in human keratinocytes: Mechanisms and implications for skin administration. *PLoS One.* 2013;8:e59632.

58. Gupta S, Mukhtar H. Chemoprevention of skin cancer through natural agents. *Skin Pharmacol Appl Skin Physiol.* 2001;14:373.

59. Ahmad N, Adhami VM, Afaq F, et al. Resveratrol causes WAF-1/p21-mediated G(1)-phase arrest of cell cycle and induction of apoptosis in human epidermoid carcinoma A431 cells. *Clin Cancer Res.* 2001;7:1466.

60. Khanna S, Roy S, Bagchi D, et al. Upregulation of oxidant-induced VEGF expression in cultured keratinocytes by a grape seed proanthocyanidin extract. *Free Radic Biol Med.* 2001;31:38.

61. Khanna S, Venojarvi M, Roy S, et al. Dermal wound healing properties of redox-active grape seed proanthocyanidins. *Free Radic Biol Med.* 2002;33:1089.

62. Sen CK, Khanna S, Gordillo G, et al. Oxygen, oxidants, and antioxidants in wound healing: An emerging paradigm. *Ann N Y Acad Sci.* 2002;957:239.

63. Pastore S, Lulli D, Fidanza P, et al. Plant polyphenols regulate chemokine expression and tissue repair in human keratinocytes through interaction with cytoplasmic and nuclear components of epidermal growth factor receptor system. *Antioxid Redox Signal.* 2012;16:314.

64. Park K, Lee JH. Protective effects of resveratrol on UVB-irradiated HaCaT cells through attenuation of the caspase pathway. *Oncol Rep.* 2008;19:413.

65. Kowalczyk MC, Walaszek Z, Kowalczyk P, et al. Differential effects of several phytochemicals and their derivatives on murine keratinocytes in vitro and in vivo: Implications for skin cancer prevention. *Carcinogenesis.* 2009;30:1008.

66. Roy P, Madan E, Kalra N, et al. Resveratrol enhances ultraviolet B-induced cell death through nuclear factor-kappaB pathway in human epidermoid carcinoma A431 cells. *Biochem Biophys Res Commun.* 2009;384:215.

67. Jagdeo J, Adams L, Lev-Tov H, et al. Dose-dependent antioxidant function of resveratrol demonstrated via modulation of reactive oxygen species in normal human skin fibroblasts in vitro. *J Drugs Dermatol.* 2010;9:1523.

68. Liu Y, Chan F, Sun H, et al. Resveratrol protects human keratinocytes HaCaT cells from UVA-induced oxidative stress damage by downregulating Keap1 expression. *Eur J Pharmacol.* 2011;650:130.

69. Osmond GW, Augustine CK, Zipfel PA, et al. Enhancing melanoma treatment with resveratrol. *J Surg Res.* 2012;172:109.

70. Jang M, Pezzuto JM. Cancer chemopreventive activity of resveratrol. *Drugs Exp Clin Res.* 1999;25:65.

71. Jang M, Pezzuto JM. Effects of resveratrol on 12-O-tetradecanoylphorbol-13-acetate-induced oxidative events and gene expression in mouse skin. *Cancer Lett.* 1998;134:81.

72. Kapadia GJ, Azuine MA, Tokuda H, et al. Chemopreventive effect of resveratrol, sesamol, sesame oil and sunflower oil in the Epstein-Barr virus early antigen activation assay and the mouse skin two-stage carcinogenesis. *Pharmacol Res.* 2002;45:499.

73. Kundu JK, Chun KS, Kim SO, et al. Resveratrol inhibits phorbol ester-induced cyclooxygenase-2 expression in mouse skin: MAPKs and AP-1 as potential molecular targets. *Biofactors.* 2004;21:33.

74. Jang JH, Surh YJ. Protective effect of resveratrol on beta-amyloid-induced oxidative PC12 cell death. *Free Radic Biol Med.* 2003;34:1100.

75. Roy P, Kalra N, Prasad S, et al. Chemopreventive potential of resveratrol in mouse skin tumors through regulation of mitochondrial and PI3K/AKT signaling pathways. *Pharm Res.* 2009;26:211.

76. Yusuf N, Nasti TH, Meleth S, et al. Resveratrol enhances cell-mediated immune response to DMBA through TLR4 and prevents DMBA induced cutaneous carcinogenesis. *Mol Carcinog.* 2009;48:713.

77. Kim KH, Back JH, Zhu Y, et al. Resveratrol targets transforming growth factor-β2 signaling to block UV-induced tumor progression. *J Invest Dermatol.* 2011;131:195.

78. Hao YQ, Huang WX, Feng HX, et al. Study of apoptosis related factors regulatory mechanism of resveratrol to human skin squamous cell carcinoma A431 xenograft in nude mice. *Zhonghua Yi Xue Za Zhi.* 2013;93:464.

79. Ash K, Lord J, Zukowski M, et al. Comparison of topical therapy for striae alba (20% glycolic acid/0.05% tretinoin versus 20% glycolic acid/10% L-ascorbic acid). *Dermatol Surg.* 1998;24:849.

80. Reagan-Shaw S, Afaq F, Aziz MH, et al. Modulations of critical cell cycle regulatory events during chemoprevention of ultraviolet B-mediated responses by resveratrol in SKH-1 hairless mouse skin. *Oncogene.* 2004;23:5151.

81. Shi X, Ye J, Leonard S, et al. Antioxidant properties of (-)-epicatechin-3-gallate and its inhibition of Cr(VI)-induced DNA damage and Cr(IV)- or TPA-stimulated NF-kappaB activation. *Mol Cell Biochem.* 2000;206:125.

82. Wei H, Zhang X, Zhao JF, et al. Scavenging of hydrogen peroxide and inhibition of ultraviolet light-induced oxidative DNA damage by aqueous extracts from green and black teas. *Free Radic Biol Med.* 1999;26:1427.

83. Nichols JA, Katiyar SK. Skin photoprotection by natural polyphenols: Anti-inflammatory, antioxidant and DNA repair mechanisms. *Arch Dermatol Res.* 2010;302:71.

84. Afaq F, Adhami VM, Ahmad N, et al. Botanical antioxidants for chemoprevention of photocarcinogenesis. *Front Biosci.* 2002;7:d784.

85. McDaniel DH, Neudecker BA, DiNardo JC, et al. Idebenone: A new antioxidant – Part I. Relative assessment of oxidative stress

protection capacity compared to commonly known antioxidants. *J Cosmet Dermatol.* 2005;4:10.

86. Giardina S, Michelotti A, Zavattini G, et al. Efficacy study in vitro: Assessment of the properties of resveratrol and resveratrol + N-acetyl-cysteine on proliferation and inhibition of collagen activity. *Minerva Ginecol.* 2010;62:195.

87. Zillich OV, Schweiggert-Weisz U, Hasenkopf K, et al. Release and in vitro skin permeation of polyphenols from cosmetic emulsions. *Int J Cosmet Sci.* 2013;35:491.

88. Brito P, Almeida LM, Dinis TC. The interaction of resveratrol with ferrylmyoglobin and peroxynitrite; protection against LDL oxidation. *Free Radic Res.* 2002;36:621.

89. Becker JV, Armstrong GO, van der Merwe MJ, et al. Metabolic engineering of Saccharomyces cerevisiae for the synthesis of the wine-related antioxidant resveratrol. *FEMS Yeast Res.* 2003;4:79.

90. Docherty JJ, Smith JS, Fu MM, et al. Effect of topically applied resveratrol on cutaneous herpes simplex virus infections in hairless mice. *Antiviral Res.* 2004;61:19.

CHAPTER 51

Flaxseed Oil

Activities:

Antioxidant, antiaging, anti-inflammatory, and anti-apoptotic

Important Chemical Components:

Linoleic acid, α-linolenic acid, oleic acid, palmitic acid, stearic acid, arachidic acid[1,2]

Origin Classification:

This ingredient is considered natural. As an ingredient used for dermatologic purposes, it is laboratory made.

Personal Care Category:

Antioxidant, antiaging

Recommended for the following Baumann Skin Types:

DSNT, DSNW, DSPT, and DSPW

SOURCE

Linum usitatissimum, an annual plant in the Linaceae family native to the eastern Mediterranean to India and better known as flax (or linseed, though the popularity of this name has waned), is grown commercially for its meal, oil, and seeds. Flaxseed oil, derived from the seeds of the plant, is thought to possess significant health properties. Indeed, flaxseed oil is one of the richest sources of ω-3 fatty acids, in particular α-linolenic acid (ALA), which represents more than 50 percent of its total fatty acid content (Table 51-1).[1,3] In addition to an abundance of ω-3 fatty acids, flaxseeds possess copious dietary fiber and lignans, which are polyphenolic phytoestrogens with antioxidant properties, linoleic acid (an ω-6 polyunsaturated fatty acid), and oleic acid (an ω-9 monounsaturated fatty acid). The only foods that contain appreciable lignan levels are flaxseed and flaxseed oil.[4,5] Most commercial supplies are produced in Argentina, Canada, North Africa, and Turkey, but it is grown widely.[6]

HISTORY

Linum usitatissimum was cultivated in ancient Egypt and Ethiopia and used for multiple purposes, including medicine, soap, hair products, and textiles (linen).[7] Its use dates back to the 23rd century BCE in Egypt and, for culinary purposes, to the

TABLE 51-1
Pros and Cons of Flaxseed Oil

Pros	Cons
Rich source of α-linolenic acid	Minimal research to establish its cutaneous efficacy
Compelling dietary benefits	May increase penetration of other ingredients

7th century BCE in Greece.[6] Flaxseed oil is one of the oldest commercial oils and was used for centuries as a drying oil in painting and varnishing.[8] In traditional medical practice it was used as a laxative and to treat urinary tract infections, colds, and lung disorders.[6,7] Currently, it is used to treat irritable bowel as well as constipation.[6]

CHEMISTRY

Antioxidant, anti-inflammatory, and antiapoptotic activities have been associated with flaxseed oil and warrant medical consideration. The substantial anti-inflammatory activity of *L. usitatissimum* has been ascribed to its primary active constituent ALA (57.38 percent), which suppresses arachidonic acid metabolism thus inhibiting the synthesis of proinflammatory n-6 eicosanoids and reducing vascular permeability.[9]

In 2011 experiments, Kaithwas et al. identified significant anti-inflammatory, analgesic, and antipyretic activities exhibited by the fixed oil of *L. usitatissimum*. The oil variably suppressed prostaglandin E_2, leukotriene-, histamine-, bradykinin-, and arachidonic acid-induced inflammation. In a mouse tail immersion model, the oil showed analgesic properties similar to aspirin against acetic acid-induced writhing. The oil was also comparable to aspirin in antipyretic activity in response to typhoid paratyphoid A/B vaccine-induced pyrexia. The investigators attributed this broad range of biological activity to the ALA rife in the herbal extract.[8]

ORAL USES

Flaxseed meal and oil have long been used for dietary purposes and as oral medications. In modern times, the anti-inflammatory activity of dietary flaxseed oil, rich in ALA, was found by Takemura et al. in 2002 to be effective in inhibiting ultraviolet (UV) B-induced skin damage to hairless mice; no such effects were observed from topical application.[10]

In 2011, Neukam et al. conducted a randomized, double-blind, 12-week intervention with two healthy 13-member groups of females with sensitive skin to assess the effect of daily supplementation with flaxseed oil and safflower seed oil. On day 0 and at weeks 6 and 12, investigators evaluated fatty acid profiles, transepidermal water loss (TEWL), as well as skin sensitivity, hydration, and surface. The flaxseed group experienced significant reductions in skin roughness, scaling, and sensitivity (after irritation provoked by nicotinate), as well as TEWL. Smoothness and hydration were augmented in this group while the ratio of ω-6 to ω-3 fatty acids in plasma declined. This ratio increased in the safflower group, which experienced a significant decrease in skin roughness and increase in hydration, but less so and at a later point than the flaxseed group and no other improvements were noted. The investigators concluded that daily consumption of flaxseed oil imparts cutaneous benefits.[11]

TOPICAL USES

In a randomized, double-blind, placebo-controlled application test in 2009, De Spirt et al. studied the cutaneous effects of supplementation with flaxseed or borage oil for 12 weeks in two groups of women (n = 45) between the ages of 18 and 65 with sensitive and dry skin. Fifteen women were in each treatment group, with 15 randomly assigned to a control group given a placebo composed of medium-chain fatty acids. ALA and linoleic acids were the primary constituents in the flaxseed oil and linoleic and γ-linolenic acids were the main constituents in the borage oil used. ALA was found to have contributed to the significant rise in total fatty acids in plasma seen in the flaxseed oil group at weeks 6 and 12. An increase in γ-linolenic acid was noted in the borage oil group. Erythema, roughness, and scaling were decreased in both treatment groups compared to baseline while skin hydration was markedly elevated after 12 weeks. In addition, TEWL was diminished by 10 percent after six weeks in both oil treatment groups, with further reductions after 12 weeks identified in the flaxseed oil group. The investigators concluded that intervention with dietary lipids can manifest in skin improvements.[1]

In 2012, Felippi et al. conducted a pilot study to ascertain the safety and efficacy of nanoparticle formulation for cosmetic application, with various antioxidants including flaxseed oil and coenzyme Q$_{10}$ among the encapsulated active ingredients in the nanoparticles. Various *in vitro* and clinical tests revealed that the nanoparticles were not comedogenic, sensitizing, or irritating and showed no potential for cytotoxicity or producing oxidative stress. Further, exposure to UVA did not result in phototoxicity. Efficacy was tested and established in healthy volunteers with varying levels of periorbital wrinkles. The nanoparticles yielded significant decreases in wrinkling after 21 days of application as compared to a control product. The investigators concluded that the antioxidant-laden nanoparticles were safe for topical application in antiaging cosmetic products.[12]

Notably, flaxseed oil is also among several natural agents developed for the diverse armamentarium used to treat psoriasis.[13] The raw oil is used as an astringent in fungicidal lotions, and for insect repellent and insecticidal activity.[8]

SAFETY ISSUES

Although too volatile to cook with, flaxseed oil is considered safe and healthy to consume.[6] There are no reports of significant adverse events associated with topically applied flaxseed products.

ENVIRONMENTAL IMPACT

Pesticides and fungicides are used in the conventional cultivation of flax. Organic farming of flaxseed mitigates the environmental toll. The use of flax as a fiber plant for clothing was largely supplanted by the cotton industry in the late 19th century, but it is still cultivated for this purpose. Oil flax is cultivated for dietary, cosmetic, and pharmaceutical purposes.[14]

FORMULATION CONSIDERATIONS

Flaxseed oil, as a calcareous liniment oil, is included in Brazil's national pharmacopeia as a treatment for burns and pruritic dermatoses.[15] It is indicated for wounds and as a moisturizer and dermal antioxidant in traditional Chinese and Ayurvedic medicine.[15,16] A test water-in-oil emulsion containing flaxseed oil, *Shorea robusta*, and *Yashada bhasma* (zinc complex) was recently shown by Datta et al. to be more effective at wound contraction, enhancing cutaneous tensile strength, and increasing collagen levels in Wistar rats as compared to a control group.[16]

USAGE CONSIDERATIONS

Oils may affect absorption of other ingredients, especially those that contain oleic acid. This should be kept in mind when choosing other ingredients to use with flaxseed oil.[17]

SIGNIFICANT BACKGROUND

Animal Studies

In 2010, Kaithwas and Majumdar evaluated the anti-inflammatory potential of flaxseed fixed oil against castor oil-induced diarrhea, turpentine oil-induced joint edema, as well as formaldehyde and Complete Freund's Adjuvant (CFA)-induced arthritis in Wistar albino rats. They found that flaxseed oil dose-dependently inhibited the adverse effects of castor oil and turpentine oil as well as CFA, and a significant inhibitory effect was also exerted by flaxseed oil against formaldehyde-induced proliferation of global edematous arthritis. Flaxseed oil also significantly diminished the secondary lesions engendered by CFA by dint of a delayed hypersensitivity reaction. The authors concluded that the significant anti-inflammatory activity imparted by *L. usitatissimum* fixed oil suggests its therapeutic viability for inflammatory conditions, such as rheumatoid arthritis.[9]

Recently, de Souza Franco et al. studied the effects on skin wounds in Wistar rats of a semisolid formulation of flaxseed oil (1, 5, or 10 percent). The investigators assessed the contraction/re-epithelialization of the wound and resistance to mechanical traction in incisional and excisional models, respectively. They found that the groups treated with flaxseed oil 1 or 5 percent largely started re-epithelialization earlier than the petroleum jelly control group and achieved complete re-epithelialization on the 14th day after injury, as compared to 33.33 percent of animals in the petroleum jelly group. The investigators concluded that flaxseed oil, at low concentrations, exhibits potential in a solid pharmaceutical preparation, for use in dermal repair.[15]

Early in 2012, Tülüce et al. set out to ascertain the antioxidant and antiapoptotic effects of flaxseed oil exerted against UVC-induced damage in Sprague-Dawley albino male rats. They divided animals into three groups: control, UVC alone, and UVC and flaxseed oil. UVC light exposure lasted for one hour twice daily for four weeks in the two exposure groups. In the flaxseed oil group, the oil was administered by gavage prior to each irradiation (4 mL/kg bw). The investigators noted that malondialdehyde and protein carbonyl levels were higher in the UVC group compared to the controls, but such levels were reduced in the flaxseed oil group compared to the UVC only group, in skin, lens, and sera. Also, the activities of glutathione peroxidase and superoxide dismutase were found to be higher in the skin, lens, and sera of the flaxseed oil group as compared to the UVC only group. In addition, retinal apoptosis was lower in the flaxseed group than the UVC group. The researchers concluded that flaxseed oil may be useful in conferring a photoprotective effect against UVC-induced damage, as manifested in protein carbonylation and reactive oxygen species generation, in rats.[2]

CONCLUSION

Flaxseed oil has gained recent attention for its salutary effects as part of the diet. Rich in ω-3 essential fatty acids and lignans, flaxseed oil has been found to improve fatty acid profiles. Significantly, emerging evidence points to beneficial cutaneous effects being derived from dietary use of flaxseed oil. Much more research is necessary to determine whether the beneficial constituents of flaxseed oil can be harnessed in topical products.

REFERENCES

1. De Spirt S, Stahl W, Tronnier H, et al. Intervention with flaxseed and borage oil supplements modulates skin condition in women. *Br J Nutr.* 2009;101:440.
2. Tülüce Y, Ozkol H, Koyuncu I. Photoprotective effect of flax seed oil (Linum usitatissimum L.) against ultraviolet C-induced apoptosis and oxidative stress in rats. *Toxicol Ind Health.* 2012;28:99.
3. Hoffmann D. *Medical Herbalism: The science and practice of herbal medicine.* Rochester, VT: Healing Arts Press; 2003:57.
4. Axelson M, Sjövall J, Gustafsson BE, et al. Origin of lignans in mammals and identification of a precursor from plants. *Nature.* 1982;298:659.
5. Scalbert A, Williamson G. Dietary intake and bioavailability of polyphenols. *J Nutr.* 2000;130:2073S.
6. Foster S. *101 Medicinal Herbs: An Illustrated Guide.* Loveland, CO: Interweave Press; 1998:88-89.
7. Grieve M. *A Modern Herbal* (Vol 1). New York: Dover Publications; 1971:317-9.
8. Kaithwas G, Mukherjee A, Chaurasia AK, et al. Anti-inflammatory, analgesic and antipyretic activities of Linum usitatissimum L. (flaxseed/linseed) fixed oil. *Indian J Exp Biol.* 2011;49:932.
9. Kaithwas G, Majumdar DK. Therapeutic effect of Linum usitatissimum (flaxseed/linseed) fixed oil on acute and chronic arthritic models in albino rats. *Inflammopharmacology.* 2010; 18:127.
10. Takemura N, Takahashi K, Tanaka H, et al. Dietary, but not topical, alpha-linolenic acid suppresses UVB-induced skin injury in hairless mice when compared with linoleic acids. *Photochem Photobiol.* 2002;76:657.
11. Neukam K, De Spirt S, Stahl W, et al. Supplementation of flaxseed oil diminishes skin sensitivity and improves skin barrier function and condition. *Skin Pharmacol Physiol.* 2011;24:67.
12. Felippi CC, Oliveira D, Ströher A, et al. Safety and efficacy of antioxidants-loaded nanoparticles for an anti-aging application. *J Biomed Nanotechnol.* 2012;8:316.
13. Rahman M, Alam K, Ahmad MZ, et al. Classical to current approach for treatment of psoriasis: A review. *Endocr Metab Immune Disord Drug Targets.* 2012;12:287.
14. GMO Compass. http://www.gmo-compass.org/eng/database/plants/11.flaxseed.html. Accessed June 25, 2013.
15. de Souza Franco E, de Aquino CM, de Medeiros PL, et al. Effect of a semisolid formulation of Linum usitatissimum L. (Linseed) oil on the repair of skin wounds. *Evid Based Complement Alternat Med.* 2012;2012:270752.
16. Datta HS, Mitra SK, Patwardhan B. Wound healing activity of topical application forms based on ayurveda. *Evid Based Complement Alternat Med.* 2011;2011:134378.
17. Naik A, Pechtold L, Potts RO, et al. Mechanism of oleic acid-induced skin penetration enhancement in vivo in humans. *J Control Release.* 1995;37:299.

CHAPTER 52

Phloretin

Activities:

Antioxidant, anti-inflammatory,[1] antibacterial,[1] anticancer,[2] penetration enhancement, photoprotection, skin lightening

Important Chemical Components:

The International Union of Pure and Applied Chemistry (IUPAC) designation is 3-(4-hydroxyphenyl)-1-(2,4,6-trihydroxyphenyl)-1-propanone.[3] It is also known as 2′,4′,6′-trihydroxy-3-(4-hydroxyphenyl)-propiophenone. Its molecular formula is $C_{15}H_{14}O_5$.

Origin Classification:

Phloretin is natural and found in various foods.

Personal Care Category:

Photoprotection

Recommended for the following Baumann Skin Types:

DRNW, DRPT, DRPW, DSNW, DSPW, ORPT, ORPW, OSPT, OSPW, and OSNW

SOURCE

Reportedly capable of demonstrating antioxidant activity, phloretin (also known as dihydronaringenin, phloretol, and naringenin chalcone) is a plant-derived dihydrochalcone polyphenol primarily found in various species of apple (in copious supply), pear, and other plants in the Rosaceae family, and recently found in much smaller quantities in various tomato species and strawberries.[2,4] Phloretin and its glucoside phloridzin have also been identified in tomatoes and are considered an important source of dietary flavonoids.[5]

HISTORY

Phloridzin was first isolated from apple tree bark in 1835 by DeKonnick.[6] Of course, the health benefits of apples and other sources of phloretin have been passed down anecdotally for centuries. In the late 1980s, botanically-derived flavonoid compounds, specifically phloretin and the structurally related compound nordihydroguaiaretic acid (NDGA), were found to strongly inhibit keratinocyte growth and were therefore thought to exhibit antipsoriatic activity.[7] The preponderance of research on phloretin and phloridzin has taken place in an *in vitro* setting.

CHEMISTRY

Phloretin occurs as a glycoside, particularly in the Rosaceae and Ericaceae families.[1] Phloridzin, the glucoside form of phloretin, has been found to display potent antioxidant activity in peroxynitrite, hydroxyl, and 1,1-diphenyl-2-picrylhydrazyl (DPPH) radical

scavenging and the suppression of lipid peroxidation.[8] Along with its glucoside phloridzin, phloretin is believed to be an important contributor to the health benefits of apples.[9] In addition, it was once used as a substitute for quinine. Notably, dihydrochalcones are among five polyphenolic groups that have been identified in apples, also including hydroxycinnamic acids, flavan-3-ols/procyanidins, anthocyanins, and flavonols.[9–11] One of the main biological actions of phloretin is the inhibition of glucose cotransporter 1.[4] It is also thought to exert antithrombotic activity.[4]

ORAL USES

Phloretin is consumed regularly as a key active ingredient in several fruits. In a study of eight different apple cultivars (Red Delicious, Golden Delicious, Cortland, Empire, Ida Red, McIntosh, Mutsu, and Northern Spy), a much greater concentration of polyphenols was found in the peel as compared to the flesh.[9]

TOPICAL USES

Phloretin has been studied as a key ingredient in a combination topical solution. In 2008, Oresajo et al. assessed the effects of a topical antioxidant formulation including 10 percent L-ascorbic acid, 2 percent phloretin, and 0.5 percent ferulic acid in mitigating ultraviolet (UV)-induced harm in 10 normal, healthy volunteers (aged 18–69 years). Biomarkers of cutaneous damage, including formation of sunburn cells and thymine dimers, and the expression of matrix metalloproteinase (MMP)-9 and p53 protein, were evaluated in the Fitzpatrick skin type II or III subjects who were randomized and treated daily for four days with the antioxidant combination or vehicle control on the lower back. Pretreatment with the antioxidant mixture effectively suppressed UV-induced damage and also prevented UV exposure from provoking immunosuppressive effects. The investigators concluded that the dual role of phloretin, as strong antioxidant and penetration enhancer, acts in this topical formulation to augment the skin availability of the other antioxidants. They also suggested that the antioxidant formulation could enhance photoprotection of human skin by serving a complementary role to sunscreens.[12]

SAFETY ISSUES

There are no specific reports of adverse effects associated with phloretin or phloridzin in the literature to the author's knowledge.

ENVIRONMENTAL IMPACT

The effects on the environment traceable to phloretin pertain to the cultivation and transport of the fruits in which the polyphenol is found.

TABLE 52-1
Pros and Cons of Phloretin

Pros	Cons
Potent antioxidant	Expensive
Cancer prevention potential	Difficult to formulate
Can penetrate the skin and interact with other antioxidants	

FORMULATION CONSIDERATIONS

Phloridzin typically displays a brown color, rendering it difficult to formulate (Table 52-1). In 2012, Baldisserotto et al. reported on the production, stability, and antimicrobial activity of a novel semi-synthetic phloridzin derivative. The product, F_2, was found to exhibit antioxidant potency comparable to phloridzin but was more stable in topical formulations.[6]

USAGE CONSIDERATIONS

No interactions with other ingredients are known by the author.

SIGNIFICANT BACKGROUND

In Vitro Studies

In 2001, phloretin was evaluated for its potential to enhance the cutaneous penetration of lignocaine hydrochloride delivered transdermally. Investigators first treated excised human skin samples with phloretin applied as a methanolic solution 12 hours before lignocaine application, at pH 4 and 7. At a pH of 4, a 3.2-fold increase in total permeation was seen as compared with the control after 24 hours. Unilamellar phosphatidylcholine liposomes were used as a vehicle for phloretin in a subsequent test, with a 5.4-fold greater permeation of lignocaine observed in pretreated skin compared with control after 24 hours. Investigators concluded that phloretin indeed demonstrated potential as a transdermal penetration enhancer for lignocaine.[13]

In 2003, Auner et al. showed that permeation of porcine skin with phloretin and 6-ketocholestanol prior to treatment with 5-aminolevulinic acid increased acid diffusion (the permeation of which was enhanced by cetylpyridinium chloride and benzalkonium chloride) at pH 7 approximately 1.7-fold.[14] In an experiment also published in April 2003, the same team studied the same compounds, phloretin and 6-ketocholestanol included in unilamellar liposomes, for the viability of enhancing the transport of sodium-fluorescein across rat, porcine, and human skin. Both compounds were used to pretreat the skin. Phloretin was found to have a significant positive effect on sodium-fluorescein diffusion in rat and porcine skin after 30 hours but no influence on human skin as compared to control; 6-ketocholestanol exhibited a positive effect on all skin types.[3]

Using various methods to evaluate membrane interactions, some of the same investigators, led by Valenta, subsequently determined that phloretin and 6-ketocholestanol interact with the lipid layer and alter the structure, rendering a greater fluidity in the membrane.[15] In addition, Auner and Valenta published a study on the effects of phloretin on the topical permeation of lidocaine using one hydrophilic and three lipophilic delivery systems. The researchers conducted standard diffusion experiments with Franz type diffusion cells through porcine skin and found that phloretin enhanced lidocaine diffusion, with permeation enhanced 1.39-fold in the hydrophilic formulation and from 1.25- to 1.76-fold in the lipophilic formulations.[16] More recently, Auner et al. have shed light on the mechanisms of action of phloretin, as well as 6-ketocholestanol. Their increase in stratum corneum (SC) intercellular lipid bilayer fluidity is thought to impart the observed penetration-enhancing effects associated with these compounds. Evaluation of the effects of these compounds on phase transition and enthalpy revealed that both compounds decrease the diffusional resistance of the SC to drugs with a hydrophilic-lipophilic equilibrium.[17]

In a 2008 examination of the phytochemicals in apples and apple juices for the purposes of ascertaining the relative contributions to potential chemopreventive properties, investigators fractionated a polyphenol-enriched apple juice extract and measured antioxidant effects, modulation of carcinogen metabolism, anti-inflammatory and antihormonal activities, and antiproliferative potential. They identified phloretin and epicatechin as the strongest inhibitors of cyclooxygenase 1, which could contribute to an anti-inflammatory effect potentially conferred by apples.[18] The researchers concluded that the combination of various constituents exhibiting complementary properties may lead to increased total chemopreventive benefits.

Earlier in 2003, investigators assessing the contribution of the major phenolic phytochemicals in apples to the total antioxidant capacity of the fruit using a 2, 2'-azinobis (3-ethylbenzothiazoline-6-sulfonic acid) radical-scavenging assay, and expressed as vitamin C equivalent antioxidant capacity, found a linear relationship between phenolic concentration and total antioxidant activity. Therefore, they estimated the greatest phenolic contribution to the total antioxidant capacity of apples to be derived from quercetin, followed in order by epicatechin, procyanidin B_2, phloretin, and chlorogenic acid, with the contribution from vitamin C falling just ahead of phloretin.[19]

In 2007, Lin et al. isolated and identified 13 compounds from the Formosan apple (*Malus doumeri*), a native Taiwanese botanical, including 3-hydroxyphloretin, which demonstrated potent antioxidant and cellular tyrosinase-reducing activities in human epidermal melanocytes. In addition, 3-hydroxyphloretin was found to be one of the two most active constituents, along with catechol, also exhibiting activity as a competitive inhibitor in a kinetic analysis of mushroom tyrosinase. The investigators concluded that both compounds display potential as cosmetic agents.[20] The tyrosinase-reducing activities associated with phloretin suggest intriguing potential as a skin-lightening agent.

Several of the same investigators earlier reported on the seven phenolic compounds isolated from the Taiwanese apple that were assessed for their potential application in skin care. Specifically, the researchers found that the compounds 3-hydroxyphloridzin, 3-hydroxyphloretin, and quercetin demonstrated the most potent free radical-scavenging properties against DPPH and superoxide radicals. The phloretin compounds (the glucoside phloridzin) also exhibited inhibitory activity against xanthine oxidase and elastase. These substances were also found to suppress MMP-1 synthesis in human fibroblast cells. This is significant because these enzymes break down key dermal constituents, contributing to cutaneous aging. The team concluded that the phloretin extracts as well as quercetin show potential for use in antiaging or other cosmetic formulations.[21]

Anticancer Activity

In 2012, Shin et al. studied the effects of phloretin in a mouse tumor model and found that topically applied phloretin significantly blocked mouse skin carcinogenesis initiated with 7,12-dimethylbenz[a]anthracene (DMBA) and promoted with 12-O-tetradecanoylphorbol 13-acetate (TPA). Further, phloretin pretreatment of dorsal skin dose-dependently suppressed TPA-induced cyclooxygenase-2 (COX-2) expression. The investigators also noted that topically applied phloretin reduced the TPA-induced DNA binding of nuclear factor-κB (NF-κB), the transcription factor that accounts for TPA-induced COX-2 expression in mouse skin. The investigators suggested that these and other inhibitory effects may partially explain the antitumor-promoting effects of phloretin on skin carcinogenesis in mice.[2] Notably, phloretin had previously been shown to selectively suppress TPA-induced calcium- and phospholipid-dependent protein kinase activity in mouse epidermis.[22] Also, phloretin derivatives have been demonstrated to inhibit croton oil-induced mouse ear edema.[23]

Interestingly, phloretin has also been found to hinder the growth of several cancer cells and to induce apoptosis of B$_{16}$ melanoma, HL60 human leukemia cells, and HT-29 human colon cancer cells, which Park et al., in an investigation of the effects of the flavonoid on the human colon cancer cell line, speculate may be mediated via mitochondrial membrane permeability alterations and activation of caspase pathways.[24]

Other Applications

Gitzinger et al. have engineered a hybrid *Pseudomonas putida*-mammalian genetic unit responsive to phloretin – the phloretin-adjustable control element (PEACE) – which, when formulated in a skin lotion, was found to have the capacity to calibrate target genes and adjust heterologous serum protein levels when topically applied to mice. The investigators believe that this new technology has potential in gene- and cell-based biopharmaceutical treatments.[25]

■ CONCLUSION

The evidence thus far compiled on the potential salutary effects of topical phloretin, a phenolic compound found most abundantly in various species of apples, and also in pears, is relatively modest. Nevertheless, data appear to suggest that phloretin exhibits antioxidant activity in oral form and a potentially significant influence on the skin, particularly in enhancing the permeation of other ingredients. While much more research is necessary, particularly randomized controlled trials, this botanical ingredient is an intriguing addition to the ever-expanding roster of naturally-derived ingredients with the potential to impart significant health benefits to the skin. Of course, it also may provide some support to the old adage "an apple a day keeps the doctor away."

REFERENCES

1. Hoffmann D. The endocrine system. In: *Medical Herbalism: The Science and Practice of Herbal Medicine*. Rochester, VT: Healing Arts Press; 2003:108.
2. Shin JW, Kundu JK, Surh YJ. Phloretin inhibits phorbol ester-induced tumor promotion and expression of cyclooxygenase-2 in mouse skin: Extracellular signal-regulated kinase and nuclear factor-κB as potential targets. *J Med Food*. 2012;15:253.
3. Auner BG, Valenta C, Hadgraft J. Influence of phloretin and 6-ketocholestanol on the skin permeation of sodium-fluorescein. *J Control Release*. 2003;89:321.
4. Stangl V, Lorenz M, Ludwig A, et al. The flavonoid phloretin suppresses stimulated expression of endothelial adhesion molecules and reduces activation of human platelets. *J Nutr*. 2005;135:172.
5. Slimestad R, Fossen T, Verheul MJ. The flavonoids of tomatoes. *J Agric Food Chem*. 2008;56:2436.
6. Baldisserotto A, Malisardi G, Scalambra E, et al. Synthesis, antioxidant and antimicrobial activity of a new phloridzin derivative for dermo-cosmetic applications. *Molecules*. 2012;17:13275.
7. Wilkinson DI, Orenberg EK. Effects of nordihydroguaiaretic acid, phloretin, and phloridzin on the activity of adenylate cyclase, lipoxygenase and hexose transport, and growth of cultured keratinocytes. *Int J Dermatol*. 1987;26:660.
8. Rezk BM, Haenen GR, van der Vijgh WJ, et al. The antioxidant activity of phloretin: The disclosure of a new antioxidant pharmacophore in flavonoids. *Biochem Biophys Res Commun*. 2002;295:9.
9. Tsao R, Yang R, Young JC, et al. Polyphenolic profiles in eight apple cultivars using high-performance liquid chromatography (HPLC). *J Agric Food Chem*. 2003;51:6347.
10. Hyson DA. A comprehensive review of apples and apple components and their relationship to human health. *Adv Nutr*. 2011;2:408.
11. Gerhauser C. Cancer chemopreventive potential of apples, apple juice, and apple components. *Planta Med*. 2008;74:1608.
12. Oresajo C, Stephens T, Hino PD, et al. Protective effects of a topical antioxidant mixture containing vitamin C, ferulic acid, and phloretin against ultraviolet-induced photodamage in human skin. *J Cosmet Dermatol*. 2008;7:290.
13. Valenta C, Cladera J, O'Shea P, et al. Effect of phloretin on the percutaneous absorption of lignocaine across human skin. *J Pharm Sci*. 2001;90:485.
14. Auner BG, Valenta C, Hadgraft J. Influence of lipophilic counterions in combination with phloretin and 6-ketocholestanol on the skin permeation of 5-aminolevulinic acid. *Int J Pharm*. 2003;255:109.
15. Valenta C, Steininger A, Auner BG. Phloretin and 6-ketocholestanol: Membrane interactions studied by a phospholipids/polydiacetylene colorimetric assay and differential scanning calorimetry. *Eur J Pharm Biopharm*. 2004;57:329.
16. Auner BG, Valenta C. Influence of phloretin on the skin permeation of lidocaine from semisolid preparations. *Eur J Pharm Biopharm*. 2004;57:307.
17. Auner BG, O'Neill MA, Valenta C, et al. Interaction of phloretin and 6-ketocholestanol with DPPC-liposomes as phospholipid model membranes. *Int J Pharm*. 2005;294:149.
18. Zessner H, Pan L, Will F, et al. Fractionation of polyphenol-enriched apple juice extracts to identify constituents with cancer chemopreventive potential. *Mol Nutr Food Res*. 2008;52(Suppl 1):S28.
19. Lee KW, Kim YJ, Kim DO, et al. Major phenolics in apple and their contribution to the total antioxidant capacity. *J Agric Food Chem*. 2003;51:6516.
20. Lin YP, Hsu FL, Chen CS, et al. Constituents from the Formosan apple reduce tyrosinase activity in human epidermal melanocytes. *Phytochemistry*. 2007;68:1189.
21. Leu SJ, Lin YP, Lin RD, et al. Phenolic constituents of Malus doumeri var. formosana in the field of skin care. *Biol Pharm Bull*. 2006;29:740.
22. Gschwendt M, Horn F, Kittstein W, et al. Calcium and phospholipid-dependent protein kinase activity in mouse epidermis cytosol. Stimulation by complete and incomplete tumor promoters and inhibition by various compounds. *Biochem Biophys Res Commun*. 1984;124:63.
23. Blazsó G, Gábor M. Effects of prostaglandin antagonist phloretin derivatives on mouse ear edema induced with different skin irritants. *Prostaglandins*. 1995;50:161.
24. Park SY, Kim EJ, Shin HK, et al. Induction of apoptosis in HT-29 colon cancer cells by phloretin. *J Med Food*. 2007;10:581.
25. Gitzinger M, Kemmer C, El-Baba MD, et al. Controlling transgene expression in subcutaneous implants using a skin lotion containing the apple metabolite phloretin. *Proc Natl Acad Sci USA* 2009;106:10638.

CHAPTER 53

Caffeic Acid

Activities:

Antioxidant, anticarcinogenic,[1] anti-inflammatory, antimicrobial,[2,3] immunostimulatory, neuroprotective,[4] photoprotective

Important Chemical Components:

Also known as 3,4-dihydroxycinnamic acid, its molecular formula is $C_9H_8O_4$.

Origin Classification:

Naturally found in a wide array of fruits, grains, and vegetables. Organic forms are available.

Personal Care Category:

Antioxidant, antiaging

Recommended for the following Baumann Skin Types:

DRNT, DRNW, DRPW, DSNT, DSNW, DSPW, ORNT, ORNW, ORPW, OSNT, OSNW, and OSPW

SOURCE

Caffeic acid (3,4-dihydroxycinnamic acid) is found in several grains, fruits, and vegetables.[5] It also occurs in *Coffea arabica* (coffee beans), particularly in its esterified form, chlorogenic acid (5-caffeoylquinic acid).[6,7] Some of the best sources of caffeic acid, besides coffee, include grapes, wine, tea, apples and apple juice, cider, blueberries, sunflower seeds, olives, olive oil, argan oil, spinach, cabbage, asparagus, and globe artichoke.[4,8–12] Caffeic acid is one of the main hydroxycinnamic acids (along with ferulic and coumaric), a major class of phenolic compounds that represent the most widely dispersed phenylpropanoids in plants.[6,8] Further, it is one of the primary constituents of *Rosmarinus officinalis* (rosemary) and *Capparis spinosa* (caper bush), which have been shown to confer cutaneous benefits.[13,14] Rosemary, in fact, is used often as a spice and is included in beverages, cosmetics, and as a therapeutic herb in traditional medicine.[13]

Caffeic acid has also been isolated in various other plants, including *Melissa officinalis* (lemon balm), and several species of Echinacea, which are known to exhibit various clinical properties.[15–20] In addition, derivatives of caffeic acid are important components in *Plantago major*, a plant used broadly in traditional folk medicines.[21] Caffeic acid phenethyl ester (CAPE), an active constituent of propolis extract, a product of honeybee hives (see Chapter 60, Honey/Propolis/Royal Jelly), specifically inhibits nuclear factor (NF)-κB and is known to display a wide array of biological activity, including antioxidant, anti-inflammatory, antiproliferative, cytostatic, and antineoplastic.[22] It has greater lipid solubility and is thought to exert greater anti-inflammatory and antibacterial activity as compared to caffeic acid.[23,24]

HISTORY

Cognizance of health benefits derived from caffeic acid dates back at least to 400 BCE, when herbal formulations including caffeic acid were administered to facilitate sleep. It is not known who first discovered caffeic acid. Notably, even though caffeic acid and caffeine are present in coffee, they are unrelated compounds.

CHEMISTRY

Along with other polyphenolic acids such as ferulic, ellagic, and tannic, caffeic acid is thought to have considerable anticarcinogenic potential,[25] and is known to confer antioxidant activity (Table 53-1).[12] Like ferulic acid, caffeic acid is also synthesized in the wide variety of plants in which it is found through the shikimate pathway from l-phenylalanine or l-tyrosine (see Chapter 54, Ferulic Acid).[8,26] Caffeic acid is conjugated with saccharides,[5,26] reacts with nitrogen oxides, and has been shown to protect phopholipidic membranes from ultraviolet (UV)-induced peroxidation by inhibiting the lipid peroxidative chain reaction.[27] More significantly, caffeic acid has also been demonstrated to protect human skin from UVB-induced erythema.[5] Caffeic acid is thought to be a stronger antioxidant than ferulic acid but not as effective at permeating the skin.[4,27]

ORAL USES

Consumed regularly through myriad foods and beverages throughout the world as the primary dietary hydroxycinnamic acid, caffeic acid is a key constituent of several vegetables, fruits, and grains and, especially, coffee. It is difficult to quantify the direct contributions of caffeic acid to skin health.

TOPICAL USES

Caffeic acid is a key constituent in kigelia fruit extract, which has shown significant anticarcinogenic activity and is used in various parts of the world, other than the United States, in products to help defend against skin cancer. Standardized water, ethanol, and dichloromethane extracts of *Kigelia pinnata* have been found to dose-dependently inhibit several melanoma cell lines.[28] In addition, caffeic acid is found as an ingredient in several multibotanical formulations.

The esterified form of caffeic acid known as CAPE has been used topically as an ingredient in sunless tanning products to provide a more natural-looking tan than previous products.[29]

TABLE 53-1
Pros and Cons of Caffeic Acid

Pros	Cons
Potent antioxidant	Limited clinical evidence for topical use
Abundant in a range of dietary sources	Usually not listed on cosmetic label
Good *in vitro* evidence of photoprotective activity	
Can penetrate the stratum corneum[27]	

SAFETY ISSUES

The author is unaware of any reports of adverse side effects or toxicity associated with caffeic acid.

ENVIRONMENTAL IMPACT

Caffeic acid appears throughout the plant kingdom. Few if any of the plants are cultivated to harness caffeic acid specifically, however. Therefore, there is no known detrimental impact on the environment from cultivating plants such as *C. arabica*.

FORMULATION CONSIDERATIONS

Noting that caffeic acid has displayed synergistically enhanced antioxidant activity when conjugated with amino acids, Kwak et al. used hydroxamic acid and prepared caffeoyl-amino acidyl-hydroxamic acid. They found that caffeoyl-prolyl-hydroxamic acid then exhibited strong antioxidant and tyrosinase-inhibitory activity in several bioassays.[30]

In 2012, Centini et al. synthesized several new multifunctional surfactants in which ferulic or caffeic acid, coupled with an amino acid, played significant roles. The surfactants meet the most recent requirements for cosmetic ingredients by displaying emulsifying, UV-protective, and radical-scavenging activity. Notably, the investigators report that these versatile surfactants have the potential to be useful in treating various skin conditions, including those related to the deleterious effects of UV exposure, free radical damage, and loss of cellular antioxidants.[4]

In a 2013 *in vitro* study of the capacity of propolis phenolic acids (including caffeic acid) from semisolid formulations to penetrate into human skin, Žilius et al. indeed showed that these acids (caffeic, ferulic, vanillic, and coumaric) demonstrated this property. Caffeic acid was found to penetrate slowly into the epidermis with dermal penetration not clearly ascertained. Deeper penetration was observed in relation to the other phenolic compounds. The investigators suggested that more research is necessary in order to devise semisolid topical application systems that can more reliably deliver antioxidants from propolis into the skin.[31]

USAGE CONSIDERATIONS

Caffeic acid is not typically seen on the cosmeceutical product label because it is usually a constituent of another ingredient in the product such as coffee or rosemary extract.

SIGNIFICANT BACKGROUND

In Vitro Studies

In 2007, Marti-Mestres et al. studied the permeation of caffeic acid, chlorogenic acid, and the natural glycoside oraposide through pig ear skin *in vitro* in order to evaluate the viability of these compounds for use in photoprotective skin formulations. After at least 48 hours of drug contact, investigators found caffeic and chlorogenic acids in all skin sections, which they thought might be attributed to systemic activity. Oraposide was found in the upper superficial skin layer, suggesting a greater facility of use for topical skin care formulation.[32]

In an *in vitro* study in five melanoma cell lines (B16-F0, B16-F10, SK-MEL-28, SK-MEL-5, and MeWo), Kudugunti et al.

demonstrated that CAPE displays significant antimelanoma efficacy and low toxicity at 10 mg/kg/day.[24]

Caffeic acid was among the ingredients tested when Chiang et al. extracted *C. arabica* leaves with methanol and hydrolyzed various concentrations of hydrochloric acid to ascertain antiphotoaging activity in 2011. Concentrations of caffeic acid and chlorogenic acid were tested for matrix metalloproteinase (MMP) and elastase inhibition and *in vitro* results showed that caffeic acid mitigated UVB irritation by suppressing MMP-1 and MMP-9 expression and both caffeic and chlorogenic acids downregulated the mitogen-activated protein kinase (MAPK) pathway. None of the extracts affected elastase. The investigators concluded that *C. arabica* and its polyphenolic constituents have potential as photodamage-preventing agents.[33]

In 2012, Pluemsamran et al. pretreated immortalized human keratinocyte (HaCaT) cells with caffeic acid or ferulic acid and found that the antioxidants suppressed UVA-induced cytotoxicity as well as the induction of MMP-1 activity and mRNA and oxidant formation. The investigators speculated that caffeic and ferulic acids delivered protection against UVA-mediated MMP-1 induction in HaCaT cells by restoring the antioxidant defense system at the cellular and molecular levels.[34]

Animal Studies

In 1988, Huang et al. assessed the effects of the topical application of curcumin as well as caffeic, chlorogenic, and ferulic acids on 12-*O*-tetradecanoylphorbol-13-acetate (TPA)-induced epidermal ornithine decarboxylase activity, epidermal DNA synthesis, and skin tumor promotion in female CD-1 mice. Although curcumin was the most successful in suppressing TPA-induced tumors, all of the hydroxycinnamic acids showed some antitumorigenic activity (see Chapter 69, Turmeric).[35]

In 2006, Staniforth et al. reported that caffeic acid inhibited UVB radiation-induced interleukin-10 (IL-10) expression and phosphorylation of MAPK as well as MAPK signal transduction pathways in mouse skin, also finding that the polyphenol significantly suppressed UVB-induced IL-10 mRNA expression and protein synthesis. In addition, the investigators noted that a contact hypersensitivity assay demonstrated attenuation of local immune suppression imparted by caffeic acid. The investigators concluded that their *in vivo* findings indicate that caffeic acid appears to offer significant protection against photocarcinogenesis and immune suppression engendered by UVB radiation. They also suggested that caffeic acid warrants consideration for its potential as a topical protective agent against UVB damage.[1]

Also in the same year, Yamada et al. showed that orally administered caffeic acid lessened the skin damage induced by UVA-induced reactive oxygen species (ROS) generation in the abdominal skin of live hairless mice. The researchers noted that caffeic acid was efficiently distributed in the skin after oral administration. Topically applied caffeic acid also inhibited ROS generation from exposure to UVA.[36]

Using skin-incised mice to analyze the wound-healing effect of caffeic acid, Song et al. found that the polyphenol exhibited significant anti-inflammatory and wound-healing properties, including collagen-like polymer production, lipid peroxidation, myeloperoxidase activity, and phospholipase A_2 activity while suppressing the silica-induced generation of ROS, melittin-induced arachidonic acid release, and PGE_2 production in Raw 264.7 cells, and melittin- or arachidonic acid-promoted histamine release in RBL 2H3 cells. The investigators concluded that their findings suggest strong antioxidant and anti-inflammatory effects imparted by caffeic acid contributing to wound healing in skin-incised mice.[37]

In 2012, Khan et al. studied the protective effects of caffeic acid against TPA-induced oxidative stress, inflammatory damage, as well as expression of NF-κB and cyclooxygenase (COX-2) in mouse skin. Pretreatment with caffeic acid at two different doses before TPA application demonstrated that the polyphenol significantly suppressed TPA-induced lipid peroxidation, inflammatory responses, and tumor necrosis factor-α release while upregulating glutathione content and various antioxidant enzymatic activity. Caffeic acid also hindered TPA-induced NF-κB and COX-2 expression.[38]

Caffeic Acid Phenethyl Ester (CAPE)

In 1993, Frenkel et al. isolated CAPE from propolis to examine the effects of the compound on TPA-induced tumor promotion in SENCAR mice. Topical treatment with low doses of CAPE (0.1–6.5 nmol/topical treatment) were found to inhibit polymorphonuclear leukocyte infiltration into mouse skin and ears, hydrogen peroxide (H_2O_2) synthesis, and formation of oxidized bases in epidermal DNA. The investigators also found that CAPE suppressed TPA-induced H_2O_2 synthesis in bovine lenses. Overall, the investigators concluded that CAPE appears to be a potent chemopreventive agent with broad potential against diseases characterized by marked inflammatory and/or oxidative stress features, including cancers and cataracts.[23]

Indeed, CAPE has been found to possess anticarcinogenic potential. In a mouse model, TPA was applied twice weekly to the backs of CD-1 mice previously initiated with 7,12-dimethylbenz[a]anthracene (DMBA), resulting in skin papillomas. Topical application of CAPE along with the tumor-promoter TPA significantly inhibited the number of skin papillomas per mouse in a dose-dependent manner and resulted in reduced tumor size, also dose dependently. Further, CAPE application decreased the level of 5-hydroxymethyl-2'-deoxyuridine (HMdU) residue in epidermal DNA that resulted from DMBA initiation.[39] CAPE was previously found to have inhibited keratinocyte proliferation in a time- and concentration-dependent fashion. Investigators making this observation 10 years ago also noted that CAPE significantly inhibited full induction of ornithine decarboxylase (ODC) by epidermal growth factor (EGF) also in a time- and concentration-dependent fashion and suppressed ODC gene expression. The researchers concluded that CAPE exhibits potential as an agent to treat hyperproliferative skin conditions.[40]

In 2007, Serarslan et al. investigated the effects of CAPE, an antioxidant and anti-inflammatory agent, on wound healing in rats by treating 20 male rats with CAPE and comparing them to an untreated control group of 20 male rats. The investigators performed linear full-thickness incisions on the backs of each rat and administered either treatment or saline. Biochemical analysis of wound tissues revealed a significant rise in glutathione and nitric oxide levels and significant reductions in malondialdehyde and superoxide dismutase levels in the group treated with CAPE as compared to controls. In the histopathological analysis, investigators reported rapid epithelium development in the wound tissues of the CAPE group compared with controls. They concluded that their findings suggest CAPE contributes to accelerating full-thickness wound healing through its antioxidant and ROS-scavenging activities.[41]

Photoprotective Activity

In 1995, Facino et al. examined the protective effects of several caffeoyl derivatives, including caffeic acid, from Echinacea family extracts on the free radical-induced degradation of type III collagen. Macromolecules were exposed to superoxide anions and hydroxyl radicals produced by the xanthine/xanthine oxidase/Fe_2+/EDTA system. The investigators found that collagen breakdown was dose-dependently suppressed by all of the Echinacea species constituents (order of potency: echinacoside ≈ chicoric acid > cynarine ≈ caffeic acid > chlorogenic acid). They concluded that Echinacea polyphenols protect collagen from free radical damage and warrant consideration for topical use to protect skin against UV-induced oxidative stress.[42] Although phenolic concentrations vary among commercial herbal Echinacea medicines, a 2004 study designed to quantify the caffeic acid concentrations in *Echinacea angustifolia*, *E. pallida*, and *E. purpurea* showed that the roots and derivatives of *E. angustifolia*, *E. pallida*, and *E. purpurea* are a good source of natural antioxidants with the concomitant potential to impart protective benefits.[43]

Caffeic, ferulic, and tannic acids were topically applied to mice along with either phorbol-12-myristate-13-acetate (PMA) or mezerein, resulting in significant protection against DMBA-induced skin tumors in a 1998 study of dietary polyphenolic acids on the tumor-promotion stage of carcinogenesis. Caffeic acid was found to be more effective than the other compounds as a tumor-promotion inhibitor. Also in this study, superoxide anion radicals, which resulted from the *in vivo* and *in vitro* treatment of murine peritoneal macrophages with the tumor promoters were potently suppressed by all three acids.[25]

In a study by Saija et al. evaluating the capacity of caffeic and ferulic acids to permeate the stratum corneum, both acids were dissolved in saturated aqueous solutions at pH 3 or 7.2, and were found to be able to permeate through excised human skin mounted in Franz cells, with ferulic acid, which is more lipophilic, performing slightly better. Investigators then based an *in vivo* experiment on their *in vitro* model to assess the capacity of the two polyphenolic acids to alleviate UVB-induced erythema in healthy human volunteers. In this experiment, both caffeic and ferulic acids, dissolved in saturated aqueous solution pH 7.2, were found to significantly protect human skin against UVB-induced erythema. Investigators concluded that both caffeic and ferulic acids are viable as agents for the topical protection of human skin against UV-induced insult and that the pH of the formulation does not influence their skin absorption.[44]

In a 2003 study by Neradil et al., caffeic acid was demonstrated to impart protection to the skin against UVC radiation. Specifically, human KF1 diploid fibroblast and A431 epidermoid carcinoma cell lines, untreated and treated with the antioxidants caffeic acid or α-tocopherol, were exposed to UVC. A potent protective effect delivered by caffeic acid was observed at both tested concentrations; the significant increase in proliferation activity after UVC irradiation was observed in both cell cultures grown in the presence of caffeic acid. In addition, the caffeic acid was more effective than α-tocopherol in countering the cytotoxic effects of UVC. Investigators ascribed the protective effect, which was more marked in transformed cells than normal diploid ones, to the antioxidant free radical-scavenging activity of caffeic acid.[12]

In 2009, Prasad et al. investigated the photoprotective effect of caffeic acid in human blood lymphocytes exposed to UVB radiation. Pretreatment of lymphocytes with the polyphenol significantly lowered the levels of lipid peroxidation markers and UVB-induced cytotoxicity while maintaining antioxidant status. The investigators also found that the largest of three doses of caffeic acid normalized UVB-induced cellular changes.[11]

Also that year, Kang et al. conducted *in vitro* and *in vivo* experiments showing that caffeic acid blocked UVB-induced skin carcinogenesis in JB6 P+ mouse skin epidermal cells by directly suppressing Fyn (a member of the non-receptor protein tyrosine kinase family) kinase activity. Caffeic acid was also more effective than chlorogenic acid in hindering UVB-induced COX-2 expression. The researchers noted that *in vivo* results from mouse skin buttressed the notion that caffeic acid inhibited UVB-induced COX-2 expression by thwarting Fyn kinase activity. They concluded that caffeic acid appears to exhibit significant potential as a strong chemopreventive agent against cutaneous cancers.[7]

Another related compound, dihydrocaffeic acid, has also been shown to exhibit photoprotective effects such as decreasing cytotoxicity and proinflammatory cytokine production (interleukin-6 and interleukin-8) in HaCaT cells after UV exposure.[45]

Anticarcinogenic Activity

An early indication of the anticarcinogenic potential of caffeic acid was seen more than a decade ago when dietary administration of several plant phenolic antioxidants including caffeic acid was performed on F344 rats to determine the effects during the initiation phase on 4-nitroquinoline-1-oxide (4-NQO)-induced tongue carcinogenesis. Consumption of the four phenolic compounds (besides caffeic, ellagic, chlorogenic, and ferulic acids were included) over the seven-week study resulted in significant decreases by 32 weeks in the incidence of tongue neoplasms (squamous cell papilloma and carcinoma) and preneoplastic lesions (hyperplasia and dysplasia). No tongue neoplasms appeared in rats fed caffeic or ellagic acids. The researchers concluded that these phenolic compounds might be suitable for use as chemopreventive agents against cancer of the tongue as well as the skin and other tissues.[46]

In a 2013 study of malignant HaCaT cells treated with caffeic acid, Yang et al. found that the polyphenol diminished the migratory ability and cancer stem cells-like phenotype, facilitating the p38-mediated downregulation of the NF-κB/snail signal pathway.[47]

■ CONCLUSION

While data are less voluminous on caffeic acid than ferulic acid, the available research is promising regarding the potential positive effects imparted to the skin by the most prolific of the dietary hyroxycinnamic acids. That said, much more research is necessary to determine the relative potency of caffeic acid within the vast family of polyphenolic acids as well as its most effective role(s) in the dermatologic armamentarium.

REFERENCES

1. Staniforth V, Chiu LT, Yang NS. Caffeic acid suppresses UVB radiation-induced expression of interleukin-10 and activation of mitogen-activated protein kinases in mouse. *Carcinogenesis.* 2006;27:1803.
2. Hoffmann D. *Medical Herbalism: The Science and Practice of Herbal Medicine.* Rochester, VT: Healing Arts Press; 2003:94.
3. Mills S, Bone K. *Principles and Practice of Phytotherapy: Modern Herbal Medicine.* London: Churchill Livingstone; 2000:25.
4. Centini M, Rossato MS, Sega A, et al. New multifunctional surfactants from natural phenolic acids. *J Agric Food Chem.* 2012;60:74.
5. Svobodová A, Psotová J, Walterová D. Natural phenolics in the prevention of UV-induced skin damage. A review. *Biomed Pap Med Fac Univ Palacky Olomouc Czech Repub.* 2003;147:137.
6. Olthof MR, Hollman PC, Katan MB. Chlorogenic acid and caffeic acid are absorbed in humans. *J Nutr.* 2001;131:66.
7. Kang NJ, Lee KW, Shin BJ, et al. Caffeic acid, a phenolic phytochemical in coffee, directly inhibits Fyn kinase activity and UVB-induced COX-2 expression. *Carcinogenesis.* 2009;30:321.
8. Rice-Evans CA, Miller NJ, Paganga G. Structure-antioxidant activity relationships of flavonoids and phenolic acids. *Free Radic Biol Med.* 1996;20:933.
9. Lutz M, Jorquera K, Cancino B, et al. Phenolics and antioxidant capacity of table grape (Vitis vinifera L.) cultivars grown in Chile. *J Food Sci.* 2011;76:C1088.
10. Mills S, Bone K. *Principles and Practice of Phytotherapy: Modern Herbal Medicine.* London: Churchill Livingstone; 2000:434.
11. Prasad NR, Jeyanthimala K, Ramachandran S. Caffeic acid modulates ultraviolet radiation-B induced oxidative damage in human blood lymphocytes. *J Photochem Photobiol B.* 2009;95:196.
12. Neradil J, Veselská R, Slanina J. UVC-protective effect of caffeic acid on normal and transformed human skin cells in vitro. *Folia Biol (Praha).* 2003;49:197.
13. al-Sereiti MR, Abu-Amer KM, Sen P. Pharmacology of rosemary (Rosmarinus officinalis Linn.) and its therapeutic potentials. *Indian J Exp Biol.* 1999;37:124.
14. Bonina F, Puglia C, Ventura D, et al. In vitro antioxidant and in vivo photoprotective effects of a lyophilized extract of Capparis spinosa L buds. *J Cosmet Sci.* 2002;53:321.
15. Cases J, Ibarra A, Feuillère N, et al. Pilot trial of Melissa officinalis L. leaf extract in the treatment of volunteers suffering from mild-to-moderate anxiety disorders and sleep disturbances. *Med J Nutrition Metab.* 2011;4:211.
16. Ibarra A, Feuillère N, Roller M, et al. Effects of chronic administration of Melissa officinalis L. extract on anxiety-like reactivity and on circadian and exploratory activities in mice. *Phytomedicine.* 2010;17:397.
17. Kennedy DO, Little W, Scholey AB. Attenuation of laboratory-induced stress in humans after acute administration of Melissa officinalis (Lemon Balm). *Psychosom Med.* 2004;66:607.
18. Cohen RA, Kucera LS, Herrmann EC Jr. Antiviral activity of Melissa officinalis (lemon balm) extract. *Proc Soc Exp Biol Med.* 1964;117:431.
19. Oh C, Price J, Brindley MA, et al. Inhibition of HIV-1 infection by aqueous extracts of Prunella vulgaris L. *Virol J.* 2011;8:188.
20. Barnes J, Anderson LA, Gibbons S, et al. Echinacea species (Echinacea angustifolia (DC.) Hell., Echinacea pallid (Nutt.) Nutt., Echinacea purpurea (L. Monench): A review of their chemistry, pharmacology and clinical properties. *J Pharm Pharmacol.* 2005;57:929.
21. Samuelsen AB. The traditional uses, chemical constituents and biological activities of Plantago major L. A review. *J Ethnopharmacol.* 2000;71:1.
22. Ozturk G, Ginis Z, Akyol S, et al. The anticancer mechanism of caffeic acid phenethyl ester (CAPE): Review of melanomas, lung and prostate cancers. *Eur Rev Med Pharmacol Sci.* 2012;16:2064.
23. Frenkel K, Wei H, Bhimani R, et al. Inhibition of tumor promoter-mediated processes in mouse skin and bovine lens by caffeic acid phenethyl ester. *Cancer Res.* 1993;53:1255.
24. Kudugunti SK, Vad NM, Ekogbo E, et al. Efficacy of caffeic acid phenethyl ester (CAPE) in skin B16-F0 melanoma tumor bearing C57BL/6 mice. *Invest New Drugs.* 2011;29:52.
25. Kaul A, Khanduja KL. Polyphenols inhibit promotional phase of tumorigenesis: Relevance of superoxide radicals. *Nutr Cancer.* 1998;32:81.
26. Bourne LC, Rice-Evans C. Bioavailability of ferulic acid. *Biochem Biophys Res Commun.* 1998;253:222.
27. Saija A, Tomaino A, Lo Cascio R, et al. Ferulic and caffeic acids as potential protective agents against photooxidative skin damage. *J Sci Food Agric.* 1999;79:476.
28. Houghton PJ, Photiou A, Uddin S, et al. Activity of extracts of Kigelia pinnata against melanoma and renal carcinoma cell lines. *Planta Med.* 1994;60:430.
29. Muizzuddin N, Maremus KD, Maes DH. Tonality of suntan vs sunless tanning with dihydroxyacetone. *Skin Res Technol.* 2000;6:199.
30. Kwak SY, Lee S, Choi HR, et al. Dual effects of caffeoyl-amino acidyl-hydroxamic acid as an antioxidant and depigmenting agent. *Bioorg Med Chem Lett.* 2011;21:5155.
31. Žilius M, Ramanauskiené K, Briedis V. Release of propolis phenolic acids from semisolid formulations and their penetration into the human skin in vitro. *Evid Based Complement Alternat Med.* 2013;2013:958717.
32. Marti-Mestres G, Mestres JP, Bres J, et al. The "in vitro" percutaneous penetration of three antioxidant compounds. *Int J Pharm.* 2007;331:139.
33. Chiang HM, Lin TJ, Chiu CY, et al. Coffea Arabica extract and its constituents prevent photoaging by suppressing MMPs expression and MAP kinase pathway. *Food Chem Toxicol.* 2011;49:309.

34. Pluemsamran T, Onkoksoong T, Panich U. Caffeic acid and ferulic acid inhibit UVA-induced matrix metalloproteinase-1 through regulation of antioxidant defense system in keratinocyte HaCaT cells. *Photochem Photobiol*. 2012;88:961.

35. Huang MT, Smart RC, Wong CQ, et al. Inhibitory effect of curcumin, chlorogenic acid, caffeic acid, and ferulic acid on tumor promotion in mouse skin by 12-O-tetradecanoylphorbol-13-acetate. *Cancer Res*. 1988;48:5941.

36. Yamada Y, Yasui H, Sakurai H. Suppressive effect of caffeic acid and its derivatives on the generation of UVA-induced reactive oxygen species in the skin of hairless mice and pharmacokinetic analysis on organ distribution of caffeic acid in ddY mice. *Photochem Photobiol*. 2006;82:1668.

37. Song HS, Park TW, Sohn UD, et al. The effect of caffeic acid on wound healing in skin-incised mice. *Korean J Physiol Pharmacol*. 2008;12:343.

38. Khan AQ, Khan R, Qamar W, et al. Caffeic acid attenuates 12-O-tetradecanoyl-phorbol-13-acetate (TPA)-induced NF-κB and COX-2 expression in mouse skin: Abrogation of oxidative stress, inflammatory responses and proinflammatory cytokine production. *Food Chem Toxicol*. 2012;50:175.

39. Huang MT, Ma W, Yen P, et al. Inhibitory effects of caffeic acid phenethyl ester (CAPE) on 12-O-tetradecanoylphorbol-13-acetate-induced tumor promotion in mouse skin and the synthesis of DNA, RNA and protein in HeLa cells. *Carcinogenesis*. 1996;17:761.

40. Zheng ZS, Xue GZ, Grunberger D, et al. Caffeic acid phenethyl ester inhibits proliferation of human keratinocytes and interferes with the EGF regulation of ornithine decarboxylase. *Oncol Res*. 1995;7:445.

41. Serarslan G, Altug E, Kontas T, et al. Caffeic acid phenethyl ester accelerates cutaneous wound healing in a rat model and decreases oxidative stress. *Clin Exp Dermatol*. 2007;32:709.

42. Facino RM, Carini M, Aldini G, et al. Echinacoside and caffeoyl conjugates protect collagen from free radical-induced degradation: A potential use of Echinacea extracts in the prevention of skin photodamage. *Planta Med*. 1995;61:510.

43. Pellati F, Benvenuti S, Magro L, et al. Analysis of phenolic compounds and radical scavenging activity of Echinacea spp. *J Pharm Biomed Anal*. 2004;35:289.

44. Saija A, Tomaino A, Trombetta D, et al. In vitro and in vivo evaluation of caffeic and ferulic acids as topical photoprotective agents. *Int J Pharm*. 2000;199:39.

45. Poquet L, Clifford MN, Williamson G. Effect of dihydrocaffeic acid on UV irradiation of human keratinocyte HaCaT cells. *Arch Biochem Biophys*. 2008;476:196.

46. Tanaka I, Kojima T, Kawamori T, et al. Inhibition of 4-nitroquinoline-1-oxide-induced rat tongue carcinogenesis by the naturally occurring plant phenolics caffeic, ellagic, chlorogenic and ferulic acids. *Carcinogenesis*. 1993;14:1321.

47. Yang Y, Li Y, Wang K, et al. P38/NF-κB/snail pathway is involved in caffeic acid-induced inhibition of cancer stem cells-like properties and migratory capacity in malignant human keratinocyte. *PLoS One*. 2013;8:e58915.

CHAPTER 54

Ferulic Acid

Activities:

Antioxidant, anticancer, anti-inflammatory,[1] antimicrobial,[2] cardioprotective, neuroprotective, hepatoprotective, photoprotective, skin lightening[3]

Important Chemical Components:

Also known as 4-hydroxy-3-methoxycinnamic acid as well as 3-(4-hydroxy-3-methoxyphenyl)-2-propenoic acid, its molecular formula is $C_{10}H_{10}O_4$.

Origin Classification:

Natural ingredient; organic forms are possible. It can also be chemically synthesized in the laboratory

Personal Care Category:

Antioxidant, antiaging, photoprotection

Recommended for the following Baumann Skin Types:

DRNW, DRPT, DRPW, DSNW, DSPT, DSPW, ORNW, ORPT, ORPW, OSNW, OSPT, and OSPW

SOURCE

Ferulic acid (4-hydroxy-3-methoxycinnamic acid) is pervasive in the plant world, present as it is in the cell walls of numerous plants, including grains, fruit, and vegetables where it is conjugated with mono-, di-, and polysaccharides and other compounds (Table 54-1).[4–7] Derived from the metabolism of phenylalanine and tyrosine,[5,8] ferulic acid is known to be prevalent in whole grains (e.g., rice, wheat, barley, oats, and sorghum), spinach, parsley, grapes, olives, rhubarb, tomatoes, asparagus, peas, artichokes, eggplant, pineapples, berries, and maize bran.[1,5,8,9] Ferulic acid is also a key component in propolis, a product of honeybee hives (see Chapter 60, Honey/Propolis/Royal Jelly).[10] In addition, it is found along with several other polyphenols in hops used in beer.[11,12] Ferulic acid is also one of the main active components in several herbs used in traditional Chinese medicine (TCM), including *Angelica sinensis*, which is used to treat various skin traumas in TCM.[1,6,13]

TABLE 54-1
Pros and Cons of Ferulic Acid

Pros	Cons
Natural ingredient	Breaks down with heat and light exposure[22]
Penetrates the stratum corneum	Difficult to formulate
Abundance of *in vitro* data	May interact with other products in a regimen
Potent antioxidant	
No reports of contact dermatitis	
Safe	
Enhances stability of vitamins C and E	

HISTORY

Ferulic acid was first isolated and identified by Hlasiwetz and Barth in Innsbruck, Austria in 1866.[8] Other than an 1891 report on the isolation of the compound from *Pinus laricio* (Corsican pine), little research on ferulic acid was published until 1925, when it was chemically synthesized from vanillin with malonic acid.[8,14] The stereochemistry of ferulic acid was determined in 1976 by nuclear magnetic resonance spectroscopy and confirmed in 1988 by X-ray crystallographic analysis.[8] Investigations, particularly *in vitro*, regarding the potential health benefits of ferulic acid have since become commonplace.

In a 1983 study on the inhibitory effects of three phenolic compounds on neoplasia in mice, ferulic acid was active against lung carcinogenesis but completely ineffective against skin tumor formation.[15] Since that time, however, much evidence has emerged regarding the oral and topical benefits of ferulic acid against skin cancer. The inhibitory effects of the topical application and oral administration of *Ixora javanica* flower extract on the growth and onset of tumors in mice was attributed, in a 1991 study, to the active compounds in the extract, namely ferulic acid.[16] In addition to its reported cutaneous benefits, ferulic acid has drawn interest for potential salutary effects in treating cardiovascular disease, diabetes, neurodegenerative conditions, and various cancers.[1,17]

CHEMISTRY

Ferulic acid, a precursor to vanillin, belongs to the family of polyphenolic compounds known as hydroxycinnamic acids, which are known to confer cutaneous benefits (Figure 54-1).[6,11,18] Other hydroxycinnamic acids include caffeic and sinapic acids, as well as the ferulic acid precursors *p*-coumaric and *p*-hydroxycinnamic acids. Hydroxycinnamic acids are produced in plants from phenylalanine or L-tyrosine through the shikimate pathway (Figure 54-2).[5]

Ferulic acid is a potent antioxidant and a strong ultraviolet (UV) absorber,[4,19] effectively protecting human skin from UVB-induced erythema in particular.[4] Phospholipid membranes are also protected by ferulic acid from UV-induced peroxidation as the lipid peroxidative chain reaction is interrupted.[4,20] The phenolic nucleus and extended side chain conjugation of ferulic acid accounts for its facility in forming a resonance-stabilized phenoxy radical, to which its antioxidant activity is attributed.[8]

ORAL USES

Ferulic acid is consumed regularly through the diet as a key constituent of numerous vegetables, fruits, and grains. While it is difficult to quantify the direct contributions of ferulic acid, it is likely that the frequent intake of such foods imparts multiple cutaneous benefits. Indeed, dietary ferulic acid is now considered a significant antioxidant substance.[21]

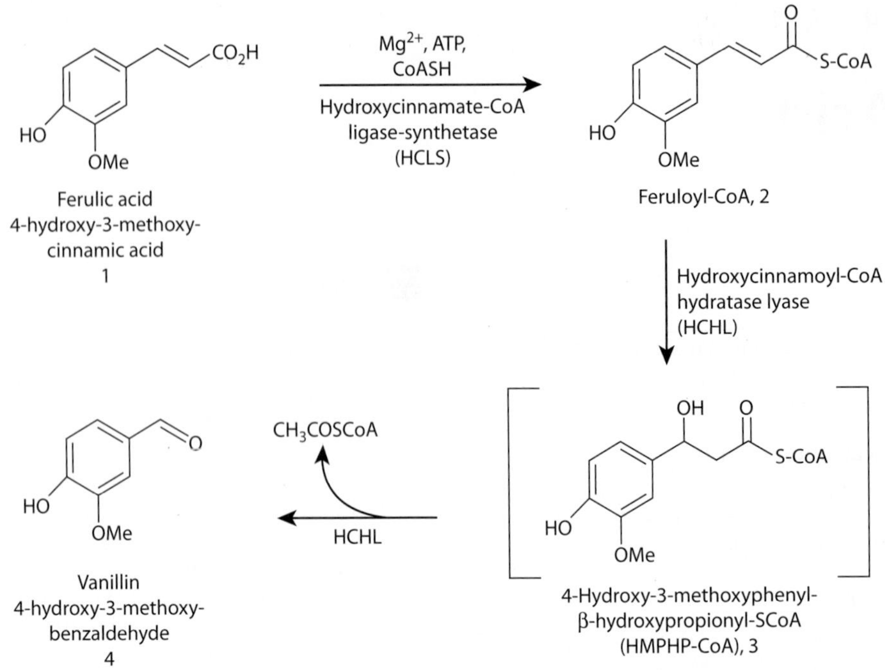

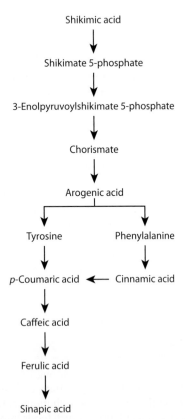

▲ **FIGURE 54-1** Ferulic acid is converted to vanillin.[42]

TOPICAL USES

Ferulic acid is known to provide photoprotection to skin when it is incorporated into cosmetic lotions,[8] and has been approved as a sunscreen agent in Japan.[22] Multiple studies have shown the utility in combining ferulic acid with vitamins C and E to enhance the antioxidant capacity and stability of the formulation.

Shikimic acid
↓
Shikimate 5-phosphate
↓
3-Enolpyruvoylshikimate 5-phosphate
↓
Chorismate
↓
Arogenic acid
↓   ↓
Tyrosine   Phenylalanine
↓   ↓
p-Coumaric acid ← Cinnamic acid
↓
Caffeic acid
↓
Ferulic acid
↓
Sinapic acid

▲ **FIGURE 54-2** Ferulic acid is formed from tyrosine or phenylalanine.

In a 2005 study by Lin et al., the addition of 0.5 percent ferulic acid to a solution of 15 percent L-ascorbic acid (vitamin C) and 1 percent α-tocopherol (vitamin E) stabilized the formulation (C E Ferulic®) and, more significantly, enhanced the skin-protective capacity of the topically-applied formulation, doubling photoprotection to skin from fourfold to eightfold.[23] The researchers found that the addition of ferulic acid imparted a synergistic effect, greatly amplifying the already synergistic effects seen in the combination of vitamins C and E, further supporting previous evidence of cooperative relationships between ferulic acid and vitamins C and E, and β-carotene.[24] Lin et al. speculated that a topical antioxidant formulation combining vitamins C and E with ferulic acid in a broad-spectrum sunscreen would be an optimal way to protect the skin from sun damage via a topically-applied product.[23]

In a subsequent study by several of the same authors, comparison of the same formulation with vitamins C and E as well as ferulic acid with a 1 percent ubiquinone, 1 percent idebenone, and 0.5 percent kinetin preparation and three different commercial creams (0.1 percent kinetin, 1 percent idebenone, and 0.5 percent idebenone) revealed that the ferulic acid-containing topical antioxidant combination was more effective at photoprotection. Results also supported the finding of eightfold photoprotection from UV conferred to the skin.[25]

Ferulic acid has also been included in a topical antioxidant formulation with vitamin C and phloretin (see Chapter 52, Phloretin). In this small study with 10 subjects, the antioxidant combination protected against all of the various harmful effects measured due to UV exposure.[26]

SAFETY ISSUES

Ferulic acid is readily absorbed and metabolized in the body.[6] It has a low toxicity with a median lethal dose (LD_{50}) of 2,445 mg/kg body weight in male and 2,113 mg/kg body weight in female rats. Because of this low toxicity it is considered safe. Ferulic acid is frequently used as a food additive and found in natural extracts of herbs, coffee, vanilla beans, and spices. It is added to foods as a Food and Drug Administration-approved antioxidant concoction.[6] There are no reports of contact dermatitis to ferulic acid in the literature.

ENVIRONMENTAL IMPACT

Ferulic acid is found throughout the plant kingdom. Few if any of the plants are cultivated to harness ferulic acid alone; therefore, there is no known impact on the environment of using this ingredient.

FORMULATION CONSIDERATIONS

Ferulic acid appears most effective for topical administration when combined with other active ingredients, particularly vitamin C because ferulic acid works synergistically with other antioxidants, stabilizing and, in turn, being stabilized in the interaction. In 2008, Anselmi et al. demonstrated that encapsulating ferulic acid with α-cyclodextrin enhanced the chemical stability of the antioxidant when exposed to UVB while increasing the bioavailability of ferulic acid on the skin.[22] The efficacy of ferulic acid is diminished by its tendency toward thermal-, air-, and photo-induced decomposition through what is thought to be a decarboxylation mechanism.[2]

In a 2011 study of the chemical stability of ferulic acid, Wang et al. evaluated the antioxidant in eight prototypical formulations, finding that the stability of the acid is related to pH and temperature. In addition, they noted that the solvent dipropylene glycol exhibited a stabilizing effect on ferulic acid.[3] The pH effects differed from the report by Saija et al., who had previously found that the efficacy of ferulic acid appears to be unaffected by the pH of the formulation in which it may be included.[19] In an attempt to improve absorption of ferulic acid, new delivery systems, such as liposomes, nanoparticles, and niosomes, have been developed.[1]

A ferulic acid-containing biodegradable polymer was prepared in 2013 through solution polymerization to chemically integrate the antioxidant into a poly(anhydride-ester). Ouimet et al. reported that *in vitro* analysis revealed that the polymer was hydrolytically degradable, allowing for the potential of controlled release of the bioactive constituents in skin care formulations. Also, polymer degradation products displayed antioxidant and antibacterial activity similar to free ferulic acid, and *in vitro* cell viability analysis showed no cytotoxicity to fibroblasts.[2]

USAGE CONSIDERATIONS

Because of the conflicting reports of the effects of pH on the stability of ferulic acid, it is possible that application at the same time or immediately after a low pH product such as glycolic acid could decrease the efficacy of the product. Studies looking at the combination of ferulic acid-containing formulations with other products in a regimen that alter pH should be conducted.

SIGNIFICANT BACKGROUND

In a 2010 study with *in vitro* and *in vivo* components, Zhang et al. assessed the efficacy and safety of the cutaneous delivery of ferulic acid and its derivatives (five total compounds) into porcine skin. The *in vitro* efficacy study revealed that ferulic acid ethyl ether (FAEE) with a pH 6 buffer achieved the greatest skin

delivery. FAEE, which occurs naturally and is more hydrophobic than ferulic acid,[27] divided readily into and penetrated across the skin via intercellular pathways. The investigators used a nude mouse model to determine the level of permeants remaining in the skin, with FAEE deposition comparable with that of coniferyl aldehyde. The safety assessment, based on transepidermal water loss, erythema, and cutaneous pH, showed no irritation after 24 hours. The investigators concluded that the topical administration of ferulic acid and its derivatives is a potentially safe and effective approach to thwart photodamage.[17]

In Vitro Studies

The vitamin E/ferulic acid compound α-tocopheryl ferulate is known to have the capacity to absorb UV radiation, thereby maintaining tocopherol in a stable state. As such, researchers investigated whether α-tocopheryl ferulate can act as a depigmenting agent and antioxidant to improve and prevent UV-induced facial hyperpigmentation. Studying the effects of α-tocopheryl ferulate using cultured human melanoma cells and normal human melanocytes *in vitro*, α-tocopheryl ferulate was found to inhibit melanization significantly better than arbutin, kojic acid, ascorbic acid, and tranexamic acid, suggesting potential as a whitening agent by, as investigators hypothesized, indirectly inhibiting tyrosine hydroxylase activity.[28] In related studies, most of the same researchers determined that α-tocopheryl ferulate inhibits the biological responses prompted by reactive oxygen species,[29] and may mitigate the damage induced by active oxygen species, thus helping to suppress or decelerate skin carcinogenesis.[28]

In a 2002 *in vitro* study by Ogiwara et al. of the free radical-scavenging abilities of ferulic acid and eugenol, ferulic acid more efficiently scavenged nitric oxide and the hydroxyl radical and was comparable to eugenol in scavenging the superoxide radical. The investigators concluded that ferulic acid exhibited the potential to be an effective antioxidant in living systems in preventing cell damage caused by free radicals such as superoxide, and especially the hydroxyl radical and nitric oxide.[30]

In 2008, Calabrese et al. showed that 25 μmol/L ferulic acid ethyl ester abrogated protein and lipid oxidation induced in human dermal fibroblasts by exposure to up 1,000 μmol/L of H_2O_2, and mitigated the loss in cell viability spurred by 500 μmol/L of H_2O_2. In addition, the nutritional antioxidant led to an increase in heme oxygenase-1 and heat shock protein-70 in the fibroblasts compared with fibroblasts treated only with H_2O_2. The investigators concluded that their findings support the protective roles of ferulic acid, and its derivatives, as well as vitagenes such as heme oxygenase-1 and heat shock protein-70 against free radical-induced skin damage.[27] In addition, the ethyl ester derivative of ferulic acid has been shown to protect skin melanocytes from UV-induced oxidative stress, lowering reactive oxygen species generation and significantly inhibiting apoptosis and other biomarkers of oxidation.[31]

In 2012, Pluemsamran et al. pretreated immortalized human keratinocyte (HaCaT) cells with caffeic acid or ferulic acid to assess the inhibitory effects of the antioxidants on UVA-induced cytotoxicity, MMP-1 activity, and mRNA level. They found that both antioxidants suppressed cytotoxicity, MMP-1 activity induction, and mRNA and oxidant formation. In addition, both hydroxycinnamic acids upregulated glutathione content, γ-glutamate cysteine ligase mRNA, and the activities as well as mRNA expression of catalase and glutathione peroxidase in UVA-exposed cells.[32]

Animal Studies

More than 20 years ago, the topical application of ferulic acid was found to inhibit by 46 percent the induction of ornithine decarboxylase activity by 12-*O*-tetradecanoylphorbol-13-acetate (TPA) in female CD-1 mice. Similar treatment of mice with ferulic acid together with TPA also dose-dependently inhibited the number of TPA-induced tumors per mouse.[33] In a 1994 study, the topical application of a dehydrogenation polymer of ferulic acid suppressed TPA-induced tumor promotion, though a monomeric ferulic acid failed to exhibit the same inhibitory effect in female ICR mice.[34]

Phenolic antioxidants including ferulic acid fed to male F344 rats were found to significantly lower the incidence of tongue neoplasms (squamous cell papilloma and carcinoma) and preneoplastic lesions (hyperplasia and dysplasia) and show promise as chemopreventive agents in tongue, skin, and other organs, researchers concluded.[35] In a study evaluating the potential of dietary polyphenols as anticarcinogenic agents, ellagic acid, tannic acid, caffeic acid, and ferulic acid were each combined with phorbol-12-myristate-13-acetate (PMA) or mezerein and topically applied to mice and showed significant protection against benzo[a]pyrene- and 7,12-dimethylbenz[a]anthracene (DMBA)-induced skin tumors in both *in vivo* and *in vitro* conditions.[36]

In 2009, Alias et al. assessed the effects of topically applied as well as orally administered ferulic acid on squamous cell carinoma induced by painting DMBA on the shaved backs of Swiss albino mice. DMBA was administered twice weekly for eight weeks to engender tumor formation. Whereas the oral administration of ferulic acid resulted in complete prevention of skin tumor formation, the topical application of the antioxidant exerted no significant chemopreventive effects. The investigators speculated that orally administered ferulic acid yielded such results through its modulatory impact in reversing lipid peroxidation byproducts and antioxidants to approximately the normal range in DMBA-treated mice.[37]

In 2012, Staniforth et al. investigated the inhibitory effects of ferulic acid on UVB-induced matrix metalloproteinase (MMP)-2 and MMP-9 activities in mouse skin, finding through histological analysis that the antioxidant diminished collagen degradation, abnormal elastic fiber accumulation, and epidermal hyperplasia. The researchers concluded that their findings pointed to a potential clinical application for ferulic acid for treating cutaneous conditions resulting from MMP-2 and MMP-9 overexpression.[38]

In an interesting 2013 comparison study using mice, Burns et al. exposed mice to UVB for 10 weeks to create skin damage. Before the appearance of cutaneous lesions, the investigators treated the animals for 15 weeks with a stable topical formula containing vitamins C and E and ferulic acid (C E Ferulic®) without additional UVB exposure. Tumor number and burden were reduced and the antioxidant combination prevented the formation of malignant skin tumors in female mice with UVB-induced damage. Female mice also chronically exposed to UVB but treated only with topical vitamin E, however, displayed increased tumor growth, cutaneous proliferation, angiogenesis, and overall DNA damage.[39]

Human Studies

Based on *in vitro* results testing the capacity of ferulic and caffeic acids to permeate through excised human skin, researchers evaluated the capacity of the same organic acids to reduce UVB-induced erythema in healthy human volunteers.

Dissolved in saturated aqueous solution (pH 7.2), both compounds conferred significant cutaneous protection. Both ferulic acid, which is more lipophilic and thus better able to penetrate the stratum corneum, and caffeic acid were assessed as worthy photoprotective agents in topical formulations and judged to be unaffected by the pH of the product into which they might be incorporated.[19]

In 2008, Murray et al. showed in a small study that a stable topical formulation of 15 percent L-ascorbic acid, 1 percent α-tocopherol, and 0.5 percent ferulic acid (CEFer) protected human skin *in vivo* from substantial solar-simulated UV radiation (SSUVR), especially lowering thymine dimer mutations, which are known to be linked to skin cancer.[40]

In 2013, Wu et al. conducted a small study with 12 healthy Chinese females to ascertain the potential photoprotective effects of a formulation containing vitamins C and E and ferulic acid against SSUVR-induced acute photodamage in human skin.[41] For four consecutive days, dorsal skin areas were treated with the topical antioxidant preparation or vehicle. On day 4, these areas along with an untreated site (positive control) were exposed to SSUVR five times the minimal erythema dose. A negative control site received neither treatment nor exposure. Using digital photographs, pre- and postexposure skin color measurements, and skin biopsies, the researchers determined that the antioxidant formulation imparted significant protection against SSUVR-induced photodamage and concluded that the topical complex has potential in the dermatologic armamentarium as a photoprotective agent.

CONCLUSION

Significant antioxidant, photoprotective, and anticarcinogenic properties have been associated with ferulic acid, with a substantial body of *in vitro* evidence. The cutaneous benefits long associated with this phenolic compound also continue to be borne out by emerging research. Ferulic acid has already been introduced into several photoprotective dermatologic products. Although good data exist to support the use of ferulic acid as a topical antioxidant, it is unstable when exposed to heat and light. Studies looking at the effects on stability of pH and combination with other ingredients in the regimen would be helpful.

REFERENCES

1. Barone E, Calabrese V, Mancuso C. Ferulic acid and its therapeutic potential as a hormetin for age-related diseases. *Biogerontology.* 2009;10:97.
2. Ouimet MA, Griffin J, Carbone-Howell AL, et al. Biodegradable ferulic acid-containing poly(anhydride-ester): degradation products with controlled release and sustained antioxidant activity. *Biomacromolecules.* 2013;14:854.
3. Wang QJ, Gao X, Gong H, et al. Chemical stability and degradation mechanisms of ferulic acid (F.A) within various cosmetic formulations. *J Cosmet Sci.* 2011;62:483.
4. Svobodová A, Psotová J, Walterová D. Natural phenolics in the prevention of UV-induced skin damage. A review. *Biomed Pap Med Fac Univ Palacky Olomouc Czech Repub.* 2003;147:137.
5. Bourne LC, Rice-Evans C. Bioavailability of ferulic acid. *Biochem Biophys Res Commun.* 1998;253:222.
6. Ou S, Kwok KC. Ferulic acid: pharmaceutical functions, preparations and applications in foods. *J Sci Food Agric.* 2004;84:1261.
7. Rice-Evans CA, Miller NJ, Paganga G. Structure-antioxidant activity relationships of flavonoids and phenolic acids. *Free Radic Biol Med.* 1996;20:933.
8. Graf E. Antioxidant potential of ferulic acid. *Free Radic Biol Med.* 1992;13:435.

9. Centini M, Rossato MS, Sega A, et al. New multifunctional surfactants from natural phenolic acids. *J Agric Food Chem.* 2012;60:74.

10. Žiliusx M, Ramanauskienex K, Briedisx V. Release of propolis phenolic acids from semisolid formulations and their penetration into the human skin in vitro. *Evid Based Complement Alternat Med.* 2013;2013:958717.

11. Chen W, Becker T, Qian F, et al. Beer and beer compounds: physiological effects on skin health. *J Eur Acad Dermatol Venereol.* 2013 Jun 27. [Epub ahead of print]

12. Arranz S, Chiva-Blanch G, Valderas-Martinez P, et al. Wine, beer, alcohol and polyphenols on cardiovascular disease and cancer. *Nutrients.* 2012;4:759.

13. Hsiao CY, Hung CY, Tsai TH, et al. A study of the wound healing mechanism of a traditional Chinese medicine, Angelica sinensis, using a proteomic approach. *Evid Based Complement Alternat Med.* 2012;2012:467531.

14. Dutt S. General synthesis of α-unsaturated acids from malonic acid. *Quart J Chem Soc.* 1925;1:297.

15. Lesca P. Protective effects of ellagic acid and other plant phenols on benzo[a]pyrene-induced neoplasia in mice. *Carcinogenesis.* 1983;4:1651.

16. Nair SC, Panikkar B, Akamanchi KG, et al. Inhibitory effects of Ixora javanica extract on skin chemical carcinogenesis in mice and its antitumor activity. *Cancer Lett.* 1991;60:253.

17. Zhang LW, Al-Suwayeh SA, Hsieh PW, et al. A comparison of skin delivery of ferulic acid and its derivatives: evaluation of their efficacy and safety. *Int J Pharm.* 2010;399:44.

18. Bonina F, Puglia C, Ventura D, et al. In vitro antioxidant and in vivo photoprotective effects of a lyophilized extract of Capparis spinosa L buds. *J Cosmet Sci.* 2002;53:321.

19. Saija A, Tomaino A, Trombetta D, et al. In vitro and in vivo evaluation of caffeic and ferulic acids as topical photoprotective agents. *Int J Pharm.* 2000;199:39.

20. Saija A, Tomaino A, Lo Cascio R, et al. Ferulic and caffeic acids as potential protective agents against photooxidative skin damage. *J Sci Food Agric.* 1999;79:476.

21. Wang X, Geng X, Egashira Y, et al. Purification and characterization of a feruloyl esterase from the intestinal bacterium Lactobacillus acidophilus. *Appl Environ Microbiol.* 2004;70:2367.

22. Anselmi C, Centini M, Maggiore M, et al. Non-covalent inclusion of ferulic acid with alpha-cyclodextrin improves photo-stability and delivery: NMR and modeling studies. *J Pharm Biomed Anal.* 2008;46:645.

23. Lin FH, Lin JY, Gupta RD, et al. Ferulic acid stabilizes a solution of vitamins C and E and doubles its photoprotection of skin. *J Invest Dermatol.* 2005;125:826.

24. Trombino S, Serini S, Di Nicuolo F, et al. Antioxidant effect of ferulic acid in isolated membranes and intact cells: synergistic interactions with alpha-tocopherol, beta-carotene, and ascorbic acid. *J Agric Food Chem.* 2004;52:2411.

25. Tournas JA, Lin FH, Burch JA, et al. Ubiquinone, idebenone, and kinetin provide ineffective photoprotection to skin when compared to a topical antioxidant combination of vitamins C and E with ferulic acid. *J Invest Dermatol.* 2006;126:1185.

26. Oresajo C, Stephens T, Hino PD, et al. Protective effects of a topical antioxidant mixture containing vitamin C, ferulic acid, and phloretin against ultraviolet-induced photodamage in human skin. *J Cosmet Dermatol.* 2008;7:290.

27. Calabrese V, Calafato S, Puleo E, et al. Redox regulation of cellular stress response by ferulic acid ethyl ester in human dermal fibroblasts: role of vitagenes. *Clin Dermatol.* 2008;26:358.

28. Ichihashi M, Funasaka Y, Ohashi A, et al. The inhibitory effect of DL-alpha-tocopheryl ferulate in lecithin on melanogenesis. *Anticancer Res.* 1999;19:3769.

29. Funasaka Y, Chakraborty AK, Komoto M, et al. The depigmenting effect of alpha-tocopheryl ferulate on human melanoma cells. *Br J Dermatol.* 1999;141:20.

30. Ogiwara T, Satoh K, Kadoma Y, et al. Radical scavenging activity and cytotoxicity of ferulic acid. *Anticancer Res.* 2002;22:2711.

31. Di Domenico F, Perluigi M, Foppoli C, et al. Protective effect of ferulic acid ethyl ester against oxidative stress mediated by UVB irradiation in human epidermal melanocytes. *Free Radic Res.* 2009;43:365.

32. Pluemsamran T, Onkoksoong T, Panich U. Caffeic acid and ferulic acid inhibit UVA-induced matrix metalloproteinase-1 through regulation of antioxidant defense system in keratinocyte HaCaT cells. *Photochem Photobiol.* 2012;88:961.

33. Huang MT, Smart RC, Wong CQ, et al. Inhibitory effect of curcumin, chlorogenic acid, caffeic acid, and ferulic acid on tumor promotion in mouse skin by 12-O-tetradecanoylphorbol-13-acetate. *Cancer Res.* 1988;48:5941.

34. Asanoma M, Takahashi K, Miyabe M, et al. Inhibitory effect of topical application of polymerized ferulic acid, a synthetic lignin, on tumor promotion in mouse skin two-stage tumorigenesis. *Carcinogenesis.* 1994;15:2069.

35. Tanaka T, Kojima T, Kawamori T, et al. Inhibition of 4-nitroquinoline-1-oxide-induced rat tongue carcinogenesis by the naturally occurring plant phenolics caffeic, ellagic, chlorogenic and ferulic acids. *Carcinogenesis.* 1993;14:1321.

36. Kaul A, Khanduja KL. Polyphenols inhibit promotional phase of tumorigenesis: relevance of superoxide radicals. *Nutr Cancer.* 1998;32:81.

37. Alias LM, Manoharan S, Vellaichamy L, et al. Protective effect of ferulic acid on 7,12-dimethylbenz[a]anthracene-induced skin carcinogenesis in Swiss albino mice. *Exp Toxicol Pathol.* 2009;61:205.

38. Staniforth V, Huang WC, Aravindaram K, et al. Ferulic acid, a phenolic phytochemical, inhibits UVB-induced matrix metalloproteinases in mouse skin via posttranslational mechanisms. *J Nutr Biochem.* 2012;23:443.

39. Burns EM, Tober KL, Riggenbach JA, et al. Differential effects of topical vitamin E and C E Ferulic® treatments on ultraviolet light B-induced cutaneous tumor development in Skh-1 mice. *PLoS One.* 2013;8:e63809.

40. Murray JC, Burch JA, Streilein RD, et al. A topical antioxidant solution containing vitamins C and E stabilized by ferulic acid provides protection for human skin against damage caused by ultraviolet irradiation. *J Am Acad Dermatol.* 2008;59:418.

41. Wu Y, Zheng X, Xu XG, et al. Protective effects of a topical antioxidant complex containing vitamins C and E and ferulic acid against ultraviolet irradiation-induced photodamage in Chinese women. *J Drugs Dermatol.* 2013;12:464.

42. Bennett JP, Bertin L, Moulton B, et al. A ternary complex of hydroxycinnamoyl-Co-A hydratase-lyase (HCHL) with acetyl-CoA and vanillin gives insights into substrate specificity and mechanism. *Biochem J.* 2008;414:281.

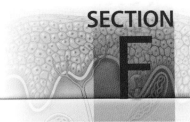

SECTION E
Vitamins

CHAPTER 55

Ascorbic Acid (Vitamin C)

Activities:

Antioxidant, anti-inflammatory, photoprotectant, depigmenting, collagen synthesis promotion, wound healing

Important Chemical Components:

Esterified forms of L-ascorbic acid, such as ascorbyl palmitate (ascorbic-6-palmitate) and magnesium ascorbyl phosphate. Its molecular formula is $C_6H_8O_6$.

Origin Classification:

Most topical formulations contain synthetic laboratory-made ascorbic acid because of the inherent obstacles in properly formulating this ingredient. Ascorbic acid is naturally occurring and organic forms are available, but their efficacy is doubtful due to instability and difficulty penetrating into the skin.

Personal Care Category:

Antioxidant, antiaging

Recommended for the following Baumann Skin Types:

DRNW, DRPT, DRPW, ORNW, ORPT, and ORPW

SOURCE

Ascorbic acid (vitamin C) is found in citrus fruits and green leafy vegetables. It is produced in most plants and animals, but a mutated gene in humans has resulted in a deficiency of L-gulono-γ-lactone oxidase, the enzyme required for its production.[1,2] Although ascorbic acid cannot be synthesized by the human body, dietary consumption renders it the most abundant antioxidant in human skin and blood, and vitamin C plays an important role in endogenous collagen production and the inhibition of collagen degradation (Table 55-1).[2–6] This essential nutrient is also a cofactor necessary for the function of numerous hydroxylases and mono-oxygenases,[7] and plays an important role in the glycosaminoglycan synthesis of proteoglycan.[5,8,9] In addition, ascorbic acid is known to regenerate α-tocopherol (vitamin E) levels and is therefore thought to protect against diseases related to oxidative stress.[10] Epidermal vitamin C can be depleted by sunlight and environmental pollution, such as ozone in urban pollution.[11,12] This

TABLE 55-1
Pros and Cons of Ascorbic Acid

PROS	CONS
Potent anti-inflammatory and antioxidant activity	Difficult to formulate
Used in a wide variety of cosmetic formulations	Topical forms are expensive
Strong safety profile	Does not readily penetrate the skin
Readily found in diet	Can increase redness in S_2 rosacea types
Most abundant antioxidant in human skin	Can cause stinging in S_3 stinging types
Increases collagen production	
Aids wound healing	
Exerts a depigmenting effect	

chapter will discuss the antiaging and antioxidant activity of vitamin C [see Chapter 40, Vitamin C (Ascorbic Acid), for information on the depigmenting activities of ascorbic acid].

HISTORY

The discovery of ascorbic acid is inextricably linked to scurvy, a disease known for several hundred years now to result from protracted vitamin C deficiency. In fact, "ascorbic" literally means "against scurvy."[13] Scurvy (derived from the Latin *scorbutus*, French *scorbut*, and German *skorbut*) was rampant among the world's navies and is believed to have afflicted as many as two million sailors by the mid-1700s.[14] The condition was actually described in writings by the ancient Egyptians, Greeks, and Romans.[5,15] Eating onions and vegetables was recommended as treatment in Egypt three millennia ago, but the first formal description of the condition is attributed to the Greek physician Hippocrates.[5,15] Several hundred years later, scurvy emerged in great numbers on the high seas as noted by the voyages of Portuguese explorer Vasco da Gama in 1498.[5,15] By 1747, as shown by James Lind,[14] sailors knew that consuming citrus fruits, oranges and lemons in particular, prevented this condition characterized by dental abnormalities, bleeding, distinctive purpuric skin lesions, and mental deterioration. Several cases of scurvy also reportedly occurred during Ireland's "great potato famine" in 1845.[14]

In 1928, Albert Szent-Györgyi isolated an organic acid from oranges, lemons, cabbage, and adrenal gland tissue from guinea pigs (which, like humans, require dietary vitamin C),[14] later dubbing it "hexuronic acid."[13,14] Researchers confirmed during the 1930s that the key constituent in citrus fruit that prevents scurvy was indeed hexuronic acid, with Walter Norman Haworth identifying its chemical structure in 1933.[14] Haworth and Szent-Györgyi ultimately decided on the name "ascorbic acid" for the compound, though it is now better known as vitamin C.[13]

In the late 1980s, Dr. Sheldon Pinnell from Duke University began looking at vitamin C as a photoprotectant. In 1987, he published a paper in the *Archives of Dermatology* demonstrating that collagen synthesis could be induced by ascorbic acid.[16] He filed a patent in 1989 on a way to stabilize vitamin C in a topical formulation that later became the basis for the company Skinceuticals. His diligence and adherence to evidence-based science made a great impact and now vitamin C is one of the ingredients most recognized by consumers in the antiaging skin care market.

Today, the role of vitamin C as a potent antioxidant is the subject of intense research. Oral vitamin C has been linked to reports of risk reduction of developing certain cancers, cardiovascular disease, and cataracts, as well as improvements in wound healing and immune modulation.[17,18] As a topical agent, vitamin C has been used to harness its antioxidant activity to prevent photodamage, and to treat melasma, striae albae, and postoperative erythema in laser patients.[19–21]

CHEMISTRY

Ascorbic acid, or ascorbate, is an α-ketolactone that functions as a hydrophilic monovalent hydroxyl anion. The active portion of ascorbic acid includes a carbon double bond with two hydroxyl groups attached. This structure, called an enediol, donates two electrons, which can bond with the unpaired electrons of a free radical.[22] Ascorbate and glutathione are among the antioxidants found in hydrophobic areas of the cell and the serum. The addition of one electron to ascorbate results in the ascorbate free radical, a transient compound more stable than other free radicals and capable of accepting other electrons. This renders it an effective free radical scavenger, and therefore a significant antioxidant. If the transient form cannot accept an electron, it will surrender its unpaired electron to an enzymatic reaction, thereby becoming an electron donor. Vitamin C is known as an effective scavenger of superoxide and hydroxyl radicals, in particular, as well as singlet oxygen, and has been shown *in vitro* to protect plasma lipids and low-density lipoproteins against peroxidative damage.[5]

The addition of two electrons to ascorbic acid results in the formation of dehydro-L-ascorbic acid (DHAA). Under physiological conditions, vitamin C exists primarily in its reduced form, ascorbic acid; in trace quantities, it is also present in the oxidized form of DHAA. This substance can be converted back into ascorbate, but if the lactone ring irreversibly opens, yielding diketogulonic acid, the compound is rendered inactive. When vitamin C formulations are oxidized, diketogulonic acid is often one of the results. Such solutions are ineffective and useless in terms of delivering any vitamin C benefits.[23,24]

Essentially, when vitamin C preparations are exposed to ultraviolet (UV) radiation or air, the molecule rapidly adds two electrons and transforms into DHAA, which contains an aromatic ring. With additional oxidation, the ring irreversibly opens and the vitamin C solution is left permanently inactive. For this reason, vitamin C formulations are best preserved in opaque airless containers with no exposure to light or air during storage, use, and application.

Ascorbyl palmitate is a fat-soluble ester of vitamin C with increased stability. It is effective at a neutral pH and its lipid solubility greatly enhances penetration versus polar L-ascorbic acid.

Hydrolysis of ascorbyl palmitate yields L-ascorbic acid and palmitic acid in the skin; however, ascorbyl palmitate is also effective as an intact molecule,[22] and has been shown to decrease inflammation and deliver beneficial effects to patients with dermatologic conditions including psoriasis and eczema.[25]

ORAL USES

A small study in 2002 compared the skin of eight untreated volunteers to the skin of 12 volunteers who were treated with oral vitamin C supplements (500 mg/day) for eight weeks. Those given oral vitamin C showed significant rises in plasma and cutaneous vitamin C content.[26] This study demonstrated that ingested vitamin C will increase ascorbic acid levels in the skin. However, when the ascorbic acid-treated subjects were given a broadband UVB (peak 310 nm, range 270–400 nm) challenge of 120 mJ/cm^2, there was no difference in UVB-induced erythemal response between the two groups. Surprisingly, reduction in the skin content of total glutathione was seen in the vitamin C-treated group versus the untreated group.

A much more recent study measured skin radical-scavenging activity with electron paramagnetic resonance spectroscopy and showed that after four weeks of orally ingested vitamin C, 100 mg vitamin C/day and 180 mg vitamin C/day resulted in a significant increase in the radical-scavenging activity by 22 percent and 37 percent, respectively.[27] Oral doses of ascorbyl palmitate have been shown to exhibit nearly 10-fold the absorption of oral L-ascorbic acid.[28] Similarly, oral supplementation with a 5 percent pelleted form of ascorbyl palmitate was shown to have an 80 percent inhibition on 12-*O*-tetradecanoylphorbol-13-acetate (TPA)-induced tumors in a mouse model versus no improvement following a 27 g/L *ad libitum* concentration of L-ascorbic acid in drinking water.[29] At this time the belief is that oral supplements of vitamin C do help increase the skin's antioxidant capacity but food sources of vitamin C are preferred when possible.

Vitamin C has also been shown in combination to exert a significant antioxidant effect from oral administration. In 2007, Cho et al. investigated the effects on UVB-induced wrinkle formation in female SKH-1 hairless mice of an orally administered antioxidant compound containing vitamins C and E, Pycnogenol, and evening primrose oil (see Chapter 49, Pycnogenol). Mice were exposed to three weekly doses of UVB over 10 weeks, during which they were administered the antioxidant mixture or vehicle control. Wrinkle formation and epidermal thickness were significantly lower in the antioxidant group. The investigators concluded that the significant inhibition of UVB-induced wrinkle formation delivered by the oral antioxidant cocktail resulted from the active constituents hindering matrix metalloproteinase activity engendered by UVB exposure, thus allowing collagen production to proceed.[30]

TOPICAL USES

The preponderance of data supporting beneficial effects of vitamin C stem from investigations of oral vitamin C or vitamin C applied to tissue cultures. There are no studies that indicate that the ingestion of oral vitamin C increases cutaneous vitamin C levels, however. Manufacturers have seized on this gap in knowledge by developing topical vitamin C preparations, which have become quite popular. Ascorbic acid can be formulated into water- or lipid-soluble products.[31] Unfortunately, few of the currently available topical vitamin C preparations can penetrate the stratum corneum because they are not formulated properly. Absorption of vitamin C is critically dependent on formulation characteristics such as a pH of 2 to 2.5 and the percentage of ascorbic acid in the formulation.[2] Some manufacturers claim that their products are nonionic and less lipophobic, which improves the chances for percutaneous absorption.[32]

Another challenge in creating effective topical ascorbic acid products is achieving stability with this volatile ingredient at a pH that is optimal for vitamin C absorption. The low pH that is required for absorption is easily obtained in the acidic stomach but on the skin can lead to stinging, which makes this a poor ingredient choice for individuals with S_3 type sensitive skin (also known as "stingers"). Exposure to air or UV light will cause the lactone ring to irreversibly open, yielding diketogulonic acid, and then the compound is rendered inactive. Because few topical vitamin C preparations are packaged in airtight containers that are protected from UV radiation, most preparations are rendered inactive within hours of opening the bottle. Nevertheless, vitamin C has been found to be effective in combination with other antioxidants, such as vitamin E and ferulic acid in one case and ferulic acid and phloretin in another, in topical formulations that exert photoprotective activity (see Chapter 52, Phloretin, and Chapter 54, Ferulic Acid).[33–35]

A lipid form of vitamin C, topical ascorbyl palmitate, is nonirritating as well as reportedly photoprotective and anti-inflammatory.[25] Its stability at nonacidic pH decreases potential irritation and its ester form increases penetration and stability. In patch testing on human skin, areas pretreated with 3 percent ascorbyl palmitate (vs. non-pretreated patches) have been shown to decrease erythema following exposure to one to three times the minimal erythema dose (MED). Further, application of a 5 percent solution of ascorbyl palmitate following exposure to one to two times MED decreased the duration of erythema in some patients.[25] In 1991, two topical forms of vitamin C (L-ascorbic acid and ascorbyl palmitate, an ascorbic acid ester) were compared using a TPA-induced tumor model in mice to determine their ability to reduce reactive oxygen species (ROS). TPA-induced tumor progression is largely enhanced by reactive oxygen superoxide ions and protein kinase C. In this study, topical ascorbyl palmitate was found to be over 30-fold more effective than L-ascorbic acid at inhibiting tumor progression with efficacy at substantially lower concentrations. Much of this benefit is attributed to the fact that ascorbyl palmitate is an amphipathic molecule with a polar ascorbic head and a long hydrophobic side chain. This means that it is both lipid- and water-soluble, leading to superior penetration into the skin. In addition, palmitic acid, a product of hydrolysis of ascorbyl palmitate in the skin, was also found to reduce tumor production in the mouse model indicating that its efficacy was not only due to its antioxidant characteristics.[29]

SAFETY ISSUES

Type 3 sensitive skin ("stingers") patients often experience stinging and mild irritation from topically applied vitamin C formulations, especially those that contain L-ascorbic acid. Ascorbyl palmitate may be associated with a lower incidence of skin irritation than L-ascorbic acid, which must be formulated at a low pH to be effective. Some type 2 (rosacea) sensitive skin types experience increased redness from low-pH preparations. The major disadvantages of these products include high cost when formulated properly, questionable

efficacy when not formulated properly, and a plethora of useless products on the market that confuse consumers. The Cosmetic Ingredient Review Expert Panel identified L-ascorbic acid and various esters, including ascorbyl palmitate, calcium ascorbate, magnesium ascorbate, magnesium ascorbyl phosphate, sodium, ascorbate, and sodium ascorbyl phosphate as safe as incorporated in topical cosmetic formulations.[36] For individuals that cannot tolerate topical vitamin C, oral vitamin C at 500 mg twice daily is recommended. Of course, the best source of oral vitamin C is through vitamin C-rich foods, including citrus fruits, berries, chili peppers, Brussels sprouts, broccoli, and many other fruits and vegetables.[37]

ENVIRONMENTAL IMPACT

Organic forms of vitamin C are widely available. It is unlikely that the synthesis of topical products featuring ascorbic acid exacts an environmental toll. More likely, of course, is the potential of ambient toxins, particularly pesticides, affecting ascorbic acid-containing plants. As of the time this text was printed, there were no properly formulated organic forms of topical vitamin C.

FORMULATION CONSIDERATIONS

To be effective, topical vitamin C products and L-ascorbic acid, in particular, must be formulated properly and stored in airtight, light-resistant containers. Pinnell et al. found that L-ascorbic acid must be formulated at a pH less than 3.5 to permeate the skin.[2] Because few topical vitamin C preparations are packaged in airtight containers that are protected from UV radiation, most preparations are rendered inactive within hours of opening the container, and appear yellowish due to the oxidation byproduct dehydroascorbic acid.[4] Nevertheless, as noted above, vitamin C has been found to have increased stability and efficacy in combination with other antioxidants, such as vitamin E, ferulic acid, phloretin, and Pycnogenol. Topical formulations containing these combinations have been shown to exert photoprotective activity.[33,34]

Ascorbic acid derivatives such as ascorbyl-6-palmitate and magnesium ascorbyl phosphate are used in topical formulations as more stable forms of the vitamin.[33] Of these, magnesium ascorbyl phosphate has been found to be the most stable in solution as well as emulsion and L-ascorbic acid, the least stable.[4,38] However, little of the antioxidant potency of magnesium ascorbyl phosphate is maintained on the skin and absorption is difficult. It is more popularly used as a depigmenting ingredient [see Chapter 40, Vitamin C (Ascorbic Acid)].[2,33]

USAGE CONSIDERATIONS

Oral ingestion of vitamin C does not increase vitamin C levels in the skin to the same extent that can be achieved with the appropriate use of topical formulations. Use of vitamin C both orally (preferably in the diet) and topically twice daily is recommended to prevent photoaging and collagen loss, although this has not been proven in human trials.

SIGNIFICANT BACKGROUND

Ascorbic acid is known to exhibit a wide range of biologic activity. Antibacterial, antimycotic, and antiviral properties were reported by Wahlqvist in 1958.[39] In 1995, Hovi et al.

conducted a randomized, double-blind, placebo-controlled trial in 43 women and 3 men with recurrent mucocutaneous herpes to evaluate the effects of Ascoxal, an ascorbic acid-containing formulation. They found that the brief topical treatment attenuated symptom intensity and persistence.[39]

Antioxidant and Antiaging Activity

Vitamin C is unique among antioxidants because of its ability to increase collagen production in addition to its free radical-scavenging "antioxidant" activity. It is also one of the most recognized antioxidants by consumers. Due to its capacity to interfere with the UV-induced generation of ROS by reacting with the superoxide anion or the hydroxyl radical, vitamin C has become a popular addition to "after-sun" products.[40,41] The nutrient is also known to delay the incidence of UV-induced neoplasms in mice.[42] In a study of the photoprotective properties of vitamin C, histologic examination revealed that pigs treated with topical ascorbic acid exhibited fewer sunburn cells than those treated with vehicle alone when exposed to both UVA and UVB irradiation.[43] Investigators also noted a significant reduction in erythema in areas treated with vitamin C and decreases in the amount of vitamin C remaining on the skin after UV exposure. In a subsequent study, the same researchers found that topical vitamin C combined with either a UVA or UVB sunscreen improved sun protection as compared to the sunscreen alone.[44] Also, the combination of vitamins C and E delivered protection from UVB insult, though the bulk of protection was attributable to vitamin E. But vitamin C alone has been demonstrated in other studies to mitigate the effects of UVB, such as erythema and signs of photoaging, on porcine and human skin.[2,45,46]

In 1999, Traikovich reported on improvements in fine wrinkles, roughness, coarse rhytides, skin tone, and sallowness delivered by topical vitamin C (Cellex-C) in a small three-month, double-blind, randomized, vehicle-controlled trial with 19 subjects.[4,47] In 2003, Humbert et al. conducted a six-month, double-blind, vehicle-controlled trial with 20 healthy female volunteers showing that patients treated with 5 percent vitamin C cream experienced significant improvements in deep furrows on the neck and forearms.[4,48]

In a 2001 study in 10 postmenopausal women, Nusgens et al. found that daily topical application of 5 percent L-ascorbic acid enhanced the levels of procollagen types I and III, their posttranslational maturation enzymes, and tissue inhibitor of matrix metalloproteinase (TIMP)-1.[7] This led to increased levels of collagen in the skin.

Several studies indicate that mice treated with topical vitamin C have less erythema, fewer sunburn cells, and diminished tumor formation in treated skin after UV exposure.[49] As noted above, vitamin C reduces (and therefore recycles) oxidized vitamin E back into its active form so the antioxidant potency of vitamin E is regenerated.[50] Potent anti-inflammatory activities have also been associated with vitamin C.[4]

In 2003, Lin et al. developed a stable aqueous solution of 15 percent L-ascorbic acid and 1 percent α-tocopherol and applied it daily to pig skin, finding that while each antioxidant alone conferred a protective effect against erythema and sunburn cell formation, the combination yielded an antioxidant protection factor of fourfold.[51] Subsequently, they combined the antioxidant ferulic acid with 15 percent L-ascorbic acid and 1 percent α-tocopherol to improve the chemical stability of the vitamins and found that this solution also acted synergistically, doubling photoprotection from fourfold to eightfold as measured by erythema and sunburn cell formation in porcine skin (see Chapter 54, Ferulic Acid). Further, the antioxidant preparation efficiently diminished thymine dimer formation and inhibited apoptosis. The investigators concluded that this combination of potent antioxidants should provide protection against skin cancer and photoaging.[35]

In 2008, Murray et al. investigated whether a stable topical preparation of 15 percent L-ascorbic acid, 1 percent α-tocopherol, and 0.5 percent ferulic acid could protect human skin *in vivo* from UV-induced damage. In this small study with nine adults with Fitzpatrick skin types II or III, they found that the antioxidant formulation, with a mechanism of action differing from sunscreens, supplemented the antioxidant pool of the skin and imparted significant photoprotection, guarding the skin against erythema and apoptosis as well as effectively inhibiting p53 activation and diminishing thymine dimer mutations known to be linked to skin cancer.[33]

In 2012, Xu et al. assessed the efficacy and safety of topical 23.8 percent L-ascorbic acid on photoaged skin in a split-face study in 20 Chinese women. Significant improvements in fine lines, dyspigmentation, and surface roughness were noted, without adverse side effects.[52]

Also that year, Taniguchi et al. assessed a stable ascorbic acid derivative, 2-O-α-glucopyranosyl-L-ascorbic acid (AA-2G), and compared it with ascorbic acid for its protective effect on human dermal fibroblasts against cellular damage and senescence spurred by hydrogen peroxide (H_2O_2). They found that pretreatment with AA-2G for 72 hours fostered the proliferation of normal human dermal fibroblasts and protected against H_2O_2-induced cell damage. The same results were achieved with ascorbic acid only when the culture medium was replenished every 24 hours. The derivative product was also found to be stronger than ascorbic acid in downregulating senescence-associated-β-galactosidase (SA-β-gal) activity, a cellular aging biomarker. In addition, the expression of the antiaging factor sirtuin 1 (SIRT1) was markedly reduced in H_2O_2-exposed normal fibroblasts compared to untreated cells. Pretreatment with AA-2G prior to H_2O_2 exposure significantly blunted the decrease in SIRT1 expression while ascorbic acid exerted no effect, however (see Chapter 81, Overview of Aging). Pretreatment with AA-2G also prevented the increase of p53 and p21 expression levels due to H_2O_2 exposure. The investigators concluded that the stable ascorbic acid derivative 2-O-α-glucopyranosyl-L-ascorbic acid protects against oxidative stress and cellular senescence, suggesting a potential role as an antiaging agent.[53]

In a blinded, 35-subject, split-face study conducted by the Baumann Cosmetic and Research Institute, subjects applied a 7 percent ascorbyl palmitate solution with dimethylaminoethanol, hyaluronic acid, and vitamin E (C-ESTA Face Serum, Jan Marini Skin Research) on one side of their face and a 15 percent L-ascorbic acid, 1 percent vitamin E, 0.5 percent ferulic acid (C E Ferulic, Skinceuticals) on the opposite side of the face for two weeks. A notably higher rate of irritation was observed on the L-ascorbic acid side of the face versus the ascorbyl palmitate side of the face (29 percent noted greater irritation vs. 11 percent). A significant number of subjects also perceived superior improvement in texture on the ascorbyl palmitate side of the face versus the L-ascorbic acid side of the face (43 percent noted greater improvement vs. 14 percent). Results trended higher on the ascorbyl palmitate side for additional antiaging concerns, but differences were not significant given the sample size and study duration. Overall, subjects indicated a statistically significant preference for the ascorbyl palmitate product.[54]

CONCLUSION

As a result of dietary consumption, ascorbic acid is the most abundant antioxidant found in human skin. It plays a critical role in multiple biologic functions, including wound healing, collagen production, and replenishing other antioxidants thereby acting against diseases and other processes, such as aging, that are mediated through oxidative stress. Though orally administered ascorbic acid is readily bioavailable, ascorbic acid in the skin is rapidly depleted and oral supplementation alone does not result in optimal skin levels; therefore, topical use is desirable. In order for ascorbic acid to be effective, it must be produced and packaged away from UV light and air to prevent the irreversible opening of the lactone ring, which generates diketogulonic acid that renders the compound inactive and useless. Numerous formulation considerations are involved in the stabilization and effective penetration of ascorbic acid into the skin. Issues such as packaging, exposure to air or light during use, skin sensitivity, and user preference factor into selection of a vitamin C product. The process of developing, manufacturing, and packaging effective, stable vitamin C formulations is expensive. In combination with other antioxidants, vitamin C has been demonstrated to be an integral constituent in topical antioxidant and antiaging formulations that show promise in the dermatologic armamentarium, particularly against photoaging.

REFERENCES

1. Nishikimi M, Fukuyama R, Minoshima S, et al. Cloning and chromosomal mapping of the human nonfunctional gene for L-gulono-gamma-lactone oxidase, the enzyme for L-ascorbic acid biosynthesis missing in man. *J Biol Chem.* 1994;269:13685.
2. Pinnell SR, Yang H, Omar M, et al. Topical L-ascorbic acid: Percutaneous absorption studies. *Dermatol Surg.* 2001;27:137.
3. Shindo Y, Witt E, Han D, et al. Enzymic and non-enzymic antioxidants in epidermis and dermis of human skin. *J Invest Dermatol.* 1994;102:122.
4. Farris PK. Topical vitamin C: A useful agent for treating photoaging and other dermatologic conditions. *Dermatol Surg.* 2005;31:814.
5. Sauberlich HE. Pharmacology of vitamin C. *Annu Rev Nutr.* 1994;14:371.
6. Burgess C. Topical vitamins. *J Drugs Dermatol.* 2008;7:s2.
7. Nusgens BV, Humbert P, Rougier A, et al. Topically applied vitamin C enhances the mRNA level of collagens I and III, their processing enzymes and tissue inhibitor of matrix metalloproteinase 1 in the human dermis. *J Invest Dermatol.* 2001;116:853.
8. Bird TA, Schwartz NB, Peterkofsky B. Mechanism for the decreased biosynthesis of cartilage proteoglycan in the scorbutic guinea pig. *J Biol Chem.* 1986;261:11166.
9. Peterkofsky B. Ascorbate requirement for hydroxylation and secretion of procollagen: Relationship to inhibition of collagen synthesis in scurvy. *Am J Clin Nutr.* 1991;54:1135S.
10. Lin JY, Selim MA, Shea CR, et al. UV photoprotection by combination topical antioxidants vitamin C and vitamin E. *J Am Acad Dermatol.* 2003;48:866.
11. Shindo Y, Witt E, Han D, et al. Dose-response effects of acute ultraviolet irradiation on antioxidants and molecular markers of oxidation in murine epidermis and dermis. *J Invest Dermatol.* 1994;102:470.
12. Thiele JJ, Traber MG, Tsange KG, et al. In vivo exposure to ozone depletes vitamins C and E and induces lipid peroxidation in epidermal layers of murine skin. *Free Radic Biol Med.* 1997;23:85.
13. De Tullio MC. Beyond the antioxidant: The double life of vitamin C. *Subcell Biochem.* 2012;56:49.
14. Carpenter KJ. The discovery of vitamin C. *Ann Nutr Metab.* 2012;61:259.
15. Magiorkinis E, Beloukas A, Diamantis A. Scurvy: Past, present and future. *Eur J Intern Med.* 2011;22:147.
16. Pinnell SR, Murad S, Darr D. Induction of collagen synthesis by ascorbic acid. A possible mechanism. *Arch Dermatol.* 1987;123:1684.
17. Gey KF. Vitamins E plus C and interacting conutrients required for optimal health. A critical and constructive review of epidemiology and supplementation data regarding cardiovascular disease and cancer. *Biofactors.* 1998;7:113.
18. McLauren S. Nutrition and wound healing. *Wound Care.* 1992;1:45.
19. Kameyama K, Sakai C, Kondoh S, et al. Inhibitory effect of magnesium L-ascorbyl-2-phosphate (VC-PMG) on melanogenesis in vitro and in vivo. *J Am Acad Dermatol.* 1996;34:29.
20. Ash K, Lord J, Zukowski M, et al. Comparison of topical therapy for striae alba (20% glycolic acid/0.05% tretinoin versus 20% glycolic acid/10% L-ascorbic acid). *Dermatol Surg.* 1998;24:849.
21. Alster TS, West TB. Effect of topical vitamin C on postoperative carbon dioxide laser resurfacing erythema. *Dermatol Surg.* 1998;24:331.
22. Perricone NV. Topical vitamin C ester (ascorbyl palmitate). *J Geriatr Dermatol.* 1997;5:162.
23. Bush JA, Cheung KJ Jr., Li G. Curcumin induces apoptosis in human melanoma cells through a Fas receptor/caspase-8 pathway independent of p53. *Exp Cell Res.* 2001;271:305.
24. Jee SH, Shen SC, Tseng CR, et al. Curcumin induces a p53-dependent apoptosis in human basal cell carcinoma cells. *J Invest Dermatol.* 1998;111:656.
25. Perricone NV. The photoprotective and anti-inflammatory effects of topical ascorbyl palmitate. *J Geriatric Derm.* 1993;1:5.
26. McArdle F, Rhodes LE, Parslew R, et al. UVR-induced oxidative stress in human skin in vivo: Effects of oral vitamin C supplementation. *Free Radic Biol Med.* 2002;33:1355.
27. Lauer AC, Groth N, Haag SF, et al. Dose-dependent vitamin C uptake and radical scavenging activity in human skin measured with in vivo electron paramagnetic resonance spectroscopy. *Skin Pharmacol Physiol.* 2013;26:147.
28. Pokorski M, Marczak M, Dymecka A, et al. Ascorbyl palmitate as a carrier of ascorbate into neural tissues. *J Biomed Sci.* 2003;10:193.
29. Smart RC, Crawford CL. Effect of ascorbic acid and its synthetic lipophilic derivative ascorbyl palmitate on phorbol ester-induced skin-tumor promotion in mice. *Am J Clin Nutr.* 1991;54:1266S.
30. Cho HS, Lee MH, Lee JW, et al. Anti-wrinkling effects of the mixture of vitamin C, vitamin E, pycnogenol and evening primrose oil, and molecular mechanisms on hairless mouse skin caused by chronic ultraviolet B irradiation. *Photodermatol Photoimmunol Photomed.* 2007;23:155.
31. Colven RM, Pinnell SR. Topical vitamin C in aging. *Clin Dermatol.* 1996;14:227.
32. Darr D, Pinnell S. U. S. Patent no. 5,140,043, 1992.
33. Murray JC, Burch JA, Streilein RD, et al. A topical antioxidant solution containing vitamins C and E stabilized by ferulic acid provides protection for human skin against damage caused by ultraviolet irradiation. *J Am Acad Dermatol.* 2008;59:418.
34. Oresajo C, Stephens T, Hino PD, et al. Protective effects of a topical antioxidant mixture containing vitamin C, ferulic acid, and phloretin against ultraviolet-induced photodamage in human skin. *J Cosmet Dermatol.* 2008;7:290.
35. Lin FH, Lin JY, Gupta RD, et al. Ferulic acid stabilizes a solution of vitamins C and E and doubles its photoprotection of skin. *J Invest Dermatol.* 2005;125:826.
36. Elmore AR. Final report of the safety assessment of L-Ascorbic Acid, Calcium Ascorbate, Magnesium Ascorbate, Magnesium Ascorbyl Phosphate, Sodium Ascorbate, and Sodium Ascorbyl Phosphate as used in cosmetics. *Int J Toxicol.* 2005;24(Suppl 2):51.
37. Baumann L. Nutrition and the skin. In: Baumann L, Saghari S, Weisberg E, eds. *Cosmetic Dermatology: Principles and Practice.* 2nd ed. New York: McGraw-Hill; 2009:53–59.
38. Austria R, Semenzato A, Bettero A. Stability of vitamin C derivatives in solution and topical formulations. *J Pharm Biomed Anal.* 1997;15:795.
39. Hovi T, Hirvimies A, Stenvik M, et al. Topical treatment of recurrent mucocutaneous herpes with ascorbic acid-containing solution. *Antiviral Res.* 1995;27:263.
40. Scarpa M, Stevanato R, Viglino P, et al. Superoxide ion as active intermediate in the autoxidation of ascorbate by molecular oxygen. Effect of superoxide dismutase. *J Biol Chem.* 1983;258:6695.
41. Cabelli DE, Bielski BH. Kinetics and mechanism for the oxidation of ascorbic acid/ascorbate by HO2/O2 radicals: A pulse radiolysis and stopped flow photolysis study. *J Phys Chem.* 1983;87:1805.
42. Dunham WB, Zuckerkandl E, Reynolds R, et al. Effects of intake of L-ascorbic acid on the incidence of dermal neoplasms induced in mice by ultraviolet light. *Proc Natl Acad Sci U S A.* 1982;79:7532.

43. Knekt P, Aromaa A, Maatela J, et al. Vitamin E and cancer prevention. *Am J Clin Nutr*. 1991;53:283S.
44. Darr D, Dunston S, Faust H, et al. Effectiveness of antioxidants (vitamin C and E) with and without sunscreens as topical photoprotectants. *Acta Derm Venereol*. 1996;76:264.
45. Darr D, Combs S, Dunston S, et al. Topical vitamin C protects porcine skin from ultraviolet radiation-induced damage. *Br J Dermatol*. 1992;127:247.
46. Murray J, Darr D, Reich J, et al. Topical vitamin C treatment reduces ultraviolet B radiation-induced erythema in human skin. *J Invest Dermatol*. 1991;96:587.
47. Traikovich SS. Use of topical ascorbic acid and its effects on photodamaged skin topography. *Arch Otolaryngol Head Neck Surg*. 1999;125:1091.
48. Humbert PG, Haftek M, Creidi P, et al. Topical ascorbic acid on photoaged skin. Clinical, topographical and ultrastructural evaluation: Double-blind study vs. placebo. *Exp Dermatol*. 2003;12:237.
49. Werninghaus K. The role of antioxidants in reducing photodamage. In: Gilchrest B, ed. *Photodamage*. London: Blackwell Science; 1995:249.
50. Chan AC. Partners in defense, vitamin E and vitamin C. *Can J Physiol Pharmacol*. 1993;71:725.
51. Lin JY, Selim MA, Shea CR, et al. UV photoprotection by combination topical antioxidants vitamin C and vitamin E. *J Am Acad Dermatol*. 2003;48:866.
52. Xu TH, Chen JZ, Li YH, et al. Split-face study of topical 23.8% L-ascorbic acid serum in treating photo-aged skin. *J Drugs Dermatol*. 2012;11:51.
53. Taniguchi M, Arai N, Kohno K, et al. Anti-oxidative and anti-aging activities of 2-O-α-glucopyranosyl-L-ascorbic acid on human dermal fibroblasts. *Eur J Pharmacol*. 2012;674:126.
54. Baumann L, Schirripa MJ, Duque D. C-ESTA serum and CE Ferulic split-face vitamin C comparison study. *J Drugs Dermatol*, submitted for publication.

CHAPTER 56

Tocopherol (Vitamin E)

Activities:

Antioxidant, photoprotection, wound healing

Important Chemical Components:

Vitamin E is actually a family of eight fat-soluble isomers that include four tocopherols and four tocotrienols. The molecular formula of α-tocopherol, the most active form of vitamin E, is $C_{29}H_{50}O_2$. By contrast, the molecular formula of α-tocotrienol is $C_{29}H_{44}O_2$. The molecular formula for γ-tocopherol, the most frequently consumed form of vitamin E in the U.S. is $C_{28}H_{48}O_2$.[1]

Origin Classification:

Vitamin E is found naturally in many vegetables, oils, seeds, nuts, and other foods. Most topical formulations contain synthetic laboratory-made α-tocopherol or one of its many esters or ethers.

Personal Care Category:

Antioxidant, moisturizing, antiaging

Recommended for the following Baumann Skin Types:

DRNW, DRPW, DSNW, DSPW, ORNW, ORPW, OSNW, and OSPW

SOURCE

Obtained in the diet through fresh vegetables (especially green leafy vegetables), vegetable oils, seeds, nuts, grains, corn, soy, whole wheat flour, margarine, and in some meat and dairy products, vitamin E, or tocopherol, is the main lipid-soluble antioxidant found in human skin (via sebum), membranes, plasma, and tissues that protects cells from oxidative stress (Table 56-1).[2–5] Meeting the definition of a vitamin, it is not synthesized by humans. Vitamin E is frequently used to treat minor burns, surgical scars, and other wounds, although its use for dermatoses has not been approved by the United States Food and Drug Administration (USFDA). The use of vitamin E

TABLE 56-1
Pros and Cons of Tocopherol

Pros	Cons
Potent antioxidant activity and primary lipophilic antioxidant	Dearth of evidence in controlled trials to support use for dermatologic conditions
Synergistically interacts with other antioxidants	Risk of contact dermatitis
Exhibits emollient activity	
Easy to formulate	
Can be regenerated back into its reduced form by hydrophilic antioxidants vitamin C and glutathione	

is thought to mitigate lipid peroxidation and protect against cardiovascular disease.[6] Similarly, it protects cutaneous cell membranes from peroxidation. In addition to its antioxidant activity, it is now understood to regulate cell signaling and gene expression.[7] The main biologically active form of vitamin E is α-tocopherol.[8]

Tocopherols, unlike tocotrienols, are found in olive, peanut, sunflower, and walnut oils.[9] One of the most abundant sources of tocotrienols is palm oil, which is free of *trans*-fatty acids, accounting for its increasingly widespread popularity, particularly in the United States.[9,10] Tocotrienols are also found in edible sources such as rice bran, coconut oil, cocoa butter, soy bean, barley, and wheat germ, as well as inedible ones such as latex (*Hevea brailiensis*).[9–11]

HISTORY

Herbert Evans and Katherine Bishop are credited with discovering vitamin E in 1922.[12–14] After inducing sterility in rats, they found that feeding the animals lettuce or wheat germ oil, but not cod liver oil or wheat flour or chaff, restored fertility. Initially, they labeled an essential dietary ingredient as "factor X."[13] They adopted the expression "vitamin E," as suggested by Sure, in 1924.[7,13] The first description of the antioxidant activity of vitamin E is attributed to Olcott and Mattill in 1931, with the first recorded isolation of α-tocopherol occurring in 1936.[13,14] Also in 1936, George Calhoun, professor of Greek at the University of California, Berkeley, suggested the name "tocopherol" based on the Greek words *tokos* (offspring or childbirth) and *phero* or *phérein* (to bear or to bring forth), to Evans and colleagues, who also worked at Berkeley; the "-ol" indicates the alcohol characteristics of the compound.[7,13] In 1938, Karrer, Fritzche, Ringier, and Salomon became the first to synthesize α-tocopherol.[9,13] In the 1940s, vitamin E became known as a "chain-breaking" antioxidant for its role in suppressing the chain reaction induced by free radicals.[14]

CHEMISTRY

Vitamin E is a family of compounds called tocopherols, including, α-, β-, γ-, and δ-tocopherol, of which α-tocopherol is the most active form, and four tocotrienols (α-, β-, γ-, and δ-tocotrienol). Tocotrienols, with three unsaturated bonds in the carbon side chain with one chiral center, have an isoprenoid instead of a phytyl side chain (long saturated carbon side chain with a chiral center).[3,9] The four forms differ by the number of methyl groups found on the chromanol nucleus (α- has three; β- and γ- each have two; and δ- has one).[3] The side chain is linked to position 2 of the chroman ring in all cases.[7] The chemical names for all vitamin E types begin with either "d" for the natural form or "dl" (or "all-*rac*") for the synthetic form. Natural vitamin E is more active and better absorbed. Synthetic vitamin E supplements contain only α-tocopherol, while food sources contain various tocopherols, including α-, δ-, and γ-tocopherol. Forms of vitamin E are labeled as either "tocopherol" or the esterified "tocopheryl" followed by the name of the substance to which it is attached, as in "tocopheryl acetate."

Although less studied than tocopherols (approximately one percent of the literature on vitamin E addresses tocotrienols),[10] tocotrienols have been reported to act as stronger antioxidants but exhibit lower biovailability;[9,15–17] the δ-tocotrienol form is thought to be especially effective in combating actinic damage.[18] Of note, some believe that α-tocotrienol is a more potent antioxidant than α-tocopherol.[9] Tocotrienols are not only members of the vitamin E family based on structure, but function as well. For instance, tocotrienols can alleviate symptoms engendered by α-tocopherol deficiency.[10] In addition, tocotrienols reportedly display hypocholesterolemic, anticancer, and neuroprotective activity seldom associated with tocopherols.[10] Tocopherols are much more widely dispersed in the plant kingdom than are tocotrienols.[10,19]

Vitamin E, CoQ_{10}, curcumin, and feverfew are among the antioxidants found in the lipophilic portion of the cell membrane (see Chapter 57, Coenzyme Q_{10}; Chapter 66, Feverfew; and Chapter 69, Turmeric). Other fat-soluble antioxidants include carotenoids, particularly lycopene, and idebenone, the synthetic analog of CoQ_{10} (see Chapter 61, Idebenone). But several investigations have shown that vitamin E is the predominant antioxidant in the skin barrier.[20] One of the primary functions of α-tocopherol is the scavenging of lipid peroxyl radicals (one molecule of tocopherol has the capacity to scavenge two molecules of peroxyl radicals); γ-tocopherol is better at scavenging reactive nitrogen oxide species (up to six times the reactivity).[7,14,21–23] In addition, α-tocopherol has twice the capacity of γ-tocopherol in scavenging oxygen radicals; γ-tocopherol has 10 percent of the biological activity of α-tocopherol.[7] Concentrations of vitamin E are found to be highest in the lowest layers of the stratum corneum (SC).[24] Exogenous factors such as ultraviolet (UV) exposure are known to deplete the stores of vitamin E in the skin.

ORAL USES

Oral vitamin E has been used in a wide range of cutaneous conditions as a treatment or prophylaxis, including skin cancer, dystrophic epidermolysis bullosa, discoid lupus erythematosus, atopic dermatitis, yellow nail syndrome, granuloma annulare, pemphigus, and lichen sclerosus et atrophicus.[25] Results have varied significantly. Vitamin E has also been used in oral form to treat cutaneous ulcers, vibration disease, as well as claudication, and to stimulate collagen synthesis and wound healing.[3,26]

In 2002, Tsoureli-Nikita et al. conducted a single-blind clinical study in 96 patients with atopic dermatitis randomly divided into a group given 400 international units (IU) of natural vitamin E or a placebo, once daily for eight months. The subjects in the vitamin E group experienced significantly better results than those on placebo, with nearly complete remission in seven of the 50 vitamin E subjects and none on placebo. Great improvement was observed in 23 of the 50 using vitamin E and only one in the placebo group. Slight improvement was seen in 10 using vitamin E and four in the placebo group, with no changes recorded in six of the vitamin E group and five in the placebo cohort. Thirty-six patients using the placebo experienced an exacerbation of their symptoms, compared to four patients using vitamin E. A reduction of 62 percent in serum immunoglobulin E levels was noted in the vitamin E patients who exhibited great improvement and near remission. The difference was approximately 34.4 percent

in those taking placebo. The investigators reported significant improvements in facial erythema, lichenification, and the appearance of normal-looking skin, concluding that vitamin E is promising as a therapeutic agent for atopic dermatitis.[27]

Some authors have reported that the use of oral vitamin E will reduce the side effects of retinoids;[28] however, other studies have not shown this benefit.[29]

Thiele and Ekanayake-Mudiyanselage note that oral vitamin E doses ranging from 50 to 1000 IU have been well tolerated in human beings with minimal or no side effects.[30] Oral supplementation with tocotrienols has been shown to protect against stroke.[31,32] When incorporated into oral supplements tocotrienols are typically processed into softgel capsules.[9]

Several studies have demonstrated a protective effect against prostate cancer purportedly delivered by α-tocopherol supplementation.[33,34] However, in a 2007 prospective study analyzing the relationship of vitamin E supplementation and dietary consumption of α-, δ-, γ- and δ-tocopherol to prostate cancer risk in 295,344 men (between 50 and 71 years old) free of cancer at enrollment in 1995–1996, investigators found that α-tocopherol did not impart protection but higher intake of γ-tocopherol was associated with a lowered risk of clinically relevant disease.[21]

A 2013 study suggests a role for argan oil improving the vitamin E profile and attenuating the symptoms of disorders seen more often in postmenopausal women. In a study of 151 menopausal women in Morocco, serum level of vitamin E was increased in women consuming edible argan oil but not in women in an olive oil group. Investigators suggested that an argan-rich diet increases antioxidant status and may contribute to the prevention of some postmenopausal disorders (see Chapter 10, Argan Oil).[35]

TOPICAL USES

Vitamin E is generally used in 1 to 5 percent concentrations as α-tocopherol or tocopherol acetate in over-the-counter products.[24] When topically applied, vitamin E has been shown to hydrate the SC and improve water-binding capacity.[24]

In a 2005 study with 13 volunteers, Ekanayake-Mudiyanselage et al. examined whether a one-time use of an α-tocopherol-enriched rinse-off product could yield effective deposition of α-tocopherol on the SC. The α-tocopherol-enriched product or an α-tocopherol-free vehicle control was applied. Skin surface lipids were analyzed after extraction from all volunteers, including a group subjected to irradiation of their forearms with low-dose UVA (8 J/cm²). The investigators found that the α-tocopherol product increased α-tocopherol levels in surface lipids whereas such levels were decreased in the control group. Deposition levels remained consistent for at least 24 hours. The α-tocopherol rinse-off product also significantly suppressed photooxidation of squalene. The researchers concluded that α-tocopherol-enriched rinse-off products can contribute skin barrier integrity maintenance by protecting it at the surface lipid level against photooxidative insult.[8]

In a small study of nine patients in 2008, Murray et al. found that a stable topical preparation of 15 percent L-ascorbic acid, 1 percent α-tocopherol, and 0.5 percent ferulic acid protected human skin in vivo from UV-induced damage, specifically erythema and apoptosis [see Chapter 54, Ferulic Acid, and Chapter 55, Ascorbic Acid (Vitamin C)]. The formulation also suppressed p53 activation and limited thymine dimer mutations, which are associated with skin cancer.[36]

Topically applied vitamin E is considered an effective ingredient for conferring skin protection and to treat atopic dermatitis.[3,37]

Wound Healing

Oxygen radicals form in response to injury and further inhibit recovery by attacking DNA, cellular membranes, proteins, and lipids. It is believed that antioxidants act to ameliorate wounds by reducing the damage induced by free oxygen radicals, which are released by neutrophils in the inflammatory phase of the healing process.[38] In the late 1960s, Kamimura et al. performed quantitative research demonstrating that topically applied vitamin E penetrates into the deep dermis and subcutaneous tissue.[39] Numerous scientists, as well as many laypersons, have interpreted this to mean that topically applied vitamin E may improve wound healing. Contradictory results have emerged from animal studies undertaken to evaluate the effects of vitamin E on wound healing, however. This may be explained by the fact that unlike other vitamins, tocopherols exhibit species-specific mechanisms of action.[26]

In a prospective, double-blind, randomized study on humans, Jenkins et al. tried to diminish scarring in burn patients following reconstructive surgery by applying topical vitamin E. The researchers observed no difference between the control and treatment groups, however, and nearly 20 percent of the patients reported local reactions to the vitamin E cream.[40] In another study, Baumann et al. assessed the cosmetic benefit resulting from the use of topically applied vitamin E to surgical scars.[37] In a double-blind fashion, patients applied 320 IU of D-α-tocopheryl/g of Aquaphor to one side of the scar and Aquaphor alone to the other side of the scar. The patients were followed for six months. At the conclusion of the study, the vitamin E preparation failed to improve the cosmetic appearance of surgical scars, and resulted in contact dermatitis in a few subjects.

Skin Lightening

In 1999, Funasaka et al. showed in a pigmented human melanoma cell line that α-tocopherol and ferulic acid, connected by an ester bond in the compound α-tocopheryl ferulate, appears to be a viable facial skin-whitening agent, inhibiting melanogenesis as well as biological responses to reactive oxygen species (see Chapter 54, Ferulic Acid).[41] In addition, the compound more efficiently hindered melanin formation than the well-known skin-lightening agents arbutin, kojic acid, magnesium-L-ascorbyl 2-phosphate (esterified vitamin C), and tranexamic acid [see Chapter 35, Arbutin; Chapter 37, Kojic Acid; and Chapter 40, Vitamin C (Ascorbic Acid)].[41]

Skin Cancer Protection

In 2013, Burns et al. demonstrated in female SKH-1 hairless mice that topical treatment with a combination of vitamins C (15 percent L-ascorbic) and E (1 percent α-tocopherol) and 0.5 percent ferulic acid (C E Ferulic®) for 15 weeks reduced squamous cell cancer (SCC) tumor burden and inhibited the development of new tumors after 10 weeks of exposure to UVB. They also found that treatment with topical 5 percent α-tocopherol alone may actually augment SCC formation.[42]

SAFETY ISSUES

The incidence of contact dermatitis elicited by topical vitamin E application may be relatively high for certain forms of tocopherol,[37,40] particularly tocopherol acetate,[43] with allergy to dl-α-tocopheryl nicotinate also reported.[44] Contact urticaria, eczematous dermatitis, and erythema multiforme-like reactions have also been reported in association with the topical application of vitamin E.[45] In 1994, Swiss researchers evaluated 1,000 cases of an atypical papular and follicular contact dermatitis provoked by vitamin E linoleate used as an additive to cosmetics. They concluded that oxidized vitamin E derivatives can operate synergistically *in vivo* as haptens or as irritants and were responsible for the allergic reaction, not the vitamin E ester.[3,46] Reports of allergic contact dermatitis or irritation in response to topical vitamin E are rare overall, though, and it is considered safe for use in topical skin care products.

Bendich and Machlin conducted a comprehensive literature review in 1988, finding extended use of oral vitamin E up to 3,000 mg/d to be safe.[47] Kappus and Diplock later established as absolutely safe vitamin E doses up to 400 mg/d, with doses between 400 mg and 2,000 mg deemed as unlikely to cause adverse reactions, and doses greater than 3,000 mg/d over a prolonged period as a potential source of side effects.[48] Patients on anticoagulant therapy are advised to avoid high doses of vitamin E (>4,000 IU) because the nutrient can contribute to blood thinning.[49] In addition, patients are often counseled to suspend vitamin E supplementation, although a clinically significant reduction in platelet aggregation in those with normal platelets is unlikely. Such a suspension is necessary for patients who have abnormal platelets or vitamin K deficiency, or who are taking antiplatelet agents.[50]

Tocopherol is used in concentrations up to 5 percent in cosmetic formulations, with tocopheryl acetate and tocopheryl linoleate used in concentrations up to 36 and 2 percent, respectively.[51] The Cosmetic Ingredient Review (CIR) Expert Panel has found that tocopherol and its ester and ether derivatives, tocopheryl acetate, tocopheryl linoleate, tocopheryl linoleate/oleate, tocopheryl nicotinate, tocopheryl succinate, dioleyl tocopheryl methylsilanol, potassium ascorbyl tocopheryl phosphate, and tocophersolan are safe as used in skin care formulations.[51]

ENVIRONMENTAL IMPACT

Organic forms of vitamin E are widely available. It is unlikely that the synthesis of topical products featuring tocopherols exacts an environmental toll. More likely, as in the case of vitamin C, is the potential of ambient toxins, particularly pesticides, affecting plants that contain forms of vitamin E. However, the cultivation and extraction of the oil palm fruit (*Elaeis guineensis*) for palm oil (a semi-solid fat rich in palmitic and oleic acids) should not be ignored insofar as vitamin E (30 percent tocopherols, 70 percent tocotrienols) is a significant minor component in palm oil and the oil palm is the highest yielding oil crop in the world.[9,52,53] The desire to cultivate and capitalize on the economic potential of the two oils derived from *E. guineensis* (native to West Africa but grown for commercial purposes mainly in Southeast Asia, particularly Malaysia), palm oil (primarily used for edible qualities in food preparation and processing) and palm kernel oil (used for commercial food preparation as well as oil and chemistry industries), has contributed to widespread and continuing deforestation and threats to biodiversity in Southeast Asia.[52,54-56]

FORMULATION CONSIDERATIONS

The lipophilic nature of vitamin E renders it conducive to topical application and percutaneous absorption through the skin.[57,58] The form of vitamin E used in formulation is a key factor in its potential efficacy in a skin care product. Because vitamin C can restore oxidized vitamin E, the combination of the antioxidants is a stabilizing factor in topical formulations [see Chapter 55, Ascorbic Acid (Vitamin C)].[42,59] Further, ferulic acid has been shown to stabilize both vitamins, with the topical combination exerting photoprotective effects against UVB exposure, including the significant reduction in thymine dimer formation (see Chapter 54, Ferulic Acid).[42,58,60] Vitamin E is often incorporated in its esterified forms, typically as acetates and succinates, as these compounds are more stable.[61]

USAGE CONSIDERATIONS

Oral ingestion of tocotrienols sufficient to achieve biologic activity is exceedingly difficult. Dietary supplements are therefore recommended. The highest bioavailability among the natural vitamin E isomers is exhibited by α-tocopherol and is the standard by which other forms of vitamin E are compared.[10]

Tocopherol displays better absorption, while tocopheryl exhibits slightly better shelf life. The most common oral supplementation forms of vitamin E are D-α tocopherol, D-α-tocopheryl acetate, and α-tocopheryl succinate. In cosmetic products, the most common vitamin E forms are α-tocopheryl acetate and α-tocopheryl linoleate, which are less likely to provoke contact dermatitis than D-α-tocopheryl and more stable at room temperature. Notably, the tocopherol esters are less well absorbed by the skin than tocopherols,[62] and may not render as much photoprotection. In one study, α-tocopheryl acetate or α-tocopheryl succinate may have actually enhanced photocarcinogenesis, rather than protected against it.[63] Such α-tocopherol esters are included in many skin lotions, cosmetics, and sunscreens; therefore, more research is necessary to determine if esterified vitamin E forms indeed foster photocarcinogenesis.

SIGNIFICANT BACKGROUND

Dietary deficiency of vitamin E has been correlated with an increase in oxidative stress and cell injury.[2] In 1993, Tanaka et al. observed that reactive oxygen species induce alterations in the biosynthesis of collagen and glycosaminoglycans (GAGs) in cultured human dermal fibroblasts.[64] The addition of α-tocopherol to the fibroblasts prevented such changes. Vitamin E has also been demonstrated to decrease prostaglandin E$_2$ production,[65] and increase interleukin (IL)-2 production, yielding anti-inflammatory and immunostimulatory activity. This stabilizing effect is thought to potentially play a role in collagen biosynthesis.[66] However, *in vivo* attempts to measure and correlate changes in collagen production with vitamin E concentration changes have not yet yielded conclusive results.

Animal Studies

In 1992, Trevithick et al. noted that topical D-α-tocopherol acetate diminished erythema due to sunburn, edema, and skin sensitivity in mice when application occurred following exposure to UVB radiation.[67] In a study in which tocopherol 5 percent was applied to mice prior to UVB exposure, Bissett et al. observed a 75 percent decrease in skin wrinkling, a rise in tumor latency, and a reduction of cutaneous tumors; however, vitamin E failed to affect UVA-induced skin sagging.[68] Indeed, the topical application of α-tocopherol to animal skin has been repeatedly shown to be effective in reducing sunburn cell production,[69,70] attenuating chronic UVB-induced damage,[71,72] and

inhibiting photocarcinogenesis.[73] Specifically, oral and topical vitamin E supplementation in certain animals diminishes the effects of photoaging, inhibits skin cancer formation, and reverses UV-induced immunosuppression.[74–76] In mice, the topical application of D-α-tocopherol has been demonstrated to be much more effective than D-α-tocopheryl succinate in protecting against acute and chronic UV-induced damage.[4]

As mentioned in the previous chapter, Cho et al. found that female SKH-1 hairless mice orally administered an antioxidant formulation containing vitamins C and E, Pycnogenol, and evening primrose oil (see Chapter 49, Pycnogenol), given during a 10-week period that included three weekly doses of UVB, exhibited significantly reduced wrinkle formation and epidermal thickness compared to controls.[77]

Antioxidant Activity and Photoprotection

Depletion of cutaneous vitamin E is considered an early indication of extrinsically caused oxidative damage.[20,37] Studies on elderly subjects that exhibit high plasma tocopherol levels reveal a lower incidence of infectious disease and cancer than in the age-matched population.[78–80] Therefore, vitamin E is thought by many to be a potent and essential antioxidant. As an ingredient in skin care agents, significant evidence has been amassed to suggest its effectiveness as a photoprotective agent. It also appears to deliver photoprotection when taken orally or applied topically.

In a study in which subjects facially applied tocopherol 5 to 8 percent cream for four weeks, observations included diminished skin roughness, shorter length of facial lines, and reduced wrinkle depth as compared to placebo.[81] In addition, in a study in which vitamin E (5 percent) was applied to human skin under light-tight occlusion 24 hours before UV treatment, UV-induced expression of human macrophage metalloelastase, a member of the matrix metalloproteinase family involved in degradation of elastin, appeared to be inhibited.[82]

There are studies that cast doubt on the efficacy of vitamin E alone in imparting photoprotective effects, however. A double-blind, placebo-controlled six-month study of the protective effects of orally administered vitamin E (400 IU/day) against UV-induced epidermal damage in humans considered minimal erythema dose (MED) and histologic response at baseline, one month, and six months. There was no significant difference between the placebo group and those treated with vitamin E and the researchers concluded that daily ingestion of 400 IU of oral α-tocopherol daily yielded no meaningful photoprotection.[83] Other authors have suggested that if vitamin E provides any photoprotection at all, it may do so only in cooperation with other antioxidants, such as vitamin C.[59] In fact, Lin et al., in a study with Yorkshire pigs, demonstrated that the combined application of 1 percent α-tocopherol with 15 percent L-ascorbic acid rendered superior protection against erythema and sunburn cell development compared to either 1 percent α-tocopherol or 15 percent L-ascorbic acid alone.[58] Of note, some data suggest a cumulative benefit derived from using oral and topical antioxidant products in combination, including vitamins C and E in particular.[84–86]

Sorg et al., who noted that vitamins A and E absorb UV radiation in the solar spectrum range most responsible for photodamage, suggested that these vitamins perform complementary functions in the skin, with topical vitamin E shown in mice to prevent UV-induced oxidative stress as well as cutaneous and systemic immunosuppression. Topical vitamin A has been demonstrated in mice to prevent epidermal hypovitaminosis engendered by UV exposure. The authors contend that combining these topical agents can reinforce the activities of each.[87]

Nevertheless, a 2009 six-month study in healthy human volunteers with actinic keratoses revealed that while topically applied dl-α-tocopherol, of which cutaneous levels were significantly increased at the conclusion of the study, did not markedly change already present lesions, changes in polyamine metabolism indicated that squamous cell carcinogenesis potential was significantly reduced.[88]

Overall, several studies using topical E have yielded evidence of photoprotective activity against erythema, edema, sunburn cell formation, and additional indicators of acute UV-induced damage as well as responses to chronic UVA and UVB exposure, including skin wrinkling and skin cancer.[3,58,68,74,89–91]

CONCLUSION

Antioxidant activity emerges as the primary but not exclusive reason for research into the dermatologic use of vitamin E. Combination with other antioxidants appears to enhance the potency of vitamin E and, likely, the other interacting antioxidants. The potential therapeutic benefits of vitamin E in the prevention and treatment of skin cancer and photoaging remain an important focus of research. As an ingredient in topical antiaging skin care preparations, vitamin E exhibits emollient properties and is stable, easy to formulate, and relatively inexpensive, rendering it a popular additive. Much more research, in the form of randomized controlled trials, is necessary, though, to establish the role of vitamin E in treating various dermatoses. Tocotrienols have gained increasing attention in the last two decades and warrant much more investigation to elucidate a fuller role of the vitamin E family in dermatology.

REFERENCES

1. Jiang Q, Christen S, Shigenaga MK, et al. Gamma-tocopherol, the major form of vitamin E in the US diet, deserves more attention. *Am J Clin Nutr*. 2001;74:714.
2. Nachbar F, Korting HC. The role of vitamin E in normal and damaged skin. *J Mol Med (Berl)*. 1995;73:7.
3. Thiele JJ, Hsieh SN, Ekanayake-Mudiyanselage S. Vitamin E: Critical review of its current use in cosmetic and clinical dermatology. *Dermatol Surg*. 2005;31:805.
4. Burke KE. Photodamage of the skin: Protection and reversal with topical antioxidants. *J Cosmet Dermatol*. 2004;3:149.
5. Thiele JJ. Oxidative targets in the stratum corneum. A new basis for antioxidative strategies. *Skin Pharmacol Appl Skin Physiol*. 2001;14(Suppl 1):87.
6. Halliwell B. The antioxidant paradox. *Lancet*. 2000;355:1179.
7. Pfluger P, Kluth D, Landes N, et al. Vitamin E: Underestimated as an antioxidant. *Redox Rep*. 2004;9:249.
8. Ekanayake-Mudiyanselage S, Tavakkol A, Polefka TG, et al. Vitamin E delivery to human skin by a rinse-off product: Penetration of alpha-tocopherol versus wash-out effects of skin surface lipids. *Skin Pharmacol Physiol*. 2005;18:20.
9. Wong RS, Radhakrishnan AK. Tocotrienol research: Past into present. *Nutr Rev*. 2012;70:483.
10. Sen CK, Khanna S, Roy S. Tocotrienols in health and disease: The other half of the natural vitamin E family. *Mol Aspects Med*. 2007;28:692.
11. Theriault A, Chao JT, Wang Q, et al. Tocotrienol: A review of its therapeutic potential. *Clin Biochem*. 1999;32:309.
12. Evans HM, Bishop KS. On the existence of a hitherto unrecognized dietary factor essential for reproduction. *Science*. 1922;56:650.
13. Bell EF. History of vitamin E in infant nutrition. *Am J Clin Nutr*. 1987;46:183.
14. Niki E, Traber MG. A history of vitamin E. *Ann Nutr Metabl*. 2012;61:207.
15. Packer L, Weber SU, Rimbach G. Molecular aspects of alpha-tocotrienol antioxidant action and cell signaling. *J Nutr*. 2001;131:369S.

16. Serbinova EA, Packer L. Antioxidant properties of alpha-tocopherol and alpha-tocotrienol. *Methods Enzymol*. 1994;234:354.
17. Serbinova E, Kagan V, Han D, et al. Free radical recycling and intramembrane mobility in the antioxidant properties of alpha-tocopherol and alpha-tocotrienol. *Free Radic Biol Med*. 1991;10:263.
18. Rona C, Vailati F, Berardesca E. The cosmetic treatment of wrinkles. *J Cosmet Dermatol*. 2004;3:26.
19. Horvath G, Wessjohann L, Bigirimana J, et al. Differential distribution of tocopherols and tocotrienols in photosynthetic and non-photosynthetic tissues. *Phytochemistry*. 2006;67:1185.
20. Thiele JJ, Schroeter C, Hsieh SN, et al. The antioxidant network of the stratum corneum. *Curr Probl Dermatol*. 2001;29:26.
21. Wright ME, Weinstein SJ, Lawson KA, et al. Supplemental and dietary vitamin E intakes and risk of prostate cancer in a large prospective study. *Cancer Epidemiol Biomarkers Prev*. 2007;16:1128.
22. Christen S, Woodall AA, Shigenaga MK, et al. Gamma-tocopherol traps mutagenic electrophiles such as NO(X) and complements alpha-tocopherol: Physiological implications. *Proc Natl Acad Sci U S A*. 1997;94:3217.
23. Cooney RV, Franke AA, Harwood PJ, et al. Gamma-tocopherol detoxification of nitrogen dioxide: Superiority to alpha-tocopherol. *Proc Natl Acad Sci U S A*. 1993;90:1771.
24. Manela-Azulay M, Bagatin E. Cosmeceuticals vitamins. *Clin Dermatol*. 2009;27:469.
25. Keller KL, Fenske NA. Uses of vitamins A, C, and E and related compounds in dermatology: A review. *J Am Acad Dermatol*. 1998;39:611.
26. Pehr K, Forsey RR. Why don't we use vitamin E in dermatology? *CMAJ*. 1993;149:1247.
27. Tsoureli-Nikita E, Hercogova J, Lotti T, et al. Evaluation of dietary intake of vitamin E in the treatment of atopic dermatitis: A study of the clinical course and evaluation of the immunoglobulin E serum levels. *Int J Dermatol*. 2002;41:146.
28. Dimery IW, Hong WK, Lee JJ, et al. Phase I trial of alpha-tocopherol effects on 13-cis-retinoic acid toxicity. *Ann Oncol*. 1997;8:85.
29. Strauss JS, Gottlieb AB, Jones T, et al. Concomitant administration of vitamin E does not change the side effects of isotretinoin as used in acne vulgaris: A randomized trial. *J Am Acad Dermatol*. 2000;43:777.
30. Thiele JJ, Ekanayake-Mudiyanselage S. Vitamin E in human skin: Organ-specific physiology and considerations for its use in dermatology. *Mol Aspects Med*. 2007;28:646.
31. Khanna S, Roy S, Slivka A, et al. Neuroprotective properties of the natural vitamin E alpha-tocotrienol. *Stroke*. 2005;36:2258.
32. Khanna S, Roy S, Parinandi NL, et al. Characterization of the potent neuroprotective properties of the natural vitamin E alpha-tocotrienol. *J Neurochem*. 2006;98:1474.
33. Rodriguez C, Jacobs EJ, Mondul AM, et al. Vitamin E supplements and risk of prostate cancer in U.S. men. *Cancer Epidemiol Biomarkers Prev*. 2004;13:378.
34. Chan JM, Stampfer MJ, Ma J, et al. Supplemental vitamin E intake and prostate cancer risk in a large cohort of men in the United States. *Cancer Epidemiol Biomarkers Prev*. 1999;8:893.
35. El Monfalouti H, Charrouf Z, El Hamdouchi A, et al. Argan oil and postmenopausal Moroccan women: Impact on the vitamin E profile. *Nat Prod Commun*. 2013;8:55.
36. Murray JC, Burch JA, Streilein RD, et al. A topical antioxidant solution containing vitamins C and E stabilized by ferulic acid provides protection for human skin against damage caused by ultraviolet irradiation. *J Am Acad Dermatol*. 2008;59:418.
37. Baumann LS, Spencer J. The effects of topical vitamin E on the cosmetic appearance of scars. *Dermatol Surg*. 1999;25:311.
38. Martin A. The use of antioxidants in healing. *Dermatol Surg*. 1996;22:156.
39. Kamimura M, Matsuzawa T. Percutaneous absorption of alpha-tocopheryl acetate. *J Vitaminol (Kyoto)*. 1968;14:150.
40. Jenkins M, Alexander JW, MacMillan BG, et al. Failure of topical steroids and vitamin E to reduce postoperative scar formation following reconstructive surgery. *J Burn Care Rehabil*. 1986;7:309.
41. Funasaka Y, Chakraborty AK, Komoto M, et al. The depigmenting effect of alpha-tocopheryl ferulate on human melanoma cells. *Br J Dermatol*. 1999;141:20.
42. Burns EM, Tober KL, Riggenbach JA, et al. Differential effects of topical vitamin E and C E Ferulic® treatments on ultraviolet light B-induced cutaneous tumor development in Skh-1 mice. *PLoS One*. 2013;8:e63809.
43. Matsumura T, Nakada T, Iijima M. Widespread contact dermatitis from tocopherol acetate. *Contact Dermatitis*. 2004;51:211.

44. Oshima H, Tsuji K, Oh-I T, et al. Allergic contact dermatitis due to DL-alpha-tocopheryl nicotinate. *Contact Dermatitis*. 2003;48:167.

45. Hunter D, Frumkin A. Adverse reactions to vitamin E and aloe vera preparations after dermabrasion and chemical peel. *Cutis*. 1991;47:193.

46. Perrenoud D, Homberger HP, Auderset PC, et al. An epidemic outbreak of papular and follicular contact dermatitis to tocopheryl linoleate in cosmetics. Swiss Contact Dermatitis Research Group. *Dermatology*. 1994;189:225.

47. Bendich A, Machlin LJ. Safety of oral intake of vitamin E. *Am J Clin Nutr*. 1988;48:612.

48. Kappus H, Diplock AT. Tolerance and safety of vitamin E: A toxicological position report. *Free Radic Biol Med*. 1992;13:55.

49. Bendich A. Safety issues regarding the use of vitamin supplements. *Ann N Y Acad Sci*. 1992;669:300.

50. Petry JJ. Surgically significant nutritional supplements. *Plast Reconstr Surg*. 1996;97:233.

51. Zondlo Fiume M. Final report on the safety assessment of Tocopherol, Tocopheryl Acetate, Tocopheryl Linoleate, Tocopheryl Linoleate/Oleate, Tocopheryl Nicotinate, Tocopheryl Succinate, Dioleyl Tocopheryl Methylsilanol, Potassium Ascorbyl Tocopheryl Phosphate, and Tocophersolan. *Int J Toxicol*. 2002;21(Suppl 3):51.

52. Sundram K, Sambanthamurthi R, Tan YA. Palm fruit chemistry and nutrition. *Asia Pac J Clin Nutr*. 2003;12:355.

53. Persson UM, Azar C. Preserving the world's topical forest—a price on carbon may not do. *Environ Sci Technol*. 2010;44:210.

54. Wilcove DS, Koh LP. Addressing the threats to biodiversity from oil-palm agriculture. *Biodivers Conserv*. 2010;19:999.

55. Koh LP, Wilcove DS. Is oil palm agriculture really destroying tropical biodiversity? *Conserv Lett*. 2008;1:60.

56. Rudel TK, Defries R, Asner GP, et al. Changing drivers of deforestation and new opportunities for conservation. *Conserv Biol*. 2009;23:1396.

57. Krol ES, Kramer-Strickland KA, Liebler DC. Photoprotective actions of topically applied vitamin E. *Drug Metab Rev*. 2000;32:413.

58. Lin JY, Selim MA, Shea CR, et al. UV photoprotection by combination topical antioxidants vitamin C and vitamin E. *J Am Acad Dermatol*. 2003;48:866.

59. Chan AC. Partners in defense, vitamin E and vitamin C. *Can J Physiol Pharmacol*. 1993;71:725.

60. Lin FH, Lin JY, Gupta RD, et al. Ferulic acid stabilizes a solution of vitamins C and E and doubles its photoprotection of skin. *J Invest Dermatol*. 2005;125:826.

61. Burke KE. Interaction of vitamins C and E as better cosmeceuticals. *Dermatol Ther*. 2007;20:314.

62. Alberts DS, Goldman R, Xu MJ, et al. Disposition and metabolism of topically administered alpha-tocopherol acetate: A common ingredient of commercially available sunscreens and cosmetics. *Nutr Cancer*. 1996;26:193.

63. Gensler HL, Aickin M, Peng YM, et al. Importance of the form of topical vitamin E for prevention of photocarcinogenesis. *Nutr Cancer*. 1996;26:183.

64. Tanaka H, Okada T, Konishi H, et al. The effect of reactive oxygen species on the biosynthesis of collagen and glycosaminoglycans in cultured human dermal fibroblasts. *Arch Dermatol Res*. 1993;285:352.

65. Diplock AT, Xu G, Yeow C, et al. Relationship of tocopherol structure to biological activity, tissue uptake, and prostaglandin synthesis. In: Diplock AT, Machlin LJ, Packer L, et al. eds. *Vitamin E: Biochemistry and Health Implications*. New York: New York Academy of Sciences; 1989:72-84.

66. Palmieri B, Gozzi G, Palmieri G. Vitamin E added silicone gel sheets for treatment of hypertrophic scars and keloids. *Int J Dermatol*. 1995;34:506.

67. Trevithick JR, Xiong H, Lee S, et al. Topical tocopherol acetate reduces post-UVB, sunburn-associated erythema, edema, and skin sensitivity in hairless mice. *Arch Biochem Biophys*. 1992;296:575.

68. Bissett DL, Chatterjee R, Hannon DP. Photoprotective effect of superoxide-scavenging antioxidants against ultraviolet radiation-induced chronic skin damage in the hairless mouse. *Photodermatol Photoimmunol Photomed*. 1990;7:56.

69. Darr D, Combs S, Dunston S, et al. Topical vitamin C protects porcine skin from ultraviolet radiation-induced damage. *Br J Dermatol*. 1992;127:247.

70. Pathak MA, Carbonare MD. Photoaging and the role of mammalian skin superoxide dismutase and antioxidants. *Photochem Photobiol*. 1988;47:7S.

71. Pinnell SR, Murad S. Vitamin C and collagen metabolism. In: Kligman AM, Takase Y, eds. *Cutaneous Aging*. Tokyo: University of Tokyo Press; 1988:275-292.

72. Bissett DL, Majeti S, Fu JJ, et al. Protective effect of topically applied conjugated hexadienes against ultraviolet radiation-induced chronic skin damage in the hairless mouse. *Photodermatol Photoimmunol Photomed*. 1990;7:63.

73. Gensler HL, Magdaleno M. Topical vitamin E inhibition of immunosuppression and tumorigenesis induced by ultraviolet irradiation. *Nutr Cancer*. 1991;15:97.

74. Jurkiewicz BA, Bissett DL, Buettner GR. Effect of topically applied tocopherol on ultraviolet radiation-mediated free radical damage in skin. *J Invest Dermatol*. 1995;104:484.

75. Slaga TJ, Bracken WM. The effects of antioxidants on skin tumor initiation and aryl hydrocarbon hydroxylase. *Cancer Res*. 1977;37:1631.

76. Meydani SN, Barklund MP, Liu S, et al. Vitamin E supplementation enhances cell-mediated immunity in healthy elderly subjects. *Am J Clin Nutr*. 1990;52:557.

77. Cho HS, Lee MH, Lee JW, et al. Anti-wrinkling effects of the mixture of vitamin C, vitamin E, pycnogenol and evening primrose oil, and molecular mechanisms on hairless mouse skin caused by chronic ultraviolet B irradiation. *Photodermatol Photoimmunol Photomed*. 2007;23:155.

78. Knekt P, Aromaa A, Maatela J, et al. Vitamin E and cancer prevention. *Am J Clin Nutr*. 1991;53:283S.

79. Menkes MS, Comstock GW, Vuilleumier JP, et al. Serum beta-carotene, vitamins A and E, selenium, and the risk of lung cancer. *N Engl J Med*. 1986;315:1250.

80. Chevance M, Brubacher G, Herbeth B, et al. Immunological and nutritional status among the elderly. In: Chandra RK, eds. *Nutrition, Immunity, and Illness in the Elderly*. New York: Pergamon Press; 1985:137-142.

81. Mayer P. The effects of vitamin E on the skin. *Cosmet Toiletries*. 1993;108:99.

82. Chung JH, Seo JY, Lee MK, et al. Ultraviolet modulation of human macrophage metalloelastase in human skin in vivo. *J Invest Dermatol*. 2002;119:507.

83. Werninghaus K, Meydani M, Bhawan J, et al. Evaluation of the photoprotective effect of oral vitamin E supplementation. *Arch Dermatol*. 1994;130:1257.

84. Greul AK, Grundmann JU, Heinrich F, et al. Photoprotection of UV-irradiated human skin: An antioxidative combination of vitamins E and C, carotenoids, selenium and proanthocyanidins. *Skin Pharmacol Appl Skin Physiol*. 2002;15:307.

85. Passi S, De Pita O, Grandinetti M, et al. The combined use of oral and topical lipophilic antioxidants increases their levels both in sebum and stratum corneum. *Biofactors*. 2003;18:289.

86. Burgess C. Topical vitamins. *J Drugs Dermatol*. 2008;7:s2.

87. Sorg O, Tran C, Saurat JH. Cutaneous vitamins A and E in the context of ultraviolet- or chemically-induced oxidative stress. *Skin Pharmacol Appl Skin Physiol*. 2001;14:363.

88. Foote JA, Ranger-Moore JR, Einspahr JG, et al. Chemoprevention of human actinic keratoses by topical DL-alpha-tocopherol. *Cancer Prev Res (Phila)*. 2009;2:394.

89. Ritter EF, Axelrod M, Minn KW, et al. Modulation of ultraviolet light-induced epidermal damage: Beneficial effects of tocopherol. *Plast Reconstr Surg*. 1997;100:973.

90. Darr D, Dunston S, Faust H, et al. Effectiveness of antioxidants (vitamin C and E) with and without sunscreens as topical photoprotectants. *Acta Derm Venereol*. 1996;76:264.

91. Bissett DL, Hillebrand GG, Hannon DP. The hairless mouse as a model of skin photoaging: Its use to evaluate photoprotective materials. *Photodermatol*. 1989;6:228.

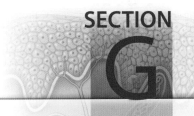

CHAPTER 57

Coenzyme Q$_{10}$

Activities:

Antioxidant, anti-inflammatory, antiaging, ATP energy producing

Important Chemical Components:

Also known as ubiquinone or 2,3-dimethoxy-5-methyl-6-decaprenyl-1,4-benzoquinone. Its molecular formula is $C_{59}H_{90}O_4$.

Origin Classification:

This nutrient or vitamin-like compound is found in most eukaryotic cells in the human body.[1] It is also synthesized for oral supplementation and topical application.

Personal Care Category:

Antiaging, moisturizing

Recommended for the following Baumann Skin Types:

DRNW, DRPW, DSNW, DSPW, ORNW, ORPW, OSNW, and OSPW

SOURCE

Coenzyme Q$_{10}$ (CoQ$_{10}$) is a fat-soluble compound found in all cells in the lipophilic portion of the cell membrane. It is the only lipid-soluble antioxidant synthesized endogenously and, as such, is not a vitamin.[2] CoQ$_{10}$ acts as a cofactor in numerous biological processes and contributes to the electron transfer chain responsible for energy production, playing an essential role for electron transport in the mitochondrial respiratory chain (Table 57-1).[3] CoQ$_{10}$ is thought to contribute 95 percent of the body's adenosine triphosphate (ATP) or energy needs.[4] It also plays a critical role in endogenous free radical scavenging.[1] In addition to its natural presence in human cells, CoQ$_{10}$ can be obtained through the diet, with fish and shellfish known to be good sources. As a supplement, the recommended oral dose is 90 to 150 mg daily, though some doctors recommend 200 to 400 mg daily. CoQ$_{10}$ has a caffeine-like effect and therefore supplements should be taken in the morning to prevent insomnia.

TABLE 57-1
Pros and Cons of Coenzyme Q$_{10}$

PROS	CONS
Plays integral role in electron transport in the mitochondrial respiratory chain	More clinical studies are needed to substantiate reported capacity to prevent DNA damage
Potent antioxidant	Formulation is often yellow
Acts as a network antioxidant, as it recycles vitamins C and E[12]	Expensive
Does not negatively affect other ingredients	
Well tolerated with a low risk of sensitivity	

HISTORY

CoQ$_{10}$ and related compounds have, as Hoppe et al. suggested, developed with biological evolution through millions of years.[5] It is now known to be widely distributed among humans and animals.[6] But CoQ$_{10}$ was first discovered by Crane et al. in 1957, when they identified and isolated the compound from beef heart mitochondria.[7] The chemical structure was subsequently determined and Peter Mitchell elucidated the role of CoQ$_{10}$ in oxidative phosphorylation and the electron transport chain in 1961, work for which he was awarded the Nobel Prize in Chemistry in 1978.[8] A great deal of the literature since that period, and stemming from seminal work by Folkers and Littarru in 1972 on the role of CoQ$_{10}$ deficiency in human heart disease, has focused on its oral administration for atherosclerosis, muscle contractility, congestive heart failure, and other cardiovascular issues.[2,9,10] A year earlier, Littarru, Folkers, and colleagues reported on CoQ$_{10}$ deficiency in the gingival tissue of adults with periodontal disease.[11] In recent years, the potential application of CoQ$_{10}$ in the treatment of various health conditions, including neurodegenerative disorders such as Parkinson's disease and Huntington's disease, migraine headaches, memory loss, inflammation, and skin aging has garnered considerable research attention.[9,12]

CHEMISTRY

CoQ$_{10}$ is a 1,4-benzoquinone compound. It is also known as ubidecarenone as well as ubiquinone, because it is known to be ubiquitous in all biological systems.[12,13] The "Q" in CoQ$_{10}$ refers to its inclusion in the quinone family; the "10" identifies the number of isoprenoid units on its side chain, a number that renders the compound highly lipophilic.[14] Its chemical structure consists of a p-benzoquinone ring with a polyisoprenoid side chain.[14] The biosynthesis of CoQ$_{10}$, which primarily involves 4-hydroxybenzoate and the polyprenyl chain,[6] is a complex process that depends on an abundance of essential amino acids, such as tyrosine, and numerous vitamins and trace elements. Several studies on the use of CoQ$_{10}$ in cardiology appear in the literature,[15] and CoQ$_{10}$ has also been found to exhibit antioxidant properties, with the reduced form of CoQ$_{10}$ (ubiquinol, Q$_{10}$H$_2$) known to be particularly effective as an antioxidant in biological membranes.[3] In its oxidized state, as ubiquinone, CoQ$_{10}$ can accept electrons from free radicals but not donate them.[9] Multiple *in vitro* and *in vivo* studies suggest that CoQ$_{10}$ imparts protective effects on various markers of oxidative DNA damage and genomic stability.[3] CoQ$_{10}$ has also exhibited a direct antiatherogenic effect in a mouse model.[2]

In addition, CoQ$_{10}$ has been demonstrated to influence the production of some key cutaneous proteins and to reduce the expression of some matrix metalloproteinases (MMPs) such as collagenase.[8] Further, it has been shown to regenerate another potent lipophilic antioxidant, α-tocopherol.[6] The ability to synthesize CoQ$_{10}$ endogenously declines after the age of 35 to 40, as does the quantity of CoQ$_{10}$ in human sebum, deficiencies which can be exacerbated by poor eating habits, stress, and infection; therefore, supplementation is thought to contribute to various health metrics to compensate for the reduced CoQ$_{10}$ levels that emerge with age.[1,16]

ORAL USES

Commercial CoQ$_{10}$ has the reputation of poor intestinal absorption.[17] Bhagavan and Chopra showed that total plasma CoQ$_{10}$ and net increase over baseline CoQ$_{10}$ concentrations gradually rise with increasing doses of orally ingested CoQ$_{10}$, with the absorption efficiency declining with increasing dose.[12] Extended supplementation of CoQ$_{10}$ in humans has been shown by Ashida et al. to diminish periocular wrinkle formation. Daily oral supplementation with CoQ$_{10}$ (0, 1, 100 mg/kg p.o.) for two weeks in adult hairless mice has also been associated with significantly higher levels of CoQ$_{10}$ in the epidermis, but not in the dermis. The researchers speculated that this might be a precondition for wrinkle reduction and other benefits related to the potent antioxidant and energizing effects of CoQ$_{10}$ in skin.[18] Notably, CoQ$_{10}$ is known to be present in humans at 10-fold higher levels in the epidermis than the dermis.[19]

In 2010, López et al. studied the *in vitro* effects of CoQ$_{10}$, CoQ$_2$, the synthetic CoQ$_{10}$ analog idebenone (see Chapter 61, Idebenone), and vitamin C, finding that primary CoQ$_{10}$ deficiencies can be treated sufficiently with CoQ$_{10}$ supplementation but not with short-tail analogs (e.g., idebenone and CoQ$_2$).[20] Oral supplementation with CoQ$_{10}$ has gained in popularity in recent years and such dietary supplements are readily available.[12]

TOPICAL USES

In an early study of the topical application of CoQ$_{10}$, Giovannini et al. suspended CoQ$_{10}$ in olive oil and administered it to rats at two different concentrations. Subsequent CoQ$_{10}$ levels were directly proportional to the concentrations and contact times. They concluded that the topical use of CoQ$_{10}$ might warrant consideration for use in the dermatologic realm.[21]

In 1999, Hoppe et al. showed that CoQ$_{10}$ penetrated into the viable layers of the epidermis, and lowered oxidation levels as measured by weak photon emission. They also measured decreases in wrinkle depth after CoQ$_{10}$ application. Further, the researchers observed that the antioxidant inhibited the expression of collagenase in human dermal fibroblasts after ultraviolet (UV) A exposure and prevented oxidative DNA damage as well as UVA-mediated oxidative stress in keratinocytes. The investigators considered their findings good evidence that CoQ$_{10}$ displays the capacity to prevent several sequelae of photoaging.[5]

In 2003, Passi et al. set out to ascertain the combined effect of topical and oral lipophilic antioxidants on the antioxidant content of sebum and the stratum corneum (SC). For two months, 50 female volunteers, aged 21 to 40, were treated daily on the face and back with a base cream containing CoQ$_{10}$, vitamin E, and squalene. To half of the volunteers, an oral preparation including the same ingredients was administered. While the daily topical application resulted in a significant boost in the levels of the lipophilic antioxidants and squalene in the sebum without affecting SC or plasma concentrations, the concomitant oral administration in the one group led to significantly higher lipophilic antioxidant measurements in the SC and plasma but no such increase in sebum levels. The investigators concluded that topically applying the antioxidants raised their levels in sebum and concomitant oral administration increased CoQ$_{10}$ and vitamin E levels in the SC as well.[16,22]

In 2010, Liu and Artmann conducted a double-blind, parallel-design, controlled, single-dose (120 mg) bioavailability study in 20 healthy male and female volunteers to compare a novel colloidal-Q$_{10}$ delivery system based on new and patented technology with three commercially available CoQ$_{10}$ products. The colloidal-Q$_{10}$ formulation was associated with the highest plasma concentrations throughout the 24-hour period along with the greatest relative bioavailability, with statistically significant differences seen in both metrics. The researchers concluded that their novel CoQ$_{10}$ delivery system enhanced enteral absorption and bioavailability.[17]

Also that year, Lee and Tsai demonstrated the efficacy of a liposomal formulation of soybean phosphatidylcholine and α-tocopherol to encapsulate CoQ$_{10}$ for topical delivery. They found that it augmented CoQ$_{10}$ accumulation in rat skin over twofold in comparison with an unencapsulated suspension. In addition, lengthening the treatment time and elevating CoQ$_{10}$ content in the formulation increased CoQ$_{10}$ levels in rat skin, with inadequate treatment time limiting accumulation. The investigators concluded that their liposomal CoQ$_{10}$ formulation shows promise as a topical delivery agent for CoQ$_{10}$ given sufficient treatment duration.[14] It is important to note that topical products containing CoQ$_{10}$ as the main ingredient should appear to have a yellow tint.

In 2010, Yue et al. developed a novel CoQ$_{10}$ topical delivery system using a nano-structured lipid carrier to enhance photoprotection. The *in vitro* protection of fibroblasts against UVA radiation afforded by a CoQ$_{10}$-loaded nano-structured lipid carrier (CoQ$_{10}$-NLC) was greater than that provided by a CoQ$_{10}$ emulsion. In cells treated with CoQ$_{10}$-NLC, malondialdehyde concentration was reduced by 61.5 percent as compared to the CoQ$_{10}$ emulsion cells. The presence of CoQ$_{10}$-NLC also yielded significant increases in the antioxidant enzymes superoxide dismutase and glutathione peroxidase. CoQ$_{10}$-NLC also exhibited better penetration into the SC and dermis after topical application in Sprague-Dawley rats as compared to the CoQ$_{10}$ emulsion.[23]

In 2012, Gokce et al. investigated CoQ$_{10}$-loaded liposomes and solid lipid nanoparticles as delivery systems of the compound for antioxidant purposes into the skin, finding that the liposome system exhibited the capacity to promote cell proliferation and the solid lipid nanoparticle system failed to protect against the accumulation of reactive oxygen species.[24]

Felippi et al. conducted a pilot study in 2012 on the safety and efficacy of a nanoparticle formulation encapsulating various active ingredients, including CoQ_{10}, retinyl palmitate, tocopheryl acetate, grape seed oil, and linseed oil. The nanoparticles demonstrated no irritating, sensitizing, or comedogenic properties and phototoxicity was not evident after exposure to UVA light. In the efficacy assessment with volunteers, significant decreases in wrinkles were observed as compared to controls after 21 days of treatment. The investigators concluded that the antioxidant-loaded nanoparticle formulation is safe for topical administration and, having displayed *in vivo* antiaging activity, warrants consideration as a cosmetic agent for such purposes.[25]

In 2013, Chen et al. formulated a CoQ_{10}-NLC using high-pressure microfluidics and assessed it *in vitro* for epidermal targeting effects. The CoQ_{10}-NLC displayed fast release through the first three hours and extended release subsequently. The accumulation of CoQ_{10} in rat epidermis was over 10-fold higher with the CoQ_{10}-NLC as compared to a CoQ_{10} emulsion in an *in vitro* skin permeation study. Further, the CoQ_{10} level in CoQ_{10}-NLC fell 5.59 percent as compared to reductions of 24.61 percent in the CoQ_{10} emulsion and 49.74 percent in a CoQ_{10} ethanol solution after 24 hours of UV exposure. The investigators concluded that their CoQ_{10}-NLC formulation demonstrated a significant epidermal targeting effect, establishing itself as a potential carrier for the topical application of CoQ_{10}.[26]

Recent *in vivo* studies have shown reductions in the symptoms of photoaging through the use of topically applied CoQ_{10}, though bioavailability of CoQ_{10} has remained poor.[14] In 1999, Blatt et al. showed through *in vivo* studies that the long-term application of CoQ_{10} could reduce crow's feet.[27]

CoQ_{10} in Combination Therapy

In 2009, Kharaeva et al. assessed the clinical effects of supplementation of a combination of CoQ_{10}, vitamin E, and selenium in the treatment of 58 patients with severe erythrodermic and arthropathic psoriasis. Patients were randomized into four groups with two groups receiving the antioxidant combination dissolved in soy lecithin for 30 to 35 days. The placebo groups received soy lecithin. The investigators reported that supplementation yielded significant improvements in clinical conditions, correlating with a quicker normalization of oxidative stress markers as compared to the placebo groups. They concluded that the use of these antioxidants merits consideration for managing severe psoriasis.[28]

Several of the same investigators conducted two controlled clinical trials in 2012 to compare a nutraceutical approach to standard therapy for two mucocutaneous chronic DNA-virus infections. The nutraceutical, containing CoQ_{10}, vitamin E, selenium, and methionine, or a placebo was administered for 180 days to 68 patients with relapsing human papillomavirus skin warts treated with cryotherapy in the first trial. In the second trial, the combination of acyclovir followed by 90 days of nutraceutical administration was compared to acyclovir alone in 60 patients with recurrent herpes or 29 patients with herpes zoster. The nutraceutical was found to provoke significantly more rapid healing with lower relapse incidence in comparison to control groups. In addition, plasma antioxidant capacity was found to be higher in the nutraceutical group as compared to controls.[29]

SAFETY ISSUES

Oral CoQ_{10} supplementation can elicit nervousness or a jittery feeling not unlike one of the side effects of caffeine. CoQ_{10} should be taken during the day to reduce the risk of causing insomnia. Other reported side effects include appetite loss, diarrhea, and mild nausea.[30] Overall, the safety of orally administered CoQ_{10}, even at high doses (up to 900 mg/day), has been established.[17,31] No contact dermatitis or any other side effects have been associated with the topical application of CoQ_{10}, which is photostable and well tolerated.[5] However, the synthetic analog of CoQ_{10}, known as idebenone, has been reported to cause contact dermatitis (see Chapter 61, Idebenone).

ENVIRONMENTAL IMPACT

There is no environmental impact of commercial CoQ_{10} production known by the author.

FORMULATION CONSIDERATIONS

Low aqueous solubility and the high molecular weight of this compound limit the topical delivery of CoQ_{10} to deeper skin layers.[24,32] It is a lipophilic compound and to increase penetration must be formulated in liposomes and other formulations designed to increase penetration. Orally ingested solubilized formulations of CoQ_{10} (both ubiquinone and ubiquinol, the predominant form – 95 percent – of circulating CoQ_{10}) exhibit superior bioavailability to nonsolubilized powder-based products as indicated by their enhanced plasma CoQ_{10} responses.[12]

USAGE CONSIDERATIONS

CoQ_{10} is stable in topical formulations. It does not, to the author's knowledge, interact with other ingredients in a skin care regimen. Products that contain a significant amount of CoQ_{10} appear yellow.

SIGNIFICANT BACKGROUND

Reduced levels of CoQ_{10} in humans have been associated with aging as well as with various pathologies (e.g., cardiac disorders, neurodegenerative diseases, AIDS, and cancer).[6,16]

Network Antioxidants

Vitamin C and CoQ_{10} exhibit the ability to recycle vitamin E, donating electrons to return vitamin E to its antioxidant state. The antioxidants identified as acting cooperatively in this fashion have been called network antioxidants.[33] The five compounds designated as network antioxidants are vitamins C and E, glutathione, lipoic acid, and CoQ_{10}. Network antioxidants are a staple in cosmetic preparations, but it is likely that many antioxidants work synergistically, and that the expression "network antioxidant" is actually applicable to many more antioxidants than the five identified as the "network." For example, in 2013, Wölfle et al. demonstrated that the addition of low concentrations of antioxidants such as CoQ_{10} and vitamin E synergistically amplified the potent antioxidant and photoprotective activity of the flavonoid luteolin in solar simulator-irradiated human skin fibroblasts.[34] One of the same researchers previously demonstrated that a topically applied cream containing luteolin, CoQ$_{10}$, and vitamin E, in the same ratio as in the *in vitro* study (4:4:1, luteolin, vitamin E, CoQ$_{10}$, respectively), was effective in protecting the skin from chemical-induced irritation.[35]

Antiaging Activity

An age-related decline of CoQ$_{10}$ levels has been reported in animals and humans.[36] Consequently, the antioxidant activities of CoQ$_{10}$ have been targeted for potential applications in treating aged skin. Hoppe et al. showed that CoQ$_{10}$ penetrated into the viable layers of the skin and significantly inhibited collagenase expression in human dermal fibroblasts following UVA exposure.[5]

In 2006, Fuller et al. found that CoQ$_{10}$ has the capacity to inhibit the inflammatory response in dermal fibroblasts induced by UV radiation (UVR) or interleukin (IL)-1. In addition, they observed that CoQ$_{10}$ suppressed UVR-induced MMP-1 synthesis. In combination with the colorless carotenoids phytoene and phytofluene, CoQ$_{10}$ enhanced inflammation suppression. The investigators concluded that combining CoQ$_{10}$ and carotenoids in a topical skin care formulation may render dual protection against photoaging and inflammation.[9]

In 2008, Prahl et al. took skin biopsies of young and old donors and observed marked age-dependent differences in the mitochondrial function of the sampled keratinocytes. This led them to conclude that aging skin is functionally anaerobic, conducted mainly through a nonmitochondrial pathway. They suggested that the topical application of CoQ$_{10}$ quickly enhances mitochondrial function in skin *in vivo*, thus conferring antiaging activity.[37] Insofar as CoQ$_{10}$ preserves mitochondrial functioning, thus contributing to energy level maintenance, it acts to prevent aging skin from employing anaerobic energy production mechanisms.[8]

Inui et al. demonstrated *in vitro* that UVB-induced IL-6 production of normal human keratinocytes was reduced in the presence of CoQ$_{10}$. MMP-1 synthesis of cultured fibroblasts was also significantly diminished. In the investigators' clinical study of 31 female subjects aged 27 to 61 years, 1 percent CoQ$_{10}$ cream used for five months resulted in wrinkle score decreases as noted by a dermatologist. They concluded that CoQ$_{10}$ appears to rejuvenate wrinkled skin by virtue of suppressing IL-6 production, which spurs fibroblasts in the dermis to upregulate MMP production thus contributing to dermal fiber degradation.[38,39]

In an *in vitro* study in 2012, Zhang et al. considered the effects of CoQ$_{10}$ on primary human dermal fibroblasts. They showed that CoQ$_{10}$ exerted a broad array of effects in embryonic and adult cells, including the spurring of fibroblast proliferation, augmenting type IV collagen expression, and lowering the levels of MMPs induced by UV radiation. CoQ$_{10}$ also dose-dependently fostered elastin gene expression in cultured fibroblasts and markedly reduced IL-1α synthesis in keratinocytes induced by UVR. In addition, they found that the antioxidant inhibited tyrosinase activity similarly to ascorbic acid, suggesting the potential for imparting depigmenting effects. Overall, they concluded that CoQ$_{10}$ demonstrated activity against intrinsic aging as well as photoaging.[40]

Coenzyme Q$_{10}$ and Skin Cancer

Patients with breast, lung, or pancreatic cancer have been found to have abnormally low plasma levels of CoQ$_{10}$.[41] A study by Rusciani et al. examined the usefulness of CoQ$_{10}$ plasma levels in predicting the risk of metastasis and the length of the metastasis-free interval in melanoma patients. They found that CoQ$_{10}$ levels were significantly lower in melanoma patients than in control subjects and in patients who experienced metastases as compared to the metastasis-free subgroup. The investigators concluded that baseline plasma CoQ$_{10}$ levels can serve as a prognostic factor to estimate the risk for melanoma progression.[42]

Large quantities of ATP are essential for an immune response initiated by interferon (IFN) to be effective in the adjuvant therapy of melanoma. Accordingly, some have theorized that the failure of some patients to respond to IFN therapy may be the result of an inability to meet the excess demand for ATP engendered by this medication. However, CoQ$_{10}$ is known to play a significant role in the mitochondrial respiratory cycle and ATP synthesis.[43,44] In 2007, Rusciani et al. conducted a clinical trial in stages I and II melanoma patients investigating a postsurgical adjuvant therapy with recombinant IFN α-2b combined with CoQ$_{10}$ vs. IFN α-2b alone for the control group. In the three-year trial, reported in 2007, patients were given twice-daily administrations of low-dose recombinant IFN α-2b and CoQ$_{10}$ (400 mg/day). The control group received only low-dose recombinant IFN α-2b in the same dosage and administration. Treatment efficacy was assessed as incidence of recurrences at five years. The risk of developing metastases was found to be about 10 times lower in the IFN + CoQ$_{10}$ patients compared with the IFN-alone group.[45] A 10-year follow-up will be needed to yield more significant results.

Gingivitis and Retinopathy

CoQ$_{10}$ has garnered attention for an increasingly broad array of health conditions. In 2012, Chatterjee et al. conducted a randomized, controlled split-mouth trial with 30 subjects with plaque-induced gingivitis to identify the effects of a solitary application of CoQ$_{10}$ after 28 days. Significant reductions in gingivitis, bleeding, and plaque scores were observed in areas where the antioxidant was topically applied.[46]

That same year, Hans et al. performed a split-mouth clinical evaluation of topically applied CoQ$_{10}$, in the form of Perio-Q gel, in 12 patients with chronic gingivitis and periodontitis. The CoQ$_{10}$ gel was associated with similar clinical results to subgingival mechanical debridement. The researchers concluded that there was insufficient clinical support to indicate the superiority of the gel to basic mechanical approaches, but suggested the potential additive effect of CoQ$_{10}$ while calling for long-term clinical studies to assess the antioxidant.[47] Previously, Hanioka et al., in a study with 10 male patients in whom 30 periodontal pockets were selected for examination, observed that the topical application of CoQ$_{10}$ ameliorated adult periodontitis alone as well as in combination with traditional nonsurgical treatment.[48]

Topical applications of CoQ$_{10}$ have also been emerging in the ophthalmologic armamentarium. For example, Lulli et al. showed that CoQ$_{10}$ eye drops protected retinal cells from apoptosis in a mouse model of kainite-induced retinal damage, prompting them to conclude that topical CoQ$_{10}$ be further considered for apoptosis-driven retinopathy therapies.[49]

In a 2011 investigation of the potential of N-trimethyl chitosan (TMC)-coated liposomes containing CoQ$_{10}$ as an ophthalmic drug delivery system, Wang et al. found that CoQ$_{10}$ concentration-dependently raised the viability of human lens epithelial cells and lowered oxidative damage. They concluded that the CoQ$_{10}$-containing liposomes were effective in protecting human lens epithelial cells against hydrogen peroxide-induced oxidative harm and appear to have potential as a suitable ophthalmic drug delivery agent.[50]

In 2013, Fogagnolo et al. assessed the postoperative effects of topical CoQ$_{10}$ (and vitamin E D-α-tocopheryl polyethylene glycol 1,000) in 40 consecutive patients who were randomized to receive

CoQ$_{10}$ or saline solution twice daily for nine months after uneventful cataract surgery with a temporal port. They found that the antioxidant contributed to restoring the anatomy of the subbasal nerve plexus of the cornea as well as ocular surface stability.[51]

CONCLUSION

CoQ$_{10}$, like melatonin (see Chapter 62, Melatonin), is intriguing insofar as it is found naturally in humans, plays multiple biological roles, and is associated with age-related decline. Indeed, the increased cellular oxidation seen with age may be due, in part, to a decrease in the endogenous synthesis of such antioxidants. Both antioxidants also appear to engage other antioxidants synergistically and are associated with multiple benefits when supplied exogenously through oral supplementation or topical administration. There is a wealth of research on the role of endogenous CoQ$_{10}$ in the human body and the broad effects of oral administration of this essential substance. While the body of research on the topical administration of CoQ$_{10}$ is not scant by any means, there remains the need for more randomized, double-blind, placebo-controlled trials, preferably on a larger scale than has been seen thus far, to clearly delineate its potential in the dermatologic armamentarium. The potential for CoQ$_{10}$ does appear to be vast, though.

REFERENCES

1. Hojerová J. Coenzyme Q10 – Its importance, properties and use in nutrition and cosmetics. *Ceska Slov Farm*. 2000;49:119.
2. Littarru GP, Tiano L. Bioenergetic and antioxidant properties of coenzyme Q10: Recent developments. *Mol Biotechnol*. 2007;37:31.
3. Schmelzer C, Döring F. Micronutrient special issue: Coenzyme Q(10) requirements for DNA damage prevention. *Mutat Res*. 2012;733:61.
4. Ernster L, Dallner G. Biochemical, physiological and medical aspects of ubiquinone function. *Biochim Biophys Acta*. 1995;1271:195.
5. Hoppe U, Bergemann J, Diembeck W, et al. Coenzyme Q10, a cutaneous antioxidant and energizer. *Biofactors*. 1999;9:371.
6. Siemieniuk E, Skrzydlewska E. Coenzyme Q10: Its biosynthesis and biological significance in animal organisms and in humans. *Postepy Hig Med Dosw (Online)*. 2005;59:150.
7. Crane FL, Hatefi Y, Lester RL, et al. Isolation of a quinone from beef heart mitochondria. *Biochim Biophys Acta*. 1957;25:220.
8. Blatt T, Littarru GP. Biochemical rationale and experimental data on the antiaging properties of CoQ(10) at skin level. *Biofactors*. 2011;37:381.
9. Fuller B, Smith D, Howerton A, et al. Anti-inflammatory effects of CoQ10 and colorless carotenoids. *J Cosmet Dermatol*. 2006;5:30.
10. Folkers K, Littarru GP, Ho L, et al. Evidence for a deficiency of coenzyme Q10 in human heart disease. *Int Z Vitaminforsch*. 1970;40:380.
11. Littarru GP, Nakamura R, Ho L, et al. Deficiency of coenzyme Q10 in gingival tissue from patients with periodontal disease. *Proc Natl Acad Sci U S A*. 1971;68:2332.
12. Bhagavan HN, Chopra RK. Plasma coenzyme Q10 response to oral ingestion of coenzyme Q10 formulations. *Mitochondrion*. 2007;7(Suppl):S78.
13. Hoffmann D. *Medical Herbalism: The Science and Practice of Herbal Medicine*. Rochester, VT: Healing Arts Press; 2003:167.
14. Lee WC, Tsai TH. Preparation and characterization of liposomal coenzyme Q10 for in vivo topical application. *Int J Pharm*. 2010;395:78.
15. Greenberg S, Frishman WH. Co-enzyme Q10: A new drug for cardiovascular disease. *J Clin Pharmacol*. 1990;30:596.
16. Passi S, De Pità O, Puddu P, et al. Lipophilic antioxidants in human sebum and aging. *Free Radic Res*. 2002;36:471.
17. Liu ZX, Artmann C. Relative bioavailability comparison of different coenzyme Q10 formulations with a novel delivery system. *Altern Ther Health Med*. 2009;15:42.
18. Ashida Y, Yamanishi H, Terada T, et al CoQ10 supplementation elevates the epidermal CoQ10 level in adult hairless mice. *Biofactors*. 2005;25:175.
19. Shindo Y, Witt E, Han D, et al. Enzymic and non-enzymic antioxidants in epidermis and dermis of human skin. *J Invest Dermatol*. 1994;102:122.
20. López LC, Quinzii CM, Area E, et al. Treatment of CoQ(10) deficient fibroblasts with ubiquinone, CoQ analogs, and vitamin C: Time- and compound-dependent effects. *PLoS One*. 2010;5(7):e11897.
21. Giovannini L, Bertelli AA, Scalori V, et al. Skin penetration of CoQ10 in the rat. *Int J Tissue React*. 1988;10:103.
22. Passi S, De Pità O, Grandinetti M, et al. The combined use of oral and topical lipophilic antioxidants increases their levels both in sebum and stratum corneum. *Biofactors*. 2003;18:289.
23. Yue Y, Zhou H, Liu G, et al. The advantages of a novel CoQ10 delivery system in skin photo-protection. *Int J Pharm*. 2010;392:57.
24. Gokce EH, Korkmaz E, Tuncay-Tanriverdi S, et al. A comparative evaluation of coenzyme Q10-loaded liposomes and solid lipid nanoparticles as dermal antioxidant carriers. *Int J Nanomedicine*. 2012;7:5109.
25. Felippi CC, Oliveira D, Ströher A, et al. Safety and efficacy of antioxidants-loaded nanoparticles for an anti-aging application. *J Biomed Nanotechnol*. 2012;8:316.
26. Chen S, Liu W, Wan J, et al. Preparation of Coenzyme Q10 nanostructured lipid carriers for epidermal targeting with high-pressure microfluidics technique. *Drug Dev Ind Pharm*. 2013;39:20.
27. Blatt T, Mundt C, Mummert C, et al. Modulation of oxidative stresses in human aging skin. *Z Gerontol Geriatr*. 1999;32:83.
28. Kharaeva Z, Gostova E, De Luca C, et al. Clinical and biochemical effects of coenzyme Q(10), vitamin E, and selenium supplementation to psoriasis patients. *Nutrition*. 2009;25:295.
29. De Luca C, Kharaeva Z, Raskovic D, et al. Coenzyme Q(10), vitamin E, selenium, and methionine in the treatment of chronic recurrent viral mucocutaneous infections. *Nutrition*. 2012;28:509.
30. Feigin A, Kieburtz K, Como P, et al. Assessment of coenzyme Q10 tolerability in Huntington's disease. *Mov Disord*. 1996;11:321.
31. Ikematsu H, Nakamura K, Harashima Sh, et al. Safety assessment of coenzyme Q10 (Kaneka Q10) in healthy subjects: A double-blind, randomized, placebo-controlled trial. *Regul Toxicol Pharmacol*. 2006;44:212.
32. Teeranachaideekul V, Souto EB, Junyaprasert VB, et al. Cetyl palmitate-based NLC for topical delivery of Coenzyme Q(10) – Development, physicochemical characterization and in vitro release studies. *Eur J Pharm Biopharm*. 2007;67:141.
33. Packer L, Colman C. *The Antioxidant Miracle*. New York: John Wiley & Sons, Inc.; 1999:9.
34. Wölfle U, Haarhaus B, Schempp CM. The photoprotective and antioxidative properties of luteolin are synergistically augmented by tocopherol and ubiquinone. *Planta Med*. 2013;79:963.
35. Schempp CM, Meinke MC, Lademann J, et al. Topical antioxidants protect the skin from chemical-induced irritation in the repetitive washing test: A placebo-controlled, double-blind study. *Contact Dermatitis*. 2012;67:234.
36. Beyer R, Ernster L. The antioxidant role of Coenzyme Q10. In: Lenaz G, Barnabei O, Rabbi A, eds. *Highlights in Ubiquinone Research*. London: Taylor & Francis; 1990:191–213.
37. Prahl S, Kueper T, Biernoth T, et al. Aging skin is functionally anaerobic: Importance of coenzyme Q10 for anti aging skin care. *Biofactors*. 2008;32:245.
38. Inui M, Ooe M, Fujii K, et al. Mechanisms of inhibitory effects of CoQ10 on UVB-induced wrinkle formation in vitro and in vivo. *Biofactors*. 2008;32:237.
39. Littarru GP, Tiano L. Clinical aspects of coenzyme Q10: An update. *Nutrition*. 2010;26:250.
40. Zhang M, Dang L, Guo F, et al. Coenzyme Q(10) enhances dermal elastin expression, inhibits IL-1α production and melanin synthesis in vitro. *Int J Cosmet Sci*. 2012;34:273.
41. Folkers K, Ostemborg A, Nylander M, et al. Activities of vitamin Q10 in animal models and serious deficiency in patients with cancer. *Biochem Biophys Res Commun*. 1997;234:296.
42. Rusciani L, Proietti I, Rusciani A, et al. Low plasma coenzyme Q10 levels as an independent prognostic factor for melanoma progression. *J Am Acad Dermatol*. 2006;54:234.
43. Crane FL. Biochemical functions of coenzyme Q10. *J Am Coll Nutr*. 2001;20:591.

44. Beyer RE, Nordenbrand K, Ernster L. The role of coenzyme Q as a mitochondrial antioxidant: A short review. In: Folkers K, Yamamura Y, eds. *Biomedical and Clinical Aspects of Coenzyme Q.* Amsterdam: The Netherlands, Elsevier Science Publishers B V (Biomedical Division); 1986:17–24.

45. Rusciani L, Proietti I, Paradisi A, et al. Recombinant interferon alpha-2b and coenzyme Q10 as a postsurgical adjuvant therapy for melanoma: A 3-year trial with recombinant interferon-alpha and 5-year follow-up. *Melanoma Res.* 2007;17:177.

46. Chatterjee A, Kandwal A, Singh N, et al. Evaluation of Co-Q10 anti-gingivitis effect on plaque induced gingivitis: A randomized controlled trial. *J Indian Soc Periodontol.* 2012;16:539.

47. Hans M, Prakash S, Gupta S. Clinical evaluation of topical application of perio-Q gel (Coenzyme Q(10)) in chronic periodontitis patients. *J Indian Soc Periodontol.* 2012;16:193.

48. Hanioka T, Tanaka M, Ojima M, et al. Effect of topical application of coenzyme Q10 on adult periodontitis. *Mol Aspects Med.* 1994;15(Suppl):s241.

49. Lulli M, Witort E, Papucci L, et al. Coenzyme Q10 instilled as eye drops on the cornea reaches the retina and protects retinal layers from apoptosis in a mouse model of kainite-induced retinal damage. *Invest Ophthalmol Vis Sci.* 2012;53:8295.

50. Wang S, Zhang J, Jiang T, et al. Protective effect of Coenzyme Q(10) against oxidative damage in human lens epithelial cells by novel ocular drug carriers. *Int J Pharm.* 2011;403:219.

51. Fogagnolo P, Sacchi M, Ceresara G, et al. The effects of topical coenzyme Q10 and vitamin E D-α-tocopheryl polyethylene glycol 1000 succinate after cataract surgery: A clinical and in vivo confocal study. *Ophthalmologica.* 2013;229:26.

CHAPTER 58

Coffeeberry

Activities:

Antioxidant, anti-inflammatory, photoprotective

Important Chemical Components:

Chlorogenic acid, caffeic acid, condensed proanthocyanidins, quinic acid, ferulic acid, *p*-coumaric acid, phenolic diterpenes (kahweol, cafestol), α-tocopherol

Origin Classification:

Coffeeberry is a legal trademark for a process of harvesting subripe fruit from the plant *Coffea arabica* and processing it to accentuate its antioxidant ingredients while eliminating microbial contaminants.[1–3] Thus, its origin is natural but marketed standardized Coffeeberry® extract products are synthesized and processed in the laboratory.

Personal Care Category:

Antiaging, moisturizing

Recommended for the following Baumann Skin Types:

DRNW, DRPW, DSNW, DSPW, ORNW, ORPW, OSNW, and OSPW

SOURCE

The coffee plant *Coffea arabica*, a member of the Rubiaceae family, is cultivated throughout the world and is, of course, a source of the globally popular beverage. Extracts of the coffee plant have been demonstrated to display antioxidant activity (Table 58-1).[4]

While much attention has been focused on coffee beans, particularly once roasted, the fruit of the coffee plant has been long ignored, and usually discarded, because it decays rapidly.[1] The fruit that grows on *C. arabica*, however, is suffused with polyphenols, especially chlorogenic acid (the primary phenolic substance in coffee), condensed proanthocyanidins, quinic acid, caffeic acid, and ferulic acid (see Chapter 53, Caffeic Acid, and Chapter 54, Ferulic Acid).[1,5,6] It is also believed to exhibit higher antioxidant activity than green tea, white tea, pomegranate, blueberries, strawberries, and raspberries (see Chapter 47, Green Tea). Polyphenols, which are secondary metabolites in plants, play an integral role in a healthy human diet, as these

TABLE 58-1
Pros and Cons of Coffeeberry

Pros	Con
Strong antioxidant activity	Dearth of clinical evidence
Superlative ORAC assay data suggest greater antioxidant potency than many standard antioxidants	

compounds are active constituents in various fruits, vegetables, grains, green and black tea, and coffee beans.[7–11] In addition, copious research during the last several years has shown that polyphenols represent a wealth of potential health benefits, typically related to anti-inflammatory and antioxidant properties. Consequently, manufacturers have targeted the activity of polyphenols for medical and cosmetic applications in several pharmaceutical and cosmeceutical products.

The Coffeeberry fruit, which is harvested subripe from the *C. arabica* plant, has been traditionally ignored, as mentioned above, but a method to translate its claimed prodigious properties has been developed and given the proprietary name Coffeeberry®. Analogous to the patented trade name for the antioxidant Pycnogenol® (see Chapter 49, Pycnogenol), derived from French maritime pine bark, Coffeeberry is a proprietary blend of antioxidants harvested from a natural botanical source.

HISTORY

C. arabica actually comes from Ethiopia and is thought to have been introduced into Arabia before or early in the 1400s, into Java before 1700, and into the West Indies as well as Central and South America in the 1700s.[12,13]

CHEMISTRY

Extracts of the beans of *C. arabica* have demonstrated antioxidant activity after roasting.[4] In addition to the beans of the coffee plant, the fruit, especially when harvested in a subripened state, also displays peak antioxidant activity.[14] This is due to its constituent polyphenols, particularly chlorogenic acid, condensed proanthocyanidins, quinic acid, caffeic acid, and ferulic acid. Indeed, polyphenols, which are also found in green, white, and black tea, various fruits, vegetables, as well as grains, are known to confer multiple health benefits, mainly due to their anti-inflammatory and antioxidant properties.[15,16]

Chlorogenic acid, an ester formed between caffeic and quinic acids (see Chapter 53, Caffeic Acid), is one of the most broadly consumed polyphenols as it is ubiquitous in food and coffee.[17] Both chlorogenic and caffeic acids have been found to inhibit ultraviolet (UV) B-induced skin tumor promotion in mouse skin.[17]

ORAL USES

The coffee plant *C. arabica* is cultivated throughout the world as the source of the widely popular coffee beverage. Only the seeds of the fruit are used to produce the popular beverage. The Coffeeberry fruit is available as an oral supplement as well as in topical cosmetic formulations.

In 2008, Ostojic et al. examined the changes in total antioxidant capacity and aerobic and anaerobic performance in 20 college athletes (14 males, 6 females) engendered by supplementation with an oral Coffeeberry formulation for four weeks. After the trial, total antioxidant capacity was significantly higher in the group supplementing with Coffeeberry as compared to the placebo group. No adverse effects were observed in either group and there were no other significant differences between the groups. The investigators concluded that Coffeeberry supplementation yielded a slight increase in antioxidant capacity, and minimal effects in terms of recovery after exercise.[18]

TOPICAL USES

The *C. arabica* plant is used in some botanical formulations intended to treat cellulite. The caffeine used in this context as an active ingredient is extracted from the leaves, however, not the berries.[19] Green *C. arabica* seed oil is also being broadly used as an ingredient in cosmetic formulations.[20] Therefore, multiple parts of the plant are now under investigation and in active use in the dermatologic realm. Preliminary data on the use of the proprietary fruit suggest that Coffeeberry extract has the potential to ameliorate overall appearance, hyperpigmentation, as well as fine lines and wrinkles.[21]

In 2008, Draelos conducted a double-blind, randomized clinical trial in 50 subjects over age 30 with mild symptoms of photoaging to assess the cutaneous benefits of Coffeeberry extract. Over the 12-week period, both groups used a Coffeeberry facial cleanser twice daily. Afterwards, one group would apply a Coffeeberry day cream in the morning and a Coffeeberry night cream in the evening to the whole face. The other group applied control creams. Compared to the control group, significant improvements were observed in the Coffeeberry extract group along all parameters considered (i.e., erythema, roughness, scaling, wrinkling, and global assessment). Transepidermal water loss decreased from baseline in the Coffeeberry group and increased in the control group. Draelos concluded that the Coffeeberry extract system of facial cleanser and morning and evening creams was well tolerated and led to significant improvements in diminishing multiple symptoms of photoaged skin.[22,23]

In a six-week pilot study conducted by McDaniel and sponsored by Stiefel Laboratories, 30 female patients (31–71 years old) with moderate actinic damage used an antioxidant system composed of 0.1 percent Coffeeberry extract facial cleanser as well as 1 percent Coffeeberry extract night and day creams (the latter of which contained octinate and oxybenzone with an SPF of 15).[14,24] Twenty subjects applied all three products to the whole face and 10 subjects applied each to half the face and vehicle on the other half. Compared to vehicle, split-face patients experienced significant improvements in fine lines and wrinkles, pigmentation, and overall appearance. Patients treated on the whole face displayed improvements in all parameters (including fine lines and wrinkles, roughness and dryness, pigmentation, and overall appearance) compared to baseline, with marked changes in pigmentation as the most salient improvement. McDaniel also reported that skin biopsies revealed that the use of Coffeeberry extract led to an increase in key structural dermal proteins (i.e., collagen types I and IV) as well as a decrease in collagenase and inflammatory mediators.[24]

In late 2010, Palmer and Kitchin reported on their 12-week, double-blind, randomized, controlled clinical usage study of the efficacy and tolerance of a new *C. arabica*-containing topical high-antioxidant skin care system (facial wash, day lotion, night cream and eye serum) to ameliorate photoaging in 40 Caucasian females. One group of participants used the test system, including twice-daily facial wash, application of the antioxidant day lotion each morning, and nightly application of the antioxidant night cream and eye serum, with the second group using the control products according to the same protocol. The authors observed statistically significant improvements in the appearance of photodamaged skin in the subjects using the test regimen.[25]

Coffeeberry extract has also been shown, in preclinical and small clinical trials, to confer protection from oxidative damage, UVB-induced pyrimidine dimer formation and inflammation, and to facilitate accelerated recovery from UVB exposure.[26]

SAFETY ISSUES

Topical products that contain *C. arabica*, or Coffeeberry extract in particular, are generally regarded as safe, though extensive data are not available.

Some safety studies have been performed on the oral use of Coffeeberry. In 2010, Heimbach et al. conducted a series of genotoxicity studies, three short-term oral toxicity studies, and a 90-day dietary toxicity study of Coffeeberry products, including a ground whole powder, a water extract, and a water-ethanol extract. None of the products exhibited genotoxic or mutagenic potential in murine peripheral cells. Although palatability issues emerged, rats displayed a tolerance for the whole powder and ethanol extracts, with females showing a higher tolerance for both. Finally, no adverse effects were seen in Sprague-Dawley rats fed the ethanol extract for 90 days at concentrations up to 5 percent.[1]

In the few preclinical or small clinical trials thus far performed, no serious adverse events have been reported as treatments have been well tolerated.[27]

ENVIRONMENTAL IMPACT

A significant environmental impact is exacted by *C. arabica* cultivation, including deforestation, water pollution and other effects of agrochemical use, soil quality degradation, loss of biodiversity, and changes in forest cover and structure.[28–32] The details and depth of the full range of actual and potential effects of industrial coffee growth as well as sustainable management approaches are beyond the scope of this text.

FORMULATION CONSIDERATIONS

Harvesting *C. arabica* fruit in a subripened state is essential to both optimize antioxidant potency and attenuate the risk of contamination with mycotoxins, which is typical later in the ripening process. The whole berry fruit is crushed and processed for its antioxidant components.[27]

USAGE CONSIDERATIONS

Coffeeberry®, a proprietary ingredient for the antioxidant derived from the fruit of *C. arabica*, is the fundamental component in the RevaléSkin™ line of cosmetic products intended to reverse various signs of photodamage and photoaging and to impart photoprotection.[33] The hydroxycinnamic acid ferulic acid, another potent antioxidant, is also an important active ingredient in these products (see Chapter 54, Ferulic Acid). In the oxygen radical absorbance capacity assay (ORAC), Coffeeberry® exhibited greater antioxidant activity than green tea, pomegranate extract, and vitamins C and E [see Chapter 55, Ascorbic Acid (Vitamin C), and Chapter 56, Tocopherol (Vitamin E)].[14] Of note, the proprietary Coffeeberry® technology associated with the cultivation, harvesting, and processing of the whole coffee fruit eliminates the risk of contamination by bacteria or fungi and the potential for generating mycotoxins.[1–3]

Antioxidant Activity

Two recent studies point to the antioxidant properties of roasted *C. arabica*. In one, in which coffee model systems were prepared from combinations of compounds, including chlorogenic acid, sucrose, and cellulose, various tests revealed that antioxidant activity exhibited a positive, nonlinear relationship with the level of chlorogenic acid, a known antioxidant, after roasting.[4]

In the other study, both *C. arabica* and *C. robusta* (*Coffea canephora*) demonstrated potent antiradical activity against the hydroxyl radical in an *in vitro* assay and *ex vivo* in IMR32 cells. The investigators concluded that both green and roasted coffee exhibit antiradical activity, with 5-*O*-caffeoyl-quinic acid, a chlorogenic acid isomer, as the most active constituent, and that the roasting process stimulates high molecular weight components to display antiradical activity in coffee. The authors speculated that these findings could account for the neuroprotective effects associated with coffee consumption in several epidemiologic studies.[34] In fact, a number of such studies have provided evidence linking regular coffee and caffeine consumption with a lower incidence or reduced risk of developing Parkinson's disease.[35,36]

Coffea Arabica in Skin Care Research

In 2009, green coffee oil was shown through *in vitro* studies and in *ex vivo* human skin models to dose-dependently promote the production of the key dermal constituents collagen, elastin, and glycosaminoglycans, as well as stimulate a greater release of the growth factors transforming growth factor-β1 and granulocyte-macrophage colony-stimulating factor. In addition, green coffee oil spurred the expression of aquaporin-3 (AQP-3) mRNA, up to 6.5-fold higher than levels seen in control cultures. The investigators concluded that green coffee oil has potential to contribute to the formation of new connective tissue and improving cutaneous function by mitigating wrinkles and preventing xerosis by raising levels of AQP-3 (see Chapter 29, Aquaporin). Consequently, they suggested that including green coffee oil in cosmetic formulations merits consideration.[20]

In early 2011, Chiang et al. reported on their investigation of the antiphotoaging effects of *C. arabica* leaf extract, its hydrolysates, chlorogenic acid, and caffeic acid. The various polyphenol-containing test compounds were subjected to matrix metalloproteinase (MMP) and elastase inhibition tests. They found that *C. arabica* leaf extracts stimulated type I procollagen expression, suppressed MMP-1, MMP-3, and MMP-9 expression, and hindered the phosphorylation of JNK, ERK and p38. They concluded that the extracts of *C. arabica* leaves can prevent photodamage by inhibiting MMP expression and the MAP kinase pathway.[37]

Given the widespread cultivation of the *Coffea arabica* plant, and the growing scientific interest in exploring the ramifications of its use, it would certainly be cost-effective if companies that harvest the plant also made use of its fruit in some capacity. Accordingly, the manufacturers of Coffeeberry® and their researchers deserve credit for resourcefulness and innovative thinking at the very least. In addition, preliminary evidence suggests that Coffeeberry warrants consideration for its strong antioxidant potential. However, claims that Coffeeberry improves wrinkles are likely due to a moisturizing effect as it is well established that antioxidants can *prevent* wrinkles from developing *but do not eliminate wrinkles* that are already present. The effects seen on improved hyperpigmentation are not unexpected as antioxidants play a role in the pigmentation process. In the author's opinion, the "superior antioxidant protection" that any product claims cannot be proven, because there is no consensus on the ideal test to evaluate antioxidant activity. Much more research, preferably in the form of randomized, double-blind, placebo-controlled clinical trials, is necessary to determine the true potential impact of Coffeeberry in the dermatologic arsenal.

REFERENCES

1. Heimbach JT, Marone PA, Hunter JM, et al. Safety studies on products from whole coffee fruit. *Food Chem Toxicol.* 2010;48:2517.
2. Miljkovic D, Duell B, Miljkovic V. Low-mycotoxin coffee cherry products. Int Patent App Publ. WO 2004/098303.
3. Miljkovic D, Duell B, Miljkovic V. Methods for coffee cherry products. Int Patent App Publ. WO 2004/098320.
4. Charurin P, Ames JM, del Castillo MD. Antioxidant activity of coffee model systems. *J Agric Food Chem.* 2002;50:3751.
5. Del Rio D, Stalmach A, Calani L, et al. Biovailability of coffee chlorogenic acids and green tea flavan-3-ols. *Nutrients.* 2010;2:820.
6. Olthof MR, Hollman PC, Katan MB. Chlorogenic acid and caffeic acid are absorbed in humans. *J Nutr.* 2001;131:66.
7. Ross JA, Kasum CM. Dietary flavonoids: Bioavailability, metabolic effects, and safety. *Annu Rev Nutr.* 2002;22:19.
8. Hertog MG, Hollman PC, Katan MB, et al. Intake of potentially anticarcinogenic flavonoids and their determinants in adults in The Netherlands. *Nutr Cancer.* 1993;20:21.
9. Birt DF, Hendrich S, Wang W. Dietary agents in cancer prevention: Flavonoids and isoflavonoids. *Pharmacol Ther.* 2001;90:157.
10. Rechner AR, Spencer JP, Kuhnle G, et al. Novel biomarkers of the metabolism of caffeic acid derivatives in vivo. *Free Radic Biol Med.* 2001;30:1213.
11. Svobodová A, Psotová J, Walterová D. Natural phenolics in the prevention of UV-induced skin damage. A review. *Biomed Pap Med Fac univ Palacky Olomouc Czech Repub.* 2003;147:137.
12. Morton JF. *Major Medicinal Plants.* Springfield, IL: C.C. Thomas; 1977.
13. Grieve M. *A Modern Herbal* (Vol 1). New York: Dover Publications; 1971:210.
14. Farris P. Idebenone, green tea, and Coffeeberry extract: New and innovative antioxidants. *Dermatol Ther.* 2007;20:322.
15. Chen D, Milacic V, Chen MS, et al. Tea polyphenols, their biological effects and potential molecular targets. *Histol Histopathol.* 2008;23:487.
16. Halder B, Bhattacharya U, Mukhopadhyay S, et al. Molecular mechanism of black tea polyphenols induced apoptosis in human skin cancer cells: Involvement of Bax translocation and mitochondria mediated death cascade. *Carcinogenesis.* 2008;29:129.
17. Kang NJ, Lee KW, Shin BJ, et al. Caffeic acid, a phenolic phytochemical in coffee, directly inhibits Fyn kinase activity and UVB-induced COX-2 expression. *Carcinogenesis.* 2009;30:321.
18. Ostojic SM, Stojanovic MD, Djordjevic B, et al. The effects of a 4-week coffeeberry supplementation on antioxidant status, endurance, and anaerobic performance in college athletes. *Res Sports Med.* 2008;16:281.
19. Hexsel D, Orlandi C, Zechmeister do Prado D. Botanical extracts used in the treatment of cellulite. *Dermatol Surg.* 2005;31:866.
20. Velazquez Pereda Mdel C, Dieamant Gde C, Eberlin S, et al. Effect of green Coffea arabica L. seed oil on extracellular matrix components and water-channel expression in vitro and ex vivo human skin models. *J Cosmet Dermatol.* 2009;8:56.
21. Berson DS. Natural antioxidants. *J Drugs Dermatol.* 2008;7:s7.
22. Draelos Z. A double-blind, randomized clinical trial evaluating the dermatologic benefits of coffee berry extract. *J Am Acad Dermatol.* 2008;58(Suppl 2):AB64.
23. Draelos ZD. Optimal skin care for aesthetic patients: Topical products to restore and maintain healthy skin. *Cosmet Dermatol.* 2009;22:S1.
24. McDaniel DH. Clinical safety and efficacy in photoaged skin with coffeeberry extract, a natural antioxidant. *Cosmet Dermatol.* 2009;22:610.

25. Palmer DM, Kitchin JS. A double-blind, randomized, controlled clinical trial evaluating the efficacy and tolerance of a novel phenolic antioxidant skin care system containing Coffea arabica and concentrated fruit and vegetable extracts. *J Drugs Dermatol.* 2010;9:1480.

26. Leyden JJ, Shergill B, Micali G, et al. Natural options for the management of hyperpigmentation. *J Eur Acad Dermatol Venereol.* 2011;25:1140.

27. Lupo MP, Draelos ZD, Farris PK, et al. CoffeeBerry: A new, natural antioxidant in professional antiaging skin care. *Cosmet Dermatol.* 2007;20:2.

28. Natural Resources Defense Council. Environmental Issues: Health. Coffee, Conservation, and Commerce in the Western Hemisphere: How Individuals and Institutions Can Promote Ecologically Sound Farming and Forest Management in Northern Latin America. http://www.nrdc.org/health/farming/ccc/chap4.asp#note54. Accessed October 3, 2013.

29. Hylander K, Nemomissa S, Delrue J, et al. Effects of coffee management on deforestation rates and forest integrity. *Conserv Biol.* 2013;27:1031.

30. Hundera K, Aerts R, Fontaine A, et al. Effects of coffee management intensity on composition, structure, and regeneration status of Ethiopian moist evergreen afromontane forests. *Environ Manage.* 2013;51:801.

31. Takahashi R, Todo Y. The impact of a shade coffee certification program on forest conservation: A case study from a wild coffee forest in Ethiopia. *J Environ Manage.* 2013;130C:48.

32. Philpott SM, Arendt WJ, Armbrecht I, et al. Biodiversity loss in Latin American coffee landscapes: Review of the evidence on ants, birds, and trees. *Conserv Biol.* 2008;22:1093.

33. Beer K, Kellner E, Beer J. Cosmeceuticals for rejuvenation. *Facial Plast Surg.* 2009;25:285.

34. Daglia M, Racchi M, Papetti A, et al. In vitro and ex vivo antihydroxyl radical activity of green and roasted coffee. *J Agric Food Chem.* 2004;52:1700.

35. Ascherio A, Zhang SM, Hernán MA, et al. Prospective study of caffeine consumption and risk of Parkinson's disease in men and women. *Ann Neurol.* 2001;50:56.

36. Ross GW, Abbott RD, Petrovitch H, et al. Association of coffee and caffeine intake with the risk of Parkinson's disease. *JAMA.* 2000;283:2674.

37. Chiang HM, Lin TJ, Chiu CY, et al. Coffea arabica extract and its constituents prevent photoaging by suppressing MMPs expression and MAP kinase pathway. *Food Chem Toxicol.* 2011;49:309.

CHAPTER 59

Ginger

Activities:

Antioxidant, anticarcinogenic, anti-inflammatory, anti-nausea, wound healing

Important Chemical Components:

Terpenes, phenolic vanilloids ([6]-gingerol and other gingerols; the structurally related [6]-paradol, and other paradols), shogaols, [10]-shogaol and other shogaols, zingerone, β-carotene, ascorbic acid, rutin

Origin Classification:

This ingredient is considered natural. As an ingredient used for dermatologic purposes, it is laboratory made.

Personal Care Category:

Antioxidant, analgesic, photoprotectant

Recommended for the following Baumann Skin Types:

DRNW, DRPW, ORNW, and ORPW

SOURCE

Ginger, the tuberous root or rhizome of *Zingiber officinalis*, is one of the most widely used species of the tropical and subtropical Zingiberaceae family, particularly as a condiment and spice for many foods and beverages.[1] Indeed, the use of ginger rhizomes, commonly referred to as ginger, in culinary spices and as medicine to treat various conditions has a long-standing and widespread tradition throughout Asia (Table 59-1). The designation *ginger* is thought to be derived from the Sanskrit word *singabera*, meaning "horn-shaped," which alludes to the knobby protuberances of ginger's rhizomes. It is now cultivated in China, India, Southeast Asia, Mexico, Africa, Fiji, and Australia.[2] Traditional uses of the herb, to treat nausea, indigestion, joint inflammation, fever and infection, continue today, but the list of indications is expanding as research reveals a wider variety of potential applications.

In fact, ginger is known as one of the most effective herbal remedies for nausea and has a longstanding reputation as a gastroprotective, carminative agent. Its antiemetic properties are attributed to an effect on gastric activity rather than a central nervous system mechanism. Ginger is also touted for its

TABLE 59-1
Pros and Cons of Ginger

Pros	Con
Long and varied history of traditional uses	More clinical evidence is needed to substantiate topical antioxidant and other benefits
Vast spectrum of biologic activity	
One of the top botanical ingredients in terms of the number of medical indications	
Compelling evidence related to skin cancer	

antioxidant, antiviral, antifungal, and antibacterial activity.[3,4] It is thought to be effective against the growth of both Gram-positive and Gram-negative microbes.

Ginger has also been cited as an effective element in treating stomach ulcers, arthritis, rheumatism, and migraines.[5] Its purported ability to improve circulation and to act as an antioxidant has led to research into its viability as an ingredient in skin care products aimed at enhancing facial complexion. Evidence is gathering, also, of the chemopreventive, antineoplastic activity of ginger.[6]

HISTORY

Native to much of Asia, ginger, dubbed *Zingiber officinale* in 1807 by English botanist William Roscoe, appears in records of its use in ancient Sanskrit and Chinese writings as well as Greek, Roman, and Arabic medical texts.[2] Ginger has been used as a traditional herb for over 2,500 years and long considered a universal remedy.[1,7] Generally, it has been employed in traditional Chinese medicine (TCM), Ayurveda, and Tibb-Unani herbal medicine to treat various illnesses involving inflammation and oxidative stress.[8] In these ancient medical systems as well as Sri Lankan, Arabic, and African traditional medicine, ginger has been used to treat a wide range of ailments, including common colds, fever, sore throats, vomiting, motion sickness, indigestion, constipation, arthritis, rheumatism, sprains, muscular aches, cramps, hypertension, dementia, helminthiasis, and infectious diseases, and continues to be used for such indications as well as asthma, allergy, headaches, diabetes, gingivitis, and stroke in TCM and other Eastern medical practices.[5,6,9-12]

In a 2010 study to ascertain the ethnopharmacological application of medicinal plants used to treat skin diseases and in folk cosmetics in northwestern Pakistan, Abbasi et al. identified *Zingiber officinale* as one of 15 mostly wild and rare plant species used for various skin and hair conditions.[13]

CHEMISTRY

Ginger is widely used as an herbal medicine, particularly due to the presence of homologous phenolic ketones, of which [6]-gingerol (1-[4'-hydroxy-3'-methoxyphenyl]-5-hydroxy-3-decanone) is the primary and most abundant.[14,15] The chemistry of ginger is complicated, though. In fact, the chief components found in ginger oil vary according to the region in which it was grown. An oleoresin, known as "ginger oil," and terpenes are the major active components of ginger; however, pungent phenolic substances, such as [6]-gingerol and [6]-paradol, are considered the source of the discrete antioxidative and anti-inflammatory action of ginger.[16,17] In addition, ginger has been found to exert anticancer activity, which is also ascribed to [6]-gingerol and [6]-paradol, as well as shogaols (the main dehydration products of gingerols) and zingerone.[1,16,18]

Several animal studies have demonstrated the antioxidant capacity of ginger. More than a decade ago, ginger was found to inhibit lipid peroxidation in rat liver microsomes.[19] Researchers also showed that ginger effectively scavenges superoxide anions.[20] A study on SENCAR mice demonstrated the antioxidant, anti-inflammatory and anticarcinogenic properties of ginger extracts. Ginger oil placed directly on the skin of mice prevented the development or growth of skin cancer after the mice were exposed to chemicals that promote cancer.[21] The anti-inflammatory effect is thought to be due to inhibition of cyclooxygenase (COX) and 5-lipoxygenase.[22] Further, ginger has been shown to inhibit fibroblast-derived elastase, suggesting a significant role in the prevention of wrinkle formation.[23]

ORAL USES

Ginger is commonly used as a condiment for foods and in beverages, particularly tea, throughout the world; it is one of the most frequently and heavily consumed of all the spices.[17] The distinctive, spicy taste of fresh ginger is attributed to the lipid-soluble [6]-gingerol, one of its main phenolic constituents; the pungency of dry ginger is linked to the shogaols.[11,24] In addition to its wide use in foods and beverages, ginger is available as a dietary supplement.

TOPICAL USES

Knee Osteoarthritis

Ginger is one among several adjuvant or secondary options in the treatment of knee osteoarthritis, which affects more than one-third of individuals over the age of 65.[25] In a 2011 double-blind, randomized controlled trial with 92 patients, an herbal ointment containing ginger, cinnamon, mastic, and sesame oil was clinically effective and comparable to a salicylate ointment in reducing pain, morning stiffness, and motion limitations.[26] Previously, among 247 patients who could be evaluated from an original 261 in a randomized, double-blind, placebo-controlled, multicenter, parallel-group, six-week study, 63 percent of responders in the ginger extract group experienced diminished knee pain as compared to 50 percent in the control group.[27] However, a systematic review of the literature to assess the safety and effectiveness of ginger to treat osteoarthritis in adults yielded weak evidence of its effectiveness as a lone therapy.[28]

Hair Care

Although ginger is used in East Asia in various products touted to stem hair loss and promote growth, Miao et al. pointed out that supportive evidence is lacking. In 2013, they investigated the effects of [6]-gingerol on hair shaft growth and human dermal papilla cells in vitro and in vivo. The researchers found that the ginger constituent inhibited hair growth as well as the proliferation of dermal papilla cells in culture as well as in mice. They concluded that contrary to popular usage in East Asia, [6]-gingerol appears better suited for hair removal than stimulating hair growth.[29]

SAFETY ISSUES

Ginger is listed by the Food and Drug Administration as generally recognized as safe (GRAS).[30] It can be irritating to the skin and should not be used in sensitive skin types, particularly S_2 rosacea types. Contact dermatitis to ginger has been reported.[31]

ENVIRONMENTAL IMPACT

Z. officinale is abundant in tropical regions throughout the world and its harvesting is not known to damage the local environment as it is easily cultivated.[32] In fact, ethanol extracts of ginger have shown sufficient antifungal activity to suggest potential for use in agriculture as one of several natural alternatives to conventional synthetic pesticides, which would protect the environment and human health.[33] Nevertheless, in an industry in which there is much money to be made by growers from a cash crop such as ginger, environmental concerns are often supplanted by bottom-line financial interests.

FORMULATION CONSIDERATIONS

The constituents of ginger vary by region and whether the rhizomes are fresh or dry.[11] The CO_2 extracts of ginger have the most abundant polyphenolic content and most closely resemble the composition of the Z. officinale rhizome.[32]

USAGE CONSIDERATIONS

Ginger is one of the several commonly used herbs, including feverfew, garlic, ginkgo, and ginseng, which may contribute to bleeding during surgical procedures.[34]

SIGNIFICANT BACKGROUND

Ginger is one of the most widely used herbs on the planet as a flavoring agent in food and for numerous medical indications. It exerts potent antioxidant activity, attenuating or preventing the formation of reactive oxygen species (ROS) and is known to impart anti-inflammatory, antiapoptotic, antitumorigenic, antihyperglycemic, antilipidemic, antiemetic, and immunomodulatory activity.[11]

Antioxidant and Anti-inflammatory Activity

The phenol [6]-gingerol displayed strong antioxidant activity in 1994 as ascertained by Aeschbach et al., who showed that the compound inhibited phospholipid peroxidation brought on by the $FeCl_3$-ascorbate system.[17,35]

In a 2010 study by Dugasani et al. of the in vitro activities of [6]-gingerol, [8]-gingerol, [10]-gingerol, and [6]-shogaol in scavenging 1,1-diphenyl-2-picyrlhydrazyl (DPPH), superoxide, and hydroxyl radicals, suppression of N-formyl-methionyl-leucyl-phenylalanine (f-MLP)-induced ROS synthesis in human polymorphonuclear neutrophils (PMN), and the hindering of lipopolysaccharide-induced nitrite and prostaglandin E_2 production in RAW 264.7 cells, [6]-shogaol displayed the strongest antioxidant and anti-inflammatory characteristics, with [10]-gingerol exhibiting the greatest potency among the gingerols. The researchers concluded that their findings buttress the use of dry ginger in traditional medical systems.[8]

Also that year, Ghasemzadeh et al. investigated the antioxidant activities of methanol extracts from the leaves, stems, and rhizomes of two Z. officinale varieties. Using various assays, they determined that Halia Bara possessed higher phenolic and flavonoid concentrations and exhibited higher antioxidant activity than Halia Bentong. Their findings supported the potential medical applications of Z. officinale (Halia Bara) leaves and young rhizomes.[32]

Previously, Minghetti et al. investigated the *ex vivo* skin permeation and *in vivo* topical anti-inflammatory activity of a commercial ginger dry extract and a gingerols-enriched dry extract in mice. Both extracts dose-dependently reduced ear edema induced by Croton oil, though the enriched extract was slightly less potent. Medicated plasters, with 1 mg/cm^2 of either extract, displayed anti-inflammatory properties and the enriched extract permeated through mouse skin (22.1 μg/cm^2) as well as human epidermis (6.9 μg/cm^2). The investigators concluded that the anti-inflammatory effects of the extracts noted in mice could also be delivered in human skin.[18]

In addition, crude extracts of *Z. officinale* have been shown to diminish rat paw and skin edema provoked by carrageenan, 48/80 compound, and serotonin.[36] The substantial antioxidant potency and anti-inflammatory properties ascribed to ginger are thought to play important roles in exerting photoprotective and chemopreventive activity.

Photoprotection

In 2006, Tsukahara et al. studied the role of elastase in UV-induced wrinkle formation by evaluating the effects of ginger extract. They found that topically applying the extract to rat hind limb skin or hairless mouse dorsal skin strongly suppressed wrinkle development engendered by chronic ultraviolet B (UVB) exposure at a suberythemal dose. The concomitant reduction in skin elasticity that accompanies such exposure was also significantly prevented, as the elasticity of rat hind limb skin was maintained. The authors concluded that herbal extracts with the demonstrated capacity to hinder fibroblast-derived elastase, which is key in UVB-induced wrinkle formation, represent potentially effective antiwrinkling agents.[23]

In vitro and *in vivo* experiments were conducted by Kim et al. in 2007 to characterize the antioxidant, anti-inflammatory, and antiapoptotic activities of the ginger extract [6]-gingerol. Pretreatment with the phenolic lowered, *in vitro*, UVB-induced intracellular ROS levels, as well as the activation of caspase-3, caspase-8, and caspase-9, Fas expression, and the expression and transactivation of COX-2. *In vivo*, the topical application of [6]-gingerol to hairless mice before UVB exposure led to the suppression of COX-2 mRNA induction and nuclear factor-κB (NF-κB) translocation. The researchers concluded that [6]-gingerol shows potential as a photoprotective agent against cutaneous disorders caused by UVB exposure.[15] In a separate study, by Pan et al., [6]-shogaol was shown to downregulate inflammatory inducible nitric oxide synthase (iNOS) and COX-2 gene expression in murine macrophages by suppressing the activation of NF-κB.[37]

The next year, Imokawa reported that a one-year clinical study on human facial skin revealed that a water-soluble ginger extract blocked the UV-induced reduction in skin elasticity, by inhibiting fibroblast-derived elastase, and prevented or diminished wrinkle formation in periorbital skin without altering stratum corneum water content.[38]

In 2010, Guahk et al. reported that *Z. officinale* exerts protection of the human keratinocyte cell line HaCaT *in vitro* and C57BL/6 mice *in vivo* from inflammation induced by UVB exposure and, therefore, warrants consideration as a photoprotective anti-inflammatory agent.[39]

In a 2013 study of the protection conferred against UVB-induced DNA damage and cytotoxicity by 15 Thai herb species, Thongrakard et al. found that the greatest UV absorption was associated with the dichloromethane extract of ginger and ethanol extract of turmeric (see Chapter 69, Turmeric). Both extracts promoted the production of the antioxidant protein thioredoxin 1 and the investigators concluded that the herbs exhibit potential to protect human keratinocytes from UV-induced harm thus warranting use in photoprotective cosmetic agents.[40]

Anticarcinogenic Activity

The anticarcinogenic activity of ginger has emerged as the most compelling area of investigation. The pungent phenolic substance [6]-paradol (1-[4'-hydroxy-3'-methoxyphenyl]-3-decanone) has been identified as the component most responsible for inhibiting tumor activity in skin cancer of mice. Other structurally-related derivatives, in addition to [6]-paradol, have been shown to induce apoptosis through a mechanism dependent on caspase-3.[17,41] Both [6]-paradol and the structurally-related [6]-gingerol, acting through different mechanisms, have been shown to inhibit epidermal growth factor (EGF)-induced cell transformation.[42]

In one of the earlier investigations into the effects of ginger extract on skin tumorigenesis in mice, Katiyar et al. topically applied an ethanol extract of ginger to the skin of SENCAR mice, which significantly and dose-dependently suppressed 12-*O*-tetradecanoylphorbol-13-acetate (TPA)-induced epidermal ornithine decarboxylase (ODC), COX, and lipoxygenase activities as well as ODC mRNA expression. Ginger extract pretreatment also led to substantial suppression of TPA-generated epidermal edema and hyperplasia. Ginger-treated mice also displayed significantly lower tumor incidence than controls after 7,12-dimethylbenz[a]anthracene (DMBA) tumor initiation and TPA tumor promotion. These findings, the investigators concluded, represented the first clear evidence that ginger extract protects against skin tumor promotion.[21]

In a two-stage mouse model, Park et al. showed in 1998 that the topical application of [6]-gingerol onto the shaved backs of female ICR mice before topical doses of the tumor promoter TPA significantly suppressed skin papillomagenesis induced by DMBA. TPA-induced epidermal ODC activity and inflammation were also inhibited by the ginger constituent.[17] Many of the same investigators reported on similar findings the following year, also including [6]-paradol along with [6]-gingerol as exhibiting potential chemopreventive properties. In this study, both ginger substances were topically applied to female ICR mice in the two-stage carcinogenesis model using TPA and DMBA and were found to suppress TPA-stimulated inflammation, tumor necrosis factor (TNF)-α synthesis, as well as epidermal ODC activity. In a separate investigation by the same team, both compounds also inhibited superoxide production spurred by TPA in differentiated HL-60 cells.[41]

In 2001, Bode et al. offered the first evidence that [6]-gingerol and [6]-paradol hinder EGF-induced cell transformation, thus blocking a critical pathway in tumor formation.[42] Two years later, Bode et al. reported a chemopreventive effect after administering 500 mg of [6]-gingerol or a placebo to athymic nude mice three times weekly for two weeks before injecting them with human colon cancer cells. Administering the ginger extract or placebo was resumed then, with the investigators finding that it took longer for tumors to emerge and grow in the gingerol-treated animals.[43]

In 2004, Kim et al. demonstrated that the topical application of [6]-gingerol blocks phorbol 12-myristate 13-acetate (also known as 12-*O*-tetradecanoylphorbol-13-acetate)-induced COX-2 expression, which is targeted by several anti-inflammatory and chemopreventive agents. In addition, [6]-gingerol inhibited NF-κB DNA binding activity in mouse skin as well as the phosphorylation of p38 mitogen-activated protein (MAP) kinase, which the authors cited as a possible explanation for the impact of [6]-gingerol on NF-κB and its inhibition of COX-2 expression.[24] In 2005, many of the same investigators showed that [6]-gingerol suppressed TPA-induced COX-2 expression in TPA-treated mouse skin *in vivo* by hindering the p38 MAP kinase-NF-κB signaling pathway.[7]

In 2009, Nigam et al. found that [6]-gingerol evinced significant cytotoxicity in human epidermoid carcinoma A431 cells, engendering ROS increases that provoked reductions in mitochondrial membrane potential and apoptosis. Treatment with [6]-gingerol also yielded an upregulation of cytochrome-c and apoptotic protease-activating factor (Apaf)-1, spurring the caspase cascade, which plays an essential role in apoptosis. The investigators concluded that [6]-gingerol warrants attention as a potentially effective agent in treating skin cancer.[14] In a study the following year, Nigam et al. topically treated mice with [6]-gingerol before inducing skin tumorigenesis through 32 weeks of exposure to benzo[a]pyrene (B[a]P). Pretreatment with the ginger component yielded delays in the onset of tumorigenesis, decreased cumulative tumors, and lower tumor volume. B[a]P-suppressed p53 levels were augmented by [6]-gingerol, which also aided in the release of cytochrome-c, activation of caspases, and the increase in Apaf-1, thus inducing apoptosis. These results further support the investigators' claims regarding the chemopreventive activity of [6]-gingerol.[44]

Other components of ginger have also been investigated. In 2004, Murakami et al. showed that zerumbone, a sesquiterpene present in the tropical ginger species *Zingiber zerumbet*, inhibits skin tumor initiation with DMBA and promotion by TPA in ICR mice by inducing antioxidative and phase II drug metabolizing enzymes and interrupting proinflammatory signaling pathways.[45] In 2011, Shin et al. investigated the effects on mice of topically applied zerumbone, previously found to block chemically-induced papilloma formation in mouse skin. They found that the ginger component upregulated the expression of the protein heme oxygenase-1 (HO-1) through activation of NF-E2-related factor 2 (Nrf2) signaling, which the researchers suggested provided an explanation for the inhibitory effect on skin carcinogenesis exhibited by zerumbone in mice.[46]

In addition, the tropical ginger-derived compound 1'-acetoxychavicol acetate has exhibited the capacity to inhibit skin tumorigenesis in K5.Stat3C mice.[47]

The anticarcinogenic effects of ginger have also been seen in Chinese herbal medicine. The methanolic extract of *Alpinia oxyphylla*, a member of the Zingiberaceae family, has been found to suppress mouse skin tumor promotion and noted for inducing apoptosis in cultured human promyelocytic leukemia cells.[48] It is speculated that the antitumor activity of the phenolic diarylheptanoids derived from *A. oxyphylla* are linked to its anti-inflammatory characteristics.[48]

Wound Healing

In 2009, Bhagavathula et al. topically treated hairless rats for a 21-day period with a combination of 10 percent curcumin and 3 percent ginger extract or with each agent alone. For another 15 days, investigators treated the animals with the corticosteroid Temovate. Superficial abrasions were then induced in treated skin, with healing occurring sooner in skin pretreated with either curcumin or ginger extract alone or in combination as compared to skin treated only with the corticosteroid and vehicle alone. The investigators analyzed skin samples taken at wound closure, finding an increase in collagen production and

decrease in matrix metalloproteinase-9 in the skin treated with the herbal ingredients compared to the skin treated with corticosteroid and vehicle. The investigators concluded that a combination of curcumin and ginger extract may have an adjuvant role to play in wound healing.[30]

In 2012, Chen et al. demonstrated that 10-shogaol, an active ingredient in ginger, exhibited potent radical scavenging activity when tested with the DPPH radical. It was also shown to foster human normal epidermal keratinocyte and dermal fibroblast production as well as the synthesis of multiple growth factors and the migration of keratinocytes and fibroblasts in an *in vitro* wound-healing assay.[9]

Skin Lightening

Ginger may have yet another indication. Huang et al. showed in 2011 that [6]-gingerol dose-dependently inhibited murine tyrosinase activity and lowered melanin as well as ROS levels. They concluded that [6]-gingerol is an effective suppressor of melanogenesis of B_{16}-F_{10} melanoma cells and merits attention as a skin-lightening agent.[49]

◼ CONCLUSION

The long history of traditional use and well-established safety profile of ginger make the herb a strong candidate for extensive research regarding its inclusion in drugs and cosmeceuticals. New data on the anticarcinogenic potential of ginger appears especially promising, but the overall antitoxic properties of the perennial herb may very well position ginger to be a key new ingredient in a wider array of skin care products. As is often the case, more randomized, placebo-controlled studies are needed to substantiate the dermatologic uses of popular botanical ingredients such as ginger. Nevertheless, its broad biologic activity has been clearly demonstrated and the antioxidant, anti-inflammatory, and chemopreventive properties manifested by ginger extracts indicate potential for topical dermatologic uses.

REFERENCES

1. Shukla Y, Singh M. Cancer preventive properties of ginger: A brief review. *Food Chem Toxicol.* 2007;45:683.
2. Mills S, Bone K. *Principles and Practice of Phytotherapy: Modern Herbal Medicine.* London: Churchill Livingstone; 2000:394.
3. Ficker CE, Arnason JT, Vindas PS, et al. Inhibition of human pathogenic fungi by ethnobotanically selected plant extracts. *Mycoses.* 2003;46:29.
4. Akoachere JF, Ndip RN, Chenwi EB, et al. Antibacterial effect of Zingiber officinale and Garcinia kola on respiratory tract pathogens. *East Afr Med J.* 2002;79:588.
5. Hoffmann D. *Medical Herbalism: The Science and Practice of Herbal Medicine.* Rochester, VT: Healing Arts Press; 2003:493, 501, 502, 520, 597.
6. Baliga MS, Haniadka R, Pereira MM, et al. Update on the chemopreventive effects of ginger and its phytochemicals. *Crit Rev Food Sci Nutr.* 2011;51:499.
7. Kim SO, Kundu JK, Shin YK, et al. [6]-Gingerol inhibits COX-2 expression by blocking the activation of p38 MAP kinase and NF-kappaB in phorbol ester-stimulated mouse skin. *Oncogene.* 2005;24:2558.
8. Dugasani S, Pichika MR, Nadarajah VD, et al. Comparative antioxidant and anti-inflammatory effects of [6]-gingerol, [8]-gingerol, [10]-gingerol and [6]-shogaol. *J Ethnopharmacol.* 2010;127:515.
9. Chen CY, Cheng KC, Chang AY, et al. 10-Shogaol, an antioxidant from Zingiber officinale for skin cell proliferation and migration enhancer. *Int J Mol Sci.* 2012;13:1762.

10. Afzal M, Al-Hadidi D, Menon M, et al. Ginger: An ethnomedical, chemical and pharmacological review. *Drug Metabol Drug Interact.* 2001;18:159.

11. Ali BH, Blunden G, Tanira MO, et al. Some phytochemical, pharmacological and toxicological properties of ginger (Zingiber officinale Roscoe): A review of recent research. *Food Chem Toxicol.* 2008;46:409.

12. Haghighi M, Khalvat A, Toliat T, et al. Comparing the effects of ginger (Zingiber officinale) extract and ibuprofen on patients with osteoarthritis. *Arch Iran Med.* 2005;8:267.

13. Abbasi AM, Khan MA, Ahmad M, et al. Ethnopharmacological application of medicinal plants to cure skin diseases and in folk cosmetics among the tribal communities of North-West Frontier Province, Pakistan. *J Ethnopharmacol.* 2010;128:322.

14. Nigam N, Bhui K, Prasad S, et al. [6]-Gingerol induces reactive oxygen species regulated mitochondrial cell death pathway in human epidermoid carcinoma A431 cells. *Chem Biol Interact.* 2009;181:77.

15. Kim JK, Kim Y, Na KM, et al. [6]-Gingerol prevents UVB-induced ROS production and COX-2 expression in vitro and in vivo. *Free Radic Res.* 2007;41:603.

16. Surh Y. Molecular mechanisms of chemopreventive effects of selected dietary and medicinal phenolic substances. *Mutat Res.* 1999;428:305.

17. Park KK, Chun KS, Lee JM, et al. Inhibitory effects of [6]-gingerol, a major pungent principle of ginger, on phorbol ester-induced inflammation, epidermal ornithine decarboxylase activity and skin tumor promotion in ICR mice. *Cancer Lett.* 1998;129:139.

18. Minghetti P, Sosa S, Cilurzo F, et al. Evaluation of the topical anti-inflammatory activity of ginger dry extracts from solutions and plasters. *Planta Med.* 2007;73:1525.

19. Reddy AC, Lokesh BR. Studies on spice principles as antioxidants in the inhibition of lipid peroxidation of rat liver microsomes. *Mol Cell Biochem.* 1992;111:117.

20. Krishnakantha TP, Lokesh BR. Scavenging of superoxide anions by spice principles. *Indian J Biochem Biophys.* 1993;30:133.

21. Katiyar SK, Agarwal R, Mukhtar H. Inhibition of tumor promotion in SENCAR mouse skin by ethanol extract of Zingiber officinale rhizome. *Cancer Res.* 1996;56:1023.

22. Kiuchi F, Iwakami S, Shibuya M, et al. Inhibition of prostaglandin and leukotriene biosynthesis by gingerols and diarylheptanoids. *Chem Pharm Bull (Tokyo).* 1992;40:387.

23. Tsukahara K, Nakagawa H, Moriwaki S, et al. Inhibition of ultraviolet-B-induced wrinkle formation by an elastase-inhibiting herbal extract: Implication for the mechanism underlying elastase-associated wrinkles. *Int J Dermatol.* 2006;45:460.

24. Kim SO, Chun KS, Kundu JK, et al. Inhibitory effects of [6]-gingerol on PMA-induced COX-2 expression and activation of NF-kappaB and p38 MAPK in mouse skin. *Biofactors.* 2004;21:27.

25. Ringdahl E, Pandit S. Treatment of knee osteoarthritis. *Am Fam Physician.* 2011;83:1287.

26. Zahmatkash M, Vafaeenasab MR. Comparing analgesic effects of a topical herbal mixed medicine with salicylate in patients with knee osteoarthritis. *Pak J Biol Sci.* 2011;14:715.

27. Altman RD, Marcussen KC. Effects of a ginger extract on knee pain in patients with osteoarthritis. *Arthritis Rheum.* 2001;44:2531.

28. Leach MJ, Kumar S. The clinical effectiveness of ginger (Zingiber officinale) in adults with osteoarthritis. *Int J Evid Based Healthc.* 2008;6:311.

29. Miao Y, Sun Y, Wang W, et al. 6-Gingerol inhibits hair shaft growth in cultured human hair follicles and modulates hair growth in mice. *PLoS One.* 2013;8:e57226.

30. Bhagavathula N, Warner RL, DaSilva M, et al. A combination of curcumin and ginger extract improves abrasion wound healing in corticosteroid-impaired hairless rat skin. *Wound Repair Regen.* 2009;17:360.

31. Kanerva L, Estlander T, Jolanki R. Occupational allergic contact dermatitis from spices. *Contact Dermatitis.* 1996;35:157.

32. Ghasemzadeh A, Jaafar HZ, Rahmat A. Antioxidant activities, total phenolics and flavonoids content in two varieties of Malaysia young ginger (Zingiber officinale Roscoe). *Molecules.* 2010;15:4324.

33. Al-Samarrai G, Singh H, Syarhabil M. Evaluating eco-friendly botanicals (natural plant extracts) as alternatives to synthetic fungicides. *Ann Agric Environ Med.* 2012;19:673.

34. Pribitkin ED, Boger G. Herbal therapy: What every facial plastic surgeon must know. *Arch Facial Plast Surg.* 2001;3:127.

35. Aeschbach R, Löliger J, Scott BC, et al. Antioxidant actions of thymol, carvacrol, 6-gingerol, zingerone and hydroxytyrosol. *Food Chem Toxicol.* 1994;32:31.

36. Penna SC, Medeiros MV, Aimbire FS, et al. Anti-inflammatory effect of the hydralcoholic extract of Zingiber officinale rhizomes on rat paw and skin edema. *Phytomedicine.* 2003;10:381.

37. Pan MH, Hsieh MC, Hsu PC, et al. 6-Shogaol suppressed lipopolysaccharide-induced up-expression of iNOS and COX-2 in murine macrophages. *Mol Nutr Food Res.* 2008;52:1467.

38. Imokawa G. Recent advances in characterizing biological mechanisms underlying UV-induced wrinkles: A pivotal role of fibroblast-derived elastase. *Arch Dermatol Res.* 2008;300(Suppl 1):7.

39. Guahk GH, Ha SK, Jung HS, et al. Zingiber officinale protects HaCaT cells and C57BL/6 mice from ultraviolet B-induced inflammation. *J Med Food.* 2010;13:673.

40. Thongrakard V, Ruangrungsi N, Ekkapongpisit M, et al. Protection from UVB toxicity in human keratinocytes by Thailand native herbs extracts. *Photochem Photobiol.* 2013 Aug 12. [Epub ahead of print].

41. Surh YJ, Park KK, Chun KS, et al. Anti-tumor-promoting activities of selected pungent phenolic substances present in ginger. *J Environ Pathol Toxicol Oncol.* 1999;18:131.

42. Bode AM, Ma WY, Surh YJ, et al. Inhibition of epidermal growth factor-induced cell transformation and activator protein 1 activation by [6]-gingerol. *Cancer Res.* 2001;61:850.

43. Burton A. Chemoprevention: Eat ginger, rub on pomegranate. *Lancet Oncol.* 2003;4:715.

44. Nigam N, George J, Srivastava S, et al. Induction of apoptosis by [6]-gingerol associated with the modulation of p53 and involvement of mitochondrial signaling pathway in B[a]P-induced mouse skin tumorigenesis. *Cancer Chemother Pharmacol.* 2010;65:687.

45. Murakami A, Tanaka T, Lee JY, et al. Zerumbone, a sesquiterpene in subtropical ginger, suppresses skin tumor initiation and promotion stages in ICR mice. *Int J Cancer.* 2004;110:481.

46. Shin JW, Ohnishi K, Murakami A, et al. Zerumbone induces heme oxygenase-1 expression in mouse skin and cultured murine epidermal cells through activation of Nrf2. *Cancer Prev Res (Phila).* 2011;4:860.

47. Batra V, Syed Z, Gill JN, et al. Effects of the tropical ginger compound, 1'-acetoxychavicol acetate, against tumor promotion in K5.Stat3C transgenic mice. *J Exp Clin Cancer Res.* 2012;31:57.

48. Chun KS, Park KK, Lee J, et al. Inhibition of mouse skin tumor promotion by anti-inflammatory diarylheptanoids derived from Alpinia oxyphylla Miquel (Zingiberaceae). *Oncol Res.* 2002;13:37.

49. Huang HC, Chiu SH, Chang TM. Inhibitory effect of [6]-gingerol on melanogenesis in B16F10 melanoma cells and a possible mechanism of action. *Biosci Biotechnol Biochem.* 2011;75:1067.

CHAPTER 60

Honey/Propolis/Royal Jelly

Activities:

Analgesic, antioxidant, anti-inflammatory, antimicrobial, antitumor, antiseptic, antipyretic, antiulcer,[1] hepatoprotective, immunomodulatory[2]

Important Chemical Components:

Honey: Hydrogen peroxide, lysozyme, polyphenols, phenolic acids, flavonoids, methylglyoxal, ascorbic acid, α-tocopherol, carotenoids, glucose oxidase, catalase, and bee peptides[3]

Propolis: Flavonoids (e.g., galangin, chrysin, pinocembrin, quercetin),[4] phenolic acids and their esters (particularly caffeic acid phenethyl ester),[5] cinnamic acid derivatives (i.e., drupanin, baccharin, and artepillin C), sesquiterpene quinones, coumarins, amino acids, and steroids[1]

Royal Jelly: 10-hydroxy-2-decenoic acid (10-HDA), water, proteins, free amino acids, carbohydrates, lipids, minerals, and vitamins

Origin Classification:

All of these ingredients used in skin care are natural products of bees.

Personal Care Category:

Antioxidant, antiaging, photoprotection, antiseptic, wound healing

Recommended for the following Baumann Skin Types:

DRNT, DRNW, DRPT, DRPW, DSNW, DSPW, ORNT, ORNW, ORPT, ORPW, OSNW, and OSPW

SOURCE

Honeybees, *Apis mellifera*, play an important but often underappreciated role in our lives (Figure 60-1). Human beings rely on bees for pollinating approximately one-third of our crops, including numerous fruits, vegetables, nuts, and seeds.[6,7] Of course, they also play a pivotal role in the propagation of other plants, flower nectar, and flower pollen. *A. mellifera*, the European honeybee, is the primary pollinator in Europe and North America but other species, including *A. cerana*, *A. dorsata*, *A. floria*, *A. andreniformis*, *A. koschevnikov*, and *A. laborisa* produce honey.[8] Further, the honeybee is the only insect that produces food consumed by human beings.[3]

Honey is a sweet food product produced by honeybees from flower nectar. It contains over 180 substances and is supersaturated in sugar, though it also contains phenolic acids, flavonoids, ascorbic acid, α-tocopherol, carotenoids, the enzymes glucose oxidase and catalase, organic and amino acids, and proteins.[9] In Ayurvedic medicine, honey has been used to treat diabetes since ancient times.[8] It has also been used for millennia to treat infected

wounds.[10] For dermatologic purposes, honey has and continues to be used in Ayurvedic medicine to treat acne, and is also used in cosmetic formulations such as facial washes, skin moisturizers, and hair conditioners.[8]

Propolis is a yellowish-green to dark brown resinous material that originates in the buds and barks of various plant sources, mostly poplar trees,[1,11,12] and is gathered by honeybees and used in the construction and maintenance of their hives.[13,14] The sources of propolis can vary widely by region and even season, however. In all cases, propolis, used to seal holes and trap predators, stabilizes bee hives and honeycombs and protects bees against cold weather and potential intruders.[11] Also known as bee glue, this extract from bee hives has been used for hundreds of years in naturopathic medicine and is known to display biologic and pharmacologic properties. In traditional medicine, it has been used for its purported antioxidant, anticancer, anti-inflammatory, and immunomodulatory effects.[15] Currently, some radiation therapists use propolis to treat actinic stomatitis and mucositis,[11] but this bee product is used more often for wound care and minor cutaneous indications as well as a dietary supplement. It is believed to contain as many as 300 constituents, including resin, wax, essential oils, pollen, and organic substances such as phenolic acids and their esters, particularly caffeic acid phenethyl ester (CAPE), flavonoids, terpenes, β-steroids, aromatic aldehydes and alcohols, sesquiterpenes, and stilbene terpenes.[1,9]

Royal jelly, a yellowish, viscous secretion from the hypopharyngeal and mandibular glands of worker bees that nourishes bee larvae of all kinds (i.e., drones, workers, queens) after which it becomes the exclusive nourishment for queens throughout their development, has been used by humans for centuries for its health-promoting characteristics.[16–18] Antitumor, antihypercholesterolemic, antibacterial, anti-inflammatory, antioxidant, antiangiogenetic, collagen production-promoting, estrogenic, hypotensive, immunomodulatory, vasodilative, and wound-healing activity have been linked to royal jelly.[9,18–22]

HISTORY

Honey, propolis, and royal jelly have all been used for medicinal purposes since ancient times, with honey, the earliest bee product discovered, particularly known for its use in wound healing.[3,9,11,12,14,23,24] In fact, the topical application of honey for various conditions has been a common traditional medical practice for at least 2,700 years, which many researchers have retrospectively attributed to its antibacterial properties.[3,25] Of course, the antiseptic and antimicrobial properties of honey are recent discoveries,[3] with the antibacterial properties of honey reported in 1892 (as cited by Dustmann in 1919).[26]

In folk remedies, honey has served as a potent anti-inflammatory and antibacterial agent and its use dates back to ancient Egypt [it was even found in the tomb of King Tutankhamun (better known as King Tut)], Greece, and Rome, with the bee products mentioned in writings in Egypt, India, and China dating back to 5500 BCE.[3,11,12,27,28] Honey has been used in Ayurvedic

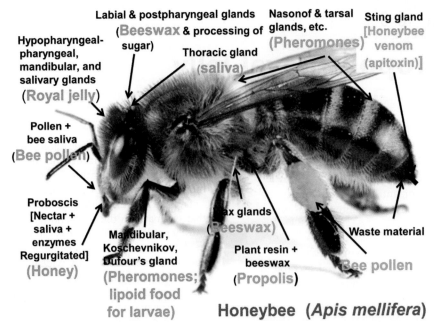

▲ FIGURE 60-1 Glandular secretions of the honeybee. Reprinted with permission from Israili Z. Antimicrobial properties of Honey. *Am J Ther* 2013. doi: 10.1097/MJT.0b013e318293b09b, accessed May 2014.

medicine for at least 4,000 years.[3] The use of honey to treat wounds was practiced in China during the Xin dynasty (circa 2000 BCE), and ancient physicians (the Greeks Hippocrates and Dioscorides, Romans Celsus and Galen, and Arabs El Mad Joussy and El Basry) are said to have cited the healing qualities of honey.[3] Abu Ali bin Sina (Latinized as Avicenna), a leading Persian doctor and scholar circa 11th century CE, wrote of using cooked honey and myrrh to decrease exudates from wounds contributing to partial tissue loss.[1,29] More recent uses of honey in medicine hewed to wound treatment, including gunshot wounds in the 17th and 18th centuries (it was an official drug in London pharmacopoeias in the 17th century)[5,30] and through World War I usage by the Russians and Germans.[29,31,32] Not until the discovery of antibiotics in the 1940s did the traditional medical use of honey begin to wane.[29,33]

The word "propolis" is derived from the Greek words *pro* (before) and *polis* (city), which reflects the ancient observation that bees built walls of the substance near the entrance of their hives.[5,12,14,34,35] It was considered the third natural product of bees (in addition to honey and wax). Ancient Egyptians, making use of the antiputrefactive activity of bee glue, used propolis to embalm their dead.[34,35] The Greek philosopher Aristotle wrote about the basic characteristics of propolis in his work *Historia Animalium* over 2,000 years ago, with recordings of its use dating back to at least 300 BCE; its use in medical applications was covered by Alexander of Tralles in the 6th century CE.[11,14,34]

Propolis has been used for centuries in folk medicine in Europe, the Americas, China, and Japan.[1] In traditional medicine, propolis was most successful in treating a wide range of wounds because of its antiedematous and anti-infectious properties. Propolis was also used in the ancient world for muscle, tendon, and joint pain. In addition, bee glue was used to treat cutaneous conditions such as lichens and condylomata.[11] In more recent times, propolis was used to treat wounds during the Anglo-Boer war between 1899 and 1902 as well as World War II, and was an accepted medical ingredient in the former Soviet Union as recently as 1969.[1] Other indications have included burns, sore throat, and stomach ulcers.[36] In fact, propolis has continued to be a popular therapeutic choice in the Balkan

countries of Southeast Europe for these indications and it is marketed in some European countries for the treatment of prostate hyperplasia.[37]

Modern studies of the medicinal benefits of propolis are traced to Stan Scheller in 1960s Poland, where the study of its biological characteristics by way of a novel approach to delivering hydrophobic ethanol extracts of propolis into aqueous solutions led to the identification of antioxidant, antibacterial, immunostimulating, and radioprotective qualities.[38]

The "queen substance" 9-oxo-2-decenoic acid (9-ODA), a queen honeybee pheromone, was isolated from queen honeybee mandibular glands by Butler et al. in 1961.[39,40] Johnston et al. found in 1965 that this minor component of royal jelly rapidly metabolizes into 9-hydroxy-2-decenoic acid (9-HDA), a precursor to royal jelly that stabilizes swarm activity.[39,41,42] Royal jelly is now used in cosmetics, dietary supplements, and beverages. Particularly in Asia, it is deployed as a health tonic.[17,43] Royal jelly has also exhibited effectiveness in alleviating chilliness in young women.[44].

CHEMISTRY

The myriad biological functions associated with honey (e.g., antibacterial, antioxidant, antitumor, anti-inflammatory, antibrowning, and antiviral), propolis (e.g., antitumor, antioxidant, antimicrobial, anti-inflammatory, and immunomodulatory), and royal jelly (e.g., antibacterial, anti-inflammatory, vasodilative, hypotensive, disinfectant, antioxidant, antihypercholesterolemic, and antitumor) are chiefly ascribed to the plethora of phenolic compounds, such as flavonoids, found in these bee products (Table 60-1).[9] The flavonoid chrysin is present in honey and propolis and is thought to play a key role in conferring anti-inflammatory activity.[9]

Honey itself contains carbohydrates, proteins, 18 free amino acids (of which proline is the most abundant), vitamins (trace amounts of B_2, B_4, B_5, B_6, B_{11}, and C), minerals (e.g., calcium, chromium, iron, magnesium, manganese, phosphorus, potassium, selenium, and zinc), antioxidants (primarily flavonoids, including pinocembrin, which is found only in honey and propolis),

TABLE 60-1
Pros and Cons of Honey/Propolis/Royal Jelly

Pros	Cons
Broad biological activities	Scant data on the pharmacologic efficacy of topical royal jelly
Long history of traditional use	Both honey and propolis are challenging to standardize and formulate
Viable antibiotic alternative in cases of antibiotic-resistant bacterial infection (honey and, perhaps, propolis)	

enzymes (e.g., invertase, amylase, glucose oxidase, catalase, and acid phosphorylase), as well as acetic, butanoic, citric, formic, gluconic, lactic, malic, pyroglutamic, and succinic acids.[8,45,46] Medical-grade honeys such as manuka honey (a monofloral honey derived from *Leptospermum scoparium*, a member of the Myrtaceae family, native to New Zealand) and Medihoney® (a standardized mix of Australian and New Zealand honeys mainly originating from Leptospermum species) are rich in flavonoids.[45,47–49] Honey exhibits a pH ranging between 3.2 and 4.5, an acidity level that hinders the growth of many microorganisms.[29,50–52]

Propolis is a complex mixture of partially digested resins from trees and bees wax, containing approximately anywhere from 50 to 300 constituents including balsams, resins, waxes, essential oils, pollen, cinnamyl alcohol, flavonoids, minerals (e.g., calcium, copper, iodine, iron, magnesium, manganese, potassium, sodium, and zinc), as well as vitamins A, B (B_1, B_2, B_6), C, and E.[1,53] Interestingly, Tsai et al. have shown that while propolis acts as an antioxidant, it can also induce oxidative DNA damage by producing hydrogen peroxide (H_2O_2). But they note that propolis-treated cells display a lower level of DNA damage when challenged with another oxidative compound (e.g., amoxicillin). They concluded that this adaptive response may play a role in the beneficial results associated with propolis.[4] Overall, propolis is thought to confer significant antioxidant activity. Phenolic compounds (particularly vanillic, coumaric, rosmarinic, chlorogenic, caffeic, and ferulic acids) and flavonoids such as quercetin are thought to account for these propolis properties, which has been found, according to *in vitro* and *in vivo* studies, to protect skin against ultraviolet (UV)-induced damage.[1,35,54–58]

Royal jelly, which bees produce from pollen, contains water, proteins (82–90 percent of which are known as the major royal jelly proteins, with five primary members), lipids, sugars, carbohydrates, free amino acids, vitamins, and minerals.[8,9,19] Its primary unsaturated fatty acid is 10-hydroxy-2-decenoic acid (10-HDA), which is uniquely found in royal jelly.[59] The benefits to human health associated with royal jelly can be partly attributed to the activity of constituent lipids, primarily aliphatic free fatty acids and few esters, which render the royal jelly emulsion highly acidic and therefore able to impart antimicrobial properties.[8] These royal jelly components are considered to function in ways that protect against skin aging, modulate the immune system, potentially thwart cancer development, induce neurogenesis, and alleviate symptoms of menopause.[16]

ORAL USES

Honey is the oldest sweetener and one of the oldest foods consumed by humans, having been in popular usage in the diet throughout the world for thousands of years. It never spoils and was even found in edible condition in King Tut's tomb.[45]

The preservative qualities of honey have been attributed to its antioxidant properties.[58] Darker honeys (such as buckwheat) are associated with greater antioxidant activity.[58]

Propolis is extensively used in food and beverage products to boost human health.[1,60] In 1995, the National Food Institute of Argentina recognized propolis as a dietary supplement.[1] It is typically available in capsule form.

In 1990, Fujii et al. found that orally administered royal jelly exhibited anti-inflammatory activity and wound-healing capacity in streptozotocin-diabetic rats,[61] a result supported by more recent findings.[62] For instance, in 2003, Taniguchi et al. found that the oral administration of royal jelly hinders the development of atopic dermatitis-like skin lesions in mice.[63]

TOPICAL USES

In over-the-counter cosmetic formulations, honey is used primarily as a moisturizing agent and in hair conditioning products because it has strong humectant properties. It is also used in home remedies for burns, wounds, eczema, and dermatitis, particularly in Asia.[8]

Propolis has been shown to have several potential topical dental applications worthy of investigation. In a study of the histological effects of propolis topically applied to dental sockets and skin wounds in rats, a 10 percent hydroalcoholic solution of propolis or a 10 percent hydroalcoholic solution alone were compared. Examination of cutaneous wound healing and the socket wound after tooth extraction revealed that topical application of the propolis hydroalcoholic solution accelerated epithelial repair but had no effect on socket wound healing.[64] Propolis has also been found to be effective in treating aphthous ulceration.[65–67]

There are several commercially available products such as lotions, creams, shampoos, lipsticks, toothpastes, and mouthwashes, as well as cough syrups, lozenges, and vitamins that contain propolis as an active ingredient.

Wound Healing

In 2010, Majtan et al. showed that incubation with honey activated human keratinocytes to increase production of mediators including cytokines [tumor necrosis factor-α, interleukin (IL)-1β, and transforming growth factor (TGF)-β1] and matrix metalloproteinase (MMP)-9. In addition, they demonstrated that this increased amount of epidermal MMP-9 facilitated the degradation of collagen type IV in the basement membrane, buttressing the notion that honey has the capacity to accelerate wound healing.[24]

A 2013 systematic literature review of honey in contemporary wound care included 55 studies revealing that honey does appear to stimulate healing of burns, ulcers, and other wounds. The authors were hesitant to draw many broad conclusions due to methodological concerns, but found that honey displays antibacterial activity in burn treatment and also exerts deodorizing, debridement, anti-inflammatory, and analgesic activity.[29] However, a search of the Cochrane Wounds Group Specialized Register, the Cochrane Central Register, Ovid Medline, Ovid Embase, and EBSCO CINAHL completed earlier that year of 25 randomized and quasi-randomized trials assessing honey in the treatment of acute or chronic wounds found that honey might delay healing in partial- and full-thickness burns compared to early excision and grafting, and it does not significantly enhance healing of chronic venous leg ulcers.[68] The authors suggested that while honey may, indeed, prove to be more effective than some conventional dressings, there is insufficient evidence to support this claim.

Propolis has also been found to exert a wound-healing effect. In 2002, Pachalski et al. assessed the use of propolis in treating the skin of the stumps of 156 patients rehabilitating after lower limb amputation (55 upper leg and 101 lower leg). Patients were treated twice daily with 4 percent propolis ointment for seven days. Treatment was extended to 14 days in cases of unsatisfactory improvement within one week. Patients with upper leg amputations experienced slightly better results, though both groups exhibited the best outcomes with *Staphylococcus* infections. The investigators noted that topically applied propolis improves circulation, stimulates intracellular metabolism, and alters skin reactivity. They also concluded that propolis ointment is indicated for skin disorders on stumps and local trophic conditions.[69]

Like its associated bee products, royal jelly has reportedly contributed to wound healing. In 2008, Abdelatif et al. conducted a pilot study to ascertain the safety and effectiveness of a new ointment combining royal jelly and panthenol (Pedyphar) in 60 patients with limb-threatening diabetic foot infections. By the end of week 9 and through six months of follow-up, 96 percent of the patients with full-thickness skin ulcers (Wagner grades 1 and 2) or deep tissue infection and suspected osteomyelitis (grade 3) responded well, with all grade 1 and 2 ulcers healing and 92 percent of grade 3 ulcers healing. All patients with gangrenous lesions (grades 4 and 5) healed after surgical excision, debridement, and conservative treatment with the royal jelly/panthenol formulation [see Chapter 27, Vitamin B_5 (Pantothenic Acid/Dexpanthenol)]. The investigators suggested that more double-blind, randomized controlled studies are required to confirm their promising findings that the royal jelly/panthenol combination is safe and effective.[70]

Suemaru et al. compared the effects of topically applied honey, propolis, and royal jelly on 5-fluorouracil (5-FU)-induced experimental oral mucositis in hamsters. The size of the lesions was not diminished by the use of honey (1, 10, and 100 percent) or propolis (0.3, 1, and 3 percent) in comparison to the Vaseline-treated control group. Royal jelly ointments (3, 10, and 30 percent) dose-dependently led to significant improvements and healing, suggesting its possible use in treating chemotherapy-induced moral mucositis in humans.[71] More recently, several of the same investigators furthered their study of royal jelly and its effects on 5-FU-induced oral mucositis in hamsters. Chitosan-sodium alginate film containing royal jelly was used to achieve healing. These films (10 and 30 percent) significantly ameliorated the damage caused by 5-FU, decreasing myeloperoxidase activity and proinflammatory cytokine production. In addition to such anti-inflammatory effects, the investigators noted that royal jelly displayed antioxidant activity. They attributed the healing effect from severe oral mucositis to the anti-inflammatory and antioxidant properties of royal jelly.[72]

In 2010, Kim et al. treated freshly scratched normal human dermal fibroblasts with different concentrations of royal jelly (0.1, 1, or 5 mg/mL) for up to 48 hours. They found that fibroblast migration peaked at 24 hours after wounding and that royal jelly significantly and dose-dependently accelerated the migration at the eight-hour mark. In addition, various lipids in fibroblasts involved in the wound-healing process were influenced by royal jelly treatment, with the cholesterol level lowered and sphinganines increased.[62]

The following year, Siavash et al. conducted a small study of eight patients to assess the efficacy of topically applied royal jelly in the treatment of diabetic foot ulcers. Of the eight ulcers treated, seven healed, with a mean healing duration of 41 days. The eighth ulcer improved, with significant reductions in size. The investigators concluded that a royal jelly dressing appears to be an effective alternative treatment option for diabetic foot ulcers.[73] However, in 2013, Siavash et al. assessed the efficacy of topical royal jelly on diabetic foot ulcers in a double-blind placebo-controlled clinical trial of 25 patients (6 females, 19 males). The 60 ulcers considered in the final analysis were treated with either 5 percent sterile topical royal jelly or placebo. They found no significant differences in the regimens.[21]

COLLAGEN PRODUCTION Koya-Miyata et al. have demonstrated that royal jelly fosters collagen production by skin fibroblasts in the presence of ascorbic acid-2-O-α-glucoside (AA-2G) and that its primary fatty acid constituent 10-HDA promotes the synthesis of collagen by AA-2G-treated fibroblasts by initiating the production of TGF-β1 production.[20]

Seborrheic Dermatitis/Dandruff

In 2001, Al-Waili completed a study in 30 patients (20 males, 10 females aged 15 to 60 years) with chronic seborrheic dermatitis of the scalp, face, and chest to evaluate the potential of topically applied crude honey (90 percent honey diluted in warm water). Treatment over a four-week period consisted of gentle rubbing of the ointment for two to three minutes onto lesions every other day, leaving honey on for three hours before gentle warm water rinsing. A six-month prophylactic phase split the group evenly into a once-weekly treatment group and a control group. Honey application yielded further marked improvements, with itching and scaling resolved within the first week. Within two weeks, skin lesions healed completely. Patients also reported subjective improvement in hair loss. Whereas no patients treated with honey experienced relapse, 12 of the 15 patients in the control group experienced relapse within two to four months of initial treatment cessation. The author concluded that weekly use of crude honey delivers significant improvement in seborrheic dermatitis and related hair loss.[74]

Subsequently, Al-Waili et al. conducted a review of the antimicrobial activity of honey, finding topical effectiveness in the treatment of adult and neonatal postoperative infection, boils, burns, infected and nonhealing wounds and ulcers, necrotizing fasciitis, pilonidal sinus, diabetic foot ulcers, as well as venous ulcers.[76] Internally, honey lowers prostaglandin levels while raising nitric oxide levels, and displays anti-inflammatory and prebiotic activity.[75]

■ SAFETY ISSUES

Allergic reactions to honey, propolis, and royal jelly have been reported.[76,77] Propolis is relatively innocuous, though.[34] A no-effect level (NOEL) of 1,400 mg/kg body weight/day was found in a 90-mouse study on propolis.[14] Some cases of allergic contact dermatitis as well as allergic contact cheilitis to propolis in humans have been reported.[53,78–81]

Royal jelly has been known to provoke an anaphylactic response in some people.[17,82] Asthmatic and anaphylactic reactions to the ingestion of royal jelly have been found to be true IgE-mediated hypersensitivity reactions.[83] Contact dermatitis has also been reported in reaction to topical royal jelly.[84] Indeed, although royal jelly has been linked to broad health benefits, such as promoting growth in children, improving general health, and enhancing longevity, adverse reactions ranging from contact dermatitis, acute asthma, anaphylaxis and even death have been linked to its use.[85]

A 1997 cross-sectional survey of 1,472 hospital employees in Hong Kong conducted by Leung et al. revealed that 461 subjects (31.3 percent) had taken royal jelly in the past. Adverse reactions to royal jelly, including urticaria, eczema, rhinitis, and acute asthma, were reported by nine subjects. Skin tests were conducted on 176 questionnaire respondents (13 of whom had a positive skin test to pure royal jelly) and 300 consecutive asthma clinic patients (23 of whom had positive skin tests). Thirty-five of the 36 participants with positive royal jelly skin tests were atopic to other common allergens.[86] In a retrospective evaluation of common environmental allergens in adult asthmatic patients completed later that year in Hong Kong, many of the same investigators found that royal jelly was the fifth most common allergen associated with positive skin tests (after *Dermatophagoides pteronyssinus*, *D. farinae*, cockroaches, and cat dander).[87]

In a 2008 study aimed at characterizing the major allergens of royal jelly, Rosmilah et al. identified major royal jelly protein 1 and major royal jelly protein 2 as the main allergens in royal jelly that affected the 53 human subjects with royal jelly allergy who were evaluated.[85]

In 2013, Moriyama et al. assessed the hypoallergenicity of alkaline protease-treated royal jelly *in vitro* and *in vivo*. They demonstrated that the immunoglobulin E-binding capacity of the treated royal jelly was substantially diminished via *in vitro* assays of the blood from patients sensitive to royal jelly. In 75 percent of royal jelly-sensitive patients given a skin-prick test, royal jelly did not elicit an allergic reaction.[17]

ENVIRONMENTAL IMPACT

As stated above, human beings depend on bees to pollinate approximately one-third of our crops, including a large proportion of the produce that we consume. Among global agricultural crops, the European honeybee is the most economically valuable pollinator.[88] *A. mellifera* also plays a significant role in maintaining biodiversity via pollinating several species of plants that need an obligatory pollinator to be fertilized.[88] Notably, the antibacterial activities of bee products, especially honey and propolis, place bees at an even more potentially crucial position related to human health given the alarming global increase in antibiotic resistance among several bacterial strains. Indeed, Dr. Margaret Chan, director-general of the World Health Organization, has warned of the dangers of increasingly pervasive antibiotic resistance, referring to this insidious threat as the possible "end of modern medicine as we know it."[89]

Given that honey, in particular, has been exploited since ancient times for its antibacterial properties in treating infected wounds and is currently known to exhibit broad-spectrum effectiveness against antibiotic-resistant strains, this iconic bee product would appear to merit careful consideration and study, as would propolis, along with a concerted effort to stem the overuse, abuse, and misuse of antibiotics. However, the effects of "colony collapse disorder" – the decimation of bee populations – certainly loom as a substantial threat to further exploring a natural alternative to antibiotic resistance within our midst. The etiology of this bee colony disaster has recently become less mysterious, as the use of neonicotinoid pesticides in industrial agriculture appears to account for much of the devastating impact on honeybees, though calls for more larger studies persist.[90,91] The European Commission has banned the use of three neonicotinoids based on such concerns.[92] Colony collapse disorder is a global phenomenon,[93] and poses significant worldwide risk to the produce on which human beings significantly rely. Regardless of the cause or causes, whether it is pesticide use or the parasitic Varroa mite,[94] colony collapse disorder presents a significant existential impact on honeybees and, possibly, numerous other species including humans.

The greater environmental impact related to bee products, then, is not in the harvesting and processing of these products themselves but, rather, from the marked strains that human industry places on the very existence of the honeybee. We quite possibly continue the use of neonicotinoid pesticides, now believed to have a pernicious effect on bees,[95] and overuse of antibiotics for livestock[96] at our own peril.

FORMULATION CONSIDERATIONS

Geographical location, pollen source, climate, environmental conditions, season during collection, genetic factors, and the processing methods it undergoes influence honey composition and quality.[9,33] Because honey is readily contaminated through processing, medical grade honey is sterilized through γ-radiation, which destroys various microorganisms without compromising the compound's antibacterial activity.[29,46,97–100]

Like honey, the collection location, time, and plant source affect propolis quality, chemical composition, and biologic activity, thus there is great variability in these products.[1,35,101,102] However, because of the unique ecosystems in which different honeybees live and the variety of plant sources from which bees collect ingredients, propolis does not have a specific chemical connotation or formula.[35] Given the potential for its use as a topical agent because of its antioxidant capacity, Marquele-Oliveira et al. found in 2007 that propolis formulations prepared with Polawax exhibited functional and physical stability in percutaneous studies in pig ear skin and hairless mouse skin as well as an *in vivo* study that indicated the viability of the formulation in protecting human skin from UVB photodamage.[103]

Dosage and safety are among the greatest challenges of using bee products for medical purposes.[23] Honey and royal jelly processed into formulations for wound care first pass through fine filters that remove the majority of pollen and other impurities. Some viable spores, such as clostridia, may be included in honey.[23] Bacterial sensitivity to bee products is influenced by the botanical origin of the product and there is significant variability in bacterial sensitivity to bee products.[23]

USAGE CONSIDERATIONS

Honey that is not medical grade is liable to contain viable bacterial spores (including clostridia), and may also exhibit less predictable antibacterial properties.[10] Several countries have approved of the use of medical-grade honey (e.g., manuka, Medihoney) and numerous brands of sterile, irradiated, antibacterial topical honey preparations are available.[10,33,104,105]

Royal jelly is used in cosmetics, dietary supplements, and beverages. Particularly in Asia, it is deployed as a health tonic.[43]

SIGNIFICANT BACKGROUND

Manuka honey and Medihoney are the primary forms of honey used in clinical practice. Propolis is one of the most copious sources of polyphenols, particularly flavonoids and phenolic acids, some of the most potent antioxidants yet discovered.[106,107]

Antioxidant Activity

In 2005, a study by Marquele et al. of Brazilian propolis extracts alone and in topical pharmaceutical formulations revealed that the antioxidant activity of the extracts was maintained in the topical products. The bee glue was particularly active against the superoxide radical.[108]

A 2006 study using New Zealand white rabbits revealed that topical propolis exhibited antioxidant, anti-inflammatory, and antibacterial activity against *Staphylococcus aureus* keratitis.[109]

In 2009, Nakajima et al. compared the antioxidant effects of various bee products, specifically Brazilian green propolis, water-soluble royal jelly, and a bee pollen ethanol extract against H_2O_2, superoxide anion, and hydroxyl radicals. They found water extracts of propolis to have the greatest potency, followed by ethanol extracts of propolis, and pollen. Royal jelly had no effects. Of the primary constituents of propolis, caffeic acid displayed the greatest antioxidant activity, followed by artepillin C, and drupanin.[110] Also that year, Izuta et al. found that Brazilian green propolis and Chinese red propolis and their components (CAPE and caffeoylquinic acid derivatives) acted as potent scavengers of the 1,1-diphenyl-2-picrylhydrazyl (DPPH) radical.[111]

Recent chemical analyses of Algerian propolis indicated a high content of polyphenols and diterpenes from samples in various north Algerian regions. Using the DPPH assay, Piccinelli et al. found that the polyphenol-rich samples of propolis exhibited potent antioxidant activity.[112]

In addition, propolis has been shown to lower oxidative stress, altering catalase, malondialdehyde, and nitric oxide levels, in N_ω-nitro-L-arginine methyl ester (1-NAME)-induced hypertension in rats, suggesting a modulatory impact on the antioxidant system.[113]

A 2010 study by Cole et al. showed that Sydney propolis significantly and dose-dependently protected mouse skin against edema, immunosuppression, and lipid peroxidation. The investigators concluded that Sydney propolis has the potential to protect human skin against UV-induced skin cancer and other photodamage.[114]

In 2011, Fonseca et al. showed that green and brown propolis extracts, with varying composition and properties, both effectively prevented UV-induced glutathione depletion *in vivo*. Oral administration of extracts in hairless mice yielded a higher recovery of glutathione, after reductions caused by UV exposure, in the green propolis group (30 percent vs. 22.8 percent). Topical propolis pretreatment before UV exposure netted a 14 percent recovery in both groups. The investigators concluded that both green and brown propolis extracts are promising agents for combating oxidative stress in skin.[55]

In 2013, Bolfa et al. studied the wide-ranging effects of a Romanian propolis topically applied in two concentrations (3 mg and 1.5 mg polyphenols/cm²) before or after UVB exposure in a Swiss mouse model. Both concentrations significantly decreased malondialdehyde formation and IL-6 levels while restoring the activity of glutathione peroxidase. Epidermal hyperplasia and dermal inflammation were diminished with the smaller concentration, with only dermal inflammation reduced by pretreatment with the larger concentration. Romanian propolis also decreased sunburn cell formation and exhibited an antigenotoxic effect by significantly attenuating cyclobutane pyrimidine dimer formation. In light of the antioxidant, anti-inflammatory, antiapoptotic, and antigenotoxic properties manifested in their study, the investigators concluded that Romanian propolis provides significant photoprotection in the mouse model and warrants consideration as a chemopreventive agent for mitigating several

UVB-induced cutaneous signaling pathways.[108] Also that year, Moniruzzaman et al. found that two Malaysian honeys, longan and sourwood, are good sources of antioxidants as compared to other rubber tree and manuka honeys.[115]

Antimicrobial and Anti-inflammatory Activity

Potent antibacterial activity is exhibited by honey, propolis, royal jelly, as well as bee venom, with even epidemic strains of methicillin-resistant *Staphylococcus aureus* (MRSA) and Vancomycin-resistant *Enterococcus* (VRE) showing sensitivity.[23] Among the bee products, propolis has shown the greatest antibacterial activity,[23] though clinical trials and laboratory data suggest that honey acts as an effective broad-spectrum antimicrobial agent.[3,76] These wide-ranging functions are thought to be derived from its acidity; bacteriostatic, bactericidal, and antioxidant constituents (i.e., H_2O_2, antioxidants, lysozyme, polyphenols, phenolic acids, flavonoids, methylglyoxal, and bee peptides); osmotic effect; high sugar concentration; induction of cytokine release; as well as immunomodulatory and anti-inflammatory activity.[3,76]

In a 2008 evaluation of medical grade honey (Revamil), Kwakman et al. found that within 24 hours 10 to 40 percent (vol/vol) honey eradicated antibiotic-susceptible and -resistant isolates of *Staphylococcus aureus*, *Staphylococcus epidermidis*, *Enterococcus faecium*, *Escherichia coli*, *Pseudomonas aeruginosa*, *Enterobacter cloacae*, and *Klebsiella oxytoca*. They also noted a 100-fold decline in forearm skin colonization in healthy volunteers after two days of honey application, with the number of positive skin cultures falling by 76 percent. The investigators concluded that the topical antimicrobial honey agent Revamil displays significant potential to prevent or treat infections, including those engendered by multidrug-resistant bacteria.[25] It is worth noting that honey is known to suppress 150 bacteria species, including clinical strains of MRSA and VRE, with no reports of microbial resistance.[10] In fact, honey has been shown to be clinically effective in treating various kinds of wound infections, reducing skin colonization of several bacteria (including MRSA),[25] and accelerating wound healing, without provoking adverse effects.[10] A 2009 report by Blair et al. supports the notion that medical-grade honey has the potential to lessen the strain caused by the emergence of antibiotic-resistant bacteria.[116]

In 2000, Vynograd et al. evaluated propolis for efficacy in the treatment of recurrent genital herpes simplex virus type 2. Ninety adults, all with local symptoms, participated in a randomized, single-blind, masked investigator, controlled study at seven medical centers in which Canadian propolis ointment containing natural flavonoids was compared with ointments of acyclovir and placebo, with 30 people randomized to each group. Study ointments were applied four times daily. Participants were examined on the 3rd, 7th, and 10th days of treatment for clinical symptoms, including the number and size of herpetic lesions, with lesions classified into four stages: vesicular, ulcerated, crusted, and healed. On Day 3, 15 members of the propolis group had crusted lesions as opposed to eight in the acyclovir group and none on placebo. Local symptoms were noted in three propolis group members, eight acyclovir individuals, and nine on placebo. On Day 7, healing was observed in 10 propolis patients, four acyclovir patients, and three in the placebo group. Investigators reported that 24 propolis patients and 14 acyclovir patients had healed by Day 10. Overall, the propolis ointment was considered more effective in healing lesions and reducing local symptoms.[117] In an earlier study of 65 patients, a topical ointment containing propolis, Nivcrisol-D, showed a significant therapeutic effect against recurrent herpes and zona zoster, with patients using the study drug healing from outbreaks in an average of four days while patients using placebo took an average of eight days to heal from outbreaks.[118]

In 2002, Gregory et al. assessed the purported antimicrobial, anti-inflammatory, and scar-healing capacity of a high-grade Brazilian propolis cream. Patients presenting with bilateral superficial second-degree burns over less than 20 percent of their body surface, with wounds of similar depth and quality, were admitted into the study within 48 hours of their injuries and then treated with propolis cream on one wound and silver sulfadiazene applied to a similar one on the other side. Wounds were debrided and dressings changed on the following morning. Patients returned to the clinic at three-day intervals to have their wounds checked and dressings changed, with reapplication of the ointment taking place only at these visits. In addition, investigators cultured the wounds for microbial growth and took photographs to record inflammation and scar formation. No significant differences were noted in microbial colonization, but wounds treated with the propolis cream showed less inflammation and quicker scar formation as compared to the silver sulfadiazene-treated burns. While noting the beneficial effects of propolis on burns, the researchers speculated that more frequent changing of wound dressings would have evinced antimicrobial results also.[119]

Omani propolis has been found to differ from many known propolis types, as it is derived from the resin of *Azadiracta indica* (neem tree), Acacia spp. (most probably *A. nilotica*) and *Mangifera indica*. However, like many other forms of propolis, the Omani variety contains biologically active phenolic compounds (e.g., prenylflavanones, cardols, and anacardic acids) and has exhibited antimicrobial activity.[36]

Activity Against Pruritus and Xerosis

In 2011, Duplan et al. assessed the activity of a synthetic counterpart to 10-HDA in several experiments (*in vitro*, *ex vivo*, and *in vivo*) aimed at characterizing its potential use in treating UV-induced xerosis. Hydroxydecine® induced involucrin, transglutaminase-1, and filaggrin protein production in normal human keratinoctyes and yielded increases in these compounds in topical treatment of skin equivalents. In healthy volunteers with UV-induced xerosis, Hydroxydecine cream use led to an increase of 28.8 percent in the hydration index after seven days and 60.4 percent after 21 days of treatment. In the *ex vivo* findings in a model of inflammation and barrier impairment involving human skin explants maintained alive, the formulation restored skin barrier function and lessened inflammation. The investigators concluded that the synthetic version of 10-HDA also displayed efficacy in activating keratinocyte differentiation *in vitro* as well as *in vivo* in hydrating dry human skin.[60]

In 2013, Yamaura et al. examined an experimental allergic contact dermatitis model in hairless mice to ascertain the antipruritic activity of topical royal jelly on chronic pruritus. They found that five weeks of treatment with topical royal jelly (0.01 or 1 percent) and 0.01 percent β-methasone significantly alleviated chronic pruritus induced by five weeks of repeated application of 2,4,6-trinitro-1-chlorobenzene. The level of nerve growth factor mRNA in back skin was elevated in mice with contact dermatitis, lower in those treated with β-methasone, and unchanged in mice treated with royal jelly. The investigators acknowledged the likely different mechanisms of action between royal jelly and β-methasone in suggesting that royal jelly may be a useful ingredient in cosmetics for easing chronic pruritus.[43]

Anticarcinogenic Activity

Various components of propolis have also been isolated and found to possess anticarcinogenic properties. Flavonoid aglycones are some of the significant constituents of propolis that are believed to contribute to antitumorigenic activity.[13] A study with a fractionated methanol extract of a Brazilian propolis resulted in the isolation of a tumoricidal substance characterized as a new clerodane diterpenoid, which reduced the growth and number of skin tumors induced by 7,12-dimethylbenz(a) anthracene (DMBA) application on mouse back skin by inhibition of DNA synthesis.[13]

In a study to determine whether CAPE, a propolis constituent, inhibits the tumor promoter 12-O-tetradecanoylphorbol-13-acetate (TPA)-induced processes associated with carcinogenesis, low doses of CAPE were topically applied to SENCAR mice. CAPE was found to strongly inhibit several TPA-mediated oxidative processes considered *sine qua non* for tumor promotion, including: polymorphonuclear leukocyte infiltration into mouse skin and ears; H_2O_2 production; and formation of oxidized bases in epidermal DNA. In addition, researchers noted inhibition of edema and ornithine decarboxylase induction in CD-1 and SENCAR mice after CAPE application, as well as the inhibition of TPA-induced H_2O_2 production in bovine lenses. Researchers concluded that CAPE appears to have potent chemopreventive capacity, particularly in treating disorders associated with strong inflammatory and/or oxidative stress processes, such as cancer and cataracts.[27]

In a different study on skin tumors, CD-1 mice were initiated with DMBA and then treated twice weekly with topically applied TPA, resulting in 18.8 skin papillomas per mouse. Subsequent topical application of CAPE to the backs of the mice together with TPA twice a week for 20 weeks inhibited the number of skin papillomas and reduced tumor size in a dose-dependent manner. The same combination also decreased the level of 5-hydroxymethyl-2′-deoxyuridine (HMdU) in epidermal DNA produced through the previous initiation with DMBA. In addition, *in vitro* CAPE introduction to cultured HeLa cells inhibited DNA, RNA, and protein synthesis. All of these inhibitory effects conferred by CAPE were deemed by investigators to be potent.[120]

In a 2004 study on polyphenolic compounds and antitumorigenic properties, a water-soluble derivative of propolis, caffeic acid, CAPE, and quercetin administered to mice resulted in a reduction in the number of lung tumor nodules. Researchers related the antitumor properties of the tested substances to their immunomodulatory capacity, cytotoxicity to tumor cells, and ability to induce apoptosis and necrosis, suggesting that propolis, caffeic acid, CAPE, and quercetin show promising potential for combating tumor growth.[121]

In 2011, Watanabe et al. found that propolis appears, *in vitro* and *in vivo*, to act against various tumor cells, suggesting its possible role in future anticancer drugs.[15]

Photoprotection

In 2011, Park et al. measured the 10-HDA content of royal jelly and investigated its effects on UVB-induced skin photoaging in normal human dermal fibroblasts. The tested royal jelly (0.211 percent 10-HDA) led to increased synthesis of procollagen type I and TGF-β1, without altering MMP-1 levels. The researchers concluded that due to its potential to spur collagen production, royal jelly could be used to protect the skin against UVB-induced photoaging.[122] Park et al. followed this work up the following year, finding that the synthesis of type I collagen in the dorsal skin of ovariectomized Sprague-Dawley rats was augmented by the dietary supplementation of 1 percent royal jelly extract. Although MMP-1 levels were again unchanged, the investigators suggest that royal jelly may provide an antiaging benefit by virtue of enhanced collagen production alone.[19]

In 2013, Zheng et al. studied the protective effects of the royal jelly fatty acid component 10-HDA against UVA-induced damage in human dermal fibroblasts and its inhibitory effects on UVA-induced MMP expression. They found that 10-HDA significantly protected the fibroblasts from UVA-induced cytotoxicity, reactive oxygen species, and cellular senescence. In addition, 10-HDA hindered the UVA-generated expression of MMP-1 as well as MMP-3, and stimulated the production of collagen. Activation of the c-Jun N-terminal kinase (JNK) and p38 mitogen-activated protein kinase (MAPK) pathways was also diminished due to 10-HDA treatment. The investigators concluded that this royal jelly fatty acid exhibits potential for use in the prevention and treatment of cutaneous photoaging.[22]

In 2013, Angelo et al. demonstrated that the addition of propolis protected *L. angustifolia* (lavender) essential oil from UV-induced degradation and preserved its antioxidant capacity in cell oxidative damage assessments on B$_{16}$–F$_{10}$ melanoma cells as well as *in vitro* antioxidant assays. The investigators concluded that propolis may act as an efficient UV-protective and antiradical adjuvant to sunscreens, cosmetics, and other products that contain plant extracts (see Chapter 73, Lavandula).[123]

Skin Whitening

Skin-lightening indications may also be a viable use for royal jelly. Han et al. found that royal jelly dose-dependently suppressed melanin biosynthesis in the B$_{16}$-F$_1$ mouse melanocyte cell line by lowering tyrosinase activity. Further, royal jelly decreased mRNA levels of tyrosinase. The researchers concluded that royal jelly merits consideration for inclusion as a therapeutic agent in new skin-whitening products.[18]

CONCLUSION

Honey, propolis, and royal jelly, all bee products with a long history of traditional medicinal use, have been found to exhibit sufficient biologic activity to warrant consideration in modern medicine. The antibacterial activity of these products is legendary, and the wide array of additional biologic activities, particularly their antioxidant capacity, suggest broad potential for these agents, meriting greater attention and study for dermatologic application. Indeed, more research, in the form of randomized, controlled trials, is needed prior to incorporating bee products into the armamentarium as first-line therapies, but the potential seems vast.

REFERENCES

1. Khalil ML. Biological activity of bee propolis in health and disease. *Asian Pac J Cancer Prev.* 2006;7:22.
2. Oka H, Emori Y, Kobayashi N, et al. Suppression of allergic reactions by royal jelly in association with the restoration of macrophage function and the improvement of Th1/Th2 cell responses. *Int Immunopharmacol.* 2001;1:521.
3. Israili ZH. Antimicrobial properties of honey. *Am J Ther.* 2013 Jun 18. [Epub ahead of print]
4. Tsai YC, Wang YH, Liou CC, et al. Induction of oxidative DNA damage by flavonoids of propolis: Its mechanism and implication about antioxidant capacity. *Chem Res Toxicol.* 2012;25:191.
5. Castaldo S, Capasso F. Propolis, an old remedy used in modern medicine. *Fitoterapia.* 2002;(73 Suppl 1):S1.
6. Walsh B. The plight of the honeybee: Mass deaths in bee colonies may mean disaster for farmers – And your favorite Foods. *Time Magazine,* August 19, 2013. http://content.time.com/time/magazine/article/0,9171,2149141,00.html#ixzz2nhSJwyqZ. Accessed December 16, 2013.
7. Klein AM, Vaissière BE, Cane JH, et al. Importance of pollinators in changing landscapes for world crops. *Proc Biol Sci.* 2007;274:303.
8. Ediriweera ER, Premarathna NY. Medicinal and cosmetic uses of bee's honey – A review. *Ayu.* 2012;33:178.
9. Viuda-Martos M, Ruiz-Navajas Y, Fernández-López J, et al. Functional properties of honey, propolis, and royal jelly. *J Food Sci.* 2008;73:R117.
10. Lipsky BA, Hoey C. Topical antimicrobial therapy for treating chronic wounds. *Clin Infect Dis.* 2009;49:1541.
11. Golder W. Propolis. The bee glue as presented by the Graeco-Roman literature. *Wurzbg Medizinhist Mitt.* 2004;23:133.
12. Ghisalberti EL. Propolis: A review. *Bee World.* 1979;60:59.
13. Mitamura T, Matsuno T, Sakamoto S, et al. Effects of a new clerodane diterpenoid isolated from propolis on chemically induced skin tumors in mice. *Anticancer Res.* 1996;16:2669.
14. Burdock GA. Review of the biological properties and toxicity of bee propolis (propolis). *Food Chem Toxicol.* 1998;36:347.
15. Watanabe MA, Amarante MK, Conti BJ, et al. Cytotoxic constituents of propolis inducing anticancer effects: A review. *J Pharm Pharmacol.* 2011;63:1378.
16. Li X, Huang C, Xue Y. Contribution of lipids in honeybee (Apis mellifera) royal jelly to health. *J Med Food.* 2013;16:96.
17. Moriyama T, Yanagihara M, Yano E, et al. Hypoallergenicity and immunological characterization of enzyme-treated royal jelly from Apis mellifera. *Biosci Biotechnol Biochem.* 2013;77:789.
18. Han SM, Yeo JH, Cho YH, et al. Royal jelly reduces melanin synthesis through down-regulation of tyrosinase expression. *Am J Chin Med.* 2011;39:1253.
19. Park HM, Cho MH, Cho Y, et al. Royal jelly increases collagen production in rat skin after ovariectomy. *J Med Food.* 2012;15:568.
20. Koya-Miyata S, Okamoto I, Ushio S, et al. Identification of a collagen production-promoting factor from an extract of royal jelly and its possible mechanism. *Biosci Biotechnol Biochem.* 2004;68:767.
21. Siavash M, Shokri S, Haghighi S, et al. The efficacy of topical royal jelly on healing of diabetic foot ulcers: A double-blind placebo-controlled clinical trial. *Int Wound J.* 2013 Apr 8. [Epub ahead of print]
22. Zheng J, Lai W, Zhu G, et al. 10-Hydroxy-2-decenoic acid prevents ultraviolet A-induced damage and matrix metalloproteinases expression in human dermal fibroblasts. *J Eur Acad Dermatol Venereol.* 2013;27:1269.
23. Boukraâ L, Sulaiman SA. Rediscovering the antibiotics of the hive. *Recent Pat Antiinfect Drug Discov.* 2009;4:206.
24. Majtan J, Kumar P, Majtan T, et al. Effect of honey and its major royal jelly protein 1 on cytokine and MMP-9 mRNA transcripts in human keratinocytes. *Exp Dermatol.* 2010;19:e73.
25. Kwakman PH, Van den Akker JP, Güçlü A, et al. Medical-grade honey kills antibiotic-resistant bacteria in vitro and eradicates skin colonization. *Clin Infect Dis.* 2008;46:1677.
26. Kwakman PH, Zaat SA. Antibacterial components of honey. *IUBMB Life.* 2012;64:48.
27. Frenkel K, Wei H, Bhimani R, et al. Inhibition of tumor promoter-mediated processes in mouse skin and bovine lens by caffeic acid phenthyl ester. *Cancer Res.* 1993;53:1255.
28. Toreti VC, Sato HH, Pastore GM, et al. Recent progress of propolis for its biological and chemical compositions and its botanical origin. *Evid Based Complement Alternat Med.* 2013;2013:697390.
29. Vandamme L, Heyneman A, Hoeksema H, et al. Honey in modern wound care: A systematic review. *Burns.* 2013;pii:S0305-4179(13)00197.
30. Salatino A, Fernandes-Silva CC, Righi AA, et al. Propolis research and the chemistry of plant products. *Nat Prod Rep.* 2011;28:925.
31. Bansal V, Medhi B, Pandhi P. Honey – A remedy rediscovered and its therapeutic utility. *Kathmandu Univ Med J (KUMJ).* 2005;3:305.
32. Sare JL. Leg ulcer management with topical medical honey. *Br J Community Nurs.* 2008;13:S22.
33. Khan FR, Ul Abadin Z, Rauf N. Honey: Nutritional and medicinal value. *Int J Clin Pract.* 2007;61:1705.
34. Sforcin JM. Propolis and the immune system: A review. *J Ethnopharmacol.* 2007;113:1.

35. Sforcin JM, Bankova V. Propolis: Is there a potential for the development of new drugs? *J Ethnopharmacol.* 2011;133:253.

36. Popova M, Dimitrova R, Al-Lawati HT, et al. Omani propolis: Chemical profiling, antibacterial activity and new propolis plant sources. *Chem Cent J.* 2013;7:158.

37. Popova M, Silici S, Kaftanoglu O, et al. Antibacterial activity of Turkish propolis and its qualitative and quantitative chemical composition. *Phytomedicine.* 2005;12:221.

38. Kuropatnicki AK, Szliszka E, Klósek M, et al. The beginnings of modern research on propolis in Poland. *Evid Based Complement Alternat Med.* 2013;2013:983974.

39. Kodai T, Nakatani T, Noda N. The absolute configurations of hydroxyl fatty acids from the royal jelly of honeybees (Apis mellifera). *Lipids.* 2011;46:263.

40. Butler CG, Callow RK, Johnston NC. The isolation and synthesis of queen substance, 9-oxodec-trans-2-enoic acid, a honeybee pheromone. *Proc R Soc Lond B Biol Sci.* 1962;155:417.

41. Johnston NC, Law JH, Weaver N. Metabolism of 9-ketodec-2-enoic acid by worker honeybees (Apis mellifera L.). *Biochemistry.* 1965;4:1615.

42. Kodai T, Umebayashi K, Nakatani T, et al. Compositions of royal jelly II. Organic acid glycosides and sterols of the royal jelly of honeybees (Apis mellifera). *Chem. Pharm Bull (Tokyo).* 2007;55:1528.

43. Yamaura K, Tomono A, Suwa E, et al. Topical royal jelly alleviates symptoms of pruritus in a murine model of allergic contact dermatitis. *Pharmacogn Mag.* 2013;9:9.

44. Yamada N, Yoshimura H. Determinants of chilliness among young women and their application to psychopharmacological trials. *Nihon Shinkei Seishin Yakurigaku Zasshi.* 2009;29:171.

45. Khan FR, Ul Abadin Z, Rauf N. Honey: Nutritional and medicinal value. *Int J Clin Pract.* 2007;61:1705.

46. Olaitan PB, Adeleke OE, Ola IO. Honey: A reservoir for microorganisms and an inhibitory agent for microbes. *Afr Health Sci.* 2007;7:159.

47. English HK, Pack AR, Molan PC. The effects of manuka honey on plaque and gingivitis: A pilot study. *J Int Acad Periodontol.* 2004;6:63.

48. Simon A, Traynor K, Santos K, et al. Medical honey for wound care – Still the 'latest resort'? *Evid Based Complement Alternat Med.* 2009;6:165.

49. Oelschlaegel S, Gruner M, Wang PN, et al. Classification and characterization of manuka honeys based on phenolic compounds and methylglyoxal. *J Agric Food Chem.* 2012;60:7229.

50. Bardy J, Slevin NJ, Mais KL, et al. A systematic review of honey uses and its potential value within oncology care. *J Clin Nurs.* 2008;17:2604.

51. Anderson I. Honey dressings in wound care. *Nurs Times.* 2006;102:40.

52. Stephen-Haynes J. Evaluation of a honey-impregnated tulle dressing in primary care. *Br J Community Nurs.* 2004(Suppl):S21.

53. Jacob SE, Chimento S, Castanedo-Tardan MP. Allergic contact dermatitis to propolis and carnauba wax from lip balm and chewable vitamins in a child. *Contact Dermatitis.* 2008;58:242.

54. Zilius M, Ramanauskiené K, Briedis V. Release of propolis phenolic acids from semisolid formulations and their penetration into the human skin in vitro. *Evid Based Complement Alternat Med.* 2013;2013:958717.

55. Fonseca YM, Marquele-Oliveira F, Vicentini FT, et al. Evaluation of the potential of Brazilian propolis against UV-induced oxidative stress. *Evid Based Complement Alternat Med.* 2011;2011:pii:863917.

56. Ramanauskiene K, Inkeniene AM, Savickas A, et al. Analysis of the antimicrobial activity of propolis and lysozyme in semisolid emulsion systems. *Acta Pol Pharm.* 2009;66:681.

57. Banskota AH, Tezuka Y, Kadota S. Recent progress in pharmacological research of propolis. *Phytother Res.* 2001;15:561.

58. Nagai T, Sakai M, Inoue R, et al. Antioxidative activities of some commercial honeys, royal jelly, and propolis. *Food Chem.* 2001;75:237.

59. Duplan H, Questel E, Hernandez-Pigeon H, et al. Effects of Hydroxydecine (®) (10-hydroxy-2-decenoic acid) on skin barrier structure and function in vitro and clinical efficacy in the treatment of UV-induced xerosis. *Eur J Dermatol.* 2011;21:906.

60. Búfalo MC, Ferreira I, Costa G, et al. Propolis and its constituent caffeic acid suppress LPS-stimulated pro-inflammatory response by blocking NF-κB and MAPK activation in macrophages. *J Ethnopharmacol.* 2013;149:84.

61. Fujii A, Kobayashi S, Kuboyama N, et al. Augmentation of wound healing by royal jelly (RJ) in streptozotocin-diabetic rats. *Jpn J Pharmacol.* 1990;53:331.

62. Kim J, Kim Y, Yun H, et al. Royal jelly enhances migration of human fibroblasts and alters the levels of cholesterol and sphinganine in an in vitro wound healing model. *Nutr Res Pract.* 2010;4:362.

63. Taniguchi Y, Kohno K, Inoue S, et al. Oral administration of royal jelly inhibits the development of atopic dermatitis-like skin lesions in NC/Nga mice. *Int Immunopharmacol.* 2003;3:1313.

64. Magro Filho O, de Carvalho AC. Application of propolis to dental sockets and skin wounds. *J Nihon Univ Sch Dent.* 1990;32:4.

65. Mills S, Bone K. *Principles and Practice of Phytotherapy: Modern Herbal Medicine.* London: Churchill Livingstone; 2000:174.

66. Morelli V, Calmet E, Jhingade V. Alternative therapies for common dermatologic disorders, part 2. *Prim Care.* 2010;37:285.

67. Samet N, Laurent C, Susarla SM, et al. The effect of bee propolis on recurrent aphthous stomatitis: A pilot study. *Clin Oral Investig.* 2007;11:143.

68. Jull AB, Walker N, Deshpande S. Honey as a topical treatment for wounds. *Cochrane Database Syst Rev.* 2013;2:CD005083.

69. Pachalski A, Franczuk B, Wilk M. An evaluation of the use of propolis in the treatment of skin disorders on the stumps of patients in rehabilitation following lower limb limb amputation. *Ortop Traumatol Rehabil.* 2002;4:60.

70. Abdelatif M, Yakoot M, Etmaan M. Safety and efficacy of a new honey ointment on diabetic foot ulcers: A prospective pilot study. *J Wound Care.* 2008;17:108.

71. Suemaru K, Cui R, Li B, et al. Topical application of royal jelly has a healing effect for 5-fluorouracil-induced experimental oral mucositis in hamsters. *Methods Find Exp Clin Pharmacol.* 2008;30:103.

72. Watanabe S, Suemaru K, Takechi K, et al. Oral mucosal adhesive films containing royal jelly accelerate recovery from 5-Fluorouracil-induced oral mucositis. *J Pharmacol Sci.* 2013;121:110.

73. Siavash M, Shokri S, Haghighi S, et al. The efficacy of topical Royal Jelly on diabetic foot ulcers healing: A case series. *J Res Med Sci.* 2011;16:904.

74. Al-Waili NS. Therapeutic and prophylactic effects of crude honey on chronic seborrheic dermatitis and dandruff. *Eur J Med Res.* 2001;6:306.

75. Al-Waili NS, Salom K, Butler G, et al. Honey and microbial infections: A review supporting the use of honey for microbial control. *J Med Food.* 2011;14:1079.

76. Shaw D, Leon C, Kolev S, et al. Traditional remedies and food supplements. A 5-year toxicological study (1991–1995). *Drug Saf.* 1997;17:342.

77. Lombardi C, Senna GE, Gatti B, et al. Allergic reactions to honey and royal jelly and their relationship with sensitization to compositae. *Allergol Immunopathol (Madr).* 1998;26:288.

78. Ting PT, Silver S. Allergic contact dermatitis to propolis. *J Drugs Dermatol.* 2004;3:685.

79. Walgrave SE, Warshaw EM, Glesne LA. Allergic contact dermatitis from propolis. *Dermatitis.* 2005;16:209.

80. Pasolini G, Semenza D, Capezzera R, et al. Allergic contact cheilitis induced by repeated contact with propolis-enriched honey. *Contact Dermatitis.* 2004;50:322.

81. Jensen CD, Andersen KE. Allergic contact dermatitis from cera alba (purified propolis) in a lip balm and candy. *Contact Dermatitis.* 2006;55:312.

82. Mizutani Y, Shibuya Y, Takahashi T, et al. Major royal jelly protein 3 as a possible allergen in royal jelly-induced anaphylaxis. *J Dermatol.* 2011;38:1079.

83. Thien FC, Leung R, Baldo BA, et al. Asthma and anaphylaxis induced by royal jelly. *Clin Exp Allergy.* 1996;26:216.

84. Takahashi M, Matsuo I, Ohkido M. Contact dermatitis due to honeybee royal jelly. *Contact Dermatitis.* 1983;9:452.

85. Rosmilah M, Shahnaz M, Patel G, et al. Characterization of major allergens of royal jelly Apis mellifera. *Trop Biomed.* 2008;25:243.

86. Leung R, Ho A, Chan J, et al. Royal jelly consumption and hypersensitivity in the community. *Clin Exp Allergy.* 1997;27:333.

87. Leung R, Lam CW, Ho A, et al. Allergic sensitisation to common environmental allergens in adult asthmatics in Hong Kong. *Hong Kong Med J.* 1997;3:211.

88. Le Conte Y, Navajas M. Climate change: Impact on honey bee populations and diseases. *Rev Sci Tech.* 2008;27:485.

89. Moisse K. Antibiotic resistance could bring "end of modern medicine." *ABC News,* March 16, 2012. http://abcnews.go.com/blogs/health/2012/03/16/antibiotic-resistance-could-bring-end-of-modern-medicine/. Accessed December 22, 2013.

90. Ballingall A. Neonicotinoid pesticides blamed for bee deaths could affect humans, EU agency says. *Toronto Star*, December 20, 2013. http://www.thestar.com/news/canada/2013/12/20/neonicotinoid_pesticides_blamed_for_bee_deaths_could_affect_humans_eu_agency_says.html. Accessed December 22, 2013.

91. Blacquière T, Smagghe G, van Gestel CA, et al. Neonicotinoids in bees: A review on concentrations, side-effects and risk assessment. *Ecotoxicology*. 2012;21:973.

92. European Food Safety Authority. Press release. January 16, 2013. http://www.efsa.europa.eu/en/press/news/130116.htm. Accessed December 22, 2013.

93. Marghitas LA, Dezmirean DS, Bobis O. Important developments in Romanian propolis research. *Evid Based Complement Alternat Med*. 2013;2013:159392.

94. Martin SJ, Highfield AC, Brettell L, et al. Global honey bee viral landscape altered by a parasitic mite. *Science*. 2012;336:1304.

95. Henry M, Béguin M, Requier F, et al. A common pesticide decreases foraging success and survival in honey bees. *Science*. 2012;336:348.

96. Schmidt CW. Antibiotic resistance in livestock: More at stake than steak. *Environ Health Perspect*. 2002;110:A396.

97. Snowdon JA, Cliver DO. Microorganisms in honey. *Int J Food Microbiol*. 1996;31:1.

98. Lusby PE, Coombes A, Wilkinson JM. Honey: A potent agent for wound healing? *J Wound Ostomy Continence Nurs*. 2002;29:295.

99. Molan PC. Potential of honey in the treatment of wounds and burns. *Am J Clin Dermatol*. 2001;2:13.

100. Alcaraz A, Kelly J. Treatment of an infected venous leg ulcer with honey dressings. *Br J Nurs*. 2002;11:859.

101. Sforcin JM, Orsi RO, Bankova V. Effect of propolis, some isolated compounds and its source plant on antibody production. *J Ethnopharmacol*. 2005;98:301.

102. Bankova V. Recent trends and important developments in propolis research. *Evid Based Complement Alternat Med*. 2005;2:29.

103. Marquele-Oliveira F, Fonseca YM, de Freitas O, et al. Development of topical functionalized formulations added with propolis extract: Stability, cutaneous absorption and in vivo studies. *Int J Pharm*. 2007;342:40.

104. Molan PC, Cooper RA. Honey and sugar as a dressing for wounds and ulcers. *Trop Doct*. 2000;30:249.

105. Cooper RA, Molan PC, Harding KG. The sensitivity to honey of Gram-positive cocci of clinical significance isolated from wounds. *J Appl Microbiol*. 2002;93:857.

106. Medić-Sarić M, Rastija V, Bojić M, et al. From functional food to medicinal product: Systematic approach in analysis of polyphenolics from propolis and wine. *Nutr J*. 2009;8:33.

107. Bolfa P, Vidrighinescu R, Petruta A, et al. Photoprotective effects of Romanian propolis on skin of mice exposed to UVB irradiation. *Food Chem Toxicol*. 2013;62C:329.

108. Marquele FD, Di Mambro VM, Georgetti SR, et al. Assessment of the antioxidant activities of Brazilian extracts of propolis alone and in topical pharmaceutical formulations. *J Pharm Biomed Anal*. 2005;39:455.

109. Duran N, Koc A, Oksuz H, et al. The protective role of topical propolis on experimental keratitis via nitric oxide levels in rabbits. *Mol Cell Biochem*. 2006;281:153.

110. Nakajima Y, Tsuruma K, Shimazawa M, et al. Comparison of bee products based on assays of antioxidant capacities. *BMC Complement Altern Med*. 2009;9:4.

111. Izuta H, Narahara Y, Shimazawa M, et al. 1,1-diphenyl-2-picrylhydrazyl radical scavenging activity of bee products and their constituents determined by ESR. *Biol Pharm Bull*. 2009;32:1947.

112. Piccinelli AL, Mencherini T, Celano R, et al. Chemical composition and antioxidant activity of Algerian propolis. *J Agric Food Chem*. 2013;61:5080.

113. Selamoglu Talas Z. Propolis reduces oxidative stress in l-NAME-induced hypertension rats. *Cell Biochem Funct*. 2013 Jun 21. [Epub ahead of print]

114. Cole N, Sou PW, Ngo A, et al. Topical 'Sydney' propolis protects against UV-radiation-induced inflammation, lipid peroxidation and immune suppression in mouse skin. *Int Arch Allergy Immunol*. 2010;152:87.

115. Moniruzzaman M, Sulaiman SA, Khalil MI, Gan SH. Evaluation of physicochemical and antioxidant properties of sourwood and other Malaysian honeys: A comparison with manuka honey. *Chem Cent J*. 2013;7:138.

116. Blair SE, Cokcetin NN, Harry EJ, et al. The unusual antibacterial activity of medical-greade Leptospermum honey: Antibacterial spectrum, resistance and transcriptome analysis. *Eur J Clin Microbiol Infect Dis*. 2009;28:1199.

117. Vynograd N, Vynograd I, Sosnowski Z. A comparative multicentre study of the efficacy of propolis, acyclovir and placebo in the treatment of genital herpes (HSV). *Phytomedicine*. 2000;7:1.

118. Giurcăneanu F, Crisan I, Esanu V, et al. Treatment of cutaneous herpes and herpes zoster with Nivcrisol-D. *Virologie*. 1988;39:21.

119. Gregory SR, Piccolo N, Piccolo MT, et al. Comparison of propolis skin cream to silver sulfadiazine: A naturopathic alternative to antibiotics in treatment of minor burns. *J Altern Complement Med*. 2002;8:77.

120. 120. Huang MT, Ma W, Yen P, et al. Inhibitory effects of caffeic acid phenethyl ester (CAPE) on 12-O-tetradecanoylphorbol-13-acetate-induced tumor promotion in mouse skin and the synthesis of DNA, RNA and protein in HeLa cells. *Carcinogenesis*. 1996;17:761.

121. Orsolić N, Knezević AH, Sver L, et al. Immunomodulatory and antimetastatic action of propolis and related polyphenolic compounds. *J Ethnopharmacol*. 2004;94:307.

122. Park HM, Hwang E, Lee KG, et al. Royal jelly protects against ultraviolet B-induced photoaging in human skin fibroblasts via enhancing collagen production. *J Med Food*. 2011;14:899.

123. Angelo G, Lorena C, Marta G, et al. Biochemical composition and antioxidant properties of Lavandula angustifolia Miller essential oil are shielded by propolis against UV radiations. *Photochem Photobiol*. 2013 Dec 23. [Epub ahead of print]

CHAPTER 61

Idebenone

Activities:

Antioxidant, photoprotective

Important Chemical Components:

Also known as 2,3-dimethoxy-5-methyl-6-(10′-hydroxydecyl)-1,4-benzoquinone, CV-2619, QSA-10, or hydroxydecyl ubiquinone. Its molecular formula is $C_{19}H_{30}O_5$.

Origin Classification:

Idebenone is a synthetic analog of ubiquinone (coenzyme Q_{10}).

Personal Care Category:

Antioxidant, antiaging, moisturizing

Recommended for the following Baumann Skin Types:

DRNW, DRPW, ORNW, and ORPW

SOURCE

Idebenone, also known as 2,3-dimethoxy-5-methyl-6-(10′-hydroxydecyl)-1,4-benzoquinone, CV-2619, or QSA-10, is a synthetic analog of, and similar in structure to, the potent antioxidant ubiquinone, or coenzyme Q_{10} (CoQ_{10}) (see Chapter 57, Coenzyme Q_{10}). CoQ_{10} is an integral cell membrane nutrient and contributor to the adenosine triphosphate (ATP)-producing mitochondrial electron transport chain, activity in which idebenone has also been shown to engage.[1] Idebenone has a significantly lower molecular weight and shorter carbon side chain as compared to CoQ_{10} and, therefore, greater solubility or ability to penetrate the skin than its natural counterpart (Table 61-1).[2–4]

HISTORY

Idebenone was first synthesized in 1984, and introduced as an active agent to treat age-related brain impairment in 1986.[5,6] In nearly three decades of extensive research, the preponderance of data that have emerged pertain primarily to the relative success of this benzoquinone compound in comparison to other drugs for treating patients with Alzheimer's disease; its use in organ

TABLE 61-1
Pros and Cons of Idebenone

Pros	Cons
Can penetrate the skin more readily than CoQ_{10}	Can cause contact dermatitis in sensitive skin types
Reportedly one of the most potent antioxidants	

transplant solutions; and its success in ameliorating various symptoms of Friedreich's ataxia. More recently, idebenone has been included in cosmeceutical products, such as Prevage™, as an antiaging agent.[6]

CHEMISTRY

As a potent free radical scavenger believed to be much stronger and efficient than other well-known antioxidants (e.g., vitamins C and E, CoQ_{10}, kinetin, and α-lipoic acid), idebenone also functions as an electron carrier and is not characterized by occasional activity as a strong pro-oxidant as is the case with CoQ_{10} under hypoxic conditions. In fact, under such conditions, idebenone is known to preserve ATP formation, protecting against free radical formation and cell damage.[1,7] In addition, idebenone is considered to have potential as a therapy to enhance energy and cognition, to protect organs against excitatory amino acid neurotoxicity, and to retard aging. As a CoQ_{10} analog, it is thought that idebenone works at least as well as its natural counterpart within the electron transport chain to maintain a high energy level. Idebenone was shown in a rat liver microsomal model to be more effective than CoQ_{10}, though, in protecting against lipid peroxidation.[8]

ORAL USES

Oral administration of idebenone has been demonstrated to improve mitochondrial oxidative metabolism in the brain, suggesting a therapeutic potential in the treatment of myopathy, encephalopathy, lactic acidosis, and stroke-like episodes (MELAS).[9,10] The protection imparted by idebenone to the brain's myelin sheath and energy-producing mitochondria may also position this antioxidant to play a therapeutic role in multiple sclerosis. Idebenone has been used orally in the treatment of several conditions, including Alzheimer's disease, liver disease, cerebrovascular disease, and Friedreich's ataxia.[1,11] Cutaneous benefits of idebenone are gleaned through topical administration.

TOPICAL USES

Idebenone has been used outside the United States for years as an antiaging agent and for improving cognition in patients with Alzheimer's disease and other neurologic disorders. As a topical agent, idebenone is believed to possess a much greater skin penetration potential and higher oxidative stress protection capacity than CoQ_{10}.[12] Idebenone has also reportedly displayed higher antioxidant activity than vitamins C and E, CoQ_{10}, kinetin, and α-lipoic acid [see Chapter 55, Ascorbic Acid (Vitamin C), and Chapter 56, Tocopherol (Vitamin E)].[12] Idebenone is thought by some, though, to be ineffective in conferring photoprotection to skin when compared to a topical antioxidant combination of vitamins C and E with ferulic acid (see Chapter 54, Ferulic Acid).[13] There are also reports that suggest greater antioxidant activity has been exhibited by resveratrol as well as L-ergothioneine (see Chapter 50, Resveratrol).[14,15]

In 2005, McDaniel et al. conducted a nonvehicle-controlled clinical trial to assess the topical safety and efficacy of 0.5 and 1 percent idebenone commercial formulations in 41 female subjects (from ages 30 to 65 years) with moderate photodamaged skin. Subjects were randomized to use a blind labeled (either 0.5 or 1 percent idebenone in otherwise identical lotion bases) skincare preparation twice daily for six weeks. Significant declines in skin roughness/dryness (by 26 percent) as well as fine lines and wrinkles (by 29 percent) were associated with the use of 1.0 percent idebenone, as were a 37 percent increase in skin hydration, and a 33 percent improvement in global skin assessment. Similar improvements were seen with the use of 0.5 percent idebenone. In addition, immunofluorescence staining indicated reductions in interleukin (IL)-1β, IL-6, and matrix metalloproteinase (MMP)-1 as well as an increase in collagen type I corresponding to both concentrations of idebenone.[7] As Bruce noted, though, the actual implications of the reported enhancements might have been better illustrated with the addition of a placebo arm in this study.[16] Nevertheless, the stated purpose of the study by McDaniel and colleagues was to ascertain baseline and after effects of the two concentrations of idebenone and not to evaluate the benefits of the antioxidant per se.

Idebenone has also been used along with hyaluronic acid as one of two formulations successfully incorporated into a new minimally invasive mesotherapy technique shown in a study with 50 subjects (ranging in age from 30 to 65 years) who demonstrated significant clinical improvement in terms of the brightness, texture, and firmness of their facial skin. Biopsies at baseline and after three months showed increases in collagen type I as well as decreases in MMP-1, IL-6, and IL-1β.[17]

SAFETY ISSUES

Idebenone is found in various over-the-counter topical antiaging products in concentrations ranging from 0.5 to 1 percent.[11] It is generally considered safe but there have been a few isolated reports of allergic contact dermatitis associated with idebenone-based Prevage since 2008. Specific symptoms have included erythema, scaling, severe edema, and vesicular dermatitis of the face, ears, and neck.[2,11,18,19] Some suggest that allergies to idebenone may be undetected or more widespread because this substance is not routinely included in standard patch testing.[19] This ingredient is not recommended for sensitive skin types.

ENVIRONMENTAL IMPACT

There is no environmental impact of commercial CoQ_{10} production known by the author.

FORMULATION CONSIDERATIONS

Although idebenone is considered more capable of permeating the skin barrier than CoQ_{10}, it is known to be irritating in free form.[20] In addition, it has been known to degrade and lose antioxidant potency when exposed for a protracted period in conditions with a relative humidity of 75 percent and a temperature of 40°C (104°F).[20,21] Several delivery methods have been investigated to account for such deficiencies and to facilitate its penetration and bioavailability.

In 2010, researchers developed nanoparticles based on chitosan and N-carboxymethylchitosan crosslinked with tripolyphosphate by co-drying with idebenone in different polymer-to-drug ratios with 20 percent (wt/wt) colloidal silicon dioxide and tripolyphosphate. The nanoparticles evinced a tenfold increase of drug stability as compared to the free drug and preserved the *in vitro* antioxidant activity of idebenone; the nanoparticle formulation resulted in less mucous membrane irritation as compared to the free form of idebenone. The investigators concluded that chitosan and N-carboxymethylchitosan nanoparticles warrant consideration as carriers for the topical and nasal use of hydrophobic and irritation-producing drugs such as idebenone.[20]

In 2012, Li and Ge investigated the percutaneous permeation of idebenone in *ex vivo* guinea pig skin after the application of various formulations, including nanostructured lipid carriers, nanoemulsions, and oil solutions. They found that nanostructured lipid carriers exhibited greater chemical stability and more effectively enhanced skin permeation as compared to the other vehicles (delivering nearly threefold the amount of idebenone to the epidermis and dermis) and thus have potential in topical skin care formulations.[22] Also that year, Montenegro et al. observed, after an *in vitro* evaluation, that loading idebenone in solid lipid nanoparticles appears to be an effective mode of drug delivery to the outer skin layers.[21]

In a review published in 2012 that covered the previous two decades, Carbone et al. found a wide range of delivery systems for idebenone, including cyclodextrin inclusion complexes, liposomes, microemulsions, prodrugs, and polymeric and lipid nanoparticles. While direct comparison was difficult, they maintained that these various carriers have successfully increased solubility and facilitated stability and bioavailability. They noted, also, that the controlled release and targeting of idebenone remains a goal in product development.[23]

In a particularly interesting meta-analysis regarding the prediction of responses to the use of antiaging cosmeceuticals, Sachs et al. enrolled 100 subjects with 16 to 20 participants applying one cosmeceutical (L-ascorbic acid, pentapeptide, α-lipoic acid, yeast extract, or 1 percent idebenone) to their photodamaged forearms for several weeks. Results varied widely, independent of age or gender, with some experiencing no improvement and others achieving sevenfold increases in collagenesis. Statistical analysis revealed that age, gender, and cosmeceutical type exerted no influence, with preexisting hypocollagenesis as the only factor affecting outcome (volunteers with hypocollagenesis responded 6.4 times more often than those with normal collagenesis). The authors suggested that this parameter might guide the future development of antiaging skin care product formulations.[24]

USAGE CONSIDERATIONS

In 2009, Wempe et al. investigated the inherent *in vitro* permeability, metabolism, and cytotoxicity of idebenone and compared it to the idebenone ester idebenone linoleate using pig ear skin and melanoma mouse cells. The researchers observed that idebenone permeated across the porcine tissue, but found no evidence that idebenone linoleate had after four hours. In the porcine tissue as well as mouse melanocytes, idebenone was metabolized to idebenone acid, with minimal idebenone linoleate metabolism noted. Further, no toxicity was associated with idebenone linoleate whereas idebenone exhibited delayed toxicity in melanocytes. The investigators concluded that the metabolic activation of idebenone likely accounts for the skin irritation associated with *in vivo* use of idebenone, which appears to have an inferior safety profile compared to its ester idebenone linoleate.[6]

SIGNIFICANT BACKGROUND

In studies on rats that paved the way to hypotheses regarding applications to neurologic, cardiologic, and antiaging indications, researchers ascertained that idebenone inhibited lipid peroxidation, protecting cell membranes and mitochondria from oxidative damage and, especially, brain mitochondria from swelling.[1,25,26] In addition, idebenone has been shown to improve cardiac function in patients with Friedreich's ataxia, and has been demonstrated to be effective in treating mitochondrial cardiomyopathy.[27]

Antioxidant Activity

The ability of idebenone to act as a potent free radical scavenger was demonstrated by Mordente et al. over 15 years ago. In particular, they showed that it could scavenge the organic radicals 2,2′-azinobis(3-ethylbenzothiazoline-6-sulfonic acid) and diphenylpicrylhydrazyl, the radicals peroxyl and tyrosyl, as well as peroxynitrite. They also found that idebenone suppresses microsomal lipid peroxidation engendered by adenosine diphosphate (ADP)-iron complexes or organic hydroperoxides, thus preventing cytochrome P450 elimination. In addition, the investigators observed in comparative experiments that idebenone manifested antioxidant efficiency ranging from 50 to just short of 100 percent of vitamin E or its water-soluble analog trolox.[28]

In 2005, McDaniel et al. conducted *in vitro* and *in vivo* studies to compare the oxidative stress protective properties of several frequently used antioxidants, including vitamins C and E, kinetin, α-lipoic acid, CoQ_{10}, and idebenone. After establishing a standardized method to summarize all results, including the human sunburn cell assay as well as experiments comparing antioxidant performance by photochemiluminescence, inhibition of ultraviolet B irradiation of human keratinocytes, and measurement of primary and secondary oxidation products, the researchers compiled overall oxidative protection scores of 95, 80, 68, 55, 52, and 41 for idebenone, vitamin E, kinetin, CoQ_{10}, vitamin C, and α-lipoic acid, respectively, as idebenone acted as a potent antioxidant most consistently across various experiments.[29] Further, they concluded that idebenone exhibits great potential for inclusion in topical skin protection products.

Neuroprotective Activity

In vitro and *in vivo* studies suggest that idebenone may reduce nerve cell damage induced by ischemia, repair neurotransmitter defects and/or cerebral metabolism, and enhance memory and learning.[1] Patients with mild dementia have been shown in clinical trials to be more likely to respond than those with greater functional decline.[30] In a multicenter, randomized, double-blind, placebo-controlled, parallel trial with Alzheimer's patients, idebenone was shown to be effective in enhancing memory, attention, and orientation as well as slowing disease progression.[31]

In a different study, repeated oral administration of idebenone, which stimulates nerve growth factor (NGF) synthesis, partially restored the age-related reduction of NGF in the frontal and parietal cortices. This is noteworthy because NGF is instrumental in maintaining cholinergic neurons the degeneration of which is linked to the cognitive impairment displayed by Alzheimer's patients. Authors of this study determined then that oral administration of idebenone has potential as a therapeutic agent in preventing cholinergic dysfunction.[32] A prospective, randomized, double-blind, placebo-controlled multicenter study of two doses

of idebenone in the treatment of patients with Alzheimer's disease further established the efficacy and safety of the drug for this indication.[33]

In a subsequent two-year prospective, randomized, double-blind multicenter study of the safety and efficacy of idebenone in the treatment of Alzheimer's patients, the synthetic CoQ_{10} analog exerted beneficial therapeutic effects on the course of the disease by slowing down its progression. Also, the antioxidant was found to be safe and tolerable.[34]

CONCLUSION

The synthetic coenzyme Q_{10} analog idebenone has been investigated for nearly 30 years, yielding an extensive body of research. Its antioxidant and other health benefits are well established, as is its use for various indications outside the United States. Recent research appears to validate the use of idebenone as a topical antiaging agent and its use in Prevage, introduced in 2005, represents the first skin product to contain a clinically tested and proven topical antioxidant. Responses to its use have been mostly favorable, with a few reports of allergic contact dermatitis. Nevertheless, it would be helpful to see studies comparing the results of idebenone-containing topical products and the antiaging retinoid products known to be effective for symptoms of cutaneous aging.

REFERENCES

1. Anonymous. Idebenone – Monograph. *Altern Med Rev.* 2001;6:83.
2. Fleming JD, White JM, White IR. Allergic contact dermatitis to hydroxydecyl ubiquinone: A newly described contact allergen in cosmetics. *Contact Dermatitis.* 2008;58:245.
3. Reszko AE, Berson D, Lupo MP. Cosmeceuticals: Practical applications. *Obstet Gynecol Clin North Am.* 2010;37:547.
4. Farris P. Idebenone, green tea, and Coffeeberry extract: New and innovative antioxidants. *Dermatol Ther.* 2007;20:322.
5. Suno M, Nagaoka A. Inhibition of lipid peroxidation by a novel compound, idebenone (CV-2619). *Jpn J Pharmacol.* 1984;35:196.
6. Wempe MF, Lightner JW, Zoeller EL, et al. Investigating idebenone and idebenone linoleate metabolism: In vitro pig ear and mouse melanocyte studies. *J Cosmet Dermatol.* 2009;8:63.
7. McDaniel DH, Neudecker BA, DiNardo JC, et al. Clinical efficacy assessment in photodamaged skin of 0.5% and 1.0% idebenone. *J Cosmet Dermatol.* 2005;4:167.
8. Wieland E, Schütz E, Armstrong VW, et al. Idebenone protects hepatic microsomes against oxygen radical-mediated damage in organ preservation solutions. *Transplantation.* 1995;60:444.
9. Napolitano A, Salvetti S, Vista M, et al. Long-term treatment with idebenone and riboflavin in a patient with MELAS. *Neurol Sci.* 2000;21:S981.
10. Ikejiri Y, Mori E, Ishii K, et al. Idebenone improves cerebral mitochondrial oxidative metabolism in a patient with MELAS. *Neurology.* 1996;47:583.
11. Sasseville D, Moreau L, Al-Sowaidi M. Allergic contact dermatitis to idebenone used as an antioxidant in an anti-wrinkle cream. *Contact Dermatitis.* 2007;56:117.
12. DiNardo JC et al. Antioxidants compared in a new protocol to measure protective capacity against oxidative stress – Part II. Paper presented at Annual Meeting of the American Academy of Dermatology; February 6–11, 2004; Washington, DC.
13. Tournas JA, Lin FH, Burch JA, et al. Ubiquinone, idebenone, and kinetin provide ineffective photoprotection to skin when compared to a topical antioxidant combination of vitamins C and E with ferulic acid. *J Invest Dermatol.* 2006;126:1185.
14. Baxter RA. Anti-aging properties of resveratrol: Review and report of a potent new antioxidant skin care formulation. *J Cosmet Dermatol.* 2008;7:2.
15. Dong KK, Damaghi N, Kibitel J, et al. A comparison of the relative antioxidant potency of L-ergothioneine and idebenone. *J Cosmet Dermatol.* 2007;6:183.
16. Bruce S. Cosmeceuticals for the attenuation of extrinsic and intrinsic dermal aging. *J Drugs Dermatol.* 2008;7:s17.

17. Savoia A, Landi S, Baldi A. A new minimally invasive mesotherapy technique for facial rejuvenation. *Dermatol Ther (Heidelb)*. 2013;3:83.

18. Natkunarajah J, Ostlere L. Allergic contact dermatitis to idebenone in an over-the-counter anti-ageing cream. *Contact Dermatitis*. 2008;58:239.

19. Mc Aleer MA, Collins P. Allergic contact dermatitis to hydroxydecyl ubiquinone (idebenone) following application of anti-ageing cosmetic cream. *Contact Dermatitis*. 2008;59:178.

20. Amorim Cde M, Couto AG, Netz DJ, et al. Antioxidant idebenone-loaded nanoparticles based on chitosan and N-carboxymethylchitosan. *Nanomedicine*. 2010;6:745.

21. Montenegro L, Sinico C, Castangia I, et al. Idebenone-loaded solid lipid nanoparticles for drug delivery to the skin: In vitro evaluation. *Int J Pharm*. 2012;434:169.

22. Li B, Ge ZQ. Nanostructured lipid carriers improve skin permeation and chemical stability of idebenone. *AAPS PharmSciTech*. 2012;13:276.

23. Carbone C, Pignatello R, Musumeci T, et al. Chemical and technological delivery systems for idebenone: A review of literature production. *Expert Opin Drug Deliv*. 2012;9:1377.

24. Sachs DL, Rittié L, Chubb HA, et al. Hypo-collagenesis in photoaged skin predicts response to anti-aging cosmeceuticals. *J Cosmet Dermatol*. 2013;12:108.

25. Nitta A, Hasegawa T, Nabeshima T. Oral administration of idebenone, a stimulator of NGF synthesis, recovers reduced NGF content in aged rat brain. *Neurosci Lett*. 1993;163:219.

26. Suno M, Nagaoka A. Inhibition of brain mitochondrial swelling by idebenone. *Arch Gerontol Geriatr*. 1989;8:299.

27. Lerman-Sagie T, Rustin P, Lev D, et al. Dramatic improvement in mitochondrial cardiomyopathy following treatment with idebenone. *J Inherit Metab Dis*. 2001;24:28.

28. Mordente A, Martorana GE, Minotti G, et al. Antioxidant properties of 2,3-dimethoxy-5-methyl-6-(10-hydroxydecyl)-1,4-benzoquinone (idebenone). *Chem Res Toxicol*. 1998;11:54.

29. McDaniel DH, Neudecker BA, DiNardo JC, et al. Idebenone: A new antioxidant – Part I. Relative assessment of oxidative stress protection capacity compared to commonly known antioxidants. *J Cosmet Dermatol*. 2005;4:10.

30. Gillis JC, Benefield P, McTavish D. Idebenone: A review of its pharmacodynamic and pharmacokinetic properties, and therapeutic use in age-related cognitive disorders. *Drugs Aging*. 1994;5:133.

31. Bergamasco B, Scarzella L, La Commare P. Idebenone, a new drug in the treatment of cognitive impairment in patients with dementia of the Alzheimer type. *Funct Neurol*. 1994;9:161.

32. Yamada K, Nitta A, Hasegawa T, et al. Orally active NGF synthesis stimulators: Potential therapeutic agents in Alzheimer's disease. *Behav Brain Res*. 1997;83:117.

33. Weyer G, Babej-Dölle RM, Hadler D, et al. A controlled study of 2 doses of idebenone in the treatment of Alzheimer's disease. *Neuropsychobiology*. 1997;36:73.

34. Gutzmann H, Hadler D. Sustained efficacy and safety of idebenone in the treatment of Alzheimer's disease: Update on a 2-year double-blind multicentre study. *J Neural Transm Suppl*. 1998;54:301.

CHAPTER 62

Melatonin

Activities:

Antioxidant, anticarcinogenic, antiaging, anti-inflammatory,[1] anxiolytic, immunomodulatory[2]

Important Chemical Components:

Also known as N-acetyl-5-methoxytryptamine

Origin Classification:

This ingredient is a natural hormone found in most living organisms. It is also synthesized for oral supplementation and topical application.

Personal Care Category:

Antioxidant, antiaging

Recommended for the following Baumann Skin Types:

DRNW, DSNW, ORNW, and OSNW

SOURCE

Melatonin (N-acetyl-5-methoxytryptamine), a tryptophan derivative, is a hormone produced naturally by the pineal gland in humans, and stimulated by β-adrenergic receptors. In addition, it is synthesized in mammals by the eyes, ovaries, bone marrow, gastrointestinal tract, lymphocytes, and skin, where it is also metabolized.[3–6] Additionally, melatonin has been recorded at significant levels in bile fluid, cerebrospinal fluid, and gastral mucosa.[7] Also found in most animal and plant species as well as fungi and even unicellular organisms, it follows a circadian light-dependent rhythm of secretion, and is derived from tryptophan, which is present in all organisms.[8,9] That is, melatonin is secreted during the dark phase of the light/dark cycle, and also regulates seasonal biorhythms (and is often accordingly referred to as the "hormone of darkness" and the body's chronological pacemaker).[5,9] In fact, melatonin is best known for regulating and facilitating sleep, with its "chronobiotic" characteristics justifying its use to treat sleep disorders including jet lag, shift-work sleep disruption, and insomnia in elderly and depressive patients.[5]

HISTORY

Although melatonin is a phylogenetically ancient methoxyindole, it was initially isolated from bovine pineal glands in 1958.[5,7–12] Subsequently, researchers learned that melatonin was produced nocturnally and secreted by the pineal gland and other organs in mammals including humans.[8] Melatonin and its relations to skin function have been studied since its skin-lightening effects on frogs were observed in the late 1950s.[10,13,14] The status of melatonin as a potent free radical scavenger was uncovered in 1993.[8,15,16] That same year, the first evidence emerged of the production of melatonin in the skin.[17–19]

Significantly, a melatoninergic antioxidative system that regulates cutaneous homeostasis and exhibits the potential to prevent ultraviolet (UV)-induced skin aging and skin cancer has been recently discovered.[7,8,20,21]

CHEMISTRY

Melatonin is a methoxyindole produced primarily by the pineal gland. In the skin, the essential amino acid tryptophan is the precursor; it is converted by tryptophan hydroxylase to 5-OH-Trp and then to serotonin. The acetylation of serotonin leads to the formation of N-acetylserotonin, which is transformed after the hydroxyindole-O-methyltransferase into melatonin.[9]

ORAL USES

Several plants are good sources of dietary melatonin, as it appears ubiquitously in nature and is found in almost 60 herbs used in traditional Chinese medicine.[5] Melatonin is also used as an oral supplement, primarily to restore regular sleep patterns. Prescriptions are required in some countries for melatonin supplements.

In 2008, Otálora et al., noting that melanoma is known to respond to melatonin *in vitro*, examined the effects of exogenous melatonin on hindering tumor growth and correcting impaired circadian rhythmicity. They found that melatonin administration (2 mg/kg/ BW/day) restored rhythmicity and improved survival in light-dark (12:12 cycle) conditions, but not under continuous light and circadian disruption, suggesting the need to restrict melatonin administration to the subjective night to hamper melanoma progression.[22]

TOPICAL USES

In recent years, melatonin has been gaining increased attention in antiaging medicine and dermatology because it has been found to exert potent antioxidant activity (Table 62-1), particularly against hydroxyl radicals,[5,23] and melatonin levels are known to decrease with age. In addition to its antioxidative and regulatory roles, including in seasonal reproduction control, melatonin is known to play a role in wound healing, to modulate the immune system, and to inhibit inflammation.[9,24] In addition, there is mounting evidence to suggest its viability as an agent to prevent cutaneous aging.[8] Topical application is preferable to oral administration for deriving cutaneous benefits because orally ingested melatonin is metabolized in the liver, yielding low levels in the blood and available to the skin.[8,25] Further, due to its potent lipophilicity, topical melatonin can penetrate the stratum corneum (SC) and form a reservoir, from where it is continuously released to the rest of the skin and dermal vasculature, potentially complementing and augmenting the activity of endogenous melatonin.[3,8,26]

Indeed, it is an important hormone in the dermatologic realm insofar as it is known to inhibit UV-induced erythema; implicated in skin functions such as hair growth, fur pigmentation/molting in

TABLE 62-1
Pros and Cons of Melatonin

Pros	Cons
Potent antioxidant	Small population sizes in clinical studies
One of the most potent scavengers of the hydroxyl radical(the strongest of free radicals)[27]	Much more research is needed on topical uses
Activates other endogenous antioxidants	Effect on cortisol levels in postmenopausal women not on estrogen replacement therapy
Exhibits immunomodulatory and oncostatic properties[5]	Anecdotal reports of melasma exacerbation
Extensive support for protective activity against UV-induced damage from *in vitro* studies	
Strongly lipophilic	
May strengthen the skin barrier	

various species, and melanoma control; and thought to have potential in treating various human dermatoses (e.g., atopic eczema, psoriasis, and malignant melanoma) as well as conditions such as androgenetic alopecia.[6,9,23] Of note, among the numerous plant species from which cutaneous applications are derived, feverfew is known to contain an appreciable level of melatonin (see Chapter 66, Feverfew).[28]

Androgenetic Alopecia

In 2004, Fisher et al. also investigated whether topically applied melatonin affects the anagen and telogen hair growth phases in women with androgenetic alopecia or diffuse hair loss. In their double-blind, randomized, placebo-controlled pilot study with 40 women, they instructed participants to apply 0.1 percent melatonin or a placebo preparation to the scalp once daily for six months. In the 12 women with androgenetic hair loss, melatonin contributed to a significantly greater anagen hair rate in occipital hair as compared to placebo. In the 28 participants with diffuse alopecia, melatonin application led to significant growth in frontal hair. Anagen hair growth in the occipital regions was increased in both groups, with insignificant differences. The investigators noted that while melatonin levels rose with treatment, the physiological night peak of serum melatonin was not exceeded. They concluded that their pilot study was the first to their knowledge to demonstrate *in vivo* that topically applied melatonin has the potential to impact hair growth in humans.[29]

In 2012, Fischer et al. reported on one pharmacodynamic study and four clinical pre–post studies of topically applied melatonin as a treatment for androgenetic alopecia. All five studies demonstrated positive results, with significant reductions in hair loss seen in multiple tests all of which were associated with good safety and tolerability. In the largest of the studies, a three-month, multicenter (200 centers) study with over 1,800 participants, the percentage of patients with a two- to threefold positive hair-pull test declined from 61.6 percent to 7.8 percent and those with a negative hair-pull test rose from 12.2 percent to 61.5 percent. Seborrheic dermatitis of the scalp was also found to have markedly diminished in these patients. The researchers concluded that the topical application of a cosmetic melatonin solution is a viable therapeutic option for patients with androgenetic alopecia.[30]

Antioxidant and Anticancer Activity

Melatonin receptors are expressed in several skin cell types, notably normal and malignant keratinocytes, melanocytes, and fibroblasts.[8,14]

Endogenous melatonin influences skin functions and structures through cell-surface- and putative-nuclear receptor-mediated expressions in skin cells and the broad expression and pleiotropic activity of the cutaneous melatoninergic system yields a high level of cell-specific selectivity, several investigators have found.[3,7]

The dynamic antioxidant activity of melatonin is thought to result from its capacity to scavenge free radicals, reduce free radical generation, and upregulate antioxidant enzymes.[31] Further, melatonin has been shown to counteract the effects of UV-induced solar damage, specifically thwarting mitochondrial and DNA harm.[8]

The decrease in endogenous melatonin synthesis with age is thought to significantly contribute to the gradual decline of the immune system and thus increased susceptibility to neoplastic disease development.[4]

In 2005, Slominski et al. identified the cutaneous expression of the mechanism of action in the transformation of L-tryptophan to serotonin and melatonin through detection of the corresponding genes and proteins with demonstrated enzymatic activities for tryptophan hydroxylase, serotonin N-acetyl-transferase, and hydroxyindole-O-methyltransferase in extracts from skin and skin cells. The investigators concluded that locally synthesized or topically administered melatonin has the potential to attenuate environmental or endogenous stresses and contribute to homeostasis as well as play a role in treating cutaneous disorders and acting as a photoprotectant.[14]

Melatonin has been demonstrated to augment T-helper cell response against malignancy by releasing interleukin (IL)-2, IL-10 and interferon (IFN)-γ. In addition, melatonin has been found to be effective in hindering neoplastic growth in melanoma, as well as breast, prostate, ovarian, and colorectal cancer.[4] Indeed, multiple studies have shown that melatonin possesses oncostatic activity.[5]

In 2013, Fischer et al. reported that melatonin dose- and time-dependently protected against UV-induced 8-hydroxy-2'-deoxyguanosine (8-OHdG) formation and antioxidant enzyme depletion (i.e., catalase, glutathione peroxidase, and superoxide dismutase) using *ex vivo* human full-thickness skin. They concluded that melatonin acted as a strong antioxidant and protector of DNA against oxidative skin damage.[32] Previously, Fischer et al. had shown that melatonin more strongly scavenged UV-induced reactive oxygen species in leukocytes than either vitamin C or the vitamin E analog trolox [see Chapter 55, Ascorbic Acid (Vitamin C), and Chapter 56, Tocopherol (Vitamin E)].[9,33]

Also in 2013, Sierra et al. investigated the *in vivo* and *in vitro* protective effects of a new melatonin-containing emulsion combined with UV filters against skin irradiation, finding good physical stability and melatonin permeation in an emulsion with a mixture of three UV filters. The formulation displayed significant radical-scavenging activity and a photoprotective assay revealed that skin treated with melatonin/UV filter formulation was statistically equivalent to nonirradiated control skin. The investigators concluded that melatonin acted in this formulation as a strong antioxidant and also activated endogenous enzymatic protection against oxidative stress.[34]

In Vitro Studies

In 2001, Ryoo et al. set out to elucidate the antioxidant role of melatonin in reaction to UVB exposure in cultured skin fibroblasts. Pretreatment with melatonin was found to mitigate cell membrane lipid peroxidation, yielding an increase in the absolute number of surviving cells and reducing malondialdehyde levels. Melatonin pretreatment also prevented the pre-G$_1$ arrest leading to apoptosis. The researchers concluded that melatonin was shown to be an effective inhibitor of membrane peroxidation. This is thought to be the first report on the protection of dermal fibroblasts from UVB by melatonin.[35]

Melatonin was one of the several substances found to act as a viable antioxidant agent by Trommer and Neubert in 2005. They screened 47 substances (drugs, plant extracts, plant ingredients, and polysaccharides) for new antioxidative compounds for topical administration using skin lipid *in vitro* models.[36]

In 2006, Fischer et al. examined the *in vitro* protective effects of melatonin against UV-induced cell damage in human keratinocytes. They found that pre-incubation is necessary for melatonin to display protective activity, which includes apoptosis inhibition.[37]

In a 2009 issue of *In Vivo*, Izykowska et al. reported on the effects of melatonin on melanoma cells in culture medium and after its addition to culture medium for 30 minutes prior to UVA or UVB exposure, finding that melatonin clearly protected cells from UVA and UVB activity *in vitro*.[38] In the same issue of *In Vivo*, noting previous studies showing a protective effect on cells exerted by melatonin mainly in relation to UVB, Izykowska et al. also reported on the effects of melatonin on keratinocytes and fibroblasts added to culture medium 30 minutes before exposure to UVA and UVB, again finding that melatonin affords protection to skin cells from the activity of UVA as well as UVB *in vitro*.[39]

In 2013, Rezzani et al. assessed the effects of pretreating murine fibroblast cells with melatonin before exposure to UVA radiation. They found that melatonin increased heme-degrading enzyme expression and inhibited UVA-induced photodamage, suggesting potential applications for limiting skin aging.[31]

Animal Studies

In 2006, Sener et al. studied the effects of melatonin in treating pressure ulcers in rats. Animals were treated twice daily during reperfusion periods with a locally applied ointment or given intraperitoneal administration of the antioxidant. Topical melatonin treatment was associated with suppressed malondialdehyde levels and attenuated decreases in glutathione in the skin induced by the pressure ulcers. Melatonin treatment also prevented significant increases in alanine aminotransferase, aspartate aminotransferase, blood urea nitrogen, creatinine, lactate dehydrogenase, and collagen levels. In addition, the researchers noted degenerative changes in the dermis and epidermis of the rats, with marked decreases in tissue injury in the animals that received topical melatonin. They concluded that melatonin, delivered topically or systemically, warrants consideration as a pressure ulcer treatment.[40]

Two years later, Pugazhenthi et al. used a full-thickness incisional rat model to evaluate the dermal wound and scar healing effects of melatonin (1.2 mg/kg intradermal). The investigators observed that melatonin significantly ameliorated scar quality. Treatment with melatonin also markedly reduced inducible nitric oxide synthase (iNOS) activity in the acute inflammatory phase but substantially elevated iNOS in the resolving phase. Further, melatonin raised cyclooxygenase-2, which has known anti-inflammatory properties, following wound induction and facilitated angiogenesis. Arginase activity, instrumental in collagen production by synthesizing the building block proline, was increased by melatonin treatment, which also upregulated the protein profiles of heme oxygenase-1 and

heme oxygenase-2 isoforms, which are essential in wound repair. The investigators suggested that their findings represented the first report showing that melatonin can significantly enhance wound healing and scar formation.[2]

In a 2009 study using NC/Nga mice, researchers investigated whether melatonin inhibits the development of 2,4-dinitrofluorobenzene (DNFB)-induced atopic dermatitis-like skin lesions. Topically administered melatonin hindered ear thickness increases and skin lesions engendered by DNFB treatment. Melatonin was also found to significantly inhibit IL-4 and IFN-γ secretion by activated CD4$^+$ T cells from the draining lymph nodes of DNFB-treated mice, and diminish serum total IgE levels. The investigators concluded that topically administered melatonin, by lowering total IgE in serum, and IL-4 and IFN-γ synthesis by activated CD4$^+$ T cells, inhibits atopic dermatitis-like skin lesion development provoked by DNFB treatment in NC/Nga mice.[24]

In a 2010 study comparing systemic and topical administration of melatonin in a chronic wound model in rats whose release of basal melatonin was hindered due to pinealectomy, Ozler et al. found that hydroxyproline levels were significantly lower in rats that underwent pinealectomy and wound formation compared to the controls (with wound formation only), with increased wound surface areas. Also compared to the control group, these animals exhibited increased malondialdehyde levels and decreases in superoxide dismutase and glutathione peroxidase compared to control animals. However, superoxide dismutase and glutathione peroxidase enzymes increased in the groups treated with melatonin and malondialdehyde decreased. The researchers concluded that melatonin exerts a positive effect on wound healing, as the absence of melatonin prolonged the healing process. Topical and systemic administration methods were equally effective.[41]

Recent studies have also shown that melatonin and the antidiabetes drug metformin have the capacity to suppress skin carcinogenesis as well as lipid peroxidation induced by benz(a)-pyrene in female SHR mice.[42,43]

Human Studies

In 1996, in one of the earliest studies of the effects of topically applied melatonin on UV-induced erythema, Bangha et al. conducted a double-blind, randomized study with 20 healthy volunteers. Each subject was exposed to UVB (0.099 J/cm^2) on the lower back and then treated with various concentrations of melatonin. The investigators observed a dose–response relationship between melatonin concentration and the degree of erythema, with significantly less redness found in the areas treated with 0.5 percent melatonin as compared to melatonin 0.05 percent or just the vehicle gel.[44]

The next year, Bangha et al. performed another double-blind, randomized study in 20 volunteers to examine the antierythema effects of topical melatonin and the role of the application time in exerting the effect. Investigators treated small areas of the lower back with 0.6 mg/cm^2 melatonin 15 minutes before or 1, 30, or 240 minutes after simulated UVA and UVB irradiation at twice the individual minimal erythema dose. They found that posttreatment with melatonin exerted no protective effect but pretreatment 15 minutes prior to irradiation yielded significant protective effects against erythema.[45] In a subsequent similar double-blind, randomized clinical trial with 20 healthy volunteers, this time led by Fischer, the visual score indicated that melatonin application 15 minutes before irradiation significantly hindered erythema as compared to vehicle control. Postirradiation treatment with melatonin did not yield UV inhibition.[46]

In a small study of the penetration kinetics of topical melatonin in six healthy volunteers between the ages of 26 and 34 years old, Bangha et al. found that melatonin has the potential to accumulate in the SC with extended release into the blood system through cutaneous delivery.[47]

In 1998, Dreher et al. conducted a randomized, double-blind study in 12 healthy adults (6 women and 6 men, all Caucasian, ranging in age from 29 to 49 years old) of the short-term photoprotective effects of topically applied melatonin as well as vitamins C and E, alone or in combination. All formulations were applied 30 minutes after UV exposure. A dose-dependent photoprotective effect was associated with melatonin, with modest effects seen with the vitamins alone. Photoprotective activity was clearly enhanced when using melatonin in combination with vitamins C and E. This is thought to be the first *in vivo* demonstration of a protective effect imparted by topical melatonin in combination with other antioxidants.[48] The following year, Dreher et al. performed a similar experiment to assess the short-term photoprotective effects of the same compounds. This randomized, double-blind, placebo-controlled human study entailed the topical use of each antioxidant alone or in combination after UV exposure in a single application (immediately or 30 minutes after UV exposure) or in multiple applications 30 minutes, one hour, and two hours after UV exposure (totaling three applications). Interestingly, no photoprotective effects were observed regardless of the number of applications of antioxidants. The investigators concluded that given the speed of damage to skin from UV radiation, antioxidants likely must be delivered at the appropriate site in sufficient concentrations at the outset of and during active oxidative insult.[49]

Similarly, in 2006, Howes et al. studied the effects of topical melatonin applied after solar-simulated UV exposure in 16 healthy Mantoux-positive volunteers and found that melatonin conferred no protection against sunburn or immune suppression.[50]

However, four years prior, Morganti et al. conducted an eight-week randomized, double-blind, placebo-controlled study on 30 xerotic female volunteers (between 48 and 59 years old) to determine the effects of topical and systemic antioxidant-enriched formulation administration on the skin. Subjects applied twice daily a nanocolloidal gel and/or took two capsules per day of an oral diet supplement. The antioxidant-enriched formulations included vitamins C and E, α-lipoic acid, emblica, and melatonin (see Chapter 38, Emblica Extract). Investigators found that oxidative stress and lipid peroxidation declined 30 to 40 percent in the blood serum of all participants who used the topical or systemic antioxidant formulation. Those treated with the antioxidants also experienced declines in free radicals recovered in blood serum and on skin and decreases in reactive oxygen species engendered by UVB irradiation of leukocytes (*in vitro*). The researchers concluded that the tested compounds indeed delivered topical and systemic photoprotection and represent promising ingredients for combating oxidative stress and photoaging.[51]

In 2004, Fischer et al. conducted a clinical study in 15 healthy volunteers to consider the skin penetration activity of melatonin 0.01 percent in a cream and 0.01 and 0.03 percent in a solution. In a 24-hour time window, investigators took blood samples for melatonin measurement prior to application at 9 am as well as 1, 4, 8, and 24 hours after application. Preapplication serum melatonin levels ranged from 0.6 to 15.9 pg/mL. The mean serum value 24 hours later after application of the 0.01 percent melatonin cream was 9.0 pg/mL. For the 0.01 percent solution group, the mean melatonin level was 12.7 pg/mL 24 hours after application. Melatonin levels also markedly increased just 1 and 8 hours later in the 0.03 percent solution group, with cumulative mela-

tonin noted as 7.1 pg/mL in the 0.01 percent cream subjects, 8.6 pg/mL in the 0.01 percent solution participants, and 15.7 pg/mL in the 0.03 percent group. The investigators concluded that markedly lipophilic melatonin penetrates the skin with serum blood levels increasing in a dose- and galenic-dependent manner without causing increases above the physiological range.[26]

In 2008, a single-blind, randomized study with 145 patients was conducted to ascertain the effectiveness of a formulation containing 2.5 mg melatonin and 100 mg SB-73 (a mixture of magnesium, phosphate, and fatty acids extracted from *Aspergillus* species, which exhibit activity against the herpes virus) and to compare it to treatment with Acyclovir. Seventy subjects were treated with the melatonin/SB-73 preparation and 75 received 200 mg of Acyclovir (group B). A statistically significant difference between the groups was noted by the authors. After seven days of treatment, 67 participants in the melatonin/SB-73 group (95.7 percent) reported complete symptom resolution; 64 participants (85.3 percent) of the Acyclovir reported such a result.[52]

In 2012, Morganti et al. conducted a randomized, placebo-controlled, 12-week multicenter study with 70 healthy participants to again examine melatonin in combination. In this case, they considered the combined activity of melatonin, vitamin E, and β-glucan complexed with chitin nanocrystals administered topically and orally. All skin parameters reviewed were significantly better after treatment with the melatonin, vitamin E, β-glucan combination as compared to placebo, with greater improvements observed when these ingredients were complexed with chitin nanocrystals. Specifically, the treatment yielded decreased wrinkling and enhanced skin appearance.[53]

SAFETY ISSUES

Exogenous melatonin is reported to be safe for short-term (<3 months) use for sleep-related disorders.[54,55] A fixed drug eruption has been reported with the use of oral melatonin.[56]

ENVIRONMENTAL IMPACT

Given the widespread availability of plants containing melatonin, no discrete environmental toll is exacted in the preparation of oral or topical melatonin products.

FORMULATION CONSIDERATIONS

The author has no insight on the challenges of formulating melatonin.

USAGE CONSIDERATIONS

The author has noticed that patients with melasma seem to worsen after taking melatonin supplements. For this reason, it is advised that individuals with pigmented skin (designated as "P" types in the Baumann Skin Type System) not use melatonin-containing preparations. This is due to activation of melanin production by melatonin.

SIGNIFICANT BACKGROUND

Melatonin should be used with care in postmenopausal women not on hormone replacement therapy. Menopause and aging are believed to impair the regulation of the hypothalamic-pituitary-adrenal (HPA) axis. The administration of melatonin increases cortisol levels in postmenopausal women, leading to increased serum glucose levels,[57] and glycation. Administration of estrogen improves the regulation of the HPA axis and blocks the increase of cortisol levels with melatonin administration.[58]

Kim et al. have shown that melatonin and its metabolite methoxykynuramine appear to stimulate differentiation in human epidermis, suggesting their important role in building the skin barrier.[59] Further, melatonin receptors are expressed in several skin cell types, notably normal and malignant keratinocytes, melanocytes, and fibroblasts.[8,14]

CONCLUSION

There is ample research on the biological functions of melatonin. There is also an interesting, emerging body of evidence on the dermatologic effectiveness of the topical application of this hormone. In fact, there seems to be a wide variety of potential cutaneous uses for melatonin. However, most of the clinical studies have been extremely small, including a couple of investigations that indicated no photoprotective effect associated with melatonin. The effects of melatonin on melanogenesis (skin pigmentation), the skin barrier, and cortisol levels all play a significant but poorly understood role. Clearly, much more research, preferably in the form of randomized, double-blind studies is necessary before adequate recommendations to patients about melatonin use for skin health can be issued.

REFERENCES

1. Puizina-Ivić N, Mirić L, Carija A, et al. Modern approach to topical treatment of aging skin. *Coll Antropol.* 2010;34:1145.
2. Pugazhenthi K, Kapoor M, Clarkson AN, et al. Melatonin accelerates the process of wound repair in full-thickness incisional wounds. *J Pineal Res.* 2008;44:387.
3. Slominski A, Tobin DJ, Zmijewski MA, et al. Melatonin in the skin: Synthesis, metabolism and functions. *Trends Endocrinol Metabl.* 2008;19:17.
4. Srinivasan V, Pandi-Perumal SR, Brzezinski A, et al. Melatonin, immune function and cancer. *Recent Pat Endocr Metab Immune Drug Discov.* 2011;5:109.
5. Pandi-Perumal SR, Srinivasan V, Maestroni GJ, et al. Melatonin: Nature's most versatile biological signal? *FEBS J.* 2006;273:2813.
6. Fischer TW, Slominski A, Tobin DJ, et al. Melatonin and the hair follicle. *J Pineal Res.* 2008;44:1.
7. Fischer TW, Slominski A, Zmijewski MA, et al. Melatonin as a major skin protectant: From free radical scavenging to DNA damage repair. *Exp Dermatol.* 2008;17:713.
8. Kleszczynski K, Fischer TW. Melatonin and human skin aging. *Dermatoendorinol.* 2012;4:245.
9. Kleszczyński K, Hardkop LH, Fischer TW. Differential effects of melatonin as a broad range UV-damage preventive dermatoendocrine regulator. *Dermatoendocrinol.* 2011;3:27.
10. Lerner AB, Case JD, Takahashi Y, et al. Isolation of melatonin, a pineal factor that lightens melanocytes. *J Am Chem Soc.* 1958;80:2587.
11. Lerner AB, Case JD, Takahasi Y. Isolation of melatonin and 5-methoxyindole-3-acetic acid from bovine pineal glands. *J Biol Chem.* 1960;235:1992.
12. Wetterberg L. Melatonin and clinical application. *Reprod Nutr Dev.* 1999;39:367.
13. Lerner AB, Case JD. Pigment cell regulatory factors. *J Invest Dermatol.* 1959;32(2, Part 2):211.
14. Slominski A, Fischer TW, Zmijewski MA, et al. On the role of melatonin in skin physiology and pathology. *Endocrine.* 2005;27:137.
15. Poeggeler B, Reiter RJ, Tan DX, et al. Melatonin, hydroxyl radical-mediated oxidative damage, and aging: A hypothesis. *J Pineal Res.* 1993;14:151.
16. Tan DX, Chen LD, Poeggeler B, et al. Melatonin: A potent, endogenous hydroxyl radical scavenger. *Endocr J.* 1993;1:57.
17. Gaudet SJ, Slominski A, Etminan M, et al. Identification and characterization of two isozymic forms of arylamine N-acetyltransferase in Syrian hamster skin. *J Invest Dermatol.* 1993;101:660.
18. Slominski A, Pisarchik A, Semak I, et al. Serotoninergic system in hamster skin. *J Invest Dermatol.* 2002;119:934.
19. Desotelle JA, Wilking MJ, Ahmad N. The circadian control of skin and cutaneous photodamage. *Photochem Photobiol.* 2012;88:1037.
20. Fischer TW, Sweatman TW, Semak I, et al. Constitutive and UV-induced metabolism of melatonin in keratinocytes and cell-free systems. *FASEB J.* 2006;20:1564.
21. Slominski A, Wortsman J, Tobin DJ. The cutaneous serotoninergic/melatoninergic system: Securing a place under the sun. *FASEB J.* 2005;19:176.
22. Otálora BB, Madrid JA, Alvarez N, et al. Effects of exogenous melatonin and circadian synchronization on tumor progression in melanoma-bearing C57BL6 mice. *J Pineal Res.* 2008;44:307.
23. Fischer T, Wigger-Alberti W, Elsner P. Melatonin in dermatology. Experimental and clinical aspects. *Hautarzt.* 1999;50:5.
24. Kim TH, Jung JA, Kim GD, et al. Melatonin inhibits the development of 2,4-dinitrofluorobenzene-induced atopic dermatitis-like skin lesions in NC/Nga mice. *J Pineal Res.* 2009;47:324.
25. Arendt J. Melatonin. *Clin Endocrinol (Oxf).* 1988;29:205.
26. Fischer TW, Greif C, Fluhr JW, et al. Percutaneous penetration of topically applied melatonin in a cream and an alcoholic solution. *Skin Pharmacol Physiol.* 2004;17:190.
27. Reiter RJ. The pineal gland and melatonin in relation to aging: A summary of the theories and of the data. *Exp Gerontol.* 1995;30:199.
28. Murch SJ, Simmons CB, Saxena PK. Melatonin in feverfew and other medicinal plants. *Lancet.* 1997;350:1598.
29. Fischer TW, Burmeister G, Schmidt HW, et al. Melatonin increases anagen hair rate in women with androgenetic alopecia or diffuse alopecia: Results of a pilot randomized controlled trial. *Br J Dermatol.* 2004;150:341.
30. Fischer TW, Trüeb RM, Hänggi G, et al. Topical melatonin for treatment of androgenetic alopecia. *Int J Trichology.* 2012;4:236.
31. Rezzani R, Rodella LF, Favero G, et al. Attenuation of UVA-induced alterations in NIH3T3 dermal fibroblasts by melatonin. *Br J Dermatol.* 2013 Sep 11. [Epub ahead of print]
32. Fischer TW, Kleszczyński K, Hardkop LH, et al. Melatonin enhances antioxidative enzyme gene expression (CAT, GPx, SOD), prevents their UVR-induced depletion, and protects against the formation of DNA damage (8-hydroxy-2'-deoxyguanosine) in ex vivo human skin. *J Pineal Res.* 2013;54:303.
33. Fischer TW, Scholz G, Knöll B, et al. Melatonin suppresses reactive oxygen species in UV-irradiated leukocytes more than vitamin C and trolox. *Skin Pharmacol Appl Skin Physiol.* 2002;15:367.
34. Sierra AF, Ramírez ML, Campmany AC, et al. In vivo and in vitro evaluation of the use of a newly developed melatonin loaded emulsion combined with UV filters as a protective agent against skin irradiation. *J Dermatol Sci.* 2013;69:202.
35. Ryoo YW, Suh SI, Mun KC, et al. The effects of the melatonin on ultraviolet-B irradiated cultured dermal fibroblasts. *J Dermatol Sci.* 2001;27:162.
36. Trommer H, Neubert RH. Screening for new antioxidative compounds for topical administration using skin lipid model systems. *J Pharm Pharm Sci.* 2005;8:494.
37. Fischer TW, Zbytek B, Sayre RM, et al. Melatonin increases survival of HaCaT keratinocytes by suppressing UV-induced apoptosis. *J Pineal Res.* 2006;40:18.
38. Izykowska I, Gebarowska E, Cegielski M, et al. Effect of melatonin on melanoma cells subjected to UVA and UVB radiation in In vitro studies. *In Vivo.* 2009;23:733.
39. Izykowska I, Cegielski M, Gebarowska E, et al. Effect of melatonin on human keratinocytes and fibroblasts subjected to UVA and UVB radiation In vitro. *In Vivo.* 2009;23:739.
40. Sener G, Sert G, Ozer Sehirli A, et al. Melatonin protects against pressure ulcer-induced oxidative injury of the skin and remote organs in rats. *J Pineal Res.* 2006;40:280.
41. Ozler M, Simsek K, Ozkan C, et al. Comparison of the effect of topical and systemic melatonin administration on delayed wound healing in rats that underwent pinealectomy. *Scand J Clin Lab Invest.* 2010;70:447.
42. Man'cheva TA, Demidov DV, Plotnikova NA, et al. Melatonin and metformin inhibit skin carcinogenesis and lipid peroxidation

induced by benz(a)pyrene in female mice. *Bull Exp Biol Med.* 2011;151:363.

43. Deriabina ON, Plotnikova NA, Anisimov VN. Melatonin and metformin inhibit skin carcinogenesis induced by benz(a)pyrene in mice. *Vopr Onkol.* 2010;56:583.

44. Bangha E, Elsner P, Kistler GS. Suppression of UV-induced erythema by topical treatment with melatonin (N-acetyl-5-methoxytryptamine). A dose response study. *Arch Dermatol Res.* 1996;288:522.

45. Bangha E, Elsner P, Kistler GS. Suppression of UV-induced erythema by topical treatment with melatonin (N-acetyl-5-methoxytryptamine). Influence of the application time point. *Dermatology.* 1997;195:248.

46. Fischer T, Bangha E, Elsner P, et al. Suppression of UV-induced erythema by topical treatment with melatonin. Influence of the application time point. *Biol Signals Recept.* 1999;8:132.

47. Bangha E, Lauth D, Kistler GS, et al. Daytime serum levels of melatonin after topical application onto the human skin. *Skin Pharmacol.* 1997;10:298.

48. Dreher F, Gabard B, Schwindt DA, et al. Topical melatonin in combination with vitamins E and C protects skin from ultraviolet-induced erythema: A human study in vivo. *Br J Dermatol.* 1998;139:332.

49. Dreher F, Denig N, Gabard B, et al. Effect of topical antioxidants on UV-induced erythema formation when administered after exposure. *Dermatology.* 1999;198:52.

50. Howes RA, Halliday GM, Damian DL. Effect of topical melatonin on ultraviolet radiation-induced suppression of Mantoux reactions in humans. *Photodermatol Photoimmunol Photomed.* 2006;22:267.

51. Morganti P, Bruno C, Guarneri F, et al. Role of topical and nutritional supplement to modify the oxidative stress. *Int J Cosmet Sci.* 2002;24:331.

52. Nunes Oda S, Pereira Rde S. Regression of herpes viral infection symptoms using melatonin and SB-73: Comparison with Acyclovir. *J Pineal Res.* 2008;44:373.

53. Morganti P, Fabrizi G, Palombo P, et al. New chitin complexes and their anti-aging activity from inside out. *J Nutr Health Aging.* 2012;16:242.

54. Buscemi N, Vandermeer B, Hooton N, et al. Efficacy and safety of exogenous melatonin for secondary sleep disorders and sleep disorders accompanying sleep restriction: Meta-analysis. *BMJ.* 2006;332:385.

55. Buscemi N, Vandermeer B, Hooton N, et al. The efficacy and safety of exogenous melatonin for primary sleep disorders. A meta-analysis. *J Gen Intern Med.* 2005;20:1151.

56. Bardazzi F, Placucci F, Neri I, et al. Fixed drug eruption due to melatonin. *Acta Derm Venereol.* 1998;78:69.

57. Cagnacci A, Arangino S, Renzi A, et al. Influence of melatonin administration on glucose tolerance and insulin sensitivity of postmenopausal women. *Clin Endocrinol (Oxf).* 2001;54:339.

58. Cagnacci A, Soldani R, Yen SS. Melatonin enhances cortisol levels in aged women: Reversible by estrogens. *J Pineal Res.* 1997;22:81.

59. Kim TK, Kleszczynski K, Janjetovic Z, et al. Metabolism of melatonin and biological activity of intermediates of melatoninergic pathway in human skin cells. *FASEB J.* 2013;27:2742.

CHAPTER 63

Peppermint

Activities:

Antioxidant, analgesic, anesthetic, anticarcinogenic, anti-inflammatory, antimicrobial, antipruritic, antiseptic, cooling, radioprotective[1]

Important Chemical Components:

Leaves, phenolic constituents: Rosmarinic acid, caffeic acid, eriocitrin, luteolin, rutin, and hesperidin
Other leaf components: Palmitic acid, linoelic acid, linolenic acid, and α-tocopherol
Essential oil constituents: Menthol, menthone, menthyl acetate, isomenthone, menthofuran, eucalyptol (1,8-cineole), eugenol, limonene, pulegone, carvone, β-myrcene, and β-caryophyllene[2–4]

Origin Classification:

Peppermint is natural. Menthol is an organic compound obtained from peppermint or other mint oils or produced synthetically.[5]

Personal Care Category:

Antioxidant, cooling

Recommended for the following Baumann Skin Types:

ORNW and DRNW

SOURCE

Mentha piperita, better known as peppermint, is a member of the Labiatae family and a popular herb used worldwide. A hybrid of *Mentha spicata* (spearmint) and *Mentha aquatica* (water mint), peppermint is used in numerous forms (i.e., oil, leaf, leaf extract, and leaf water), with the oil as the most versatile and most used.[2,3] In fact, peppermint oil is used in food, cosmetic, personal hygiene, and pharmaceutical products. Peppermint has long been known for its beneficial gastrointestinal effects and has a well-established record of antimicrobial, antifungal, and analgesic activity.[6,7] Topical preparations of peppermint oil are used to confer antipruritic, cooling, and calming effects to treat inflammation and cutaneous irritation.[2] Menthol ($C_{10}H_{20}O$) is a naturally occurring monocyclic terpene alcohol derived from *M. piperita* as well as other mint oils,[8] and has been associated with several health benefits. Recently, anticancer properties have been attributed to menthol.[9]

HISTORY

The use of peppermint for culinary and medical purposes dates back to ancient Greece and Rome,[10] though there is also evidence to suggest that peppermint has been cultivated for medicinal purposes in Japan for over 2,000 years (Table 63-1).[11,12] Most sources appear to point to Mediterranean

TABLE 63-1
Pros and Cons of Peppermint

Pros	Cons
Long history of traditional use	Dearth of clinical studies
Broad range of biological activity	Can act as a skin sensitizer

origins. The term *Mentha* is thought to be rooted in Greek mythology, referring to the nymph pursued by Pluto and subsequently trampled into the ground, transforming her into mint, by Pluto's jealous wife Persephone.[2] *M. piperita* was cultivated by the ancient Egyptians and was cited in the pharmacopoeias of Iceland in the 1200s.[6,10]

A perennial herb native to Mediterranean Europe but disseminated through travel, trade, and conquest and now cultivated globally, peppermint has been used in various traditional and folk medicines through Europe and Asia. Peppermint entered general medical usage in Western Europe in the 1700s, and the first commercial crops were grown in England around 1750.[6,10,13] Known for many years through traditional medicine as a stimulant as well as carminative agent effective for various gastrointestinal conditions (e.g., dyspepsia, dysentery, flatulence, nausea, vomiting, and gastritis), modern clinical trials have borne out such indications.[3,6,13,14] It has been used as a sedative and analgesic, and menthol, a key constituent, has been used as an inhalant for upper respiratory disorders.

In the West, menthol was first isolated by the German physician and chemist Gaubius in 1771.[12] In 1886, Goldscheider attributed the cooling sensation conferred by menthol to the stimulation of thermoreceptors.[12] It was not until 2002, though, that a common site of action for cold and menthol was identified in two unrelated studies.[12,15,16]

CHEMISTRY

Peppermint has been shown to exhibit significant antimicrobial and antiviral activities, strong antioxidant and antitumor actions, and some antiallergenic potential *in vitro*.[3] Its antioxidant activities are ascribed primarily to important active components such as the phenolic acids caffeic and rosmarinic acids as well as eugenol and α-tocopherol.[1,17]

ORAL USES

Peppermint or menthol is a popular flavoring agent for some foods, including confections and chewing gums, and is also a widely consumed single ingredient herbal tea, or tisane.[3] Peppermint leaf is used as a standard medicinal tea for dyspepsia in Germany and has been approved by the German Commission E for internal use to treat various gastrointestinal issues.[3] In addition, it is also used to add flavor to a wide range of oral hygiene products, including toothpastes, mouthwashes, dental floss, breath fresheners, and dissolving oral thin strips.[2] The distinctive and refreshing flavor and aroma of peppermint is attributed to its constituents menthol and menthyl acetate.[4,12] For this reason, it is also used as a fragrance, as well as therapeutic agent.[2]

TOPICAL USES

Due to its flavor, aroma, and cooling qualities, peppermint oil is used in a wide range of products, including cosmeceuticals, personal hygiene products (e.g., bath preparations, mouthwashes, toothpastes, and topical formulations), foods, pharmaceuticals, and aromatherapy products. Topical indications include pruritus, irritation, and inflammation.

In 2003, Schuhmacher et al. investigated the virucidal effect of peppermint oil and found that it imparted a direct effect against herpes simplex virus type 1 (HSV-1) and herpes simplex virus type 2 (HSV-2) as well as an acyclovir-resistant HSV-1 strain. The investigators concluded, noting the lipophilic nature of peppermint oil, that it might be an appropriate topical treatment for recurrent herpes outbreaks.[18]

In a recent examination of the antibacterial and antifungal properties as well as speculated anti-inflammatory activity of menthol as a topical treatment for diaper dermatitis, investigators conducted a pilot clinical trial in a hospital setting with 84 neonates with diagnosed candidal diaper dermatitis who required no critical care or systemic antifungal and anti-inflammatory medications. The menthol group ($n = 42$) received topical clotrimazole and topically applied menthol drops and the control group ($n = 42$) received topical clotrimazole and a placebo. Thirty-five infants in each group completed the study. The researchers found that complete healing was shorter in the menthol group, with significant relief of erythema and pustules observed in this group. They concluded that topically applied menthol may be an effective agent in the treatment of candidal diaper dermatitis.[19]

In 2011, Qiu et al. showed, through various assays, that menthol, in low concentrations, could significantly suppress the expression of α-hemolysin, enterotoxins A and B, and toxic shock syndrome toxin 1 in *Staphylococcus aureus*. The investigators concluded that menthol may warrant inclusion in the armamentarium against *S. aureus* when combined with β-lactam antibiotics, which, at subinhibitory concentrations, can actually augment *S. aureus* toxin secretion. They added that menthol may also have possible uses in novel antiviral drugs.[20] Currently, menthol is included in several over-the-counter (OTC) topical pain relief medications for its analgesic and anesthetic properties.

SAFETY ISSUES

Peppermint oil can act as a skin sensitizer, particularly in impaired and sensitive skin.[2] Some recent reports indicate that acute allergic contact dermatitis has been seen in reaction to the use of lip balm containing peppermint oil.[21] Peppermint oil and menthol have also been associated with sensitivity reactions in patients with burning mouth syndrome, oral lichenoid reactions, recurrent oral ulcers, perioral dermatitis, and stomatitis.[2,22,23] For this reason peppermint should not be used in dry or sensitive skin types. Peppermint is a frequent cause of perioral dermatitis, a recurring irritation around the mouth that is often due to flavorings in toothpaste and mints.

Although peppermint oil has been reported to be a sensitizer in isolated cases, peppermint oil 8 percent was not found to be a sensitizer in a recent test using a maximization protocol and the various forms of peppermint (i.e., oil, extract, leaves, and water) used in skin care products, in fact, have been deemed safe for use in cosmetic formulations.[24] The United States Food and Drug Administration has also approved concentrations of menthol up to 16 percent in OTC topical products.[8] It can provoke cold pain in concentrations of 30 percent and higher.[8]

ENVIRONMENTAL IMPACT

Menthol consumption is now believed to surpass 7,000 tons annually, with a raw product value approximated at $300 million as of 2005, and with demand outpacing natural resource supply.[12] Production of menthol from natural sources has reportedly led to the consumption of more fossil fuel, production of more carbon dioxide effluent, and exerted more of an environmental impact than the primary synthetic production routes.[25]

FORMULATION CONSIDERATIONS

In rinse-off products, peppermint oil is used in concentrations up to 3 percent and in leave-on formulations up to 0.2 percent.[24] The concentration of pulegone in any peppermint products should be limited to 1 percent.[3,24]

USAGE CONSIDERATIONS

Peppermint can cause stinging and irritation in individuals with sensitive skin. Those with dry skin may have an impaired skin barrier, which allows increased absorption. Consequently, individuals with dry skin should also avoid peppermint.

SIGNIFICANT BACKGROUND

Antioxidant Activity

Various Mentha species, including *M. piperita*, have exhibited significant antioxidant activity.[17,26,27] In a 2010 study of the antioxidant activity of the essential oils of six popular herbs, including lavender (*Lavendular angustifolia*), peppermint (*M. piperita*), rosemary (*Rosmarius officinalis*), lemon (*Citrus limon*), grapefruit (*Citrus paradise*), and frankincense (*Boswellia carteri*), investigators found, in testing free radical-scavenging capacity and lipid peroxidation in the linoleic acid system, that peppermint essential oil exhibited the greatest radical-scavenging activity against the 2,2′-azinobis-(3-ethylbenzothiazoline-6-sulfonic acid) ABTS radical.[28]

In 2010, Baliga and Rao showed that *M. piperita* and *M. arvensis* (wild mint) protected mice against γ-radiation-induced morbidity and mortality. Specifically, *M. piperita* protected murine testes as well as gastrointestinal and hemopoietic systems.[4] In a 2012 study of nine Mentha species, *M. piperita* was found to have the third greatest antioxidant capacity, with all species displaying antioxidant activity in scavenging the 1,1-diphenyl-2-picrylhydrazyl (DPPH) free radical.[17]

Anticancer Activity

In 2002, Ohara and Matsuhisa found that of 120 screened edible plants, peppermint was one of only eight to exhibit potent inhibitory effects against the tumor promoter okadaic acid.[3,29]

Kumar et al. showed, in a 2004 two-stage carcinogenesis model in mice, that orally administered *M. piperita* exerted inhibitory effects. Specifically, the botanical suppressed skin papilloma development induced by 7,12 dimethyl(a)anthracene and promoted by croton oil application. Significant reductions were observed in total tumor number and incidence. There was also a significant increase in the latency period of tumor formation in treated vs. control mice.[1]

Investigations by Jain et al. into the molecular mechanisms supporting the anticarcinogenic potential of *M. piperita* leaf extracts on six human cancer cell lines (HeLa, MCF-7, Jurkat, T24, HT-29, and MIAPaCa-2) in 2011 revealed that chloroform and ethyl acetate extracts dose- and time-dependently displayed anticarcinogenic activity leading to G_1 cell cycle arrest and mitochondrial-mediated apoptosis among the cascade of effects. The investigators identified their findings as the first evidence of direct anticarcinogenic activity of Mentha leaf extracts and suggested that future work might focus on isolating active constituents as a foundation for mechanistic and translational studies leading to new anticancer drugs, alone or in combination, to prevent and treat human cancers.[30] Previously, peppermint was reported to exhibit antimutagenic properties in a hamster cheek pouch model, suppressing the carcinogenicity of benzo[a]-pyrene, aflatoxin B1, methylmethane sulfonate, and an extract of shamma (a mixture of powdered tobacco, slaked lime, ash, oils, spices, and other additives, which has been correlated with oral cancer in Saudi Arabia).[4,31]

Pruritus, TRPM8, and Melanoma

Topically applied menthol, in concentrations of 1 to 3 percent, is often used to treat pruritus, particularly in the elderly.[8] In addition, recent evidence suggests that the presence of menthol can facilitate penetration of other agents in topical products.[12,24] Patel and Yosipovitch suggest that elderly patients who report diminished pruritus with cooling may stand to benefit from menthol-containing topical therapies.[8,12] In 2002, two different teams discovered that menthol acts as an agonist of a thermally sensitive receptor, formerly known as the cold- and menthol-sensitive receptor 1 (CMR1), and now known as transient receptor potential melastatin subfamily 8 (TRPM8) receptor, a member of a family of excitatory ion channels.[8,15,16] Notably, menthol engenders the same cooling sensation as low temperature, though menthol is not linked to a reduction in skin temperature.[8,12]

Although the exact mechanisms by which menthol exerts its antipruritic and analgesic effects remain to be elucidated, the discovery that the TRPM8 is its underlying receptor appears pivotal in understanding the cooling effect of the botanical.[12] There are also indications that menthol may exhibit therapeutic potential for melanoma. Specifically, melanoma expresses TRPM8 receptors, the activation of which inhibits melanoma viability. Menthol appears to mediate this response through an influx of extracellular calcium ions.[5,32]

Antibacterial Activity

In 2003, Mimica-Dukić et al. investigated the antimicrobial activity and free radical-scavenging capacity of essential oils from *M. aquatica*, *M. longifolia*, and *M. piperita*, finding that *M. piperita* displayed the greatest antibacterial potency. All three species exhibited such properties, especially against *Esherichia coli* strains, though *Shigella sonei* and *Micrococcus flavus* ATTC 10,240 were also susceptible. The investigators were especially intrigued by the finding that the essential oils were effective against bacteria known to be resistant to synthetic drugs (i.e., all tested *E. coli* species, and *Salmonella typhi* IPH-MR). All tested Mentha species also demonstrated significant fungistatic and fungicidal activity, with *M. piperita* again particularly effective against *Trichophyton tonsurans* and *Candida albicans*. Further, all Mentha species dose-dependently reduced the DPPH and OH radicals, with *M. piperita* again most effective against both radicals. Monoterpene ketones (i.e., menthone and isomenthone) were found to be the strongest scavenging ingredients in *M. piperita*. The investigators concluded that all tested species, particularly *M. piperita*, exhibited significant antibacterial, antifungal, and antioxidant activity.[33]

Three years later, in a study of the biochemical activities of *M. piperita* and *Myrtus communis*, Yadegarinia et al. reported that the oils of both species, particularly *M. piperita*, exhibited strong antimicrobial activities against *E. coli*, *S. aureus*, and *C. albicans*. The investigators also noted, after screening both species for antioxidant activity, that *M. piperita* showed greater antioxidant capacity in DPPH free radical scavenging as well as β-carotene/linoleic acid systems.[34]

CONCLUSION

Peppermint and menthol, its naturally occurring monocyclic terpene alcohol derivative, have long been used for medical and culinary purposes. Contemporary practice and continuing research continue to support various uses of *Mentha piperita* in the medical armamentarium, with its use in dermatology ubiquitous though hardly prominent. Its application for antipruritic, analgesic, antiseptic, and cooling activity may be the most compelling uses for cutaneous purposes, but its potential for wider use remains intriguing as much more research is conducted.

REFERENCES

1. Kumar A, Samarth RM, Yasmeen S, et al. Anticancer and radioprotective potentials of Mentha piperita. *Biofactors.* 2004;22:87.
2. Herro E, Jacob SE. Mentha piperita (peppermint). *Dermatitis.* 2010;21:327.
3. McKay DL, Blumberg JB. A review of the bioactivity and potential health benefits of peppermint tea (Mentha piperita L.). *Phytother Res.* 2006;20:619.
4. Baliga MS, Rao S. Radioprotective potential of mint: A brief review. *J Cancer Res Ther.* 2010;6:255.
5. Slominski A. Cooling skin cancer: Menthol inhibits melanoma growth. Focus on "TRPM8 activation suppresses cellular viability in human melanoma." *Am J Physiol Cell Physiol.* 2008;295:C293.
6. Mills S, Bone K. *Principles and Practice of Phytotherapy: Modern Herbal Medicine.* London: Churchill Livingstone; 2000:507–513.
7. Toroglu S. In-vitro antimicrobial activity and synergistic/antagonistic effect of interactions between antibiotics and some spice essential oils. *J Environ Biol.* 2011;32:23.
8. Patel T, Yosipovitch G. The management of chronic pruritus in the elderly. *Skin Therapy Lett.* 2010;15:5.
9. Kim SH, Nam JH, Park EJ, et al. Menthol regulates TRPM8-independent processes in PC-3 prostate cancer cells. *Biochim Biophys Acta.* 2009;1792:33.
10. Grieve M. *A Modern Herbal* (Vol 2). New York: Dover Publications; 1971:537.
11. Simonsen JL. *The Terpenes: The Simpler Acyclic and Monocyclic Terpenes and Their Derivatives.* Volume I (2nd ed.). Cambridge: Cambridge University Press; 1947:230–249.
12. Patel T, Ishiuji Y, Yosipovitch G. Menthol: A refreshing look at this ancient compound. *J Am Acad Dermatol.* 2007;57:873.
13. Foster S. *101 Medicinal Herbs: An Illustrated Guide.* Loveland, CO: Interweave Press; 1998:156.

14. Naghibi F, Mosaddegh M, Motamed SM, et al. Labiatae family in folk medicine in Iran: From ethnobotany to pharmacology. *Iran J Pharm Res*. 2005;2:63.

15. McKemy DD, Neuhausser WM, Julius D. Identification of a cold receptor reveals a general role for TRP channels in thermosensation. *Nature*. 2002;416:52.

16. Peier AM, Moqrich A, Hergarden AC, et al. A TRP channel that senses cold stimuli and menthol. *Cell*. 2002;108:705.

17. Ahmad N, Fazal H, Ahmad I, et al. Free radical scavenging (DPPH) potential in nine Mentha species. *Toxicol Ind Health*. 2012;28:83.

18. Schuhmacher A, Reichling J, Schnitzler P. Virucidal effect of peppermint oil on the enveloped viruses herpes simplex virus type 1 and type 2 in vitro. *Phytomedicine*. 2003;10:504.

19. Sabzghabaee AM, Nili F, Ghannadi A, et al. Role of menthol in treatment of candidial napkin dermatitis. *World J Pediatr*. 2011;7:167.

20. Qiu J, Luo M, Dong J, et al. Menthol diminishes Staphylococcus aureus virulence-associated extracellular proteins expression. *Appl Microbiol Biotechnol*. 2011;90:705.

21. Tran A, Pratt M, DeKoven J. Acute allergic contact dermatitis of the lips from peppermint oil in a lip balm. *Dermatitis*. 2010;21:111.

22. Morton CA, Garioch J, Todd P, et al. Contact sensitivity to menthol and peppermint in patients with intra-oral symptoms. *Contact Dermatitis*. 1995;32:281.

23. Wilkinson SM, Beck MH. Allergic contact dermatitis from menthol in peppermint. *Contact Dermatitis*. 1994;30:42.

24. Nair B. Final report on the safety assessment of Mentha Piperita (Peppermint) Oil, Mentha Piperita (Peppermint) Leaf Extract, Mentha Piperita (Pepperming) Leaf, and Mentha Piperita (Peppermint) Leaf Water. *Int J Toxicol*. 2001;20(Suppl 3):61.

25. Sell CS, ed. *The Chemistry of Fragrances: From Perfumer to Consumer*. 2nd ed. London: Royal Society of Chemistry; 2006:294–301.

26. Schmidt E, Bail S, Buchbauer G, et al. Chemical composition, olfactory evaluation and antioxidant effects of essential oil from Mentha x piperita. *Nat Prod Commun*. 2009;4:1107.

27. Dorman HJ, Kosar M, Baser KH, et al. Phenolic profile and antioxidant evaluation of Mentha x piperita L. (peppermint) extracts. *Nat Prod Commun*. 2009;4:535.

28. Yang SA, Jeon SK, Lee EJ, et al. Comparative study of the chemical composition and antioxidant activity of six essential oils and their components. *Nat Prod Res*. 2010;24:140.

29. Ohara A, Matsuhisa T. Anti-tumor promoting activities of edible plants against okadaic acid. *Food Sci Technol Res*. 2002;8:158.

30. Jain D, Pathak N, Khan S, et al. Evaluation of cytotoxicity and anticarcinogenic potential of Mentha leaf extracts. *Int J Toxicol*. 2011;30:225.

31. Samman MA, Bowen ID, Taiba K, et al. Mint prevents shamma-induced carcinogenesis in hamster cheek pouch. *Carcinogenesis*. 1998;19:1795.

32. Yamamura H, Ugawa S, Ueda T, et al. TRPM8 activation suppresses cellular viability in human melanoma. *Am J Physiol Cell Physiol*. 2008;295:C296.

33. Mimica-Dukić N, Bozin B, Soković M, et al. Antimicrobial and antioxidant activities of three Mentha species essential oils. *Planta Med*. 2003;69:413.

34. Yadegarinia D, Gachkar L, Rezaei MB, et al. Biochemical activities of Iranian Mentha piperita L. and Myrtus communis L. essential oils. *Phytochemistry*. 2006;67:1249.

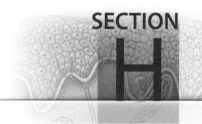

SECTION H
Anti-Inflammatory Agents

CHAPTER 64

Anti-Inflammatory Agents

In the 1st century CE, Cornelius Celsus described the signs of acute inflammation as: *calor* (heat), *dolor* (pain), *rubor* (redness) and *tumor* (swelling).[1] This accurate depiction of the sequence of events that occurs in inflammation is characteristic of all types of inflammation regardless of the provocative stimuli, which can include injury, friction, emotion, exposure to irritants or allergens, or infectious agents.[2] The initial insult to the skin causes vasodilation that is seen as redness. The endothelial lining of the blood vessels becomes more permeable and leads to extravasation. In other words, substances leak out of the vessel causing increased fluid in the tissues, which results in swelling. Inflammatory mediators such as cytokines and interleukins are released and activate multiple pathways that can lead to pain, redness, and swelling as well as serve to beckon immune cells to the area.

The process of inflammation is orchestrated by a large array of inflammatory mediators including histamines, cytokines, eicosanoids (e.g., prostaglandins, thromboxanes, and leukotrienes), complement cascade components, kinins, fibrinopeptide enzymes, and free radicals. For a more extensive review, see *Cosmetic Dermatology: Principles and Practice*, 2nd edition, Chapter 35 (McGraw-Hill, 2009).

Although the many causes of inflammation are very complicated and beyond the scope of this book, arachidonic acid (AA) and its pathways are important to understand when considering the anti-inflammatory claims of skin care products. AA production is a major cause of inflammation because AA is broken down into inflammation-causing substances such as prostaglandins and leukotrienes. Production of AA is blocked by corticosteroids, which is one of the ways that topical steroids decrease inflammation (they also cause vasoconstriction). Two important pathways involved in the breakdown of AA are worth noting (Figure 64-1).

1. Cyclooxygenase pathway: Results in the production of prostaglandins. This is the pathway in which salicylates (aspirin) and nonsteroidal anti-inflammatory drugs (NSAIDs) such as ibuprofen work.

2. Lipoxygenase pathway: Results in the production of the inflammatory mediator group leukotrienes.

Several categories of anti-inflammatory ingredients are considered in this section: salicylates, prostaglandin antagonists, leukotriene antagonists, polyphenols, and vasoconstrictors. Examples of salicylates include salicylic acid and *Aloe vera*.

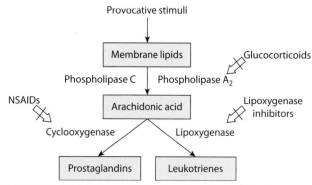

▲ **FIGURE 64-1** This simplified chart shows how arachidonic acid is broken down into prostaglandins and leukotrienes, key groups of inflammatory mediators. Many contributors to the arachidonic acid cascade have been omitted here for ease of explanation.

Prostaglandin antagonists include feverfew, licorice extract, and oatmeal, while turmeric and chamomile are leukotriene antagonists. Coumarin and its derivatives, found in tamanu oil, for example, suppress prostaglandin biosynthesis through inhibition of the lipoxygenase and cyclooxygenase systems.[3] Horse chestnut is a vasoconstrictor, as are corticosteroids such as hydrocortisone. Polyphenols are also discussed in the Antioxidants section introduction as well as several chapters in that section. Anti-inflammatory polyphenols considered here include calendula, edelweiss, and lavandula. Polyphenols decrease inflammation by neutralizing free radicals.

Inflammation is typically the common denominator for individuals with sensitive skin. The etiology varies depending on the condition. For example, in acne, the cause of inflammation is thought to result from byproducts generated by bacteria as they digest fatty acids. In rosacea, part of the observed inflammation is due to vasodilation of unknown etiology. Those with allergic skin reactions develop inflammation when the immune system cells in the skin are exposed to an allergen.

INFLAMMATION AND AGING

Inflammation is believed to play a role in aging because its activation can lead to the breakdown of skin collagen and elastin and other important cutaneous components in addition to increased glycation, lipofuscin, and free radical production. This is discussed in Chapter 81, Overview of Aging.

Botanical, natural, and organic products often exhibit potent anti-inflammatory activity. The most commonly seen ingredients in anti-inflammatory skin care include feverfew, green tea, cucumber, chamomile, and licorice extract. It is anticipated that many new ingredients will enter the market as our understanding of the causes of rosacea and other inflammatory skin conditions increases.

REFERENCES

1. Williams RH, Stedman TL. *Stedman's Medical Dictionary*. 25th ed. Philadelphia, PA: Williams & Wilkins; 1990.
2. Kimball ES. *Cytokines and Inflammation*. Boca Raton, FL: CRC Press; 1991.
3. Fylaktakidou KC, Hadjipavlou-Litina DJ, Litinas KE, et al. Natural and synthetic coumarin derivatives with anti-inflammatory/ antioxidant activities. *Curr Pharm Des*. 2004;10:3813.

CHAPTER 65

Aloe Vera

Activities:

Anti-inflammatory, antioxidant, antimicrobial,[1] immunomodulatory, laxative,[2] wound healing[3]

Important Chemical Components:

Aloe resin, aloesin (2-acetyonyl-8-glucopyranosyl-7-hydroxy-5-methylchromone), glucomannans, particularly acemannan (also known as acetylated mannose or mannose-6-phosphate),[4] and other polysaccharides (galactose, xylose, arabinose); aloe emodin and other anthraquinones, including aloin A and B (anthrone-C-glucosyls or C-glucosides of emodin and also known collectively as barbaloin);[3,5] lectin, phenols (gentisic acid, epicatechin, and quercitrin), amino acids, enzymes, lignin, minerals (selenium, zinc), salicylic acid, magnesium lactate, saponins, sterols, and vitamins A, C, and E[1,6–11]

Origin Classification:

This ingredient is natural. Organic forms exist.

Personal Care Category:

Moisturizing, soothing, cooling, burn and wound healing

Recommended for the following Baumann Skin Types:

DSNT, DSPT, DSNW, DSPW, OSNT, OSNW, OSPT, and OSPW

SOURCE

A cactus-like perennial succulent and member of the Xanthorrhoeaceae family and the subfamily Liliaceae (lily) native to North Africa and the Arabian peninsula, *Aloe vera* (also known as *Aloe barbadensis*) is the most potent of the several aloe species and one of the most widely used herbal products throughout the world (Table 65-1).[12] The plant is now widely distributed throughout Africa, Asia, southern Europe, the Americas, and other areas with tropical climates.[13] *Aloe* (from the Arabic *alloeh* for a "shining bitter substance") *vera* (Latin for "truth") thrives in warm, dry climates, but can survive

TABLE 65-1
Pros and Cons of Aloe Vera

Pros	Con
One of the main herbal agents in widespread use for dermatologic purposes	Dearth of clinical trials
Impressive anecdotal evidence of efficacy	
Broad range of reputed medicinal, and dermatologic, applications	

high temperatures and even humid conditions as long as its roots are not submerged in water.[11,14] Various cultures have used aloe to treat burns (including sunburns), wounds, abrasions, insect bites, cuts, blisters, and frostbite. *A. vera* has been used for several decades, both topically and systemically, to enhance wound repair based more on traditional and anecdotal evidence than rigorously established scientific study.[15] Its effectiveness in healing wounds and treating infections has been established in laboratory animals, though.[9]

Reputed to have potent anti-inflammatory and antimicrobial effects, the fresh or dehydrated whole aloe leaf is used for treatment of radiation injuries, ulcers, burns, eczema, and psoriasis.[13] Other anecdotal cutaneous indications may include seborrhea, acne, androgenetic alopecia, and herpes zoster (shingles). Aloe is believed to balance the pH of the skin and is used in hundreds of medicines and over-the-counter (OTC) products such as shampoos, soaps, shaving creams, deodorants, tissue paper products, sunscreens, moisturizers, and other skin creams to soothe, heal, and protect the skin. It is also believed to exhibit antioxidant properties.[16]

In fact, the medical establishment recognizes the use of *A. vera* in treating radiation and stasis ulcers and has acknowledged the antibacterial and antifungal effects of *A. vera* components.[17] Aloe is also indicated for the treatment of frostbite.[1] The vasoconstrictive effects of thromboxane have been shown to be improved with the application of *A. vera* cream such as Dermaide.[18,19] Further, *A. vera* is recognized as one of the many herbal products to contain pharmacologically active ingredients with the potential to enhance wound healing.[20] Such ingredients include salicylates and a carboxypeptidase that inactivates bradykinin *in vitro*.[17] *A. vera* is considered the most commercially important of the more than 500 species in the genus *Aloe*.[3,11,21]

The manufacturing of *A. vera* extracts represents one of the largest global botanical industries, and aloe is one of the few herbal agents used broadly in Western cultures.[22]

HISTORY

In traditional folk medicine, topical *A. vera* is used to treat inflammation, cicatrization, and dyspigmentation. Its constituent aloesin has been demonstrated to inhibit tyrosinase activity from human, murine, and mushroom sources.[23] The traditional use of *A. vera* gel dates back nearly 2,500 years to ancient Egypt (where it was known as the "the plant of immortality")[11,24], Greece, India, China (where it was dubbed an "elixir of youth")[11], Japan, and Mexico.[11,14,25] It is believed to have been included in the skin care regimens of Egyptian queens Nefertiti and Cleopatra, as well as for embalming and as an offering at funerals for pharoahs.[14,24] Egyptians, Assyrians, and others in the Mediterranean region are said to have used the gel as well as the latex (found inside the leaves).[24] Aloe was also reportedly used to treat battlefield wounds in ancient times under Alexander the Great and more than 1,500 years later under Christopher Columbus.[14] The first documentation of healing properties associated with *A. vera* is attributed to Mesopotamian clay tablets circa 2100 BCE, with medicinal properties characterized with greater detail in Egyptian writings circa 1550 BCE.[22]

Through human trade and migration, this dynamic plant became known and widely used to cure burns and wounds throughout ancient civilizations in Persia, Egypt and elsewhere in Africa, Greece, Rome, India, and China and appears in the folklore of Japan, the Philippines, and Hawaii. The Spanish used it and brought it to South America and to such Caribbean locales as Aruba, Curaçao, and Barbados (from which the alternate INCI name *Aloe barbadensis* nomenclature is derived).[26]

Aloe is believed to have been first cited in English in John Goodyew's 1655 translation of *De Materia Medica* by the Greek physician Dioscorides, who used the plant to treat sores and wounds in the first century CE.[14,22,24] It was used as a laxative in the United States (US) beginning in the early 1800s, and listed in the US pharmacopoeia in 1820 as a purgative and skin protectant.[14,22] Modern clinical use of *A. vera* began in the 1930s, when it was shown to be effective in treating chronic and severe radiation dermatitis.[14,25] Aloe products have maintained their popularity through the course of time.[27] In 1983, the US Food and Drug Administration (FDA) approved topical aloe to treat inflammation.[10] It continues to be used today primarily for anti-inflammatory applications, but several other uses are under investigation. *A. vera* is also approved as a food flavoring and oral cathartic (Aloe latex).[10] In traditional Chinese medicine, *A. vera* is used for fungal conditions; in Ayurvedic medicine, it is used to treat cutaneous and other conditions.[22]

CHEMISTRY

Rich in glucomannans and other polysaccharides, the gel and sap from the inner core of the full leaf confer healing qualities and pose no risk. Aloe is known to lessen the itching and inflammation associated with minor wounds. The gel is also thought to be effective in eliminating the yeasts, fungi, and bacteria that infiltrate and inhabit wounds and, is believed by some to accelerate collagen production. Research in recent years has determined that aloe contains three agents with significant antitumor potential: emodin, mannose, and lectin. While the use of *A. vera* has not achieved unqualified acceptance from the medical establishment, components of the plant are under serious scientific investigation.

There is a large body of anecdotal evidence attesting to the efficacy of aloe for the treatment of myriad diseases; unfortunately, exaggerated claims are not uncommon and therefore caution is warranted in the interpretation of some of the available information.[28] Explanations of aloe gel efficacy are still varied because it has, in fact, several active constituents operating through different mechanisms.[29] Indeed, aloe has been compared to honey as an exceedingly convoluted amalgam of natural components (see Chapter 60, Honey/Propolis/Royal Jelly).[30] Its action as a moisturizer is a popular use that may account for many of its effects.[31] Furthermore, aloe is reputed to exhibit potent anti-inflammatory effects, and the substances that have been proposed as its active anti-inflammatory constituents include salicylates (providing "aspirin-like effects"); magnesium lactate, which is believed to inhibit the production of histamine; bradykinin and thromboxane inhibitors, which provide pain reduction; and polysaccharides, particularly acemannan, which has reported immunomodulatory properties.[16,32,33] Another substance isolated from aloe, C-glucosyl chromone, has exhibited topical anti-inflammatory activity equivalent to that of hydrocortisone (200 µg/mouse ear).[34] A glycoprotein fraction of *A. vera* is thought to account, through cell proliferation and migration, for the wound healing effect associated with extracts of the plant.[35]

ORAL USES

Aloe is used as a functional food and an ingredient in other food products as well as health-boosting beverages.[3,11] Traditionally, for health purposes, aloe has been used orally as a purgative and antihelminthic agent.[10] In addition, it has been used systemically for ulcers and diverticulitis.[36] The oral administration of *A. vera* has recently been found to be effective in ameliorating the effects of acute radiation-delayed wound healing in rats by increasing transforming growth factor (TGF)-β1 and basic fibroblast growth factor.[37] Overall, however, oral use of aloe is thought to exacerbate some chronic conditions and to be susceptible to multiple drug interactions.[36] Therefore, despite some evidence of systemic efficacy, oral use of aloe is not recommended.[36]

Acemannan, a polysaccharide extracted from *A. vera*, has been shown to be an effective and safe alternative for treating oral aphthous ulcers for patients who prefer to avoid steroid therapy, though it is less effective than 0.1 percent triamcinolone acetonide.[38]

In 2009, Cho et al. investigated the cutaneous antiaging effects of dietary *A. vera* gel in 30 healthy females over 45 years old who received either a low-dose (1,200 mg/d) or high-dose (3,600 mg/d) supplement for 90 days, with baseline status serving as control. The researchers noted significant improvement in facial wrinkles in both groups, and facial elasticity was enhanced in the group using the low-dose supplement. Based on skin samples taken before and after supplementation, matrix metalloproteinase (MMP)-1 mRNA levels were found to be significantly diminished in the high-dose group. In both groups, type I procollagen immunostaining was significantly elevated. The investigators concluded that although no dose-response relationship was found, oral administration of aloe gel appeared to significantly improve signs of photoaged human skin, with increases noted in collagen synthesis and decreases in collagen-degrading MMP-1 gene expression.[39]

A. vera is also a featured ingredient in a multi-phytonutrient liquid dietary supplement that contains a proprietary blend of fruits, vegetables, and catechin complex from green tea (VIBE Cardiac & Life) found *in vitro* to have exerted antimutagenic, and DNA-protective effects on human epidermal cells exposed to ultraviolet (UV)-induced DNA damage.

There are indications that the oral use of gel may lower blood glucose levels in type 2 diabetes mellitus, alleviate mild-to-moderate ulcerative colitis, and even stabilize metastatic cancer. Much more research is necessary to corroborate such findings, according to Foster et al.[22]

TOPICAL USES

In 2008, Reuter et al. conducted a randomized, double-blind, placebo-controlled, Phase III study in 40 volunteers to evaluate the anti-inflammatory activity of a highly concentrated *A. vera* gel (97.5 percent). After test sites on the back were exposed to 1.5-fold minimal erythema dose (MED) of UVB, these areas were treated for the next two days with *A. vera* gel, positive controls (0.25 percent prednicarbate, 1 percent hydrocortisone in placebo gel, and 1 percent hydrocortisone cream), or a placebo gel. After 48 hours, the *A. vera* gel was found to have significantly lowered UV-induced erythema more effectively than 1 percent hydrocortisone in placebo gel, but less efficiently than 1 percent hydrocortisone cream. Nevertheless, the researchers suggested the potential use of highly concentrated A. vera gel for topically treating inflammatory skin conditions.[40]

Oyelami et al. reported in 2009, based initially on an open, non-comparative study, that the crude gel of A. vera was used successfully in Nigeria to treat five patients with scabies. Subsequently, the investigators compared the efficacy of the botanical agent (16 subjects) with that achieved with benzyl benzoate lotion (14 subjects) in 30 patients. After two courses of treatment, three of the patients using benzyl benzoate lotion and two of those using A. vera still complained of pruritus. Lesions were found to have essentially disappeared in all patients, with no detectable side effects. The researchers concluded that A. vera gel is as effective as benzyl benzoate for treating scabies.[41]

Earlier that year, Feily and Namazi performed a literature search for *in vitro*, *in vivo*, and clinical trial data on dermatologic uses of A. vera, finding 40 pertinent studies. Oral administration in mice was seen as effective in wound healing, reducing the number and size of papillomas, and lowering the incidence of tumors and leishmaniasis. The researchers found that while topically applied aloe offered no photoprotective or radioprotective activity, it was noted for efficacy in treating aphthous stomatitis, burns and other wounds, frostbite, genital herpes, human papilloma virus, inflammation, lichen planus, psoriasis, seborrheic dermatitis, and xerosis. They added that data support the use of aloe as a biological vehicle, an antimicrobial and antifungal agent, and a potential option for photodynamic therapy for some forms of cancer. Finally, the authors cautioned that while encouraging results have been obtained for A. vera for a broad range of dermatologic applications, the clinical data establishing effectiveness of oral and topical A. vera remain insufficient.[13]

Psoriasis

Aloe is rarely, if ever, mentioned among the wide array of products comprising the dermatologic armamentarium for psoriasis. There is some evidence suggesting its usefulness, however. Syed et al. performed a double-blind, placebo-controlled examination of A. vera extract 0.5 percent in a hydrophilic cream for the treatment of psoriasis vulgaris.[42] Psoriatic plaques cleared in only two of 30 subjects on placebo while the aloe group showed clearance in 25 of 30 patients, and significant improvement in desquamation, erythema, and Psoriasis Area Severity Index (PASI) score.[42,43] Inflammation remains a major indication for aloe products. Research has established the anti-inflammatory effects of A. vera gel extracts, which may also impart inhibitory activity, via cyclooxygenase, on the arachidonic acid pathway.[44] Immunomodulatory properties of the gel polysaccharides, particularly the acetylated mannans (now a proprietary compound under several patents), have been reported.[29]

In 2005, Paulsen et al. led a randomized, double-blind, placebo-controlled, right/left comparison study in 41 patients with stable plaque psoriasis to determine the efficacy of a commercial A. vera gel. Results were modest, with the gel not shown to be superior to placebo. However, the researchers suggested that the high response rate to placebo might have left the aloe gel looking less effective than it actually was.[45]

A 2010 randomized, comparative, double-blind, eight-week study of 80 patients conducted by Choonhakarn et al. suggested that A. vera may be more effective than 0.1 percent triamcinolone acetonide in the treatment of mild-to-moderate plaque psoriasis. The mean PASI score decreased from 11.6 to 3.9 over eight weeks in the A. vera group and from 10.9 to 4.3 in the triamcinolone acetonide group. The researchers noted, though,

that both treatments displayed similar efficacy in improving quality of life for psoriasis patients.[46]

In 2012, Dhanabal used a mouse tail model to assess the antipsoriatic activity of A. vera, showing that an ethanolic extract of the gel generated a significant differentiation in the epidermis as well as a significant increase in relative epidermal thickness compared to negative control and the lack of change in the standard positive control (tazarotene). The investigators concluded that A. vera exerted an overall antipsoriatic activity of 81.95 percent in the mouse tail model, as compared to 87.94 percent for tazarotene.[47]

Wound Healing

A. vera has been used for several decades, both topically and systemically, to enhance wound repair based more on traditional and anecdotal evidence than rigorously established scientific study.[15]

A few recent studies buttress the long-standing anecdotal evidence in support of aloe in the treatment of wounds. An investigation using rats showed that full-thickness wounds treated with A. vera displayed elevated biosynthesis of collagen and its degradation, suggesting that aloe affected the wound-healing process by enhancing collagen turnover in the wounded tissue.[48] In another study using rats, A. vera exhibited both anti-inflammatory and wound-healing activity when applied to second-degree burns.[49] Similar effects have been seen in studies with humans. Researchers observed that the partial thickness burn wounds of 27 patients treated with A. vera gel evinced early epithelialization and faster healing time than the area treated with Vaseline gauze. Some patients reported mild discomfort.[50]

After an exhaustive literature search in 1999 of controlled clinical trials on aloe, Vogler and Ernst sounded skeptical notes, however. They concluded that the topical application of A. vera may be effective for genital herpes and psoriasis, but its effectiveness in promoting wound healing was, as yet, unproven, and its use does not prevent radiation-induced injuries.[51]

Ten years later, topically applied A. vera gel was shown in a study in 63 male rats to reduce wound diameter significantly when administered twice daily as compared to once-daily treatment or control groups.[52]

A 2012 report by Inpanya et al. demonstrated that a blended fibroin/aloe gel film could accelerate wound healing in streptozotocin-induced diabetic rats, with wounds treated with the blended film enhancing the attachment and proliferation of skin fibroblasts compared to aloe-free fibroin film and yielding smaller wounds after day 7 compared to untreated diabetic wounds. The investigators concluded that their fibroin/aloe gel film may have potential for treating diabetic non-healing skin ulcers in humans.[53]

Also that year, in a randomized, controlled, comparative study by Tarameshloo et al., topically applied A. vera gel more rapidly accelerated the healing process than silver sulfadiazine 1 percent, thyroid hormone, or vehicle in skin wounds surgically induced in Wistar rats (see Chapter 80, Silver).[54] Hosseinimehr et al. previously found that aloe cream was significantly more effective than silver sulfadiazine in augmenting reepithelialization in burn wounds in rats.[55]

Human trials have been lacking, however. Indeed, Dat el. conducted a 2012 search of several databases (the Cochrane Wounds Group Specialized Register, the Cochrane Central Register of Controlled Trials, Ovid MEDLINE, Ovid AMED, and EBSCO CINAHL) for all randomized controlled trials assessing the effectiveness of A. vera, aloe-derived products, and dressings combining *A. vera* and other components in treating acute or chronic wounds. Seven trials, with a total of 347 subjects treated, met inclusion criteria, but were deemed to be of such poor quality that trial results should be viewed cautiously. The authors cited the paucity of high quality clinical trials on the use of *A. vera* topical products or dressings for treating acute and chronic wounds as a justification for withholding support for such treatments.[2]

Lichen Planus

In 2010, Cheng et al. conducted a comprehensive database search [the Cochrane Skin Group Specialized Register, the Cochrane Central Register of Controlled Trials (CENTRAL) in The Cochrane Library, MEDLINE (from 2005), EMBASE (from 2007), and LILACS (from 1982)] to evaluate the results of treatment for erosive lichen planus involving the anogenital, oral, and/or esophageal regions. They identified 15 randomized controlled trials (473 total subjects) pertaining to oral lichen planus only. Notably, in a study with 45 patients, *A. vera* gel was found to be six times more likely than placebo to yield at least a 50 percent decline in pain symptoms.[56]

A. vera juice and gel were shown to be effective in a case study of a 38-year-old man who was successfully treated for lichen planus of the skin and oral mucosa with a two-month course of the botanical agent.[57]

Atopic Dermatitis and Xerosis

In 2006, Dal'Belo et al. assessed the effects of cosmetic preparations containing various concentrations of freeze-dried *A. vera* extract on the skin hydration of the volar forearm of 20 female volunteers. Stratum corneum (SC) water content and transepidermal water loss (TEWL) were evaluated after a single application as well as after one and two weeks of daily use of stable formulations containing 5 percent (w/w) of a trilaureth-4 phosphate-based blend with 0.10, 0.25, or 0.50 percent (w/w) of freeze-dried *A. vera* extract. SC water content increased after one application of the formulations supplemented with 0.25 and 0.50 percent (w/w) *A. vera* extract. After two weeks, SC water content was higher as a result of using any of the formulations. When compared with vehicle, TEWL was unaltered by any of the products. The investigators concluded that freeze-dried *A. vera* extract is effective at enhancing skin hydration and would be useful in cosmetic moisturizers.[58]

In 2010, Kim et al. demonstrated in a study of the effects of *Scutellariae radix* and *A. vera* gel, alone or in combination, on NC/Nga mice that both plants modulate immunological responses in atopic dermatitis primarily by suppressing interleukin (IL)-5 and IL-10 levels.[59]

A. vera was cited as one of nine botanical extracts by Casetti et al. in a 2011 PubMed database search for botanical extracts noted for enhancing the skin barrier and/or facilitating keratinocyte differentiation *in vivo* after topical application. The researchers suggested that while further investigation is necessary, *A. vera* and the other herbs appear to have potential as dermocosmetic agents for treating dry skin.[60,61]

Aloe-coated Examination Gloves

A. vera-infused gloves were first shown to be effective in a 2003 open, contralateral comparison study by West and Zhu. This investigation involved 30 adult females with bilateral dry skin due to occupational exposure on a factory assembly line who were directed to use the dry-coated *A. vera* glove on one hand for eight hours/day and no glove on the other hand for 30 days.

The investigators reported that the gradual delivery of aloe to the skin yielded uniformly enhanced skin integrity, diminished fine wrinkling, and reduced erythema.[62] In a letter responding to West and Zhu's study, Mitchell emphasized that their study involved factory not health care workers, who must be vigilant about hand hygiene. Further, she noted that hands not decontaminated after patient contact risk serving as disease vectors, but speculated that decontaminating hands after using *A. vera* gloves would also negate any benefits of the herbal agent. Finally, she wondered whether the soothing feeling conferred to hands by the *A. vera*-infused gloves might discourage some users from decontaminating their hands after use.[63]

In a 2007 quasi-experimental pilot study of 272 health care workers as controls and 203 health care workers as test subjects, investigators working in three US hospitals and one Canadian hospital found that the use of *A. vera*-impregnated medical exam gloves improved perceived skin condition and attitudes about hand hygiene.[64] Although such gloves are available on the market in the UK, a report by Ford and Phillips earlier in 2007 suggested that it has not been established that the coating contains active aloe, whether the physical or chemical properties of the gloves are altered by aloe, and what, if any, long-term effects there are for users of the gloves. They did acknowledge that no adverse reactions had been published.[65]

Healing from Radiotherapy

In 2005, Richardson et al. systematically reviewed biomedical and alternative medicine databases for randomized controlled trials on the effectiveness of *A. vera* gel for treating radiation-induced skin reactions. In the five published trials as well as two unpublished randomized controlled trials that they identified, they found no evidence that topically applied *A. vera* is effective in preventing or attenuating radiation-induced cutaneous reactions in cancer patients.[66] Nevertheless, Wang et al. demonstrated during the previous year that aloe polysaccharides exerted radioprotective effects *in vitro* and *in vivo* in mice through suppressing apoptosis.[67]

In a literature review published after the database investigation by Richardson and colleagues, Maddocks-Jennings et al. found data to suggest that *A. vera* gel is as effective as mild steroid creams (e.g., 1 percent hydrocortisone) in mitigating reactions to radiotherapy, with the added benefit of not provoking adverse side effects.[68]

In a 2009 study with Swiss albino mice, Goyal and Gehlot showed that *A. vera* leaf extract displays radioprotective effects against the biochemical alterations engendered by whole-body γ-irradiation.[69]

Combination Therapies: In Use or Under Investigation

A. vera extract is considered a key ingredient in a formulation also containing wheat germ oil and turmeric extract found to be an effective moisturizer in a small study with human volunteers (see Chapter 69, Turmeric).[70]

In 2008, Gupta et al. found that a poly-herbal topical formulation combining the aqueous lyophilized leaf extracts of *Hippophae rhamnoides* and *A. vera* and the ethanol rhizome extract of *Curcuma longa* (in an optimized ratio of 1:7:1) accelerated wound healing in normal and diabetic rats (see Chapter 69, Turmeric).[71]

Mendonça et al. performed a study with Wistar rats in 2009 that compared the wound-healing effects of topically applied *A. vera* gel alone or not with microcurrent application. The group treated only with aloe gel experienced accelerated wound healing compared to the control group. Animals treated only with micro-current and those treated with aloe and microcurrent exhibited earlier proliferative phase activity compared to the control and aloe-only groups. The investigators concluded that *A. vera* gel and microcurrent acted synergistically in treating open wounds and has potential as a therapeutic option.[72]

A. vera extract is also an active ingredient in a cream containing Dead Sea minerals that was shown in 2009 to display antioxidant, anti-inflammatory, and photoprotective activity against UVB irradiation when topically applied to human skin organ cultures.[73]

Aloe is included in a 4 percent hydroquinone/10 percent L-ascorbic acid treatment system shown in 2011 to be effective in attenuating the early signs of photodamage in the normal to oily skin of 30 female subjects enrolled in a study by Bruce and Watson [see Chapter 36, Hydroquinone, and Chapter 55, Ascorbic Acid (Vitamin C)].[74]

In a 2012 randomized, double-blind, clinical trial with 67 patients, an *A. vera*/olive oil cream was demonstrated to be as effective as β-methasone 0.1 percent in treating sulfur mustard-induced chronic skin lesions, characterized by pruritus, xerosis, a burning sensation, and scaling.[75]

Aloe is also included in Menpentol Leche, an emulsion based on hyperoxygenated fatty acids, *A. vera*, and *Mimosa tenuiflora* that was found in a nonrandomized open clinical evaluation to be beneficial in alleviating the cutaneous symptoms prior to the appearance of ulcers in patients susceptible to vascular ulcers and diabetic foot ulcers.[76]

SAFETY ISSUES

The Cosmetic Ingredient Review Expert Panel has found that anthraquinone levels have been well characterized and understood in *A. vera* products and should not exceed 50 parts per million (ppm) in cosmetic products.[9] Further, the panel reports that the phototoxicity associated with some anthraquinone constituents of *A. vera* has been undermined by multiple clinical studies using amounts of the ingredient typical of commercial preparations that have revealed no phototoxicity, suggesting that the concentrations of anthraquinones are too low in *A. vera* preparations to cause phototoxicity.[9] Anthraquinones are found in the sap of aloe, but not the leaf gel, which is the source of most aloe ingredients used in commercial preparations.[30]

The yellow juice from the outer margins of the leaf is the traditional source for a laxative and while used by many, the FDA issued a statement in 2001 identifying the stimulant laxative aloe ingredients (aloe extract and aloe flower extract) in OTC drug products as misbranded and not generally safe and effective.[77]

Although the use of topical *A. vera* products is recognized as safe, with reports of truly adverse reactions extremely rare, dermatologic side effects, including acute eczema, contact urticaria, and dermatitis have been documented.[9,25,78] Mild discomfort has been linked to aloe use in some patients. Specifically, products containing *A. vera* (as well as vitamin E) as the major active ingredient are contraindicated in the immediate weeks after surgery for patients undergoing dermabrasion or chemical peels.[79] Application of aloe gel is not contraindicated in women who are pregnant or lactating, but no standards regarding a maximum treatment period have been established.

A. vera is considered a sensitizing ingredient in emollients, and may exacerbate xerosis, particularly in the elderly.[80]

In 2007, Xia reported on findings that suggest humans exposed to formulations that contain *A. vera* whole leaf extract may experience amplified sensitivity to UV light, likely due to the anthraquinones present in the leaf extract, which have been demonstrated to produce reactive oxygen species due to UVA exposure.[81]

ENVIRONMENTAL IMPACT

There are no significant challenges or effects on the environment imposed by *A. vera* plant cultivation known by the author, though it is one of the largest botanical industries in the world.[22] As a succulent, it actually acts against desertification.

FORMULATION CONSIDERATIONS

Cole and Heard showed in 2007 that *A. vera* juice displayed skin permeation-enhancing activity.[82]

In a 2007 study of vehicles for topically applied *A. vera* as well as *Arnica montana*, Bergamante et al. found that a gel formulation, containing Sepigel 305, had the capacity to decrease the release and permeation of aloin, a key constituent of *A. vera* extract known to exhibit antibacterial activity. Limiting aloin to surface activity was considered important because human skin fibroblasts can metabolize absorbed aloin and render the skin more sensitive to UV light.[83]

Two years later, Takahashi et al. showed that liposome encapsulation of *A. vera* leaf gel extracts significantly enhanced bioavailability and spurred proliferation and synthesis of type I collagen in normal human neonatal skin fibroblasts.[84]

Based on *in vitro* findings in 2012, Popadic et al. suggested caution regarding the use and proper labeling of aloe emodin in topical products given the capacity of this hydroxyanthraquinone constituent of *A. vera* to suppress the proliferation of adult human keratinocytes.[85] Topically applied aloe emodin has also been demonstrated to intensify cutaneous sensitivity to the effects of UV exposure.[86,87] In addition, aloe emodin has been shown to induce apoptosis in nonmelanoma skin cancer cells, with such effects accelerated by the incorporation of aloe emodin in a liposomal formulation, which enhances transdermal delivery.[88]

In 2013, Vandana et al. formulated *A. vera* gel into a base to prepare nimesulide emulgel with a higher drug-load capacity than commercial nimesulide gel (86.4 vs. 70.5 percent) and characterized by significant anti-inflammatory potential.[89]

USAGE CONSIDERATIONS

Known traditionally for its soothing and multifaceted capacity to treat a wide variety of skin lesions, *A. vera* use as an active ingredient has exploded in the lucrative field of cosmetics and cosmeceuticals. Aloe and α-hydroxy acids are the natural products and extracts used most often in skin care formulations (see Chapter 82, Hydroxy Acids). Hundreds of such products have flooded the market since the mid-1990s. Aloe is even included in a new protective garment. Quantum Labs received FDA approval in April 2002 for its SoftSkin *A. vera* gel-coated glove with vitamin E. The broad array of processed and commercially available aloe products are known to contain several ingredients, but little is known regarding the stability of the active ingredients. Some such products have so little aloe or active ingredients that the agent is rendered diluted or unstable to the point of providing no therapeutic effects. Products that list "aloe vera extract" tend to be more dilute, while those listing "aloe gel" are more likely effective, but the lack of meaningful regulation of these products makes proper selection a significant challenge for consumers. Indeed, aloe is known to be ineffective in concentrations below 50 percent; for optimal benefits, 100 percent is recommended.[6]

SIGNIFICANT BACKGROUND

A. vera is widely used in various products, including cosmetics, pharmaceuticals, food supplements, and beverages. An increasing array of biological activity has been associated with this plant long associated with the healing of minor wounds.

Antioxidant and Anti-inflammatory Activity

Aloe constituents such as salicylic acid, magnesium lactate, and several polysaccharides are instrumental in reducing levels of thromboxane A_2, thromboxane B_2, and prostaglandin E_2, thus rendering anti-inflammatory effects (see Chapter 78, Salicylic Acid).[24]

In a wide-ranging 2003 study of the anti-inflammatory and antioxidant properties of various aloe isolates, including cinnamoyl, p-coumaroyl, feruloyl, caffeoyl aloesin, and related compounds, Yagi et al. found that the involvement of the caffeoyl, feruloyl, and coumaroyl groups bound to aloesin was well established, and the contact hypersensitivity response suggested that aloesin prevented UVB-induced immune suppression. In addition, they noted that aloesin inhibited the tyrosine hydroxylase and DOPA oxidase activities of tyrosinase in normal human melanocyte cell lysates. The investigators concluded that the potent antioxidant and anti-inflammatory effects imparted by aloesin derivatives helped to explain, in part, the anti-inflammatory and wound-healing properties of A. vera.[90,91] Further, in 2013, López et al. observed in vitro antioxidant activities displayed by methanol extracts of A. vera leaf skin and flowers, using the 1,1-diphenyl-2-picrylhydrazyl (DPPH) and ferric antioxidant reducing power (FRAP) assays. The leaf skin fraction was more active, also exhibiting activity against tested microbial strains.[92]

Anticancer Activity

Aloe emodin has emerged as the focus of much of the research into the capacity of A. vera for cancer inhibition. A hydroxyanthraquinone naturally present in A. vera leaves, aloe emodin has been noted for its strong inhibition of Merkel cell carcinoma (MCC) proliferation, but has been found to be nontoxic to normal cells.[1,93] The antineuroectodermal tumor activity of aloe emodin has been noted in vitro and in vivo and may represent a significant new direction for antitumor drugs, according to some researchers.[94]

Key factors in the anticarcinogenic potential of aloe are its active constituents found to have immunomodulating activity. The small molecular weight compounds prevent UVB-induced immune suppression in the skin by repairing UVB-induced damages on epidermal Langerhans cells (LC).[95,96] These substances may also play a role in natural cancer therapy. Investigators have identified some therapeutic benefits, such as disease stabilization and survival, from natural cancer therapy with melatonin plus A. vera extracts for patients with advanced solid tumors and for whom no other standard therapies are judged appropriate.[97] Also, a combination of vitamin C and A. vera gel extract supplementation was found to be effective in reducing the severity of chemical hepatocarcinogenesis in a study using Sprague-Dawley rats.[98]

In 2007, Chaudhary et al. used a two-stage skin carcinogenesis model in mice to ascertain the chemopreventive potential of A. vera. Tumorigenesis was induced in Swiss albino mice with a single topical application of 7,12-dimethylbenz(a) anthracene (DMBA) and promoted with croton oil for 16 weeks. A. vera leaf extract was orally administered (1,000 mg/kg body weight/d) and/or aloe gel topically applied (1 mL/9 cm^2/mice/d). Combined aloe treatment was found to reduce the number and size of papillomas, with a significantly lower tumor incidence seen in animals treated with aloe compared with 100 percent tumor incidence in the DMBA-treated control group. In addition, significantly fewer papillomas were seen in aloe-treated mice as compared to controls during a 16-week observation period; a significantly longer average latency period and reduced tumor burden and tumor yield were associated with the aloe-treated animals.[99]

In a 2010 one-year study of the potential of A. vera in skin care formulations enhancing UV-induced skin cancer, the National Toxicology Program evaluated topical creams containing aloe plant extracts (aloe gel, whole leaf, decolorized whole leaf) or aloe emodin on SKH-1 hairless mice exposed to simulated solar light. A weak enhancing effect exerted by aloe gel or aloe emodin was identified in female but no male mice based on histologic analysis. There was also a weak enhancing effect rendered by whole or decolorized whole leaf in male and female SKH-1 mice as indicated by histologically-ascertained squamous cell neoplasms. No effect from the creams was seen during the in-life phase.[100]

Also that year, Saini et al. investigated the antitumor activity of aloe in a two-stage skin carcinogenesis model in Swiss albino mice, using DMBA to induce and croton oil to promote tumors. The mice were randomly divided into four groups, with the first group exposed only to DMBA and croton oil and serving as controls; the second group received topical A. vera gel; the third group was treated with oral A. vera extract; and the fourth group received both topical A. vera gel and oral A. vera extract. Tumor incidence was 100 percent in the first group, and dipped to 50, 60, and 40 percent, in the second, third, and fourth groups, respectively. The number of papillomas, tumor yield, and tumor burden in the treatment groups were also significantly diminished compared to controls, while the average latency period increased significantly as compared to controls. The investigators concluded that A. vera exerts a protective effect against DMBA-croton oil-induced skin papillomagenesis in mice due to its high concentration of beneficial constituents, including vitamins A, C, and E, glutathione peroxidase, superoxide dismutase isozymes, selenium, zinc, and polysaccharides.[8]

Antimicrobial Activity

Antibacterial, antifungal, and antiviral activities have been associated with A. vera.[1,17] A 2007 study by Habeeb et al. explored reports of antimicrobial effects associated with the plant.[17,101] Using a simple in vitro assay, they determined the effect of the inner gel of aloe on bacterial-induced proinflammatory cytokine production (namely, TNF-α and IL-1β) from human leukocytes stimulated with Shigella flexneri. Results demonstrated the suppression of both bacterial-induced cytokines with the use of aloe inner gel.[101] Further studies are still needed for a deeper and more precise understanding of aloe constituents and their varied biological activities.

A 2009 in vitro comparison of a copper biocide/A. vera-based hand rub (Xgel) revealed that the agent was less cytotoxic to human skin cells than seven commercially available products and more effective than Purell against all tested bacteria (i.e., methicillin-resistant *Staphylococcus aureus* (MRSA), *Acinetobacter baumanii*, and *Clostridium difficile*).[102]

Photoprotection

In a recent *in vitro* study, Hwang et al. demonstrated that immature aloe shoot extracts (one-month old) were more effective than adult aloe extracts in protecting normal human dermal fibroblasts from UVB-induced damage, better inhibiting MMP-1, MMP-3, and IL-6 levels. The younger shoots also contributed to increasing type I procollagen and TGF-β1 levels.[103]

CONCLUSION

For decades, the use of *A. vera* has been promoted for a seemingly limitless variety of conditions. It remains one of the most popular botanical products in mainstream usage, if not the most popular, in the US. Often patients know more than doctors about the purported benefits. Topical products that contain *A. vera* appear to be safe, but there is a scarcity of clinical evidence establishing efficacy. Aloe appears to have great potential for a wide range of medical applications. Its use in a plethora of OTC topical products, though, is likely yet another attempt by manufacturers to capitalize on deeply entrenched cultural knowledge and more casual popular awareness regarding the benefits of the aloe plant. The risks of using such products are low, but much more clinical evidence is necessary from randomized, double-blind, case-controlled studies to quantify any benefits of aloe as a primary active ingredient. Such work is clearly warranted by current findings, especially when noting the cogent evidence on natural or less dilute forms of the plant. While clinical effectiveness has not yet been sufficiently defined, promising outcomes have been seen.

REFERENCES

1. Thornfeldt C. Cosmeceuticals containing herbs: Fact, fiction, and future. *Dermatol Surg.* 2005;31:873.
2. Hoffmann D. *Medical Herbalism: The Science and Practice of Herbal Medicine.* Rochester, VT: Healing Arts Press; 2003:394.
3. Hamman JH. Composition and applications of Aloe vera leaf gel. *Molecules.* 2008;13:1599.
4. Mills S, Bone K. *Principles and Practice of Phytotherapy: Modern Herbal Medicine.* London: Churchill Livingstone; 2000:70.
5. Hoffmann D. *Medical Herbalism: The Science and Practice of Herbal Medicine.* Rochester, VT: Healing Arts Press; 2003:98.
6. Korać RR, Khambholja KM. Potential of herbs in skin protection from ultraviolet radiation. *Pharmacogn Rev.* 2011;5:164.
7. Dweck AC. Herbal medicine for the skin – their chemistry and effects on skin and mucous membranes. *Pers Care Mag.* 2002;3:19.
8. Saini M, Goyal PK, Chaudhary G. Anti-tumor activity of Aloe vera against DMBA/croton oil-induced skin papillomagenesis in Swiss albino mice. *J Environ Pathol Toxicol Oncol.* 2010;29:127.
9. Cosmetic Ingredient Review Expert Panel. Final report on the safety assessment of Aloe Andongensis Extract, Aloe Andongensis Leaf Juice, aloe Arborescens Leaf Extract, Aloe Arborescens Leaf Juice, Aloe Arborescens Leaf Protoplasts, Aloe Barbadensis Flower Extract, Aloe Barbadensis Leaf, Aloe Barbadensis Leaf Extract, Aloe Barbadensis Leaf Juice, aloe Barbadensis Leaf Polysaccharides, Aloe Barbadensis Leaf Water, Aloe Ferox Leaf Extract, Aloe Ferox Leaf Juice, and Aloe Ferox Leaf Juice Extract. *Int J Toxicol.* 2007;26(Suppl 2):1.
10. Gallagher J, Gray M. Is aloe vera effective for healing chronic wounds? *J Wound Ostomy Continence Nurs.* 2003;30:68.
11. Ahlawat KS, Khatkar BS. Processing, food applications and safety of aloe vera products: A review. *J Food Sci Technol.* 2011;48:525.
12. Dat AD, Poon F, Pham KB, et al. Aloe vera for treating acute and chronic wounds. *Cochrane Database Syst Rev.* 2012;2:CD008762.
13. Feily A, Namazi MR. Aloe vera in dermatology: A brief review. *G Ital Dermatol Venereol.* 2009;144:85.
14. Surjushe A, Vasani R, Saple DG. Aloe vera: A short review. *Indian J. Dermatol.* 2008;53:163.
15. MacKay D, Miller AL. Nutritional support for wound healing. *Altern Med Rev.* 2003;8:359.
16. Wu J. Anti-inflammatory ingredients. *J Drugs Dermatol.* 2008;7:s13.
17. Klein AD, Penneys NS. Aloe vera. *J Am Acad Dermatol.* 1988;18:714.
18. McCauley RL, Heggers JP, Robson MC. Frostbite. Methods to minimize tissue loss. *Postgrad Med.* 1990;88:67.
19. Miller MB, Koltai PJ. Treatment of experimental frostbite with pentoxifylline and aloe vera cream. *Arch Otolaryngol Head Neck Surg.* 1995;121:678.
20. Pribitkin ED, Boger G. Herbal therapy: What every facial plastic surgeon must know. *Arch Facial Plast Surg.* 2001;3:127.
21. Coopoosamy RM, Naidoo KK. A comparative study of three Aloe species used to treat skin diseases in South African rural communities. *J Altern Complement Med.* 2013;19:425.
22. Foster M, Hunter D, Samman S. Evaluation of the nutritional and metabolic effects of Aloe vera. In: Benzie IFF, Wachtel-Galor S, eds. *Biomolecular and Clinical Aspects.* 2nd ed. Boca Raton (FL): CRC Press; 2011:36-54.
23. Jones K, Hughes J, Hong M, et al. Modulation of melanogenesis by aloesin: A competitive inhibitor of tyrosinase. *Pigment Cell Res.* 2002;15:335.
24. Fowler JF Jr, Woolery-Lloyd H, Waldorf H, et al. Innovations in natural ingredients and their use in skin care. *J Drugs Dermatol.* 2010;9:S72.
25. Foster S. *An Illustrated Guide to 101 Medicinal Herbs: Their History, Use, Recommended Dosages, and Cautions.* Loveland, CO: Interweave Press, 1998:18–19.
26. Baumann LS. Aloe vera. *Skin & Allergy News.* 2003;34:32.
27. Capasso R, Laudato M, Borrelli F. Meeting report: First National Meeting on Aloe, April 20-21, 2013, Isernia, Italy. New perspectives in Aloe research: From basic science to clinical application. *Nat Prod Commun.* 2013;8:1333.
28. Marshall JM. Aloe vera gel: What is the evidence? *Pharm J.* 1990;244:360.
29. Reynolds T, Dweck AC. Aloe vera leaf gel: A review update. *J Ethnopharmacol.* 1999;68:3.
30. Davis SC, Perez R. Cosmeceuticals and natural products: Wound healing. *Clin Dermatol.* 2009;27:502.
31. Briggs C. Herbal medicine: Aloe. *Can Pharm J.* 1995;128:48.
32. Talmadge J, Chavez J, Jacobs L, et al. Fractionation of aloe vera L. inner gel, purification and molecular profiling of activity. *Int Immunopharmacol.* 2004;4:1757.
33. Lee JK, Lee MK, Yun YP. Acemannan purified from Aloe vera induces phenotypic and functional maturation of immature dendritic cells. *Int Immunopharmacol.* 2001;1:1275.
34. Hutter JA, Salman M, Stavinoha WB, et al. Antiinflammatory C-glucosyl chromone from Aloe barbadensis. *J Nat Prod.* 1996;59:541.
35. Choi SW, Son BW, Son YS, et al. The wound-healing effect of a glycoprotein fraction isolated from aloe vera. *Br J Dermatol.* 2001;145:535.
36. Goodyear-Smith F. Aloe vera – Aloe vera, Aloe barbadensis, Aloe capensis. *J Prim Health Care.* 2011;3:322.
37. Atiba A, Nishimura M, Kakinuma S, et al. Aloe vera oral administration accelerates acute radiation-delayed wound healing by stimulating transforming growth factor-β and fibroblast growth factor production. *Am J Surg.* 2011;201:809.
38. Bhalang K, Thunyakitpisal P, Rungsirisatean N. Acemannan, a polysaccharide extracted from Aloe vera, is effective in the treatment of oral aphthous ulceration. *J Altern Complement Med.* 2013;19:429.
39. Cho S, Lee S, Lee MJ, et al. Dietary Aloe vera supplementation improves facial wrinkles and elasticity and it increases the type I procollagen gene expression in human skin in vivo. *Ann Dermatol.* 2009;21:6.
40. Reuter J, Jocher A, Stump J, et al. Investigation of the anti-inflammatory potential of Aloe vera gel (97.5%) in the ultraviolet erythema test. *Skin Pharmacol Physiol.* 2008;21:106.
41. Oyelami OA, Onayemi A, Oyedeji OA, et al. Preliminary study of effectiveness of aloe vera in scabies treatment. *Phytother Res.* 2009;23:1482.
42. Syed TA, Ahmad SA, Holt AH, et al. Management of psoriasis with Aloe vera extract in a hydrophilic cream: A placebo-controlled, double-blind study. *Trop Med Int Health.* 1996;1:505.
43. Morelli V, Calmet E, Jhingade V. Alternative therapies for common dermatologic disorders, part 2. *Prim Care.* 2010;37:285.

44. Vázquez B, Avila G, Segura D, et al. Antiinflammatory activity of extracts from Aloe vera gel. *J Ethnopharmacol.* 1996;55:69.

45. Paulsen E, Korsholm L, Brandrup F. A double-blind, placebo-controlled study of a commercial Aloe vera gel in the treatment of slight to moderate psoriasis vulgaris. *J Eur Acad Dermatol Venereol.* 2005;19:326.

46. Choonhakarn C, Busaracome P, Sripanidkulchai B, et al. A prospective, randomized clinical trial comparing topical aloe vera with 0.1% triamcinolone acetonide in mild to moderate plaque psoriasis. *J Eur Acad Dermatol Venereol.* 2010;24:168.

47. Dhanabal SP, Priyanka Dwarampudi L, Muruganantham N, et al. Evaluation of the antipsoriatic activity of Aloe vera leaf extract using a mouse tail model of psoriasis. *Phytother Res.* 2012;26:617.

48. Chithra P, Sajithlal GB, Chandrakasan G. Influence of Aloe vera on collagen turnover in healing of dermal wounds in rats. *Indian J Exp Biol.* 1998;36:896.

49. Somboonwong J, Thanamittramanee S, Jariyapongskul A, et al. Therapeutic effects of Aloe vera on cutaneous microcirculation and wound healing in second degree burn model in rats. *J Med Assoc Thai.* 2000;83:417.

50. Visuthikosol V, Chowchuen B, Sukwanarat Y, et al. Effect of aloe vera gel to healing of burn wound: A clinical and histologic study. *J Med Assoc Thai.* 1995;78:403.

51. Vogler BK, Ernst E. Aloe vera: A systematic review of its clinical effectiveness. *Br J Gen Pract.* 1999;49:823.

52. Takzare N, Hosseini MJ, Hasanzadeh G, et al. Influence of Aloe vera gel on dermal wound healing process in rat. *Toxicol Mech Methods.* 2009;19:73.

53. Inpanya P, Faikrua A, Ounaroon A, et al. Effects of the blended fibroin/aloe gel film on wound healing in streptozotocin-induced diabetic rats. *Biomed Mater.* 2012;7:035008.

54. Tarameshloo M, Norouzian M, Zarein-Dolab S, et al. A comparative study of the effects of topical application of Aloe vera, thyroid hormone and silver sulfadiazine on skin wounds in Wistar rats. *Lab Animal Res.* 2012;28:17.

55. Hosseinimehr SJ, Khorasani G, Azadbakht M, et al. Effect of aloe cream versus silver sulfadiazine for healing burn wounds in rats. *Acta Dermatovenerol Croat.* 2010;18:2.

56. Cheng S, Kirtschig G, Cooper S, et al. Interventions for erosive lichen planus affecting mucosal sites. *Cochrane Database Syst Rev.* 2012;2:CD008092.

57. Patil BA, Bhaskar HP, Pol JS, et al. Aloe vera as cure for lichen planus. *N Y State Dent J.* 2013;79:65.

58. Dal'Belo SE, Gaspar LR, Maia Campos PM. Moisturizing effect of cosmetic formulations containing Aloe vera extract in different concentrations assessed by skin bioengineering techniques. *Skin Res Technol.* 2006;12:241.

59. Kim J, Lee Is, Park S, et al. Effects of Scutellariae radix and Aloe vera gel extracts on immunoglobulin E and cytokine levels in atopic dermatitis NC/Nga mice. *J Ethnopharmacol.* 2010;132:529.

60. Casetti F, Wölfle U, Gehring W, et al. Dermocosmetics for dry skin: A new role for botanical extracts. *Skin Pharmacol Physiol.* 2011;24:289.

61. Dohil MA. Natural ingredients in atopic dermatitis and other inflammatory skin disease. *J Drugs Dermatol.* 2013;12:s128.

62. West DP, Zhu YF. Evaluation of aloe vera gel gloves in the treatment of dry skin associated with occupational exposure. *Am J Infect Control.* 2003;31:40.

63. Mitchell H. Evaluation of aloe vera gel gloves in the treatment of dry skin associated with occupational exposure. *Am J Infect Control.* 2003;31:516.

64. Korniewicz DM, El Masri M. Effect of aloe-vera impregnated gloves on hand hygiene attitudes of health care workers. *Medsurg Nurs.* 2007;16:247.

65. Ford JL, Phillips P. Are aloe-coated gloves effective in healthcare? *Nurs Times.* 2007;103:40.

66. Richardson J, Smith JE, McIntyre M, et al. Aloe vera for preventing radiation-induced skin reactions: A systematic literature review. *Clin Oncol (R Coll Radiol).* 2005;17:478.

67. Wang ZW, Zhou JM, Huang ZS, et al. Aloe polysaccharides mediated radioprotective effect through the inhibition of apoptosis. *J Radiat Res.* 2004;45:447.

68. Maddocks-Jennings W, Wilkinson JM, Shillington D. Novel approaches to radiotherapy-induced skin reactions: A literature review. *Complement Ther Clin Pract.* 2005;11:224.

69. Goyal PK, Gehlot P. Radioprotective effects of Aloe vera leaf extract on Swiss albino mice against whole-body gamma irradiation. *J Environ Pathol Toxicol Oncol.* 2009;28:53.

70. Saraf S, Sahu S, Kaur CD, et al. Comparative measurement of hydration effects of herbal moisturizers. *Pharmacognosy Res.* 2010;2:146.

71. Gupta A, Upadhyay NK, Sawhney RC, et al. A poly-herbal formulation accelerates normal and impaired diabetic wound healing. *Wound Repair Regen.* 2008;16:784.

72. Mendonça FA, Passarini Junior JR, Esquisatto MA, et al. Effects of the application of Aloe vera (L.) and microcurrent on the healing of wounds surgically induced in Wistar rats. *Acta Cir Bras.* 2009;24:150.

73. Portugal-Cohen M, Soroka Y, Ma'or Z, et al. Protective effects of a cream containing Dead Sea minerals against UVB-induced stress in human skin. *Exp Dermatol.* 2009;18:781.

74. Bruce S, Watson J. Evaluation of a prescription strength 4% hydroquinone/10% L-ascorbic acid treatment system for normal to oily skin. *J Drugs Dermatol.* 2011;10:1455.

75. Panahi Y, Davoudi SM, Sahebkar A, et al. Efficacy of Aloe vera/olive oil cream versus betamethasone cream for chronic skin lesions following sulfur mustard exposure: A randomized double-blind clinical trial. *Cutan Ocul Toxicol.* 2012;31:95.

76. Puentes Sánchez J, Pardo González CM, Pardo González MB, et al. Prevention of vascular ulcers and diabetic foot. Non-randomized open clinical evaluation on the effectiveness of "Mepentol Leche." *Rev Enferm.* 2006;29:25.

77. Food and Drug Administration, HHS. Status of certain additional over-the-counter drug category II and III active ingredients. Final rule. *Fed Regist.* 2002;67:31125.

78. Ernst E. Adverse effects of herbal drugs in dermatology. *Br J Dermatol.* 2000;143:923.

79. Hunter D, Frumkin A. Adverse reactions to vitamin E and aloe vera preparations after dermabrasion and chemical peel. *Cutis.* 1991;47:193.

80. White-Chu EF, Reddy M. Dry skin in the elderly: Complexities of a common problem. *Clin Dermatol.* 2011;29:37.

81. Xia Q, Yin JJ, Fu PP, et al. Photo-irradiation of Aloe vera by UVA – formation of free radicals, singlet oxygen, superoxide, and induction of lipid peroxidation. *Toxicol Lett.* 2007;168:165.

82. Cole L, Heard C. Skin permeation enhancement potential of Aloe vera and a proposed mechanism of action based upon size exclusion and pull effect. *Int J Pharm.* 2007;333:10.

83. Bergamante V, Ceschel GC, Marazzita S, et al. Effect of vehicles on topical application of aloe vera and arnica Montana components. *Drug Deliv.* 2007;14:427.

84. Takahashi M, Kitamoto D, Asikin Y, et al. Liposomes encapsulating Aloe vera leaf gel extract significantly enhance proliferation and collagen synthesis in human skin cell lines. *J Oleo Sci.* 2009;58:643.

85. Popadic D, Savic, E, Ramic Z, et al. Aloe-emodin inhibits proliferation of adult human keratinocytes in vitro. *J Cosmet Sci.* 2012;63:297.

86. Wamer WG, Vath P, Falvey DE. In vitro studies on the photobiological properties of aloe emodin and aloin A. *Free Radic Biol Med.* 2003;34:233.

87. Vath P, Wamer WG, Falvey DE. Photochemistry and phototoxicity of aloe emodin. *Photochem Photobiol.* 2002;75:346.

88. Chou TH, Liang CH. The molecular effects of aloe-emodin (AE)/liposome-AE on human nonmelanoma skin cancer cells and skin permeation. *Chem Res Toxicol.* 2009;22:2017.

89. Vandana K, Prasanna Raju Y, Sundaresan C, et al. In-vitro assessment and pharmacodynamics of nimesulide incorporated aloe vera transemulgel. *Curr Drug Discov Technol.* 2013 Dec 2. [Epub ahead of print]

90. Yagi A, Takeo S. Anti-inflammatory constituents, aloesin and aloemannan in Aloe species and effects of tanshinon VI in Salvia miltiorrhiza on heart. *Yakugaku Zasshi.* 2003;123:517.

91. Yagi A, Kabash A, Okamura N, et al. Antioxidant, free radical scavenging and anti-inflammatory effects of aloesin derivatives in Aloe vera. *Planta Med.* 2002;68:957.

92. López A, de Tangil MS, Vega-Orellana O, et al. Phenolic constituents, antioxidant and preliminary antimycoplasmic activities of leaf skin and flowers of Aloe vera (L.) Burm. F. (syn. A. barbadensis Mill.) from the Canary Islands (Spain). *Molecules.* 2013;18:4942.

93. Wasserman L, Avigad S, Beery E, et al. The effect of aloe emodin on the proliferation of a new merkel carcinoma cell line. *Am J Dermatopathol.* 2002;24:17.

94. Pecere T, Gazzola MV, Mucignat C, et al. Aloe-emodin is a new type of anticancer agent with selective activity against neuroectodermal tumors. *Cancer Res.* 2000;60:2800.

95. Lee CK, Han SS, Mo YK, et al. Prevention of ultraviolet radiation-induced suppression of accessory cell function of Langerhans cells by Aloe vera gel components. *Immunopharmacology*. 1997;37:153.

96. Lee CK, Han SS, Shin YK, et al. Prevention of ultraviolet radiation-induced suppression of contact hypersensitivity by Aloe vera gel components. *Int J Immunopharmacol*. 1999;21:303.

97. Lissoni P, Giani L, Zerbini S, et al. Biotherapy with the pineal immunomodulating hormone melatonin versus melatonin plus aloe vera in untreatable advanced solid neoplasms. *Nat Immun*. 1998;16:27.

98. Shamaan NA, Kadir KA, Rahmat A, et al. Vitamin C and aloe vera supplementation protects from chemical hepatocarcinogenesis in the rat. *Nutrition*. 1998;14:846.

99. Chaudhary G, Saini MR, Goyal PK. Chemopreventive potential of Aloe vera against 7,12-dimethylbenz(a)anthracene induced skin papillomagenesis in mice. *Integr Cancer Ther*. 2007;6:405.

100. National Toxicology Program. Photocarcinogenesis study of aloe vera [CAS NO. 481-72-1(Aloe-emodin)] in SKH-1 mice (simulated solar light and topical application study). *Natl Toxicol Program Tech Rep Ser*. 2010;553:7.

101. Habeeb F, Stables G, Bradbury F, et al. The inner gel component of Aloe vera suppresses bacterial-induced pro-inflammatory cytokines from human immune cells. *Methods*. 2007;42:388.

102. Hall TJ, Wren MW, Jeanes A, et al. A comparison of the antibacterial efficacy and cytotoxicity to cultured human skin cells of 7 commercial hand rubs and Xgel, a new copper-based biocidal hand rub. *Am J Infect Control*. 2009;37:322.

103. Hwang E, Kim SH, Lee S, et al. A comparative study of baby immature and adult shoots of Aloe vera on UVB-induced skin photoaging in vitro. *Phytother Res*. 2013 Mar 15. [Epub ahead of print]

CHAPTER 66

Feverfew

Activities:

Anti-inflammatory, anticarcinogenic, analgesic, antiproliferative, antipyretic, antimicrobial

Important Chemical Components:

Sesquiterpene lactones (especially parthenolide), sesquiterpenes, monoterpenes (e.g., pinenes), polyacetylene compounds, essential oil (including the terpenoid camphor and chrysanthenyl acetate in both the aerial and root essential oils; bornyl acetate), flavonoids (including tanetin, quercetin, apigenin, and luteolin), coumarins (e.g., isofraxidin), and melatonin[1–4]

Origin Classification:

This ingredient is natural. Organic forms exist. There are processed formulations available using feverfew with parthenolide removed. This puts the parthenolide-removed feverfew in a category known as "Active Naturals."[5]

Personal Care Category:

Anti-inflammatory, appearance enhancing, soothing, moisturizing

Recommended for the following Baumann Skin Types:

DSNT, DSPT, DSNW, DSPW, OSNT, OSNW, OSPT, and OSPW

SOURCE

Tanacetum parthenium, an aromatic perennial herb native to the Balkan peninsula and better known as feverfew, belongs to the Asteraceae or Compositae family and has long been used in traditional medicine (Table 66-1).[6] The plant (also known by previous botanical names, including *Chrysanthemum parthenium*, *Pyrethrum parthenium*, *Matricaria pyrethrum*, and *Matricaria parthenium*)[1,4,7] is now broadly dispersed throughout the world, primarily the northern hemisphere, and is particularly prolific in Iran and Turkey.[2,3,8] The expression "feverfew" is believed to be a corruption of the word "febrifuge," derived from the Latin

TABLE 66-1
Pros and Cons of Feverfew

Pros	Cons
Long history of traditional use	May cause contact dermatitis especially in ragweed-allergic individuals
Potency and potential of its chief constituent, parthenolide, is compelling	Unknown how it reacts when exposed to other ingredients such as retinoids and skin lighteners

febris (fever) and *fugure* (to drive away) to describe the antipyretic actions of the plant.[1,2] Feverfew has long been cultivated for ornamental and medicinal purposes.[9] The term "parthenium" is derived from the ancient Greek name for the plant bestowed, according to legend, because the plant was used to save the life of a worker who had fallen from the Parthenon during its 5th century BCE construction.[6,10] Modern evidence of the anti-inflammatory properties of feverfew has been accruing over the last several decades and is now considered well established.[11]

HISTORY

For over 2,000 years, folk medicine has incorporated feverfew for internal use to regulate menstruation, assist in labor during childbirth, and treat fevers, headaches, and infertility; externally, it has been used as an analgesic.[4,6] The first century CE Greek physician Dioscorides recommended feverfew for all inflammatory conditions.[6,10] Known as *aqhovan* in Iran, the roots and rhizomes of feverfew have been used in Iranian traditional medicine to treat gastrointestinal disorders.[2] Early European herbalists also used feverfew.[9] The Kallaway people of the Andes mountains of South America have used feverfew to treat colic, stomach and kidney pain, as well as morning sickness.[4] Native Mexican peoples have, for centuries, used feverfew to treat fever, arthritis, and migraines.[12,13] The broad range of traditional medical uses of feverfew also includes therapeutic applications for allergies, arthritis, asthma, coughs and colds, constipation, depression, dermatitis, earache, edema, infant colic, inflammatory conditions, insect bites, kidney stones, labor, potential miscarriage, nausea and vomiting, psoriasis, skin wounds, spasms, tinnitus, toothache, vertigo, and worms.[4,5,9,14] Nonmedical applications have included cosmetics, balsams, dyes, preservatives, and insecticides.[3] Feverfew gained more modern, nontraditional adherents in the late 1970s and 1980s, with several reports suggesting its effectiveness as an oral agent in preventing migraine headaches.[4,15,16]

CHEMISTRY

Feverfew, vitamin E, coenzyme Q_{10}, and turmeric are among the antioxidants found in the lipophilic portion of the cell membrane [see Chapter 56, Tocopherol (Vitamin E), Chapter 57, Coenzyme Q_{10}, and Chapter 69, Turmeric]. Other fat-soluble antioxidants include carotenoids (e.g., lycopene) and idebenone, the synthetic analog of coenzyme Q_{10} (see Chapter 61, Idebenone).

T. parthenium is known to suppress the release of proinflammatory mediators from macrophages and lymphocytes.[17] In a Medline literature review of herbal agents that many people take but that might warrant discontinuing before dermatologic surgery, authors cited feverfew for its known success as a treatment for migraines,[15] and arthritis as well as its anti-inflammatory activity in blocking phospholipase breakdown of arachidonic acid into prostaglandins and leukotrienes.[18,19] They noted that platelet aggregation is also induced by the feverfew extract parthenolide and a byproduct of the arachidonic acid cascade, thromboxane A$_2$.[18,20,21]

Many of the anti-inflammatory, antioxidant, and antiproliferative characteristics of feverfew are ascribed to its primary constituent parthenolide, a hydroalcoholic extract of the aerial parts of the plant known to inhibit nuclear factor-κB (NF-κB), which contributes to anti-inflammatory activity, and to exhibit exceptional anticancer and antiproliferative properties.[11,12,14,22] In fact, the sesquiterpene lactone parthenolide (within the subclass germacranolides)[23] is the first small molecule discovered to act selectively against cancer stem cells.[5] Notably, parthenolide, which is not present in all varieties of feverfew, is thought to account for the antimigraine activity of the herb.[6] In 2011, Majdi et al. discovered that glandular trichomes of *T. parthenium* are the secretory tissues where the production and accumulation of parthenolide occur.[24] Parthenolide can be very irritating when applied topically; therefore, manufacturers have marketed topical preparations with the parthenolide component removed from the molecule. Feverfew imparts numerous benefits that are not derived from parthenolide. The strong antioxidant melatonin is also found in feverfew.[7,25] In addition, the lipophilic flavonoid tanetin, present in feverfew leaves, flowers, and seeds, has been found to inhibit prostaglandin production.[4,26,27]

Investigations of parthenolide do represent a significant portion of research into feverfew, though. In 2008, Parada-Turska et al. conducted an *in vitro* study of the effects of parthenolide on the proliferation of the rabbit synoviocytes cell line HIG-82, rheumatoid arthritis fibroblast-like synoviocytes, and human skin fibroblasts. They found that parthenolide suppressed the proliferation of HIG-82 as well as the rheumatoid arthritis fibroblast-like synoviocytes, with human skin fibroblasts inhibited but less effectively. The researchers concluded that their findings highlighted the antiproliferative potential of parthenolide, particularly in relation to rheumatoid arthritis.[28]

ORAL USES

Oral uses of feverfew have included infusions to treat arthritis, fever, migraine headaches, and stomach aches.[29] The fresh leaves can be chewed fresh, freeze-dried- or dried, and supplements containing the dried leaves are available in capsule, tablet, or liquid extract form in Europe and the United States.[4,10]

In 1999, Jain and Kulkarni demonstrated that orally administered feverfew extract dose-dependently exerted significant antinociceptive and anti-inflammatory activity against acetic acid-induced writhing in mice and carageenan-induced paw edema in rats.[9]

An orally bioavailable analog of parthenolide, dimethylaminoparthenolide (DMAPT), has been developed as a result of structure–activity relationship studies of the feverfew constituent, and may have implications pertaining to the antiproliferative properties of the compound, particularly for patients with leukemia.[5]

Headache Treatment

Cady et al. conducted a one-month, multicenter, double-blind, placebo-controlled pilot study with 60 subjects in 2011, finding that a sublingual feverfew and ginger preparation (LipiGesic™ M) was safe and effective as a first-line therapy for patients who typically experience a mild headache before the onset of a moderate-to-severe migraine (see Chapter 59, Ginger).[30] De Weerdt et al. performed a randomized, double-blind, placebo-controlled crossover trial in 1996 based on the encouraging results of two studies in the 1980s, but their results indicated that feverfew did not exert a significant prophylactic effect against migraines.[31]

In 2012, a randomized study of 69 female volunteers was conducted by Ferro et al. to examine the efficacy and tolerability of acupuncture, *T. parthenium*, or a combination for the treatment of chronic migraines. Twenty-two patients received acupuncture in 20 sessions over 10 weeks; 23 patients received 150 mg/day of feverfew; and 23 patients received combination therapy. Using the Short-Form 36 quality of life assessment score, Migraine Disability Assessment, and a visual analog scale, the investigators determined that acupuncture along with *T. parthenium* was substantially more effective than either therapy alone, with statistically significant differences in yielding a greater analgesic effect and improved quality of life.[32]

However, Loder et al. reviewed the American Headache Society and the American Academy of Neurology 2012 updated treatment guideline recommendations along with a systematic Medline search, including recent guidelines for migraine prevention from the Canadian Headache Society and the European Federation of Neurological Societies, and found significant differences of opinion regarding the use of feverfew for migraines.[33] Goodyear-Smith contends that, at present, there is insufficient data from five randomized, double-blind trials on migraine headaches and one on rheumatoid arthritis to support the use of feverfew to prevent migraines or treat rheumatoid arthritis.[34] Triptans remain the "gold standard" for first-line migraine therapy, according to Cady et al.[30]

TOPICAL USES

Topically applied feverfew is thought to improve the appearance of the skin.[35] It is included in moisturizing agents to impart a calming, soothing effect. A parthenolide-free formulation has recently been studied for treatment of acne and rosacea, with some indications of efficacy.[36,37] In fact, parthenolide-free Feverfew PFE™ is a nonsteroidal anti-inflammatory topical product found to suppress multiple pathways related to skin irritation.[38]

SAFETY ISSUES

The Compositae family (ragweed is an example) is known to cause contact dermatitis in susceptible individuals, and Compositae allergy is among the top ten contact sensitivities in Europe. Sesquiterpene lactones are considered to be the primary sensitizing constituents in these plants.[39] Nevertheless, feverfew is considered safe, with reactions typically mild to moderate and manifested by those with Compositae allergy. Indeed, feverfew has long been acknowledged as a key sensitizer in European Compositae-allergic patients due to parthenolide, which is known as a potent skin sensitizer.[16,40] In 2007, there was a report of two patients experiencing contact dermatitis from using a topical moisturizer containing feverfew.[41] Such reactions prompted the development of parthenolide-depleted formulations even though adverse reactions to feverfew are considered to be minimal and rare.

Sensitivity to parthenolide-depleted agents remains possible, nevertheless. In a small study with seven patients conducted in 2010, Paulsen et al. used patch tests to examine the tolerance of individuals with known contact allergy to topical parthenolide-depleted feverfew formulations. Subjects were patch tested with two parthenolide-depleted creams. The researchers noted that four patients tested positive to one of the agents and reactivity was linked to simultaneous positive response to parthenolide. Two years later, Paulsen and colleagues analyzed the cream, finding no parthenolide, which they ascribed to degradation of the compound.[40]

When feverfew is ingested orally for migraines, oral ulcers have been reported.[34] Use of feverfew may increase the risk of bleeding during surgical procedures.[42] Similarly, feverfew may elevate such risk for patients using warfarin or aspirin.[34] Feverfew is contraindicated in pregnant women as it acts as an emmenagogue.

ENVIRONMENTAL IMPACT

Feverfew is one of several wild medicinal plants in the Concord area of New England that have undergone accelerated flowering times due to climate change.[43]

Fonseca et al. have shown that changing environmental conditions immediately before harvest affects secondary metabolites in feverfew, with parthenolide yields higher with light and reduced water and phenolic yields higher with water and little light. They suggest that the controlled environment of a greenhouse might be the ideal setting for harnessing the optimal phytochemicals from *T. parthenium*.[27,44]

Parthenolide content in feverfew plants is recognized as high in France and Germany, but the plants in Serbia, the US, and Mexico almost completely lack parthenolide.[45] Beyond regional and geographical differences, the parthenolide content of feverfew can also be influenced by processing and extraction methods (including drying temperature and extraction solvent used).[45–47]

FORMULATION CONSIDERATIONS

Researchers have developed a form of feverfew with the parthenolide portion removed, rendering it safer as a topical ingredient.

In vitro and *in vivo* antioxidant efficacy of a parthenolide-depleted feverfew extract (PD-Feverfew) was reported by Martin et al. in 2008. The extract restored cigarette smoke-mediated depletion of cellular thiols, diminished the formation of ultraviolet (UV)-induced hydrogen peroxide, and hindered proinflammatory cytokine release *in vitro*, manifesting greater radical scavenging-potency than vitamin C. In addition, the topical formulation reduced UV-induced epidermal hyperplasia, DNA damage, and apoptosis *in vivo*. Phototoxicity and photoallergy tests for the formulation were consistently negative, and clinical tolerance testing in over 1,200 individuals showed that formulations containing PD-Feverfew did not elicit allergic reactions. The researchers also reported that a clinical study (randomized, placebo-controlled, double-blinded with 12 females and males, Fitzpatrick types II and III) revealed that treatment significantly mitigated UVB-induced erythema as compared to placebo 24 hours after exposure. They concluded that their parthenolide-depleted feverfew formulation protects the skin from exogenous oxidizing factors.[48]

In 2009, some of the same investigators assessed the anti-inflammatory capacity of the parthenolide-depleted feverfew extract that they developed. *In vitro*, the extract hindered the activity of several proinflammatory enzymes (i.e., 5-lipoxygenase, phosphodiesterase-3, and phosphodiesterase-4) as well as the release of proinflammatory mediators. *In vivo*, the extract thwarted oxazolone-induced dermatitis and was more effective than regular feverfew in treating 12-*O*-tetradecanoylphorbol-13-acetate-induced dermatitis. In a clinical assessment, the investigators found that their extract diminished erythema in a methyl nicotinate-induced vasodilation model. They concluded that PD-Feverfew exhibits strong anti-inflammatory activity but without the accompanying sensitizing activity characteristic of whole feverfew.[16]

In a three-week screening study in 2007, Jin et al. found that parthenolide is comparatively stable when the environmental pH is in the range of 5 to 7, and is unstable when the pH is less than 3 or above 7. They also found that it is compatible with frequently used excipients under stressed conditions. Further, they noted that parthenolide degradation in feverfew solution seems to be a typical first-order reaction but its degradation in the solid state fits no obvious reaction model. The degradation rate was found to be highly influenced by moisture content and temperature, with an increase from 18 percent to 32 percent degradation of parthenolide after six months of storage under 40°C at a relative humidity of 75 percent.[45]

The following year, the same researchers evaluated the flowability, hygroscopicity, compressibility, and compactibility of multiple commercial feverfew extracts, and ascertained the parthenolide content of the formulations. They found poor to very poor flowability, and highly variable hygroscopicity and compactibility among the products, with no tested products actually containing the parthenolide quantity as claimed by the labels. Parthenolide content varied even in different batches from the same manufacturers. The investigators suggested that proper quality controls are necessary for manufacturers, who should also be cognizant of inconsistent physicochemical characteristics in the feverfew provided by myriad suppliers.[49]

USAGE CONSIDERATIONS

Stability studies of feverfew products have not yet appeared in the literature.[45] It is unknown how feverfew is affected by interaction with other ingredients. Feverfew should not be used in patients with a known ragweed allergy.

SIGNIFICANT BACKGROUND

Feverfew is known to provide a broad range of biologic activity with or without its primary constituent parthenolide. The anti-inflammatory activity of feverfew is thought by some to be more potent than that of *Aloe vera*, *Camellia sinensis*, licorice extract, and other Asteraceae family members such as chamomile and echinacea (see Chapter 47, Green Tea, Chapter 65, Aloe Vera, Chapter 67, Licorice Extract, and Chapter 70, Chamomile).[50,51]

In 2013, Rodriguez et al. assessed the influence of a purified parthenolide-depleted feverfew extract on the nuclear factor erythroid 2-related factor-2 (Nrf2)/antioxidant response element (ARE) pathway and DNA repair in primary human keratinocytes or KB cells (subline of the keratin-forming tumor cell line HeLa). The investigators observed that the feverfew extract induced Nrf2 nuclear translocation and dose-dependently augmented ARE activity. Activation of this pathway is known to restore cutaneous oxidative homeostasis. The findings of this experiment led the authors to conclude that the parthenolide-depleted feverfew extract promoted skin cell DNA repair through a phosphoinositide (PI)3-kinase-dependent Nrf2/ARE pathway and may contribute to protection against environmental insult.[52]

Antibacterial Activity

Polatoglu et al. examined the water-distilled essential oils of *T. parthenium* from two different regions in Turkey in 2010. Camphor was a key ingredient in samples collected from the Davutpasa-Istanbul area as well as the remote eastern part (Savşat-Ardahan region) of the country. Camphene and *trans*-chrysanthenyl acetate were also found in the Istanbul samples; camphene was identified in the eastern sample. The oil of the Istanbul sample evinced mild antibacterial activity against *Bacillus subtilis* and methicillin-resistant *Staphylococcus aureus*. Similarly, the eastern sample demonstrated mild activity against *S. aureus*. Both oils demonstrated toxicity against *Vibrio fischeri*.[8]

In 2011, Mohsenzadeh et al. examined the components of the hydrodistilled essential oils of preflowering, flowering, and postflowering *T. parthenium* from western Iran, identifying camphor and bornyl acetate as prevalent among 29 components. They also found that the essential oils displayed appreciable activity against four Gram-positive and four Gram-negative bacteria without significant toxicity, with the antibacterial properties strongest during the flowering stage. They concluded that their findings suggest the viability of *T. parthenium* essential oil as a natural health product.[3]

Parthenolide, Skin Cancer, and Photoaging

Parthenolide has been consistently shown to exhibit *in vitro* antitumor activity.[53] In 2004, Won et al. conducted *in vitro* and *in vivo* investigations of the cancer chemopreventive potential of parthenolide using a UVB-induced skin cancer model, revealing that SKH-1 hairless mice given parthenolide exhibited later onset of papilloma, significantly fewer papillomas/mouse, and smaller lesions in comparison to mice exposed only to UVB but not fed the primary component of feverfew. The *in vitro* phase of the study, using cultured JB6 murine epidermal cells, showed that noncytotoxic concentrations of parthenolide pretreatment significantly suppressed UVB-induced activator protein-1 DNA binding and transcriptional activity as well as c-Jun-N-terminal kinase (JNK) and p38 kinase signaling activation, all of which might be crucial in the anticancer mechanism of action of parthenolide, according to the authors.[11] Three of the same investigators have also noted that parthenolide sensitizes UVB-induced apoptosis through pathways that depend on protein kinase C.[54] Further, parthenolide has been found to reduce the number of viable adherent cells in melanoma cultures.[55]

The primary constituent of feverfew has become known as an NF-κB inhibitor. In a 2005 study, parthenolide effectively blocked the gene expression mediated by NF-κB and the synthesis of basic fibroblast growth factor (bFGF) and matrix metalloproteinase-1 as well as the UVB-induced proliferation of keratinocytes and melanocytes in mouse skin, leading the authors to conclude that NF-κB inhibitors, especially parthenolide, may have a role in preventing photoaging.[56] This conclusion has since been reinforced.[57]

In 2010, Tanaka et al. found that the NF-κB inhibitors parthenolide and magnolol can effectively block NF-κB-mediated gene expression as well as UVB-induced proliferation of keratinocytes and melanocytes in murine skin, suggesting that both compounds may play a role in preventing photoaging.[57]

Also that year, Lesiak et al. studied the anticancer effects of parthenolide in melanoma cells *in vitro*, in melanoma cell lines and melanocytes, as well as melanoma cells obtained from a surgical excision, finding that the herbal compound decreased the number of viable adherent cells in melanoma cultures. The researchers also noted that preincubation of parthenolide with the thiol nucleophile N-acetyl-cysteine shielded melanoma cells from parthenolide-induced cell death, implying, as they interpreted, that the mechanism attributable to parthenolide activity is the reaction with intracellular thiols. They concluded that the apparent anticancer activity of parthenolide warrants further evaluation for melanoma therapy.[55] Parthenolide has

demonstrated potential activity *in vitro* against several other cancer types, including acute myelogenous leukemia, breast cancer, cholangiocarcinoma, and pancreatic adenocarcinoma, as well as *in vivo* in an adjuvant breast cancer metastasis model.[53,58–60]

Mathema et al. reported in 2012 that parthenolide exhibits potent NF-κB and signal transduction and activation of transcription (STAT)-mediated transcriptional inhibition of proapoptotic genes. They also suggested that the unique capacity of parthenolide to spare normal cells while provoking sensitization to extrinsic and intrinsic apoptosis signaling in cancer cells renders the compound primed for use in treating cancer and disorders involving inflammation.[22] Koprowska and Czyz have added that parthenolide also protects normal cells from UVB and oxidative stress and appears to have the potential to target some cancer stem cells. In addition, they asserted that the low toxicity and diverse biological activity of parthenolide position the sesquiterpene lactone as a promising agent with potentially vast pharmacologic applications.[29]

Other Potential Applications of Parthenolide

In addition to its potential activity against skin cancer and photoaging, the feverfew constituent parthenolide confers other benefits pertinent to dermatology. In 2005, investigators identified potent intracellular antioxidant activity displayed by parthenolide in hippocampal HT22 cells, properties that are mediated by an increase of glutathione but not found to mediate the sesquiterpene lactone's antiproliferative activities or its inhibition of NF-κB.[12] Parthenolide has also shown marked leishmanicidal activities suitable enough, according to researchers, to be considered for inclusion in the development of new drugs to treat this disease.[14] While several *in vitro* studies have indicated that parthenolide delivers anti-inflammatory effects, a recent *in vivo* study with mice demonstrated that the sesquiterpene lactone component of feverfew modestly suppressed only one gene, interleukin-6 after lipopolysaccharide-induced increases.[61] The authors concluded that more study of the effects of parthenolide and other herbal constituents on inflammatory gene expression using animal models is needed to assess the efficacy of various supplements.[61]

Parthenolide was found, in 2006, to display significant activity in suppressing hepatitis C virus (HCV), which is often a precursor to cirrhosis and hepatocellular carcinoma.[62] In addition, parthenolide has also been found to enhance in hepatoma cells the apoptosis induced by fenretinide (N-4-hydroxyphenyl retinamide, 4HPR), a synthetic anticancer retinoid and established apoptosis-inducing agent. In a study focusing on the relationship of these two compounds, parthenolide was found to up- or downregulate 35 apoptosis-related genes and its role as an adjuvant anticancer agent against hepatoma was elucidated.[63]

It is worth noting that while parthenolide has been cited as the main active ingredient in feverfew, a double-blind study revealed that it could not be the only active ingredient, and that melatonin is an antioxidant component of the plant, though its role in feverfew potency is not clearly understood.[7,31]

■ CONCLUSION

Feverfew is best known as an effective herbal alternative for treating migraine headaches. New evidence is emerging that numerous other health benefits might be derived from this plant, and particularly its chief component parthenolide. The findings regarding anticarcinogenic and anti-inflammatory capacity are promising and may soon have dermatologic implications. Cancer clinical trials using parthenolide are ongoing.

Feverfew contains parthenolide and melatonin, both of which exhibit antioxidant activity. *T. parthenium* formulations must be developed to account for the allergenic potential of parthenolide while still harnessing its strong ameliorative properties. Notably, recent success has been observed with parthenolide-depleted feverfew. It remains unclear what role melatonin plays in such formulations. The ability to take a naturally occurring ingredient and improve it by removing an undesirable part of the chemical structure appears to be an integral part of the future of "natural" skin care. While more research is needed, particularly randomized, controlled trials, cutaneous applications of feverfew are likely to proliferate.

REFERENCES

1. Mills S, Bone K. *Principles and Practice of Phytotherapy*. London: Churchill Livingstone; 2000:385–393.
2. Mojab F, Tabatabai SA, Naghdi-Badi H, et al. Essential oil of the root of Tanacetum parthenium (L.) Schulz. Bip. (Asteraceae) from Iran. *Iran J Pharm Res*. 2007;6:291.
3. Mohsenzadeh F, Chehregani A, Amiri H. Chemical composition, antibacterial activity and cytotoxicity of essential oils of Tanacetum parthenium in different developmental stages. *Pharm Biol*. 2011;49:920.
4. Pareek A, Suthar M, Rathore GS, et al. Feverfew (Tanacetum parthenium L.): A systematic review. *Pharmacogn Rev*. 2011;5:103.
5. Ghantous A, Sinjab A, Herceg Z, et al. Parthenolide: From plant shoots to cancer roots. *Drug Discov Today*. 2013;18:894.
6. Foster S. *An Illustrated Guide to 101 Medicinal Herbs: Their History, Use, Recommended Dosages, and Cautions*. Loveland, CO: Interweave Press; 1998:86–87.
7. Murch SJ, Simmons CB, Saxena PK. Melatonin in feverfew and other medicinal plants. *Lancet*. 1997;350:1598.
8. Polatoglu K, Demirci F, Demirci B, et al. Antibacterial activity and the variation of Tanacetum parthenium (L.) Schultz Bip. Essential oils from Turkey. *J Oleo Sci*. 2010;59:177.
9. Jain NK, Kulkarni SK. Antinociceptive and anti-inflammatory effects of Tanacetum parthenium L. extract in mice and rats. *J Ethnopharmacol*. 1999;68:251.
10. Setty AR, Sigal LH. Herbal medications commonly used in the practice of rheumatology: Mechanisms of action, efficacy, and side effects. *Semin Arthritis Rheum*. 2005;34:773.
11. Won YK, Ong CN, Shi X, et al. Chemopreventive activity of parthenolide against UVB-induced skin cancer and its mechanisms. *Carcinogenesis*. 2004;25:1449.
12. Herrera F, Martin V, Rodriguez-Blanco J, et al. Intracellular redox state regulation by parthenolide. *Biochem Biophys Res Commun*. 2005;332:321.
13. Heinrich M, Robles M, West JE, et al. Ethnopharmacology of Mexican asteraceae (Compositae). *Annu Rev Pharmacol Toxicol*. 1998;38:539.
14. Tiuman TS, Ueda-Nakamura T, Garcia Cortez DA, et al. Antileishmanial activity of parthenolide, a sesquiterpene lactone isolated from Tanacetum parthenium. *Antimicrob Agents Chemother*. 2005;49:176.
15. Johnson ES, Kadam NP, Hylands DM, et al. Efficacy of feverfew as prophylactic treatment of migraine. *Br Med J (Clin Res Ed)*. 1985;291:569.
16. Sur R, Martin K, Liebel F, et al. Anti-inflammatory activity of parthenolide-depleted Feverfew (Tanacetum parthenium). *Inflammopharmacology*. 2009;17:42.
17. Amirghofran Z. Herbal medicines for immunosuppression. *Iran J Allergy Asthma Immunol*. 2012;11:111.
18. Chang LK, Whitaker DC. The impact of herbal medicines on dermatologic surgery. *Dermatol Surg*. 2001;27:759.
19. Makheja AN, Bailey JM. A platelet phospholipase inhibitor from the medicinal herb feverfew (Tanacetum parthenium). *Prostaglandins Leukot Med*. 1982;8:653.
20. Groenewegen WA, Heptinstall S. A comparison of the effects of an extract of feverfew and parthenolide, a component of feverfew, on human platelet activity in-vitro. *J Pharm Pharmacol*. 1990;42:553.
21. Heptinstall S, Groenewegen WA, Spangenberg P, et al. Extracts of feverfew may inhibit platelet behaviour via neutralization of sulphydryl groups. *J Pharm Pharmacol*. 1987;39:459.
22. Mathema VB, Koh YS, Thakuri BC, et al. Parthenolide, a sesquiterpene lactone, expresses multiple anti-cancer and anti-inflammatory activities. *Inflammation*. 2012;35:560.
23. Kreuger MR, Grootjans S, Biavatti MW, et al. Sesquiterpene lactones as drugs with multiple targets in cancer treatment: Focus on parthenolide. *Anticancer Drugs*. 2012;23:883.
24. Majdi M, Liu Q, Karimzadeh G, et al. Biosynthesis and localization of parthenolide in glandular trichomes of feverfew (Tanacetum parthenium L. Schulz Bip.). *Phytochemistry*. 2011;72:1739.
25. Taylor FR. Nutraceuticals and headache: The biological basis. *Headache*. 2011;51:484.
26. Williams CA, Hoult JR, Harborne JB, et al. A biologically active lipophilic flavonol from Tanacetum parthenium. *Phytochemistry*. 1995;38:267.
27. Fonseca JM, Rushing JW, Rajapakse NC, et al. Phenolics and parthenolide levels in feverfew (Tanacetum parthenium) are inversely affected by environmental factors. *J Appl Hort*. 2008;10:36.
28. Parada-Turska J, Mitura A, Brzana W, et al. Parthenolide inhibits proliferation of fibroblast-like synoviocytes in vitro. *Inflammation*. 2008;31:281.
29. Koprowska K, Czyz M. Molecular mechanisms of parthenolide's action: Old drug with a new face. *Postepy Hig Med Dosw (Online)*. 2010;64:100.
30. Cady RK, Goldstein J, Nett R, et al. A double-blind placebo-controlled pilot study of sublingual feverfew and ginger (LipiGesic™ M) in the treatment of migraine. *Headache*. 2011;51:1078.
31. De Weerdt CJ, Bootsma HPR, Hendricks H. Herbal medicines in migraine prevention. *Phytomedicine*. 1996;3:225.
32. Ferro EC, Biagini AP, da Silva ÍE, et al. The combined effect of acupuncture and Tanacetum parthenium on quality of life in women with headache: Randomised study. *Acupunct Med*. 2012;30:252.
33. Loder E, Burch R, Rizzoli P. The 2012 AHS/AAN guidelines for prevention of episodic migraine: A summary and comparison with other recent clinical practice guidelines. *Headache*. 2012;52:930.
34. Goodyear-Smith F. Feverfew. Bachelor's buttons, Featherfew (Tanacetum parthenium L, aka Chrysanthemum parthenium L. aka Pyrethrum parthenium L.). *J Prim Health Care*. 2010;2:337.
35. Bowe WP. Cosmetic benefits of natural ingredients: Mushrooms, feverfew, tea, and wheat complex. *J Drugs Dermatol*. 2013;12:s133.
36. Fowler JF Jr, Woolery-Lloyd H, Waldorf H, et al. Innovations in natural ingredients and their use in skin care. *J Drugs Dermatol*. 2010;9:S72.
37. Wu J. Treatment of rosacea with herbal ingredients. *J Drugs Dermatol*. 2006;5:29.
38. Baumann L, Woolery-Lloyd H, Friedman A. "Natural" ingredients in cosmetic dermatology. *J Drugs Dermatol*. 2009;8:s5.
39. Jovanović M, Poljacki M. Compositae dermatitis. *Med Pregl*. 2003;56:43.
40. Paulsen E, Christensen LP, Fretté XC, et al. Patch test reactivity to feverfew-containing creams in feverfew-allergic patients. *Contact Dermatitis*. 2010;63:146.
41. Killoran CE, Crawford GH, Pedvis-Leftick A. Two cases of compositae dermatitis exacerbated by moisturizer containing feverfew. *Dermatitis*. 2007;18:225.
42. Pribitkin ED, Boger G. Herbal therapy: What every facial plastic surgeon must know. *Arch Facial Plast Surg*. 2001;3:127.
43. Cavaliere C. The effects of climate change on medicinal and aromatic plants. *HerbalGram*. 2008;81:44–57. http://cms.herbalgram .org/herbalgram/issue81/article3379.html?Issue=81&ts=1392558958&signature=9f349be3405f938bf4d897301c9e6934. Accessed February 16, 2014.
44. Fonseca JM, Rushing JW, Rajapakse NC, et al. Potential implications of medicinal plant production in controlled environments: The case of feverfew (Tanacetum parthenium). *HortScience*. 2006;41:531.
45. Jin P, Madieh S, Augsburger LL. The solution and solid state stability and excipient compatibility of parthenolide in feverfew. *AAPS PharmSciTech*. 2007;8:E105.
46. Rushing JW, Hassell RL, Dufault RJ. Drying temperature and developmental stage at harvest influence the parthenolide content of feverfew leaves and stems. *Acta Hort*. 2004;629:167.
47. Kaplan M, Simmonds MR, Davidson G. Comparison of supercritical fluid and solvent extraction of feverfew (Tanacetum parthenium). *Turk J Chem*. 2002;26:473.

48. Martin K, Sur R, Liebel F, et al. Parthenolide-depleted Feverfew (Tanacetum parthenium) protects skin from UV irradiation and external aggression. *Arch Dermatol Res.* 2008;300:69.

49. Jin P, Madieh S, Augsburger LL. Selected physical and chemical properties of feverfew (Tanacetum parthenium) extracts important for formulated product quality and performance. *AAPS PharmSciTech.* 2008;9:22.

50. Reszko AE, Berson D, Lupo MP. Cosmeceuticals: Practical applications. *Dermatol Clin.* 2009;27:401.

51. Wu J. Anti-inflammatory ingredients. *J Drugs Dermatol.* 2008;7:s13.

52. Rodriguez KJ, Wong HK, Oddos T, et al. A purified feverfew extract protects from oxidative damage by inducing DNA repair in skin cells via a PI3-kinase-dependent Nrf2/ARE pathway. *J Dermatol Sci.* 2013;72:304.

53. Sweeney CJ, Mehrotra S, Sadaria MR, et al. The sesquiterpene lactone parthenolide in combination with docetaxel reduces metastasis and improves survival in a xenograft model of breast cancer. *Mol Cancer Ther.* 2005;4:1004.

54. Won YK, Ong CN, Shen HM. Parthenolide sensitizes ultraviolet (UV)-B-induced apoptosis via protein kinase C-dependent pathways. *Carcinogenesis.* 2005;26:2149.

55. Lesiak K, Koprowska K, Zalesna I, et al. Parthenolide, a sesquiterpene lactone from the medical herb feverfew, shows anticancer activity against human melanoma cells in vitro. *Melanoma Res.* 2010;20:21.

56. Tanaka K, Hasegawa J, Asamitsu K, et al. Prevention of the ultraviolet B-mediated skin photoaging by a nuclear factor kappaB inhibitor, parthenolide. *J Pharmacol Exp Ther.* 2005;315:624.

57. Tanaka K, Asamitsu K, Uranishi H, et al. Protecting skin photoaging by NF-kappaB inhibitor. *Curr Drug Metab.* 2010;11:431.

58. Guzman ML, Jordan CT. Feverfew: Weeding out the root of leukaemia. *Expert Opin Biol Ther.* 2005;5:1147.

59. Kim JH, Liu L, Lee SO, et al. Susceptibility of cholangiocarcinoma cells to parthenolide-induced apoptosis. *Cancer Res.* 2005;65:6312.

60. Yip-Schneider MT, Nakshatri H, Sweeney CJ, et al. Parthenolide and sulindac cooperate to mediate growth suppression and inhibit the nuclear factor-kappa B pathway in pancreatic carcinoma cells. *Mol Cancer Ther.* 2005;4:587.

61. Smolinski AT, Pestka JJ. Comparative effects of the herbal constituent parthenolide (Feverfew) on lipopolysaccharide-induced inflammatory gene expression in murine spleen and liver. *J Inflamm (Lond).* 2005;2:6.

62. Hwang DR, Wu YS, Chang CW, et al. Synthesis and anti-viral activity of a series of sesquiterpene lactones and analogs in the subgenomic HCV replicon system. *Bioorg Med Chem.* 2006;14:83.

63. Park JH, Liu L, Kim IH, et al. Identification of the genes involved in enhanced fenretinide-induced apoptosis by parthenolide in human hepatoma cells. *Cancer Res.* 2005;65:2804.

CHAPTER 67

Licorice Extract

Activities:

Anti-inflammatory, antioxidant, antimicrobial, antitumor, antispasmodic, antiviral, immunomodulatory[1–3]

Important Chemical Components:

Glycyrrhiza glabra: glycyrrhizin, also known as glycyrrhizic acid or glycyrrhizinic acid (a triterpenoid saponin glycoside), 18β-glycyrrhetinic acid, polysaccharides, and various polyphenols (such as the isoflavone formononetin and the prenylated isoflavonoid glabridin as well as liquiritin, isoliquiritin, isoliquiritigenin, and liquiritigenin)[4,5]
Glycyrrhiza inflata: phenols, namely licochalcone A, licochalcone B, licochalcone C, licochalcone D, licochalcone E, echinatin, and isoliquiritigenin[5,6]
Glycyrrhiza uralensis: phenylflavonoids, such as dehydroglyasperin C, dehydroglyasperin D, isoangustone A; glycyrrhetinic acid; and the benzofuran courmarin glycyrol[7]

Origin Classification:

This ingredient is natural. Many organic choices exist.

Personal Care Category:

Anti-inflammatory, antiaging, skin lightening

Recommended for the following Baumann Skin Types:

DSNT, DSPT, DSNT, DSNW, OSNT, OSNW, OSPT, and OSPW. This ingredient is an optimal choice for sensitive pigmented types.

SOURCE

Licorice (also spelled as "liquorice") is best known in its popular confectionery form of black or red candy. Although it is not often thought of as a plant, it is derived from the roots and rhizomes of multiple Glycyrrhiza species and has been used in systemic and topical herbal medications for approximately 4,000 years (Table 67-1). In fact, licorice is one of the oldest and most popular herbs used in traditional Chinese medicine (TCM), second only to ginseng.[8–10] Members of the Fabaceae or Leguminosae family (better known as the legume, pea, or bean family), *Glycyrrhiza glabra* (also known as *Liquiritiae officinalis*)

TABLE 67-1
Pros and Cons of Licorice Extract

Pros	Cons
Long history of traditional medical applications	Several contraindications for oral use, particularly chronic oral use
Multiple bioactive ingredients in several species	More data needed regarding use in patients with rosacea
Favorable safety record	

and *G. inflata* are the species that have displayed the most therapeutic actions among the 18 known Glycyrrhiza species, with *G. glabra* the most used since antiquity. *G. inflata* is actually the Chinese licorice root, while *G. glabra* grows around the Mediterranean Sea, the Middle East, and central and southern Russia.[11] The Roman physician of Greek extraction Pedanius Dioscorides, who practiced in the 1st century CE, is credited with bestowing the botanical name of the plant based on the Greek *glukos* (sweet) and *riza* (root).[7,12,13] The Latin name "Liquiritiae" is a corruption of the Greek "Glycyrrhiza."[12]

G. glabra is a perennial herb that originated on the land surrounding the Mediterranean Sea as well as central and southern Russia and the Middle East.[11] Licorice is now cultivated throughout much of Asia, Europe, and the Middle East, though, and is also used globally as a pharmacologic agent,[14] particularly as an effective anti-inflammatory product.[15] In addition to anti-inflammatory potency, licorice root is believed to possess antiviral, antiulcer, and anticarcinogenic properties.[10] In China, licorice root has served as a folk elixir and antidote, and long been used as a demulcent (an agent that provides a soothing film over a mucous membrane).[11] One of its active components, glycyrrhetinic acid, has traditionally been used in Asian and European herbal medicine to treat skin and pulmonary diseases, hepatitis, and peptic ulcers.[2,16,17] A panel from the University of Würzburg, the World Wildlife Fund, and TRAFFIC chose licorice (*G. glabra*) as "medicinal plant of the year" for 2012 in recognition of its important roles in human health.[18]

HISTORY

Licorice has been used for medicinal and dietary purposes for thousands of years, with such use dating back to ancient Egypt, Greece, and Rome in the West and to the times of the Han Dynasty (300–200 BCE) in ancient China.[3] Asthma, dry cough, and lung disorders were described by the Roman naturalist Theophrastus (circa 372–287 BCE) as indications for licorice root.[12,19] Gastric ulcer and various forms of inflammation have also been targets of licorice root in traditional medicine.[6]

The radices of *G. uralensis* and herbal preparations containing Glycyrrhiza spp. have been used for thousands of years as an herbal medicine for the treatment of viral-induced cough, viral hepatitis, and viral skin diseases like ulcers in China.[20] At least six Glycyrrhiza species, mainly *G. uralensis* and *G. inflata*, are used in Chinese licorice *gan-cao*, or "sweet herb" (and known as *kanzo* in Japan).[19,21] *G. inflata* has a wide range of pharmaceutical and dietary applications and is related to *G. glabra*.[22]

In contemporary times, licorice remains one of the most frequently used herbs in TCM.[3,7] Licorice was introduced into Japan from China in the 8th century,[3] and is also an important herb in Kampo (the Japanese adaptation of TCM) and Ayurvedic medicine.[23,24] During the past 75 years, a glycyrrhizin formulation called Stronger Neo-Minophagen C™ (SNMC) has been used in the clinical setting in Japan as an antiallergic and antihepatitis treatment.[3] In 1946, the Dutch physician Revers recommended licorice extracts to treat gastric ulcer, but side effects led to its swift removal from the market.[3] In the United Kingdom, a licorice preparation was used to treat peptic ulcers.[3] The modern scientific investigation into the pharmacologic properties of licorice species began in earnest in the 1950s and quickly revealed a broad range of biologic activity.[24] The long history of traditional uses of licorice root and its extensive study over the last several decades make licorice one of the most widely researched plants for medicinal purposes.

CHEMISTRY

More than 400 compounds have been isolated from Glycyrrhiza species.[25] Of the six major Glycyrrhiza species, *G. glabra*, *G. uralensis*, and *G. inflata* produce glycyrrhizin as a major saponin; *G. echinata*, *G. macedonica,* and *G. pallidiflora* produce macedonoside C as a major saponin. *G. uralensis* and *G. inflata* are closely related,[26] but *G. inflata* is more often used medically and in the diet. *G. glabra*, *G. inflata*, and *G. uralensis* are the three species of licorice most often used medically, and are the focus of this discussion.

Glycyrrhiza Glabra

Extracts from this more Western species of licorice, sometimes referred to as European licorice, are increasingly found in anti-inflammatory products.[5,14] Glycyrrhizin, the primary water-soluble constituent of licorice, has been shown to confer numerous pharmacological benefits, though various derivatives also possess such properties.[11] A sweet-tasting triterpene saponin exhibiting poor blood solubility as compared with other saponins, glycyrrhizin is typically present in the root in 5 to 10 percent concentrations,[14,27] and is the source of the plant's sweetness.[28] In addition to the triterpenoid glycyrrhizin, and its aglycone form glycyrrhizic acid, licorice root contains polysaccharides and various polyphenols, such as the isoflavone formononetin, to which antioxidant characteristics have been ascribed.[10]

Glabridin, which is the main component in the hydrophobic fraction of licorice extract, was also found to exhibit inhibitory effects on melanogenesis and inflammation when evaluated using cultured murine melanoma cells and guinea pig skin.[29] A prenylated isoflavonoid of *G. glabra* roots, glabridin was first described in 1976 and has since been characterized as exhibiting broad biologic activity, including antioxidant, anti-inflammatory, antiatherogenic, energy metabolism regulating, estrogenic, neuroprotective, antiosteoporotic, and skin whitening. Its anti-inflammatory, antiatherogenic, estrogenic, and energy-regulating capacities are currently thought to be most prominent.[5]

Glycyrrhiza Inflata

The primary active ingredient isolated and extracted from Chinese licorice roots is licochalcone A, also known as 3-a, a-dimethylallyl-4,4'-dihydroxy-6-methoxychalcone, an oxygenated or reversely-constructed chalcone or "retrochalcone."[22,30,31] Licochalcone A has been shown to exhibit antiparasitic and antibacterial properties as well as antitumorigenic activity.[31–33] This extract has also demonstrated anti-inflammatory activity against arachidonic acid- and 12-O-tetradecanoylphorbol 13-acetate (TPA)-induced mouse ear edema and been reported to manifest *in vivo* antitumor properties in mouse skin papilloma initiated by 7,12-dimethylbenz(a)anthracene (DMBA) and promoted by TPA.[31] Chalcones exhibit activity against oxidative stress. A study assessing their radical-scavenging

activity revealed that licochalcones B and D potently delay superoxide anion production.[34]

Noting that the herbal formulation PC-SPES, which contains licorice root, has been shown to possess potent estrogenic activity *in vitro*, in animals, and in patients with prostate cancer, researchers investigated whether the flavonoid licochalcone A shared these characteristics. Through a range of assays, they determined that licochalcone A is a phytoestrogen, demonstrates antitumor activity, enhancing the effects of paclitaxel and vinblastine, and can affect the apoptotic protein bcl-2 in human cell lines derived from several cancers.[33]

In 2010, Cho et al. studied the capacity of the recently isolated licochalcone E to influence the synthesis of interleukin (IL)-12p40, a subunit of IL-12 and IL-23, and found that the *G. inflata* extract inhibited IL-12p40 expression and attenuated symptoms induced by oxazolone in a chronic allergic contact dermatitis model. They concluded that licochalcone E displays potential for use in treating cutaneous inflammation.[35]

Glycyrrhiza Uralensis

Li et al. used a calcineurin inhibitory test in 2010 to identify glycyrol, a benzofuran coumarin isolate, as an effective immunosuppressant in *G. uralensis*. Various assays revealed that glycyrol exerted immunosuppressive activity by blocking calcineurin activity, thus inhibiting the synthesis of IL-2 and regulating T lymphocytes. The investigators concluded that glycyrol shows promise as an immunomodulatory agent.[36] Previously, glycyrol had been shown to exert *in vitro* anti-inflammatory effects.[37]

ORAL USES

Licorice is used broadly as a natural sweetening agent in food as well as tobacco products.[7,25] Notably, glycyrrhizin is 50-fold sweeter than sugar.[19] Indeed, in the United States, it is used more often as a flavoring and sweetening agent in food products than for salutary purposes,[10] though licorice candy is typically flavored with anise oil, not licorice. Glycyrrhizin can be found in the confection, though, in concentrations ranging from 1 to 25 percent, with a minimum of 4 percent found in good quality licorice.[19] Licorice is also widely available in supplement form.[24]

Various herbal product companies provide licorice oral supplements as well as some topical preparations that contain licorice extract amid a cocktail of other botanical ingredients. Licorice extract is widely used as an anti-inflammatory in Europe and has been reported to be effective as an antiviral medication for chronic hepatitis.[27] The use of oral licorice is approved by the German Commission E for bronchitis and chronic gastritis.

G. glabra has also been shown to effectively protect against or treat oral mucositis engendered by radiation and chemotherapy for head and neck malignancies.[38]

TOPICAL USES

Modern research has shown that licorice extracts are comparably effective to corticosteroids in treating dermatitis, eczema, and psoriasis.[39] Licorice extracts are also among the compounds known to be effective in topical creams intended to repair the skin barrier.[40]

G. glabra has been used for a wide range of medical indications. Among the cutaneous indications, the extract has been used to treat dermatitis, eczema, pruritus, cysts,[41] and skin irritation.[42] In the modern pharmacopoeia, licorice is incorporated into cosmetics for acne patients as well as the treatment of sunburn.[42]

Anti-inflammatory Uses

The topical anti-inflammatory properties and antiulcer capacity of licorice root have been attributed mainly to glycyrrhetic acid, the biologically active metabolite of glycyrrhizic acid,[27,43,44] which has been used successfully to treat inflammation without secondary infection.[45] It has been reported to have anti-inflammatory activity in subacute and chronic dermatoses, and therefore has been used to treat eczema, pruritus, contact dermatitis, seborrheic dermatitis, and psoriasis.[41] In a series of animal studies in 1988, glyderinine, a derivative of glycyrrhizic acid isolated from *G. glabra*, was shown by Azimov et al. to exhibit anti-inflammatory effects as well as analgesic and antipyretic properties. The researchers concluded that glyderinine is an appropriate ointment for treating skin diseases.[46]

Studies have shown that glycyrrhetic acid is able to exert a cortisone-like effect, thus inhibiting proinflammatory prostaglandins and leukotrienes.[47] Licorice (glycyrrhetic acid) has not been demonstrated to be superior to topical corticosteroids in treating acute inflammation, such as atopic dermatitis.[41] The combination of corticosteroids with glycyrrhetic acid has been proven to be effective, however. One study displayed effective potentiation of hydrocortisone activity in skin by the addition of 2 percent glycyrrhetic acid.[48]

A 2002 study assessing the effects of five different chalcones, including licochalcone A, revealed that four of the five tested chalcones, including licochalcone A, inhibited the production of proinflammatory cytokines from monocytes and T cells. The investigators concluded that licochalcone A and some of its synthetic analogs may have immunomodulatory effects, potentially rendering them suitable agents for the treatment of infectious and other inflammatory diseases.[32]

Furuhashi et al., in 2005, studied the *in vitro* anti-inflammatory effects of licochalcone A on the formation of chemical mediators [e.g., prostaglandin E_2 (PGE_2) and cytokines) by IL-1β in human skin fibroblasts and compared it to the effects of other compounds. The steroid dexamethasone was found to inhibit PGE_2, prostaglandin F(2α) [$PGF(2\alpha)$], IL-6, and IL-8 production, and potently blocked cyclooxygenase (COX)-2 mRNA and protein expression, whereas licochalcone A, in response to IL-1β, hindered $PGF(2\alpha)$ generation and PGE_2 synthesis, but had no effect on increased levels of COX-2 mRNA and protein in cells or IL-6, and IL-8 production. The investigators concluded that the licorice isolate engenders anti-inflammatory activity by suppressing COX-2-dependent PGE_2 synthesis with a response to IL-1β that is markedly divergent from that of dexamethasone.[49]

In 2008, Kwon et al. reported on the dynamic anti-inflammatory properties of licochalcone A as demonstrated *in vitro* and in animal models. The *G. inflata* extract inhibited the generation of nitric oxide (NO), PGE_2, inflammatory cytokines such as IL-1 and IL-6, as well as the expression of inducible NO synthase (iNOS) and COX-2 induced by lipopolysaccharide (LPS) in RAW264.7 cells *in vitro*. In addition, the investigators speculated that licochalcone A may have suppressed inflammatory cytokine and NO synthesis in the process of protecting BALB/c mice from LPS-induced endotoxin shock in an animal model. They concluded that licochalcone A might be considered for use in treating various inflammatory conditions.[50]

Studies by Furusawa et al. in 2009 revealed that the anti-inflammatory activity of *G. inflata* could be attributed to potent suppression of nuclear factor (NF)-κB exerted by licochalcones A, B, and D.[6]

Funakoshi-Tago et al. have shown in mice that licochalcone A potently suppresses tumor necrosis factor-α-induced NF-κB activation and that the fixed structure of licochalcone A is pivotal in imparting its anti-inflammatory properties. They also noted, in 2010, that licochalcone A demonstrates great promise *in vivo* as an anti-inflammatory agent.[51]

In 2013, Lee et al. demonstrated that topically applied licochalcone E displayed strong anti-inflammatory properties in a TPA-induced mouse ear edema model and similar effects when the *G. inflata* extract was administered *in vitro* in an LPS-stimulated RAW 264.7 murine macrophage model. They found that licochalcone E inhibited AKT and p38 mitogen activated protein kinase (MAPK), thus suppressing NF-κB and activator protein (AP)-1 transcriptional activity, which in turn facilitates the decline of proinflammatory cytokines.[52]

Also that year, Fu et al. isolated six flavonoids from *G. inflata* and *G. uralensis*, with all six compounds [5-(1,1-dimethylallyl)-3, 4,4'-trihydroxy-2-methoxychalcone, licochalcones A and B, echinatin, glycycoumarin, and glyurallin B] found to possess varying degrees of antioxidant and anti-inflammatory characteristics.[25]

Acne

In a 2003 study of antiacne activity displayed by Asian herbal extracts, Name et al. found that *G. glabra* showed significant antibacterial activity against *Propionibacterium acnes* without inducing noteworthy resistance. The investigators suggested that a formulation combining three herbal extracts, including *G. glabra*, *Angelica dahurica*, and *Coptis chinensis*, may be suitable for preventing and treating acne.[53]

Ten years later, Angelova-Fischer et al. conducted a nine-week, randomized, double-blind, vehicle-controlled study with 60 volunteers with mild-to-moderately severe acne to evaluate and provide proof-of-concept for a formulation containing licochalcone A, L-carnitine and 1,2-decanediol. After one week for standardization of the cleansing procedure, the participants (40 females and 20 males between the ages of 14 and 40 years old) were randomized to apply either the test formulation or vehicle to the face twice daily for eight weeks. At the end of the study, the mean total lesion count and papular lesions were decreased in the active formulation group compared to baseline. Significant reductions in pustules, sebum levels, and *P. acnes* were recorded in the active formulation subjects along with improvements in Dermatology Life Quality Index (DLQI), whereas no significant improvements were observed in the vehicle group. Evidence of acne improvement associated with the licochalcone A-containing formulation was noted in both physician and patient assessments.[54]

Atopic Dermatitis

G. glabra is one among various plant constituents demonstrated to be effective in treating atopic dermatitis.[55,56] In a 2003 double-blind study over two weeks, investigators evaluated the effect of 1 and 2 percent topical licorice extract preparations on atopic dermatitis in two 30-patient groups. Results indicated that the 2 percent licorice topical gel was more effective in reducing erythema, edema, and pruritus. Significantly, the authors also concluded that licorice extract was effective in treating atopic dermatitis.[41]

In 2011, Udompataikul and Srisatwaja conducted a six-week, randomized, controlled, investigator-blinded comparative pilot study of the effects of moisturizers containing licochalcone A or hydrocortisone on children with atopic dermatitis (mean age, 5.8 years). Twenty-six patients completed the protocol, which included twice-daily application of licochalcone A on one side of the body and hydrocortisone on the other side. The response rate to both treatments was found to be 73.33 percent, with no significant differences in scoring atopic dermatitis (SCORAD) score reductions from treatment. Edema and erythema resolved more rapidly with hydrocortisone, but the relapse rate associated with hydrocortisone was higher; in both cases, the differences were not significant. The investigators concluded that licochalcone A lotion, which was found to be equally effective as hydrocortisone lotion, is an option to treat mild-to-moderate childhood atopic dermatitis in the maintenance as well as acute phases.[57]

In 2013, Wananukul et al. led a four-week, prospective, multicenter, randomized, double-blind, split-side study in 55 children (three months to 14 years of age) with mild-to-moderate atopic dermatitis to compare the efficacy of a licochalcone A-containing moisturizer and 1 percent hydrocortisone. Simultaneous treatment with either the licochalcone A preparation or 1 percent hydrocortisone on opposite sides of the lesion were administered twice daily. The SCORAD declined significantly for both treatments from baseline, with no statistically significant differences between the treatments. Transepidermal water loss was found to be significantly decreased from baseline on the side that received licochalcone A treatment. The investigators also reported that continuing treatment with licochalcone A for four weeks maintained clinical and skin barrier benefits.[58]

Hyperpigmentation

Licorice extracts are included among the array of topical tyrosinase inhibitors used to lighten hyperpigmented areas of the skin.[59–61] Glabridin, found in concentrations between 10 and 40 percent in commercial depigmenting agents, is thought to be the chief ingredient in licorice to provide skin-lightening activity.[61] Draelos has noted that the status of licorice extracts as the safest of options among skin-lightening agents while eliciting the fewest side effects accounts for its popularity for this purpose.[62,63]

In a study of 20 women between the ages of 18 and 40 with a clinical diagnosis of bilateral and symmetrical idiopathic epidermal melasma, liquiritin cream was applied on one side of the face and a vehicle cream on the other twice daily for four weeks. Liquiritin is a flavonoid component of licorice that, along with other ingredients, contributes to the natural yellow pigment. Individuals with dermal melasma, melasma with pregnancy, and those receiving hormone replacement therapy were excluded from the study. Topical sunscreen use was encouraged during the treatment period while sun exposure was discouraged. Sixteen patients (80 percent) were characterized as exhibiting excellent responses from liquiritin, with no discernible differences between the normal skin and previously pigmented areas. Two patients (10 percent) showed a good response on the liquiritin side, and two patients (10 percent) had fair responses from liquiritin, with moderate pigmentation, while moderate improvement was seen in only 20 percent on the vehicle side.[64]

Nerya et al. found in 2003 that in addition to glabridin, glabrene, and isoliquiritigenin (2′,4′,4-trihydroxychalcone), constituents of licorice root extract contributed significantly and dose-dependently in the observed potent tyrosinase-inhibiting activity displayed by the plant.[65]

In a 2010 single-blind, 60-day study with 56 women between 18 to 60 years old, Costa et al. found that a formulation combining belides, emblica, and licorice was as effective as hydroquinone 2 percent in ameliorating the effects of melasma (see Chapter 38, Emblica Extract). There were no statistically significant differences between the groups and the herbal combination was associated with fewer adverse effects.[66]

In 2008, Adhikari et al. screened 52 crude drugs traditionally used in Nepal to treat hyperpigmentation for inhibitory activity against mushroom tyrosinase, finding that methanolic extracts of G. glabra manifested the greatest inhibitory activity, with kojic acid used as a positive control.[67] Licorice extract is frequently combined with other skin-lightening ingredients (see Chapter 32, Overview of the Pigmentation Process). Vitamin C is often combined with licorice extracts or soy when deployed for skin-lightening purposes [see Chapter 40, Vitamin C (Ascorbic Acid), and Chapter 45, Soy].[68]

Psoriasis

Cassano et al. conducted a pilot, randomized, open-label, parallel-group trial in 40 patients in 2010 to assess the effects of an emollient cream containing milk proteins and G. glabra extracts in the treatment of palmar and/or plantar psoriasis treated with topical corticotherapy. Twenty patients were treated only with mometasone furoate ointment for four weeks and 20 patients received the same corticosteroid in combination with the licorice-containing emollient, which was applied twice daily during the four-week study period. Statistically significant decreases in the severity of all clinical signs of psoriasis were seen in all patients, all of whom completed the study. In the group treated with the test emollient, significantly greater reductions in desquamation, affected surface area, and subjective symptoms were reported as compared with the corticosteroid-only treatment group. The investigators concluded that their findings support the adjuvant use of this new emollient combining G. glabra extracts and milk proteins for psoriasis management.[69]

The topical application of Tuhuai, a Chinese herbal medicine that includes licorice, has also been found by Man et al. to exhibit antiproliferative and anti-inflammatory activity in murine models of inflammatory dermatoses. The investigators suggest the herbal formulation may offer an effective, relatively safe, and inexpensive option to treat inflammatory disorders such as psoriasis.[70]

Sensitive Skin/Rosacea

In 2006, Weber et al. assessed the cutaneous compatibility and efficacy of a skin care regimen containing licochalcone A in 62 patients with mild-to-moderate rosacea over eight weeks. The regimen was well tolerated and effective in reducing erythema, as indicated by clinical evaluations, subject response, and photographic review. Responses to quality-of-life questionnaires revealed subjective improvements, and average erythema scores at four and eight weeks indicated significant improvements. The investigators concluded that licochalcone A use is suitable for patients with sensitive facial skin, as characterized by rosacea, and that the tested licochalcone A-containing regimen was compatible with daily metronidazole application.[71]

That same year, Kolbe et al. showed in prospective, randomized, vehicle-controlled clinical trials that licochalcone A displays significant anti-irritative efficacy in cosmetic formulations and is thus well suited for sensitive or irritated skin. They also showed in vitro that licochalcone A-rich extracts of G. inflata as well as synthetic licochalcone A potently inhibit proinflammatory responses.[72] Licorice extract is a popular ingredient in over-the-counter skin care products designed to treat rosacea, although few studies supporting its use in rosacea are published.

SAFETY ISSUES

Most, if not all, pharmacopoeias around the world recognize and include licorice extract.[12] The United States Food and Drug Administration (FDA) bestowed generally recognized as safe (GRAS) status upon licorice in 1983.[28] The dietary ingredient licorice flavonoid oil, in which glabridin is a primary bioactive flavonoid, has been found to be safe when used once daily up to 1,200 mg/day.[73]

The rare side effects from the oral administration of licorice are dose-dependent and occur more frequently in women and with the use of oral contraceptives.[74] At doses of less than 10 mg of glycycrrhizin daily, side effects are thought to be nominal.[75] Chronic use of high doses of glycyrrhizin or glycyrrhetinic acid can result in adverse effects such as edema, hypertension, and hypokalemia. Chemical modifications to licorice formulations have been made to enhance therapeutic benefits while reducing the risk of side effects.[3] Oral licorice is contraindicated in pregnancy according to the German Commission E, though doses up to 3 g daily are thought to be safe; hypertension, cardiac or renal histories, various liver conditions, hypokalemia, and edema are also contraindications.[24,27,75]

The Cosmetic Ingredient Review (CIR) Expert Panel suggested that acute, short-term, subchronic, or chronic toxicity is minimal and deemed the use of all licorice constituents safe for skin care in the current usage and concentration practices.[17]

ENVIRONMENTAL IMPACT

The CIR Expert Panel noted that the chemicals isolated from the licorice plant may have pesticide and toxic metal residues, and advised that polychlorobiphenyl (PCB)/pesticide contamination should be no higher than 40 parts per million. They further cautioned that toxic metal levels should be limited to 3 mg/kg of arsenic, 1 mg/kg of lead, and 0.002 percent heavy metals.[17]

In 2003, Yamamoto et al. acknowledged that cultivation of *G. uralensis* had emerged to compensate for the waning supply of wild Glycyrrhiza plants in China incurred by collection restrictions spurred by over-collection of wild plants.[21,76] Six years later, Gao et al. reported on the ramifications of using *G. uralensis* seeds flown on a recoverable satellite for 18 days. After their return to earth, the seeds were planted and grown to maturity. Analysis of the content of the roots of the seeds flown in space revealed glycyrrhizic acid as 2.19 times higher than a control group and liquiritin content as 1.18 times that of the control. The investigators suggested that extraterrestrial breeding warrants attention as an approach to future breeding of what is considered an endangered medicinal plant.[76]

FORMULATION CONSIDERATIONS

The licorice derivatives glycyrrhizin and glycyrrhetinic acid occasionally cause edema, hypertension, and hypokalemia when used orally in patients treated over a long period and with higher doses. Topical use has not been associated with these side effects. Chemical modifications to the myriad compounds have enhanced the anti-inflammatory activities of the various forms of licorice extract,[3] and several products have been formulated with the intent to increase penetration of the active compounds.

Hao et al. demonstrated in 2010 that glycyrrhetinic acid, a metabolite of glycyrrhizic acid, could better penetrate the skin when combined with organic bases (triethanolamine or triethylamine) in nonaqueous solvent comprising isopropyl myristate and alcohols (ethanol, butanol, octanol, and dodecanol). Specifically, they found that an ion pair between glycyrrhizic acid and an organic base enhanced the solubility of the extract in the stratum corneum as well as its partition into the viable skin, thus fostering the penetration of the licorice component into the skin.[77]

Marianecci et al. found in 2012 that using niosomes composed of surfactants (Tween 85 and Span 20) loaded with ammonium glycyrrhizinate is potentially effective for treating various inflammatory disorders, as the delivery system was shown to exhibit good skin tolerability and no toxicity while enhancing the drug anti-inflammatory activity in mice. Skin erythema chemically induced in a human model was also found to be improved by the ammonium glycyrrhizinate-infused vesicles.[39]

Early in 2014, Mostafa et al. reported on the formulation of a stable, cost-effective, easy-to-use transdermal microemulsion system (ME3) for *G. glabra* delivery that delivers 13-fold higher *ex vivo* antioxidant capacity than the licorice extract solution itself.[78]

USAGE CONSIDERATIONS

No topical products with licorice extract as the primary active ingredient are FDA approved for the treatment of melasma, rosacea, acne, or other inflammatory skin disorders.[27] Glycyrrhetinic acid is used in many cosmeceuticals at concentrations of up to 2 percent and glycyrrhizic acid, up to 0.1 percent.[17] Studies have not been performed to investigate how other agents affect efficacy and penetration when used in combination with various forms of licorice extract.

SIGNIFICANT BACKGROUND

In some of the earlier research on licorice extract, the use of topical ointments containing active isomers of glycyrrhetic acid reportedly showed anti-inflammatory activity in subacute and chronic dermatoses, such as contact dermatitis, seborrheic dermatitis, and psoriasis. Topical corticosteroids were more effective than the glycyrrhetic acid formulation in treating acute atopic dermatitis.[79] But glycyrrhetic acid has been characterized as exerting a cortisone-like effect, rendering it viable as an anti-inflammatory agent, and has inhibited proinflammatory prostaglandins and leukotrienes.[47,80] Combining glycyrrhetic acid with corticosteroids has also been shown to be effective. Results from topical corticosteroid application were significantly improved with the addition of 2 percent glycyrrhetic acid in one study.[48]

Antioxidant Activity

Assays of physical stability and antioxidant activity of topical preparations containing various plant extracts performed by Di Mambro and Fonseca in 2005 revealed that *G. glabra* and *Ginkgo biloba* are suitable for incorporation into topical formulations intended to protect skin from the deleterious effects of free radical and reactive oxygen species.[81]

In 2011, Veratti et al. investigated the potential protective properties of glycyrrhizin, 18β-glycyrrhetinic acid, and glabridin against UVB-induced damage in human keratinocyte cultures. They found that 18β-glycyrrhetinic acid and glabridin exhibit strong antioxidant activity by blocking oxidative DNA fragmentation as well as the induction of apoptosis in human keratinocytes.[82]

Also during that year, Li et al. employed novel techniques to screen and characterize 35 radical scavengers in *G. inflata*,

G. glabra, G. pallidflora, and *G. uralensis,* with 21 identified as flavonoids.[9]

The phenolic compounds licochalcone A-D and echinatin, retrochalcones isolated from *G. inflata* roots, have exhibited activity against an array of oxidative stresses. A study assessing their inhibitory capacity on lipid peroxidation and radical-scavenging activity, specifically, revealed that licochalcones B and D potently hindered superoxide anion production in the xanthine/xanthine oxidase system, protected red cells from oxidative hemolysis, and displayed potent scavenging activity.[34] These retrochalcones have also demonstrated antimicrobial activity. Specifically, licochalcones A and C have been shown to exert potent activity against some Gram-positive bacteria and hamper oxygen consumption in vulnerable bacterial cells.[83]

Antibacterial Activity

In a study evaluating the *in vitro* activities of licochalcone A against some food contaminant microorganisms, the licorice derivative exhibited activity against all Gram-positive bacteria tested, particularly all Bacillus spp. tested, but was ineffective against tested Gram-negative bacteria and eukaryotes at 50 µg/mL. This study demonstrated the potential viability of licochalcone A as an integral constituent in antibacterial products designed to preserve food high in salts and proteases.[22]

Flavonoid extracts of several species of licorice plant have been shown to exhibit antiulcer activity for peptic ulcers. Inhibitory activity against *Helicobacter pylori* growth has also been observed *in vitro* among glabridin and glabrene (components of *G. glabra*), licochalcone A (*G. inflata*), as well as licoricidin and licoisoflavone B (*G. uralensis*). Among these licorice constituents, anti-*H. pylori* activity was also identified against a clarithromycin- and amoxicillin-resistant strain.[23]

In 2013, Long et al. showed that high concentrations of 18β-glycyrrhetinic acid, a constituent of the root of several Glycyrrhiza species, were bactericidal to methicillin-resistant *Staphylococcus aureus* (MRSA). In addition, both *in vitro* and *in vivo*, the licorice component, at sublethal doses, decreased virulent gene expression in *S. aureus.*[84]

Chemopreventive/Photoprotective Activity

Oral feeding of licorice extract to Sencar mice was shown in 1991 to protect against skin tumorigenesis caused by DMBA initiation and TPA promotion. Tumors developed in much less time in mice not fed the licorice preparation; treated mice also had significantly fewer tumors during and at the end of the study. Researchers concluded that the considerable antitumorigenic activity of licorice extract might ultimately be proved useful in protecting against some forms of human cancer.[11] Since the time that this study was published, the polyphenols in licorice have been shown to induce apoptosis in cancer cells, as licorice constituents have exhibited significant antimutagenic, anticarcinogenic, and tumor-suppressive capacity in animal models.[10] In fact, the National Cancer Institute has formally recognized the chemopreventive worth of licorice root and its primary constituent glycyrrhizin.[82,85]

In 2005, Rossi et al. assessed the effect of glycyrrhizin and its aglycone metabolite 18β-glycyrrhetinic acid on UVB-irradiated human melanoma cells, finding that glycyrrhizin has the potential to confer photoprotection, though it is ineffective on metastatic cells.[86]

Also that year, Agarwal et al. reported that 18β-glycyrrhetinic acid inhibits TPA-mediated oxidative stress and tumor promotion

in murine skin, attenuating the activity of ornithine decarboxylase, incorporation of [3H]-thymidine in DNA, and induction of oxidative stress. The licorice component also suppressed DMBA/TPA-induced skin tumor formation in mice. The researchers concluded that the antioxidant glycyrrhetinic acid may be a viable chemopreventive agent.[87]

In 2007, Rahman et al. investigated the chemopreventive effects of glycyrrhizin on TPA-induced cutaneous oxidative stress and tumor protection in Swiss albino mice. Pretreatment of animals with the licorice compound prior to TPA yielded significant reductions in cutaneous microsomal lipid peroxidation and restoration of cutaneous glutathione and its dependent enzymes. The investigators suggested that glycyrrhizin provided substantial protection to mice from pernicious TPA-induced effects.[88]

Cherng et al. showed in 2011 that oral administration of glycyrrhizic acid to SKH-1 hairless mice prior to UVB exposure (180 mJ/cm[2] per exposure) mitigates UVB-induced tumorigenesis through downregulation of cell proliferation controls (i.e., thymine dimer-positive cells, proliferative cell nuclear antigen expression, apoptosis, and transcription factor NF-κB) and inflammatory responses (i.e., COX-2, PGE$_2$, and NO) and upregulation of p53 and p21/Cip1 to preclude damage while mediating repair to DNA.[1]

Afnan et al. conducted an *in vitro* study in 2012 of the effects of glycyrrhizic acid against UVB-induced photoaging in human dermal fibroblasts, finding that treatment with the licorice extract diminished reactive oxygen species, NF-κB, cytochrome c, and caspase 3 levels and hindered hyaluronidase. The investigators speculated, though, that the botanical ingredient significantly suppressed photoaging primarily through inhibiting matrix metalloproteinase-1 activation and altering NF-κB signaling. They concluded that glycyrrhizic acid appears to have potential as a key ingredient in natural and safe products intended to protect against UVB-induced damage.[4]

Dry, Itchy Scalp

A *G. inflata* extract containing licochalcone A was included in a formulation with urea, lactate, and polidocanol that was tested by Schweiger et al. in 2013 in 30 volunteers with dry and itchy scalp conditions. Participants applied the leave-on tonic three times each week for four weeks on one side of the scalp. Investigators found that scalp moisture was significantly enhanced after treatment with the tonic, while pruritus was significantly diminished. A substantial decrease in key proinflammatory markers was also confirmed through scalp washup analyses. The investigators concluded that the formulation containing anti-inflammatory licochalcone A, urea, lactate, and polidocanol displayed great efficacy in normalizing scalp lipid disturbances and, more importantly, relieving scalp dryness, itching, and microinflammation.[89]

Infantile Seborrheic Dermatitis

In 2012, Wananukul et al. conducted a two-week, prospective, randomized, double-blind, split-side comparison study of a 0.025 percent licochalcone-containing moisturizer and 1 percent hydrocortisone in 75 infants (72 of whom completed the study) with infantile seborrheic dermatitis. Patients were treated twice daily on opposite sides of the lesion. A significantly higher clearance rate (42 percent vs. 32 percent) was recorded in the licochalcone group at days 3 to 4, with the products appearing equally effective at days 6 to 7 and 14.[90]

Other Biologic Activity

Shin et al. conducted *in vitro* and *in vivo* investigations of the antiallergic effects of *G. glabra* and its constituents in 2007, reporting that glycyrrhizin, 18β-glycyrrhetinic acid, and liquiritigenin are primarily responsible for imparting antiallergic activity that can alleviate the symptoms of immunoglobulin E-mediated allergic conditions such as dermatitis and asthma.[91]

Pellati et al. showed *in vitro* in 2009 that 18β-glycyrrhetinic acid substantially stemmed, in a pH-dependent manner, the growth of clinical isolates of *Candida albicans* strains from patients with recurrent vulvovaginal candidiasis. The researchers suggested that the constituent of Glycyrrhiza species has potential as a topical therapeutic option for patients with the condition.[92]

Peng et al. showed in 2011 that glycyrrhetinic acid extracted from *G. uralensis* induced the dose-dependent expression of Toll-like receptor 4 in Ana-1 murine macrophages and activated its downstream signaling pathway, which is involved in the regulation of the innate immune reaction to encroaching pathogens.[16]

Kato et al. studied the extracts of 25 plants used in Kampo medicine in 2012 to identify anti-UV and anti-HIV activity. Of the plants tested, licorice displayed the second highest anti-UV activity (gardenia fruit was first) and was one of only six plants to display some anti-HIV activity.[93]

In 2013, Wang et al. extracted the radices of *G. uralensis* with hot water and reported antiviral activity against enterovirus 71 and coxackievirus A16, validating the use of the botanical extract against the etiological sources of hand, foot, and mouth disease, with glycyrrhizic acid identified as the primary antiviral component of *G. uralensis*.[20]

◼ CONCLUSION

Licorice root has been used in traditional medicine in the East and West for well over two millennia. In addition, it has been evaluated in a vast range of modern scientific studies, and licorice extracts have been included in the cosmeceutical as well as medical realm. The reputed anti-inflammatory and depigmenting properties of licorice root are particularly intriguing. The great challenge in producing cosmeceutical products – harnessing the identified strengths of a given ingredient and bottling it, delivering health benefits in a topical formulation – applies here as in most cases discussed in this text. The wealth of evidence points to the benefits of several species of licorice plant, indicating that such benefits have been reaped in oral and topical preparations of the extract. Given the relative wealth of history and research supporting its use, licorice root is likely to be incorporated into an increasing number of products. Several medical applications have been derived from various species of licorice, particularly *G. glabra*, *G. inflata*, and *G. uralensis*. Overall, there appears to be ample reason for optimism regarding the role of licorice extracts in dermatology.

REFERENCES

1. Cherng JM, Tsai KD, Yu YW, et al. Molecular mechanisms underlying chemopreventive activities of glycyrrhizic acid against UVB-radiation-induced carcinogenesis in SKH-1 hairless mouse epidermis. *Radiat Res.* 2011;176:177.
2. Asl MN, Hosseinzadeh H. Review of pharmacological effects of Glycyrrhiza sp. and its bioactive compounds. *Phytother Res.* 2008;22:709.
3. Shibata S. A drug over the millennia: pharmacognosy, chemistry, and pharmacology of licorice. *Yakugaku Zasshi.* 2000;120:849.
4. Afnan Q, Adil MD, Nissar-Ul A, et al. Glycyrrhizic acid (GA), a triterpenoid saponin glycoside alleviates ultraviolet-B irradiation-induced photoaging in human dermal fibroblasts. *Phytomedicine.* 2012;19:658.
5. Simmler C, Pauli GF, Chen SN. Phytochemistry and biological properties of glabridin. *Fitoterapia.* 2013;90:160.
6. Furusawa J, Funakoshi-Tago M, Mashino T, et al. Glycyrrhiza inflata-derived chalcones, Licochalcone A, Licochalcone B and Licochalcone D, inhibit phosphorylation of NF-kappaB p65 in LPS signaling pathway. *Int Immunopharmacol.* 2009;9:499.
7. Kao TC, Wu CH, Yen GC. Bioactivity and potential health benefits of licorice. *J Agric Food Chem.* 2014 Jan. 8. [Epub ahead of print]
8. Gibson MR. Glycyrrhiza in old and new perspectives. *Lloydia.* 1978;41:348.
9. Li YJ, Chen J, Li Y, et al. Screening and characterization of natural antioxidants in four Glycyrrhiza species by liquid chromatography coupled with electrospray ionization quadrupole time-of-flight tandem mass spectrometry. *J Chromatogr A.* 2011;1218:8181.
10. Wang ZY, Nixon DW. Licorice and cancer. *Nutr Cancer.* 2001;39:1.
11. Agarwal R, Wang ZY, Mukhtar H. Inhibition of mouse skin tumor-initiating activity of DMBA by chronic oral feeding of glycyrrhizin in drinking water. *Nutr Cancer.* 1991;15:187.
12. Grieve M. *A Modern Herbal* (Vol. II). New York: Dover Publications; 1971:487-492.
13. Fiore C, Eisenhut M, Ragazzi E, et al. A history of the therapeutic use of liquorice in Europe. *J Ethnopharmacol.* 2005;99:317.
14. Aburjai T, Natsheh FM. Plants used in cosmetics. *Phytother Res.* 2003;17:987.
15. Lee O, Kang H, Han S. Oriental herbs in cosmetics. *Cosmet Toiletries.* 1997;112:57.
16. Peng LN, Li L, Qiu YF, et al. Glycyrrhetinic acid extracted from Glycyrrhiza uralensis Fisch. induces the expression of Toll-like receptor 4 in Ana-1 murine macrophages. *J Asian Nat Prod Res.* 2011;13:942.
17. Cosmetic Ingredient Review Expert Panel. Final report on the safety assessment of Glycyrrhetinic Acid, Potassium Glycyrrhetinate, Disodium Succinoyl Glycyrrhetinate, Glyceryl Glycyrrhetinate, Glycyrrhetinyl Stearate, Stearyl Glycyrrhetinate, Glycyrrhizic Acid, Ammonium Glycyrrhizate, Dipotassium Glycyrrhizate, Disodium Glycyrrhizate, Trisodium Glycyrrhizate, Methyl Glycyrrhizate, and Potassium Glycyrrhizinate. *Int J Toxicol.* 2007;26(Suppl 2):79.
18. Liquorice named "medicinal plant of the year in 2012." http://www.traffic.org/home/2011/11/21/liquorice-named-medicinal-plant-of-the-year-2012.html. Accessed March 15, 2014.
19. Foster S. *An Illustrated Guide to 101 Medicinal Herbs: Their History, Use, Recommended Dosages, and Cautions.* Loveland, CO: Interweave Press; 1998:132–133.
20. Wang J, Chen X, Wang W, et al. Glycyrrhizic acid as the antiviral component of Glycyrrhiza uralensis Fisch. against coxsackievirus A16 and enterovirus 71 of hand foot and mouth disease. *J Ethnopharmacol.* 2013;147:114.
21. Yamamoto Y, Majima T, Saiki I, et al. Pharmaceutical evaluation of Glycyrrhiza uralensis roots cultivated in eastern Nei-Meng-Gu of China. *Biol Pharm Bull.* 2003;26:1144.
22. Tsukiyama R, Katsura H, Tokuriki N, et al. Antibacterial activity of licochalcone A against spore-forming bacteria. *Antimicrob Agents Chemother.* 2002;46:1226.
23. Fukai T, Marumo A, Kaitou K, et al. Anti-Helicobacter pylori flavonoids from licorice extract. *Life Sci.* 2002;71:1449.
24. Mills S, Bone K. *Principles and Practice of Phytotherapy.* London: Churchill Livingstone; 2000:465–475.
25. Fu Y, Chen J, Li YJ, et al. Antioxidant and anti-inflammatory activities of six flavonoids separated from licorice. *Food Chem.* 2013;141:1063.
26. Hayashi H, Hosono N, Kondo M, et al. Phylogenetic relationship of six Glycyrrhiza species based on rbcL sequences and chemical constituents. *Biol Pharm Bull.* 2000;23:602.
27. Rico MJ. Rising drug costs: the impact on dermatology. *Skin Therapy Lett.* 2000;5:1.
28. Piersen CE. Phytoestrogens in botanical dietary supplements: implications for cancer. *Integr Cancer Ther.* 2003;2:120.
29. Yokota T, Nishio H, Kubota Y, et al. The inhibitory effect of glabridin from licorice extracts on melanogenesis and inflammation. *Pigment Cell Res.* 1998;11:355.
30. Friis-Møller A, Chen M, Fuursted K, et al. In vitro antimycobacterial and antilegionella activity of licochalcone A from Chinese licorice roots. *Planta Med.* 2002;68:416.

31. Shibata S, Inoue H, Iwata S, et al. Inhibitory effects of licochalcone A isolated from Glycyrrhiza inflate root on inflammatory ear edema and tumour promotion in mice. *Planta Med.* 1991;57:221.

32. Barfod L, Kemp K, Hansen M, et al. Chalcones from Chinese liquorice inhibit proliferation of T cells and production of cytokines. *Int Immunopharmacol.* 2002;2:545.

33. Rafi MM, Rosen RT, Vassil A, et al. Modulation of bcl-2 and cytotoxicity by licochalcone-A, a novel estrogenic flavonoid. *Anticancer Res.* 2000;20:2653.

34. Haraguchi H, Ishikawa H, Mizutani K, et al. Antioxidative and superoxide scavenging activities of retrochalcones in Glycyrrhiza inflata. *Bioorg Med Chem.* 1998;6:339.

35. Cho YC, Lee SH, Yoon G, et al. Licochalcone E reduces chronic allergic contact dermatitis and inhibits IL-12p40 production through down-regulation of NF-kappa B. *Int Immunopharmacol.* 2010;10:1119.

36. Li J, Tu Y, Tong L, et al. Immunosuppressive activity on the murine immune responses of glycyrol from Glycyrrhiza uralensis via inhibition of calcineurin activity. *Pharm Biol.* 2010;48:1177.

37. Shin EM, Zhou HY, Guo LY, et al. Anti-inflammatory effects of glycyrol isolated from Glycyrrhiza uralensis in LPS-stimulated RAW264.7 macrophages. *Int Immunopharmacol.* 2008;8:1524.

38. Das D, Agarwal SK, Chandola HM. Protective effect of Yashtimadhu (Glycyrrhiza glabra) against side effects of radiation/chemotherapy in head and neck malignancies. *Ayu.* 2011;32:196.

39. Marianecci C, Rinaldi F, Mastriota M, et al. Anti-inflammatory activity of novel ammonium glycyrrhizinate/niosomes delivery system: human and murine models. *J Control Release.* 2012;164:17.

40. Draelos ZD. New treatments for restoring impaired epidermal barrier permeability: skin barrier repair creams. *Clin Dermatol.* 2012;30:345.

41. Saeedi M, Morteza-Semnani K, Ghoreishi MR. The treatment of atopic dermatitis with licorice gel. *J Dermatolog Treat.* 2003;14:153.

42. Marks A. Herbal extracts in cosmetics. *Agro-Food-Industry Hi-Tech.* 1997;8:28.

43. Ploeger B, Mensinga T, Sips A, et al. The pharmacokinetics of glycyrrhizic acid evaluated by physiologically based pharmacokinetic modeling. *Drug Metab Rev.* 2001;33:125.

44. Baker ME, Fanestil DD. Liquorice as a regulator of steroid and prostaglandin metabolism. *Lancet.* 1991;337:428.

45. Olukoga A, Donaldson D. Historical perspectives on health. The history of liquorice: the plant, its extract, cultivation, commercialization and etymology. *J R Soc Promot Health.* 1998;118:300.

46. Azimov MM, Zakirov UB, Radzhapova ShD. Pharmacological study of the anti-inflammatory agent dlyderinine. *Farmakol Toksikol.* 1988;51:90.

47. Ohuchi K, Kamada Y, Levine L, et al. Glycyrrhizin inhibits prostaglandin E2 production by activated peritoneal macrophages from rats. *Prostaglandins Med.* 1981;7:457.

48. Teelucksingh S, Mackie AD, Burt D, et al. Potentiation of hydrocortisone activity in skin by glycyrrhetinic acid. *Lancet.* 1990;335:1060.

49. Furuhashi I, Iwata S, Shibata S, et al. Inhibition by licochalcone A, a novel flavonoid isolated from liquorice root, of IL-1beta-induced PGE2 production in human skin fibroblasts. *J Pharm Pharmacol.* 2005;57:1661.

50. Kwon HS, Park JH, Kim DH, et al. Licochalcone A isolated from licorice suppresses lipopolysaccharide-stimulated inflammatory reactions in RAW264.7 cells and endotoxin shock in mice. *J Mol Med (Berl).* 2008;86:1287.

51. Funakoshi-Tago M, Nakamura K, Tsuruya R, et al. The fixed structure of Licochalcone A by alpha, beta-unsaturated ketone is necessary for anti-inflammatory activity through the inhibition of NF-kappaB activation. *Int Immunopharmacol.* 2010;10:562.

52. Lee HN, Cho HJ, Lim do Y, et al. Mechanisms by which licochalcone e exhibits potent anti-inflammatory properties: studies with phorbol ester-treated mouse skin and lipopolysaccharide-stimulated murine macrophages. *Int J Mol Sci.* 2013;14:10926.

53. Nam C, Kim S, Sim Y, et al. Anti-acne effects of Oriental herb extracts: a novel screening method to select anti-acne agents. *Skin Pharmacol Appl Skin Physiol.* 2003;16:84.

54. Angelova-Fischer I, Rippke F, Fischer TW, et al. A double-blind, randomized, vehicle-controlled efficacy assessment study of a skin care formulation for improvement of mild to moderately severe acne. *J Eur Acad Dermatol Venereol.* 2013;27(Suppl 2):6.

55. Reuter J, Wölfle U, Weckesser S, et al. Which plant for which skin disease? Part 1: Atopic dermatitis, psoriasis, acne, condyloma and herpes simplex. *J Dtsch Dermatol Ges.* 2010;8:788.

56. Reuter J, Merfort I, Schempp CM. Botanicals in dermatology: an evidence-based review. *Am J Clin Dermatol.* 2010;11:247.

57. Udompataikul M, Srisatwaja W. Comparative trial of moisturizer containing licochalcone A vs. hydrocortisone lotion in the treatment of childhood atopic dermatitis: a pilot study. *J Eur Acad Dermatol Venereol.* 2011;25:660.

58. Wananukul S, Chatproedprai S, Chunharas A, et al. Randomized, double-blind, split-side, comparison study of moisturizer containing licochalcone A and 1% hydrocortisone in the treatment of childhood atopic dermatitis. *J Med Assoc Thai.* 2013;96:1135.

59. Davis EC, Callender VD. Postinflammatory hyperpigmentation: a review of the epidemiology, clinical features, and treatment options in skin of color. *J Clin Aesthet Dermatol.* 2010;3:20.

60. Zhu W, Gao J. The use of botanical extracts as topical skin-lightening agents for the improvement of skin pigmentation disorders. *J Investig Dermatol Symp Proc.* 2008;13:20.

61. Leyden JJ, Shergill B, Micali G, et al. Natural options for the management of hyperpigmentation. *J Eur Acad Dermatol Venereol.* 2011;25:1140.

62. Draelos ZD. Skin lightening preparations and the hydroquinone controversy. *Dermatol Ther.* 2007;20:308.

63. Cronin H, Draelos ZD. Top 10 botanical ingredients in 2010 anti-aging creams. *J Cosmet Dermatol.* 2010;9:218.

64. Amer M, Metwalli M. Topical liquiritin improves melasma. *Int J Dermatol.* 2000;39:299.

65. Nerya O, Vaya J, Musa R, et al. Glabrene and isoliquiritigenin as tyrosinase inhibitors from licorice roots. *J Agric Food Chem.* 2003;51:1201.

66. Costa A, Moisés TA, Cordero T, et al. Association of emblica, licorice and belides as an alternative to hydroquinone in the clinical treatment of melasma. *An Bras Dermatol.* 2010;85:613.

67. Adhikari A, Devkota HP, Takano A, et al. Screening of Nepalese crude drugs traditionally used to treat hyperpigmentation: in vitro tyrosinase inhibition. *Int J Cosmet Sci.* 2008;30:353.

68. Sheth VM, Pandya AG. Melasma: a comprehensive update: part II. *J Am Acad Dermatol.* 2011;65:699.

69. Cassano N, Mantegazza R, Battaglini S, et al. Adjuvant role of a new emollient cream in patients with palmar and/or plantar psoriasis: a pilot randomized open-label study. *G Ital Dermatol Venereol.* 2010;145:789.

70. Man MQ, Shi Y, Man M, et al. Chinese herbal medicine (Tuhuai extract) exhibits topical anti-proliferative and anti-inflammatory activity in murine disease models. *Exp Dermatol.* 2008;17:681.

71. Weber TM, Ceilley RI, Buerger A, et al. Skin tolerance, efficacy, and quality of life of patients with red facial skin using a skin care regimen containing Licochalcone A. *J Cosmet Dermatol.* 2006;5:227.

72. Kolbe L, Immeyer J, Batzer J, et al. Anti-inflammatory efficacy of Licochalcone A: correlation of clinical potency and in vitro effects. *Arch Dermatol Res.* 2006;298:23.

73. Aoki F, Nakagawa K, Kitano M, et al. Clinical safety of licorice flavonoid oil (LFO) and pharmacokinetics of glabridin in healthy humans. *J Am Coll Nutr.* 2007;26:209.

74. Bernardi M, D'Intino PE, Trevisan F, et al. Effects of prolonged ingestion of graded doses of licorice by healthy volunteers. *Life Sci.* 1994;55:863.

75. Hoffmann D. *Medical Herbalism: The Science and Practice of Herbal Medicine.* Rochester, VT: Healing Arts Press; 2003:555.

76. Gao W, Li K, Yan S, et al. Effects of space flight on DNA mutation and secondary metabolites of licorice (Glycyrrhiza uralensis Fisch.). *Sci China C Life Sci.* 2009;52:977.

77. Hao J, Sun Y, Wang Q, et al. Effect and mechanism of penetration enhancement of organic base and alcohol on glycyrrhetinic acid in vitro. *Int J Pharm.* 2010;399:102.

78. Mostafa DM, Ammar NM, Abd El-Alim SH, et al. Transdermal microemulsions of Glycyrrhiza glabra L.: characterization, stability and evaluation of antioxidant potential. *Drug Deliv.* 2014;21:130.

79. Evans FQ. The rational use of glycyrrhetinic acid in dermatology. *Br J Clin Pract.* 1958;12:269.

80. Okimasu E, Moromizato Y, Watanabe S, et al. Inhibition of phospholipase A2 and platelet aggregation by glycyrrhizin, an antiinflammation drug. *Acta Med Okayama.* 1983;37:385.

81. Di Mambro VM, Fonseca MJ. Assays of physical stability and antioxidant activity of a topical formulation added with different plant extracts. *J Pharm Biomed Anal.* 2005;37:287.

82. Veratti E, Rossi T, Giudice S, et al. 18beta-glycyrrhetinic acid and glabridin prevent oxidative DNA fragmentation in UVB-irradiated human keratinocyte cultures. *Anticancer Res*. 2011;31:2209.

83. Haraguchi H, Tanimoto K, Tamura Y, et al. Mode of antibacterial action of retrochalcones from Glycyrrhiza inflata. *Phytochemistry*. 1998;48:125.

84. Long DR. Mead J, Hendricks JM, et al. 18β-Glycyrrhetinic acid inhibits methicillin-resistant Staphylococcus aureus survival and attenuates virulence gene expression. *Antimicrob Agents Chemother*. 2013;57:241.

85. Craig WJ. Health-promoting properties of common herbs. *Am J Clin Nutr*. 1999;70:491S.

86. Rossi T, Benassi L, Magnoni C, et al. Effects of glycyrrhizin on UVB-irradiated melanoma cells. *In Vivo*. 2005;19:319.

87. Agarwal MK, Iqbal M, Athar M. Inhibitory effect of 18beta-glycyrrhetinic acid on 12-O-tetradecanoyl phorbol-13-acetate-induced cutaneous oxidative stress and tumor promotion in mice. *Redox Rep*. 2005;10:151.

88. Rahman S, Sultana S. Glycyrrhizin exhibits potential chemopreventive activity on 12-O-tetradecanoyl phorbol-13-acetate-induced cutaneous oxidative stress and tumor promotion in Swiss albino mice. *J Enzyme Inhib Med Chem*. 2007;22:363.

89. Schweiger D, Baufeld C, Drescher P, et al. Efficacy of a new tonic containing urea, lactate, polidocanol, and glycyrrhiza inflata root extract in the treatment of a dry, itchy, and subclinically inflamed scalp. *Skin Pharmacol Physiol*. 2013;26:108.

90. Wananukul S, Chatproedprai S, Charutragulchai W. Randomized, double-blind, split-side comparison study of moisturizer containing licochalcone vs. 1% hydrocortisone in the treatment of infantile seborrhoeic dermatitis. *J Eur Acad Dermatol Venereol*. 2012;26:894.

91. Shin YW, Bae EA, Lee B, et al. In vitro and in vivo antiallergic effects of Glycyrrhiza glabra and its components. *Planta Med*. 2007;73:257.

92. Pellati D, Fiore C, Armanini D, et al. In vitro effects of glycyrrhetinic acid on the growth of clinical isolates of Candida albicans. *Phytother Res*. 2009;23:572.

93. Kato T, Horie N, Matsuta T, et al. Anti-UV/HIV activity of Kampo medicines and constituent plant extracts. *In Vivo*. 2012;26:1007.

CHAPTER 68

Colloidal Oatmeal

Activities:

Anti-inflammatory, antipruritic, antioxidant, antimicrobial, anticholesterolemic, antidiabetic, immunomodulatory, neurotonic, wound healing[1]

Important Chemical Components:

Polysaccharides (particularly β-glucan), lipids, polyphenols (i.e., hydroxycinnamic acids such as caffeic, ferulic, p-coumaric, and sinapic acids; and avenanthramides), proteins, vitamin E, vitamin B complex, phytic acid[2–4]

Origin Classification:

This ingredient is natural. Organic forms exist. Derivatives of avenanthramides have been synthesized in the laboratory.

Personal Care Category:

Anti-inflammatory, moisturizer, cleanser, buffer, barrier protection, soothing agent

Recommended for the following Baumann Skin Types:

DSNW, DSPW, DSNT, and DSPT

SOURCE

Avena sativa (also known as oatstraw or wild oats, and *Jai* or *Javi* on the Indian subcontinent)[5] has a long history of traditional folk use, particularly as a poultice or soak, to alleviate pruritus and irritation related to dry skin conditions (Table 68-1).[6,7] As a cultivated plant, this annual cereal grain and member of the Poaceae (also known as Gramineae or true grasses) family, is grown for its seeds for multiple uses. In recent decades, colloidal oatmeal (CO), dehulled oats ground into a fine powder, has been used, typically in a bath, for purposes similar to the traditional ones, namely lessening the irritation and mild pruritus characteristic of eczema, insect bites, rashes, poison ivy, and other contact allergens.[8] CO has also been used for decades as an adjunct in the treatment of atopic dermatitis.[9]

TABLE 68-1
Pros and Cons of Colloidal Oatmeal

Pros	Con
Long history of traditional medical use	More research and clinical studies are necessary to ascertain full range of skin-protective properties (particularly against UV radiation)
One of the few natural products approved by the FDA for skin indications	
Published clinical trials support therapeutic use	

Generally, better benefits are seen with the use of oat fractions than whole oatmeal.[10]

Evidence suggests that CO, the modern version of the traditional elixir, is effective in protecting and repairing skin and hair damaged from environmental insults such as ultraviolet (UV) radiation, smoke, bacteria, and free radicals as well as alleviating cutaneous inflammation and discomfort.[10] In addition, CO appears to have the capacity to repair damage from other chemicals such as α-hydroxy acids, surfactants, and bleaches.[11]

A. sativa is also believed to promote the release of luteinizing hormone, which is integral in the production and release of sex hormones such as testosterone. This might account for its traditional use as an aphrodisiac and the origin of the expression "sowing wild oats."

HISTORY

The skin care application of *A. sativa* dates back earlier than 2000 BCE to its native Mediterranean region, particularly Egypt and the Arabian Peninsula, and oatstraw was widely cultivated in Europe by 2000 BCE.[6] Early references to the medical application of oats were made by Hippocrates (circa 460–370 BCE) and, later, by Dioscorides, Galen, and Pliny the Elder in the 1st century CE.[12–14] The use of oats as a food source has been traced to the 1st century CE.[10] As teas, food, and in baths, oats were used for centuries to treat anxiety, insomnia, and various cutaneous conditions, including burns and eczema.[15] Consumption of whole grain oats is now associated with a lower risk for coronary heart disease.[5,16]

In the 19th and early 20th centuries, oatmeal baths were frequently used for the treatment of pruritic inflammatory skin conditions, such as eczema and burns. A ready-to-use CO preparation, created by finely grinding and then boiling the oat to extract the colloidal substance, became available in 1945.[2,14] In the late 1950s, Dick and Sompayrac reported separately that CO baths were demonstrably effective in the management of pediatric atopic dermatitis.[17,18] As a component of the modern dermatologic armamentarium, CO has replaced rolled oats and plain oatmeal, and has been used for decades to ameliorate inflammatory and pruritic conditions. CO is composed of dehulled oats ground to a fine powder that retains the moisturizing effects of the whole oat grain and disperses more easily in bath water. It can also be added to creams and lotions for use in topical products.

CHEMISTRY

CO consists primarily of polysaccharides (60–85 percent), proteins and enzymes, such as superoxide dismutase (10–20 percent), lipids (3–11 percent), β-glucan (5 percent), fiber (5 percent), and avenanthramides (0.03 percent).[2,13] The remaining constituents include saponins, vitamins, flavonoids, and inhibitors of prostaglandin synthesis. Oat lipids contribute to the viscosity of CO and help decrease transepidermal water loss, a key factor in skin dryness.[19,20] Phenols in oatmeal contribute to the antioxidant and anti-inflammatory activity of the extract, and some oat phenols exhibit potent UV-absorbing properties.[14] Constituent saponins are responsible for most of the cleansing activity of oat.[14] In addition, oatmeal proteins exhibit emulsification, hydration, and antioxidant activity along with low foaming potential. CO proteins and polysaccharides bind to skin and provide a protective barrier to external insults. The proteins further act as a buffer against strong acids and bases.[21] The protective and water-retaining properties of CO are thought to result from its high concentration of starches (polysaccharides), particularly β-glucan.[14] Oat β-glucan is believed to be immunomodulatory.CO lotion application is also known to affect arachidonic acid, cytosolic phospholipase A_2, and tumor necrosis factor (TNF)-α pathways in exerting potent anti-inflammatory activity.[22] The biologic activity of oat compounds appears to be quite dynamic. The activity of whole oat flour is characterized as antioxidant, prostaglandin synthesis-inhibiting, cleansing, and protective in nature.

Avenanthramides

The therapeutic and cosmetic uses of oatmeal have been enhanced by the isolation and identification of specific oat components. Oatmeal has been found to contain 20 unique polypenolic alkaloids, avenanthramides, which act as phytoalexins, exhibiting antimicrobial properties that serve to protect the plant.[13] Found exclusively in oats, avenanthramides, which are substituted N-cinnamoylanthranilic acids with hydroxycinnamic acid and anthranilic acid moieties, have exhibited potent antioxidant activity *in vitro* and *in vivo* as well as anti-inflammatory, antiproliferative, and antipruritic activity.[4,16] This is not surprising insofar as phenolics, as a group, display a broad range of biologic activities including prevention of inflammation and oxidation.[23] In fact, phenolics are the strongest antioxidants found in nature,[24] although within this class of compounds, individual substances exert varying levels of antioxidant activity. Oat phenolic compounds including avenanthramides have been identified as potent antioxidants that scavenge reactive oxygen and nitrogen species.[23] Of the oat phenolics, avenanthramides are thought to manifest 10 to 30 times the antioxidant activity of other oat phenolics such as caffeic acid or vanillin.[25] Furthermore, they have been reported to inhibit prostaglandin biosynthesis nearly as well as the synthetic anti-inflammatory agent indomethacin.[26] Indeed, avenanthramides are now being credited with imparting many of the beneficial effects of CO.[27]

A 2007 study by Wallo et al. provided more evidence that avenanthramides evince potent anti-inflammatory activity. The investigators incubated keratinocytes with an inducer of proinflammatory interleukin (IL)-8 in the presence of vehicle or avenanthramides. The phenolic compounds diminished the release of the proinflammatory cytokine IL-8 by 10 to 25 percent.[28] Avenanthramides in topical formulations have also been shown in multiple preclinical and preliminary clinical studies to suppress the activity of nuclear factor-κB (NF-κB) and the release of proinflammatory cytokines and histamine, thus blocking the activation of inflammatory pathways in the skin.[20,27] In addition, avenanthramides have been demonstrated to mitigate skin irritation and erythema induced by exposure to UVB irradiation.[20]

After previously showing that avenanthramides significantly inhibited IL-1β-stimulated secretion of proinflammatory cytokines, such as IL-6, IL-8, and monocyte chemotactic protein (MCP)-1, by human aortic endothelial cells, Guo et al. showed in 2008 that oat polyphenols reduce the expression of endothelial proinflammatory cytokines, in part, via blocking NF-κB activation by suppressing the phosphorylation of the inhibitor of nuclear factor κB (IκB) complex (IKK) and IκB, and hindering proteasome activity.[3]

In 2008, Sur et al. found that avenanthramides, typically present in oats at approximately 300 parts per million (ppm), suppressed the degradation of IκB-α in keratinocytes in concentrations as low as 1 part per billion. In this *in vitro* study, they also found that avenanthramide-treated cells significantly inhibited TNF-α-induced NF-κB luciferase activity as well as IL-8 release. In murine models, the investigators showed that topically applied avenanthramides (in concentrations of 1–3 ppm) attenuated inflammation and diminished scratching. They concluded that avenanthramides are strong anti-inflammatory compounds that account for the anti-irritant activity manifested by oats.[13]

A year later, Lee-Manion et al. used assays to assess the antioxidant and antigenotoxic activity of synthetic avenanthramides, hydroxycinnamic acids, Tranilast, and ascorbic acid. They observed that N-(3',4'-dihydroxy-(E)-cinnamoyl)-5-hydroxyanthranilic acid, an avenanthramide compound found in copious amounts in oats, displayed the highest activity, indicating that avenanthramides possess antioxidant and antigenotoxic characteristics similar to those of ascorbic acid with the potential to deliver beneficial physiological effects.[4]

ORAL USES

A. sativa and oat products have been consumed since the 1st century CE.[10] Oatmeal is known for its calming effects when taken internally, and remains a staple typically among breakfast options particularly among health-conscious consumers.

TOPICAL USES

The combination of components and properties of CO renders it suitable for various uses in the care of inflammatory skin conditions, such as cleaning, moisturizing, protecting (i.e., barrier preservation), and relieving pruritus in inflamed skin. In fact, oatmeal is one of the few natural products recognized by the United States Food and Drug Administration (FDA) as an effective skin protectant.[29] As a consequence, CO is one of the few botanicals subject to FDA regulation.[29] The range of dermatologic applications for CO is extensive and includes adjunctive therapy in inflammatory and pruritic skin conditions such as atopic dermatitis; allergic and irritant contact dermatitis including contact to poison ivy, oak, and sumac; chicken pox; cercarial dermatitis; diaper dermatitis; epidermolysis bullosa; ichthyosis; insect bites; pediatric and senile dermatoses; prickly heat; pruritic conditions; psoriasis; rashes; sunburn; urticaria; and xerosis.[15,17,21,30,31] CO also prevents and repairs damage caused by environmental insults such as UV radiation, smoke, bacteria, and free radicals.[10] In addition, oatmeal baths are included in the accepted treatment arsenal for erythroderma, also known as exfoliative dermatitis, which affects the majority of the cutaneous surface.[32] Oatmeal extracts also confer modulating effects in the sodium lauryl sulfate skin irritancy model.

In a small study with 20 patients in 2007, the application of topical CO lotion (derived from *A. rhealba*®, which is a white oat cultivar of *A. sativa*) was shown to be effective in treating acneiform eruptions associated with the use of small-molecule tyrosine-kinase inhibitors in treating epidermal growth factor (EGFR)-positive cancers, thus facilitating continued neoplastic therapy.[22]

Further, Wu contends that CO is well suited as a treatment option for rosacea due to its barrier and skin-protective, antipruritic, anti-inflammatory, and antioxidant properties.[33]

Atopic Dermatitis

Several studies have shown that the daily use of CO-containing moisturizers and/or cleansers has significantly improved the symptoms of patients, from infants to those in their 60s, with mild-to-moderate atopic dermatitis and proven to be safe and well tolerated.[34]

In 2007, Grimalt et al. conducted a six-week randomized controlled study in 173 infants treated for inflammatory lesions with moderate- or high-potency topical corticosteroids to assess the effects of an oat extract-containing emollient on the amount of steroid needed for treatment. While the 7.5 percent lower use of moderate-strength corticosteroids in the emollient group compared to the control group was not significant, the oatmeal emollient treatment significantly decreased the use of high-potency topical corticosteroid use in infants with atopic dermatitis by 42 percent compared to controls.[35]

Also that year, Boussault et al. reported findings from a study of 302 prospectively recruited children with atopic dermatitis who were referred for allergy testing between June 2001 and December 2004. Various sensitivity tests revealed that oat sensitization in atopic children under the age of two who were seen for allergy testing was higher than the investigators expected. They speculated that repeated applications of oat-containing cosmetics on an already susceptible epidermal barrier may account for this phenomenon, concluding that such oat products should be avoided in infants with atopic dermatitis.[36]

SAFETY ISSUES

In 1997, the FDA, based on evidence that consumption of oatmeal or oat bran decreased low-density lipoproteins and total plasma cholesterol (largely attributed to its constituent β-glucan), approved the heart-health benefit claim on labels of food containing oat-soluble fiber.[5,16] Oatmeal is also one of the few natural products or ingredients acknowledged by the FDA as an effective skin protectant. Indeed, CO has been found to be safe, cosmetically stable, and nonirritating. With the issuance of its Over-The-Counter Final Monograph for Skin Protectant Drug Products issued in June 2003, the FDA began regulating CO as a skin protectant and its preparation is standardized in the United States Pharmacopeia.[14,37] It is also approved for use in Germany for inflammatory skin conditions.[6]

While rare, cases of allergic contact dermatitis and urticaria have been reported in reaction to the use of CO preparations.[38] No adverse drug interactions have been reported in association with CO.[39] Overall, oatmeal has an excellent safety profile in the treatment of dermatologic disorders.

In 2012, Criquet et al. performed a series of studies to examine the safety and efficacy of personal care products (i.e., creams, cleansers, and lotions) containing CO. They found a very low potential in these agents for engendering irritation and allergenic sensitization. Of 2,291 participants, one subject developed a persistent but dubious (because it was confirmed with the product but not with A. sativa) mild edema during the challenge phase in a test of 12 personal care products containing CO. In the induction phase of insult patch testing, 1 percent of subjects experienced similarly low-level reactions. The investigators also reported that skin moisturization was sustained in subjects with dry skin, extending to two weeks beyond discontinuation of the product. They noted that no allergies were documented in the 80 subjects observed following patch testing after in-use application or by consumers of 445,820 products sold during a three-year

period. Criquet and colleagues concluded that personal care products containing CO are safe and effective.[40]

ENVIRONMENTAL IMPACT

The environmental impact from the cultivation and commercial use of A. sativa is not well documented to the author's knowledge.

FORMULATION CONSIDERATIONS

Most oatmeal products come in the form of colloidal baths, but shampoos, soaps, body washes, shaving gels, and moisturizing lotions and creams are also prepared with oatmeal.[14]

USAGE CONSIDERATIONS

As part of a daily skin care regimen, CO is appropriate for cleansing (especially dry, sensitive, or atopic skin), moisturizing, and providing protection to the skin.

SIGNIFICANT BACKGROUND

In a literature review of in vitro, in vivo, and clinical studies of oatmeal preparations in 2012, Pazyar et al. found that oatmeal exhibits antioxidant and anti-inflammatory activity in its effective medical use for conditions including acneiform eruptions, atopic dermatitis, pruritus, and viral infections as well as in cosmetic formulations in providing photoprotection to the skin.[2] Cerio et al. have noted that CO has also demonstrated effectiveness in treating psoriasis and drug-induced rashes.[2,27]

Human Studies

In a 1997 double-blind, randomized patch study of two concentrations of colloidal oat and rice grains (0.007 and 0.7 percent), the products were applied topically to the backs of 65 Italian children between 6 months and 2 years old (of whom 43 were atopic and 22 were normal). Both topical colloidal grains showed efficacy as adjuncts in the treatment of mild atopic dermatitis, with no evidence of inducing sensitization.[9]

In a 2001 10-month assessor-blind clinical study to identify an adequate treatment to alleviate pruritus experienced by 35 acute burn patients, the comparative effectiveness of two shower and bath oils, one containing liquid paraffin with 5 percent CO and the other containing liquid paraffin, was evaluated. Analysis of patient assessments of pain (recorded twice daily) and the daily number of their antihistamine requests showed that the CO group reported significantly less pruritus and requested significantly less antihistamine.[41]

In an influential study on 12 healthy individuals, researchers evaluated the anti-inflammatory activity of two topically applied oatmeal extracts, A. sativa and A. rhealba®, using the sodium lauryl sulfate irritation model, finding that both extracts displayed preventive effects on skin irritation.[42]

Further, Boisnic et al. developed a clinical model of cutaneous inflammation involving the effects of an oatmeal extract oligomer on skin tissue fragments exposed to vasoactive intestinal peptide, a proinflammatory neuromediator. The application of the peptide augmented inflammation, which was significantly reduced by treatment with the oatmeal extract.[43]

Antioxidant Activity

In 2013, Feng et al. investigated the protective effect of oat bran extract by enzymatic hydrolysates on hydrogen peroxide (H_2O_2)-induced human dermal fibroblast injury. They found, using a 1,1-diphenyl-2-picrylhydrazyl (DPPH) radical-scavenging assay that peptide-rich oat bran extracts concentration-dependently exhibited direct antioxidant activity. Further, they showed that incubating human dermal fibroblasts with oat bran extracts for 24 hours prior to exposure led to the significant suppression of H_2O_2-induced damage, but simultaneously applying oat peptides with H_2O_2 did not yield a similar result. However, the oat pretreatment also markedly reversed the H_2O_2-induced reduction of superoxide dismutase as well as malondialdehyde inhibition. The investigators concluded that oat peptides have potent antioxidant properties and that oat peptide-rich extract warrants further study and consideration as an antioxidant functional food with the capacity to prevent or mitigate cutaneous aging when incorporated into skin care products.[44]

CONCLUSION

Oatmeal has a surprisingly long tradition in skin care and rare recognition by the FDA as a skin protectant. Over the last several decades, the amassed research and clinical evidence appear to bear out the anti-inflammatory and other protective activities ascribed to oats in folk medicine.

REFERENCES

1. Singh R, De S, Belkheir A. Avena sativa (Oat), a potential neutraceutical and therapeutic agent: An overview. *Crit Rev Food Sci Nutr.* 2013;53:126.
2. Pazyar N, Yaghoobi R, Kazerouni A, et al. Oatmeal in dermatology: A brief review. *Indian J Dermatol Venereol Leprol.* 2012;78:142.
3. Guo W, Wise ML, Collins FW, et al. Avenanthramides, polyphenols from oats, inhibit IL-1beta-induced NF-kappaB activation in endothelial cells. *Free Radic Biol Med.* 2008;44:415.
4. Lee-Manion AM, Price RK, Strain JJ, et al. In vitro antioxidant activity and antigenotoxic effects of avenanthramides and related compounds. *J Agric Food Chem.* 2009;57:10619.
5. Sadiq Butt M, Tahir-Nadeem M, Khan MK, et al. Oat: Unique among the cereals. *Eur J Nutr.* 2008;47:68.
6. Foster S. *An Illustrated Guide to 101 Medicinal Herbs: Their History, Use, Recommended Dosages, and Cautions.* Loveland, CO: Interweave Press; 1998:146–147.
7. Mills S, Bone K. *Principles and Practice of Phytotherapy.* London: Churchill Livingstone; 2000:154.
8. Reszko AE, Berson D, Lupo MP. Cosmeceuticals: Practical applications. *Dermatol Clin.* 2009;27:401.
9. Pigatto P, Bigardi A, Caputo R, et al. An evaluation of the allergic contact dermatitis potential of colloidal grain suspensions. *Am J Contact Dermat.* 1997;8:207.
10. Aburjai T, Natsheh FM. Plants used in cosmetics. *Phytother Res.* 2003;17:987.
11. Hart J, Polla C, Hull JC. Oat fractions. *Cosmet Toiletries.* 1998;113:45.
12. Wickens GE. *Economic Botany: Principles and Practice.* Norwell, MA: Kluwer Academic Publishers; 2001:168.
13. Sur R, Nigam A, Grote D, et al. Avenanthramides, polyphenols from oats, exhibit anti-inflammatory and anti-itch activity. *Arch Dermatol Res.* 2008;300:569.
14. Kurtz ES, Wallo W. Colloidal oatmeal: History, chemistry and clinical properties. *J Drug Dermatol.* 2007;6:167.
15. Baumann LS. Less-known botanical cosmeceuticals. *Dermatol Ther.* 2007;20:330.
16. Meydani M. Potential health benefits of avenanthramides of oats. *Nutr Rev.* 2009;67:731.
17. Dick LA. Colloidal emollient baths in pediatric dermatoses. *Arch Pediatr.* 1958;75:506.
18. Sompayrac LM, Ross C. Colloidal oatmeal in atopic dermatitis of the young. *J Fla Med Assoc.* 1959;45:1411.
19. Baumann L, Woolery-Lloyd H, Friedman A. "Natural" ingredients in cosmetic dermatology. *J Drugs Dermatol.* 2009;8:s5.
20. Castanedo-Tardan MP, Baumann L. Anti-inflammatory Agents. In Baumann L., Saghari S., Weisberg E. eds. *Cosmetic Dermatology: Principles and Practice.* 2nd ed. New York: McGraw-Hill; 2009:320–1.
21. Grais ML. Role of colloidal oatmeal in dermatologic treatment of the aged. *AMA Arch Derm Syphilol.* 1953;68:402.
22. Alexandrescu DT, Vaillant JG, Dasanu CA. Effect of treatment with a colloidal oatmeal lotion on the acneform eruption induced by epidermal growth factor receptor and multiple tyrosine-kinase inhibitors. *Clin Exp Dermatol.* 2007;32:71.
23. Chen CY, Milbury PE, Kwak HK, et al. Avenanthramides and phenolic acids from oats are bioavailable and act synergistically with vitamin C to enhance hamster and human LDL resistance to oxidation. *J Nutr.* 2004;134:1459.
24. Tsao R, Akhtar MH. Neutraceuticals and functional foods: I. Current trend in phytochemical antioxidant research. *J Food Agric Environ.* 2005;3:10.
25. Dimberg LH, Theander O, Lingnert H. Avenanthramides – A group of phenolic antioxidants in oats. *Cereal Chem.* 1993;70:637.
26. Saeed SA, Butt NM, McDonald-Gibson WJ, et al. Inhibitors of prostaglandin biosynthesis in extracts of oat (Avena sativa) seeds. *Biochem Soc Trans.* 1981;9:444.
27. Cerio R, Dohil M, Jeanine D, et al. Mechanism of action and clinical benefits of colloidal oatmeal for dermatologic practice. *J Drugs Dermatol.* 2010;9:1116.
28. Wallo W, Nebus J, Nystrand G. Agents with adjunctive potential in atopic dermatitis. *J Am Acad Dermatol.* 2007;56(Suppl 2):AB70. tract P712.
29. U.S. Food and Drug Administration. Title 21: Food and Drugs, Chapter 1: Food and Drug Administration Department of Health and Humans Services, Subchapter D: Drugs for human use, Part 347: Skin protectant drug products for over-the-counter human use. U.S. Dept of Health and Human Services, FDA;21 CFR347. April 1, 2007.
30. Smith GC. The treatment of various dermatoses associated with dry skin. *JSC Med Assoc.* 1958;54:282.
31. Dick LA. Colloidal emollient baths in geriatric dermatoses. *Skin (Los Angeles).* 1962;1:89.
32. Rothe MJ, Bernstein ML, Grant-Kels JM. Life-threatening erythroderma: Diagnosing and treating the "red man." *Clin Dermatol.* 2005;23:206.
33. Wu J. Treatment of rosacea with herbal ingredients. *J Drugs Dermatol.* 2006;5:29.
34. Fowler JF, Nebus J, Wallo W, et al. Colloidal oatmeal formulations as adjunct treatments in atopic dermatitis. *J Drugs Dermatol.* 2012;11:804.
35. Grimalt R, Mengeaud V, Cambazard F, et al. The steroid-sparing effect of an emollient therapy in infants with atopic dermatitis: A randomized controlled study. *Dermatology.* 2007;214:61.
36. Boussault P, Léauté-Labrèze C, Saubusse E, et al. Oat sensitization in children with atopic dermatitis: Prevalence, risks and associated factors. *Allergy.* 2007;62:1251.
37. Food and Drug Administration HHS. Skin protectant drug products for over-the-counter human use; final monograph. Final rule. *Fed Regist.* 2003 Jun 4;68(107):33362–81.
38. De Paz Arranz S, Pérez Montero A, Remón LZ, et al. Allergic contact urticaria to oatmeal. *Allergy.* 2002;57:1215.
39. Hoffmann D. *Medical Herbalism: The Science and Practice of Herbal Medicine.* Rochester, VT: Healing Arts Press; 2003:532.
40. Criquet M, Roure R, Dayan L, et al. Safety and efficacy of personal care products containing colloidal oatmeal. *Clin Cosmet Investig Dermatol.* 2012;5:183.
41. Matheson JD, Clayton J, Muller MJ. The reduction of itch during burn wound healing. *J Burn Care Rehabil.* 2001;22:76.
42. Vié K, Cours-Darne S, Vienne MP, et al. Modulating effects of oatmeal extracts in the sodium lauryl sulfate skin irritancy model. *Skin Pharmacol Appl Skin Physiol.* 2002;15:120.
43. Boisnic S, Branchet-Gumila MC, Coutanceau C. Inhibitory effect of oatmeal extract oligomer on vasoactive intestinal peptide-induced inflammation in surviving human skin. *Int J Tissue React.* 2003;25:41.
44. Feng B, Ma LJ, Yao JJ, et al. Protective effect of oat bran extracts on human dermal fibroblast injury induced by hydrogen peroxide. *J Zhejiang Univ Sci B.* 2013;14:97.

CHAPTER 69

Turmeric

Activities:

Antioxidant, anti-inflammatory, anticarcinogenic, antiviral, antibacterial, antifungal immunomodulatory, wound healing[1,2]

Important Chemical Components:

Curcuminoids (curcumin, the key constituent of which is diferuloylmethane, demethoxycurcumin, bisdemethoxycurcumin, cyclocurcumin); volatile oils (tumerone, atlantone, and zingiberone); heptanoids; turmerin, sugars, proteins, and resins[3-8]

Origin Classification:

This ingredient is natural. Organic forms exist. Curcumin can be isolated from *Curcuma longa* or synthesized in the laboratory.[9]

Personal Care Category:

Anti-inflammatory, anticancer

Recommended for the following Baumann Skin Types:

DRNW, DRPW, DSNW, DSPW, ORNW, ORPW, OSNW, and OSPW

TABLE 69-1
Pros and Cons of Turmeric

PROS	CONS
Long history of traditional medical use	Not easy to formulate in topical products without transferring yellowish pigment and strong smell
One of the most thoroughly researched of the spices	Poor oral bioavailability
Potent anti-inflammatory and antioxidant (at neutral or low – acidic – pH) activity	Poor solubility
Compelling anticancer evidence from *in vitro* and *in vivo* animal studies	Poor stability at alkaline, or high, pH
	Controlled clinical trials are needed to establish the topical efficacy of turmeric or curcumin in rosacea and photoaging

SOURCE

Native to the Indian subcontinent and Southeast Asia, turmeric (*Curcuma longa*), a member of the Zingiberaceae (ginger) family, is best known as a spice and coloring agent used primarily in Asian cuisine, particularly curry, and in prepared mustard, margarine, as well as carbonated and other beverages.[10] Turmeric is one of the best researched spices for pharmacologic application.[11] It is used as a preservative, aromatic, cosmetic ingredient, and in some traditional Indian communities as a topical burn treatment.[12] In fact, turmeric has long been used as an anti-inflammatory agent in various traditional medical systems (Table 69-1). Specifically, turmeric has been deployed in Ayurvedic medicine to treat sprains and edema due to injury.[11,13-15] It has also been used topically, orally, and by inhalation for anti-inflammatory action.[16] The rhizome of the curcuma plant is the portion used for medicinal purposes.[14]

In Samoa, the powdered rhizome of *C. longa* is sprinkled on newborn infants to mend the belly button after severing the umbilical cord; to prevent diaper rash; to maintain skin softness and resilience; and to treat, as a paste or poultice, skin ulcers and eruptions.[14] The wide array of modern dermatologic uses of turmeric and its principal active ingredient curcumin also includes prevention or treatment of psoriasis, acne, wounds, burns, eczema, photodamage, and photoaging.[17] The turmeric rhizome is used topically in Thailand to treat wounds, insect bites, ringworm, and bleeding.[11,18] It is also a popular medicinal plant in Nepal, and one of the top two medicinal plants for use in skin ailments and cosmetics in the northeastern Indian state of Assam.[19,20] Notably, curcumin is incorporated into cosmetics, particularly for those used in Hindu rituals and ceremonies.[10,21]

HISTORY

The turmeric rhizome has been used for medicinal purposes for thousands of years, with documented uses dating to 600 BCE in Assyria, where it was used in herbal therapy, and to ancient Rome, where the Greece-born physician Dioscorides (circa 40–90 CE) was said to have cited it.[22] Turmeric is believed to have been used for therapeutic purposes in Ayurvedic medicine as early as 1900 BCE and its use in traditional Chinese medicine dates back to ancient times.[2] The traditional uses in these medical systems, as well as Unani medicine, included treatment for inflammation, skin wounds, acne, skin rashes, warts, and liver disorders.[23,24] Turmeric was introduced into Europe during the 14th century.[25]

In 1815, Vogel and Pelletier were the first in modern history to report extracting a "yellow coloring-agent" from *C. longa*, which they named "curcumin."[10,26,27] In 1842, Vogel became the first to isolate curcumin, but he did not document its formula.[3,26] Although several scientists, including Daube and Ivanov, reported on possible structures in the ensuing decades, Lampe and Milobedzka, in 1910, became the first to identify the structure of curcumin ($C_{21}H_{20}O_6$) as diferuloylmethane.[3,26,28] Three years later, they became the first to synthesize the compound.[26] The first article to address the medical use of curcumin, specifically considering the effects on patients with biliary diseases, was published in *The Lancet* in 1937.[10,27] In a *Nature* article in 1949, Schraufstatter and Bernt identified antibacterial activity against *Mycobacterium tuberculosis*, *Salmonella paratyphi*, *Staphylococcus aureus*, and *Tricophyton gypseum* displayed by curcumin.[26,29] Over the ensuing 20 years, only five papers were published, but during the 1970s, antidiabetic, antioxidant, and anti-inflammatory properties of the polyphenolic compound were observed, and anticancer activity was displayed by curcumin and documented based on *in vitro* and *in vivo* models in the 1980s by Kuttan and colleagues.[26,30] In 1995, Singh and Aggarwal were the first to report that curcumin evinced anti-inflammatory activity by inhibiting nuclear factor (NF)-κB.[26,31] Over 6,400 research articles had been published on curcumin and included in the National Institutes of Health PubMed database as of early 2014, dating back to Schraufstatter and Bernt's 1949 article, with more than 6,000 published since 1980.

CHEMISTRY

Turmeric tubers contain curcuminoids: the most abundant (~77 percent) curcumin I [diferuloylmethane or bis(4-hydroxy-3-methoxyphenyl)-1,6-heptadiene-3,5-dione], curcumin II, or demethoxycurcumin (6–17 percent), curcumin III, or bisdemethoxycurcumin (0.3–3 percent), and curcumin IV, or cyclocurcumin (typically less abundant than curcumin III).[5,6,32] The key biologically active constituent of turmeric, curcumin I, or simply curcumin, is a small-molecular-weight naturally-occurring polyphenol found in the root of *C. longa* that confers a distinctive flavor and yellow color to food.[14,33–36] Curcumin is the lipid-soluble component of turmeric; turmerin is its water-soluble component.[8,37] Curcumin displays more acute anti-inflammatory effects when compared to the volatile oil fraction of turmeric.[38] Indeed, it has displayed great potency against acute inflammation,[13] and is associated with few adverse effects.[39] It is an exceedingly pleiotropic molecule with multiple disease targets related to the skin.[40]

Evidence compiled over the last several decades reveals that curcumin exhibits a broad array of biologic activities, such as anti-inflammatory, anticarcinogenic, antioxidant, antimicrobial, and wound healing.[15,41–44] These effects are mediated through the regulation of numerous signaling pathways, transcription factors, growth factors, inflammatory cytokines, protein kinases, adhesion molecules, apoptotic genes, angiogenesis regulators, and enzymes, such as cyclooxygenase (COX) and glutathione S-transferases.[45–47] But inhibition of NF-κB is thought to be the linchpin of the anti-inflammatory and antioxidant activity of the curcuminoid.[24] Curcumin is also known, at various levels, to suppress other signaling pathways such as transforming growth factor (TGF)-β and the mitogen-activated protein kinase pathway, in particular.[24,47] Further, it affects angiogenesis and cell–cell adhesion, and exerts immunomodulatory activity.[47] This broad range of biologic activity forms the basis for additional study of the potential applications of curcumin to prevent or treat photoaging and photocarcinogenesis.[48]

The anticarcinogenic characteristics of curcumin are particularly well documented as are its demonstrated antioxidant and lipid peroxidation properties.[8,21,44,49–52] Antibacterial, antiparasitic, and anti-HIV activities have also reportedly been manifested by turmeric or curcumin.[53] In 1987, an ethanol extract of turmeric and an ointment with curcumin as its active ingredient demonstrated efficacy in relieving patients of pruritus associated with external cancerous lesions.[54] In addition, curcumin reportedly has greater anti-inflammatory capacity than ibuprofen.[13,55] More importantly, it has been shown to protect against ultraviolet (UV)-induced photodamage by inhibiting inflammation and attenuating oxidative stress.[48] Curcumin is also a selective inhibitor of phosphorylase kinase, which fosters photocarcinogenesis in photodamaged skin by activating NF-κB signaling pathways and suppressing apoptosis of photodamaged cells.[56,57]

ORAL USES

Turmeric is consumed regularly in the diet, particularly in the Indian subcontinent. It is approved in Germany for the treatment of dyspepsia.[11] The systemic and topical use of turmeric for medicinal purposes is also officially sanctioned in Thailand.[11,18]

Curcumin is available in oral supplement form throughout the world.[10] When used orally, curcumin inhibits leukotriene formation as well as platelet aggregation and stabilizes neutrophilic lysosomal membranes, thus inhibiting inflammation at the cellular level.[58] Notably, it produces varying dose-dependent effects: at low dose curcumin can be a prostaglandin inhibitor, while at higher levels it stimulates the adrenal glands to secrete cortisone.[59] Overall, though, it is known to exhibit poor systemic bioavailability after oral administration, except in the gastrointestinal tract, where biologically active levels have been recorded in animal and human studies.[60,61] Low curcumin bioavailability to organs such as the skin partially accounts for the impetus for investigations into transdermal and other modes of delivery (see the Formulation Considerations section below).

In 2013, Ryan et al. conducted a randomized, double-blind, placebo-controlled clinical trial to evaluate the effects of oral curcumin on radiation dermatitis in 30 adult female breast cancer patients. They found that 6 g of daily intake of curcumin during radiotherapy mitigated radiation dermatitis.[61]

TOPICAL USES

A limited number of cosmetic products contain curcumin at the present time as its distinct and pungent aroma and color render it especially challenging to formulate into a cosmetically elegant product. More clinical trials are required to assess the influence of topical curcumin on human skin. Bioavailability in topical products has also been problematic. A recent examination of the inhibitory activity of encapsulated curcumin on UV-induced photoaging in mice represents the first clinical support for the topical delivery of curcumin to minimize the effects of photoaging.[62]

In 2013, Heng showed that the topical application of curcumin gel in the clinical setting yielded rapid healing of burns, nominal or no scarring, and also ameliorated various signs of photodamage, such as hyperpigmentation, solar elastosis, advanced solar lentigines, actinic poikiloderma, and actinic keratoses.[57] Curcumin is also thought to have a therapeutic role in eczema and scleroderma.[63]

SAFETY ISSUES

No adverse effects, drug interactions, or general contraindications have been reported in association with the oral use of turmeric.[11] Allergic reactions are thought to be rare. It has also been found to be safe in human trials.[16] The United States Food and Drug Administration, the Natural Health Products Directorate of Canada, and the Expert Joint Committee of the Food and Agriculture Organization/World Health Organization on food additives have deemed turmeric and curcumin food products safe for consumption.[10,64] Even at high doses, curcumin is characterized by a favorable safety profile for oral and cutaneous use.[65] The German Commission E does claim that the use of turmeric is contraindicated in patients whose biliary tract is obstructed.[22] Oral curcumin has been shown in animal models to inhibit the activity of some chemotherapy drugs and enhance the activity of others.[3] The National Cancer Institute in the United States has listed curcumin as one among approximately 35 plant-based foods [including genistein from soybeans, epigallocatechin gallate (ECGC) from green tea, resveratrol from grapes, and gingerol from ginger] to have cancer-preventive characteristics (see Chapter 45, Soy, Chapter 47, Green Tea, Chapter 50, Resveratrol, and Chapter 59, Ginger).[64]

ENVIRONMENTAL IMPACT

As a perennial spice plant, *C. longa* is cultivated extensively throughout India and Southeast Asia.[3] In fact, much of the world's turmeric is grown by India, which consumes approximately 90 to 95 percent of what is produced, with the remainder exported.[10] For investigations into its potential medical applications or incorporation into topical formulations, it is likely that a significant majority of the turmeric, and curcumin in particular, can be attributed to synthesis in the laboratory. Therefore, the environmental impact of turmeric in skin care products is likely not substantial.

FORMULATION CONSIDERATIONS

Topical curcumin is inexpensive, nontoxic, and safe.[12,28,66] However, given the undesirability of the yellow pigment and the strong smell being transferred to the skin via topical application, turmeric and curcumin have posed formulation challenges, though some authors believe new technologies may soon remedy this problem.[13] In fact, there are cosmetics containing curcumin available throughout the world, particularly India and Japan.[67] In addition, extensive research into more cosmetically elegant and biologically active delivery systems to achieve skin permeability is well underway. These options also address the instability of curcumin when exposed to light or heat, and loss of activity in storage.[68]

The myriad technologies, which merit continuing attention, include various forms of nanoencapsulation: β-cyclodextrin-curcumin nanoparticle complex in a hydrophilic matrix gel to foster skin permeability and enhanced bioavailability[60]; curcumin-loaded monoolein aqueous dispersions (for extended curcumin activity) and lecithin organogels for conditions requiring rapid curcumin activity, as percutaneous delivery systems[69,70]; curcumin-loaded micelles and thermosensitive hydrogels[71]; curcumin/xanthan:galactomannan hydrogels[72]; curcumin-loaded oleic acid-based polymeric bandages[73]; curcumin-loaded proniosomal gel bases[74]; *C. longa*-loaded vesicular systems (niosomes, liposomes, ethosomes, and transferomes) incorporated in cream formulations or carbopol gel or other curcuminoid niosomes[75–78]; turmeric oil in chitosan-alginate nanocapsules[79]; and curcumin in eucalyptol microemulsions.[80]

In 2012, Basnet et al. also showed that liposomal delivery of curcumin appears to have potential as an appropriate formulation for treating vaginal inflammation.[81] During the same year, Liu et al. found that curcumin-loaded myristic acid microemulsions were capable of inhibiting the growth of *Staphylococcus epidermidis* on neonate pig skin. They suggested that this combination of curcumin and myristic acid in a microemulsion carrier has potential as an option for treating conditions associated with *S. epidermidis* as well as acne.[82]

USAGE CONSIDERATIONS

Curcumin, in the form of a mouthwash used twice daily, was found in a small 2013 study of seven pediatric and young adult oncology patients to be safe, well tolerated, and effective in lowering pain scale scores associated with oral mucositis.[83] Over-the-counter products such as Johnson & Johnson's Band-Aids™ include turmeric for the Indian market.[25]

SIGNIFICANT BACKGROUND

In vitro studies have demonstrated that curcumin dose-dependently increases tumor cell apoptosis, slows cell growth, and lowers the number of clonogenic cells.[12] Topical curcumin has also been identified as one of the only safe therapies for radiation exposure and appears to be one of the only chemicals known to protect skin after exposure to radiation or during radiotherapy.[12] Also, curcumin is known, along with other curcuminoids, to inhibit fibrosis and has recently been shown to have potential as a chemopreventive agent to prevent or treat keloids.[84]

Antifungal activity was displayed by curcumin in a 2013 murine model study of oral candidiasis. Dovigo et al. showed that the phenolic substance worked as a photosensitizer in the photoinactivation of *Candida albicans*. They found that curcumin-mediated photodynamic therapy exerted antifungal effects without damaging the murine host tissue.[85]

In 2012, Takahashi et al. set out to identify plants with bioactive potential for dermatologic purposes by screening methanol extracts of 47 medical and edible plants cultivated in Okinawa, Japan. In testing for proliferative effects on skin fibroblast cells *in vitro*, the investigators reported that *C. longa* led to higher fibroblast proliferation than the control and augmented collagen production. They noted that, as compared to the positive control (ascorbic acid), expression of the collagen synthesis marker TGF-β1 was higher after *C. longa* treatment.[86] The ability of *C. longa* to increase fibroblast proliferation and increase collagen production could have implications for the use of curcumin in wound healing and photoprotection.

Curcumin has also been reported to hinder melanogenesis in B16 melanoma cells and been shown *in vitro* to inhibit melanogenesis in human melanocytes by activating the Akt/glycogen synthase kinase 3 (GSK 3β), extracellular signal-regulated kinase (ERK) or p38 MAPK signaling pathways. While more research is needed according to the authors Tu et al., their findings suggest the potential application of curcumin as a whitening agent for hyperpigmentation.[87]

Curcumin and Wound Healing

Wound closure was shown by Sidhu et al. to occur significantly faster in curcumin-treated normal and genetically diabetic animals as compared to controls. The improvement of neovascularization and reepithelialization, the increase of TGF-β1 and fibronectin expression and synthesis, and the reduction of apoptosis were cited as the mechanisms by which curcumin contributed to this enhanced healing effect.[88,89] Collagen deposition and fibroblast and vascular density have also been bolstered by curcumin treatment, enhancing normal as well as impaired wound healing. The observed proangiogenic effect of curcumin in wound healing has been attributed to the induction of TGF-β, which in turn spurs angiogenesis and the accumulation of extracellular matrix.[90]

In a study using Swiss albino mice, researchers assessed the effects on wound contraction of pretreatment with doses of 25, 50, 100, 150, or 200 mg/kg body weight of curcumin before exposure to 6 Gy whole-body γ-radiation. While irradiation resulted in delayed wound healing, curcumin pretreatment was associated with a dose-dependent increase in wound contraction in comparison to control, with optimal contraction noted with the 100 mg/kg dose. The authors concluded that curcumin shows great potential as a therapeutic agent for wound repair, particularly in reducing healing delays caused by radiation and involving combined injuries.[36]

A 2005 study by Kundu et al. compared the wound-healing capacity of fresh turmeric paste to that of honey and a control in full-thickness circular wounds in 18 rabbits (see Chapter 60, Honey/Propolis/Royal Jelly). The investigators found that compared to the control group, wound healing in animals in the turmeric and honey treatment groups was considerably more rapid, with statistically significant differences in healing time.[91]

C. longa was included in another polyherbal formulation that Gupta et al. investigated in 2008 for its effects in treating diabetic wound healing in rats. The preparation combined the aqueous lyophilized leaf extracts of *Hippophae rhamnoides* and *Aloe vera* along with the ethanol rhizome extract of *C. longa* (optimized ratio of 1:7:1) (see Chapter 65, Aloe Vera). The investigators found that the topically applied polyherbal formulation augmented cellular proliferation and collagen production at the wound site in normal rats as compared to positive controls. Wound contraction was accelerated in normal and streptozotocin-induced diabetic rats, and the formulation was found to have fostered angiogenesis.[92]

In 2009, Bhagavathula et al. examined the effects of a combination of topical curcumin and ginger extracts on wound healing in corticosteroid-impaired hairless rats (see Chapter 59, Ginger). For 21 days, the researchers treated animals with a combination of 10 percent curcumin and 3 percent ginger extract or each herbal agent alone, followed by a 15-day period of topical application of the corticosteroid Temovate. Superficial abrasions were induced in the treated skin after the treatment period. Healing was more rapid in the skin of control animals compared to animals treated only with Temovate, and in all of the groups pretreated with botanicals compared to animals treated with Temovate and vehicle alone. Skin samples obtained at wound closure revealed that collagen synthesis was higher and matrix metalloproteinase (MMP)-9 synthesis lower in rats treated with the herbal combination as opposed to those treated with Temovate and vehicle.[93]

In 2011, López-Jornet et al. conducted a prospective, randomized study with mice to evaluate the effects of topical curcumin on skin wounds induced by CO_2 laser. Three groups of 30 mice, each given three wounds, were divided into a control group that received no treatment, a vehicle group (which received 5 mg/day per wound of vehicle), and the treatment group that received 5 mg/day per wound of topical curcumin. After seven days, 73.33 percent of the curcumin-treated wounds displayed complete reepithelialization whereas 41.67 percent in the vehicle group and 37.50 percent in the control group showed such improvement. All wounds in the curcumin group were healed after 14 days.[94]

The topical application of curcumin was shown by Kulac et al. to be effective in accelerating wound healing of burns in Wistar albino rats, with enhanced collagen deposition, angiogenesis, granulation tissue formation, and epithelialization.[95]

C. longa is one of four herbs combined in a Thai herbal phytopharmaceutical agent that Chusri et al. found in 2013 to exert strong antibacterial activities *in vitro* against methicillin-resistant *Staphylococcus aureus* (MRSA) isolates as well as anti-inflammatory and antioxidant activities and low toxicity on Vero cells. They concluded that given such potent properties, this formulation is suitable for use in treating wounds.[96]

Also that year, Chereddy et al. demonstrated using a mouse excisional wound model that a combination of poly(lactic-co-glycolic) acid (PLGA) and curcumin nanoparticles exhibited twofold greater wound-healing activity compared to PLGA or curcumin alone.[97]

Psoriasis

The anti-inflammatory potency of curcumin is considered a potential source for psoriasis therapy. A small study with 12 patients taking curcumin orally showed a low response rate.[98,99] Nevertheless, curcumin has displayed effectiveness in treating psoriasis.[28,66,100]

An *in vitro* study in 2011 by Saelee et al., who had previously shown that three Thai medicinal herbs, including *C. longa*, had antipsoriatic activity, considered the psoriasis-inhibiting potential of these herbs through the regulation of NF-κB signaling biomarkers. Specifically, they analyzed the influence of *C. longa*, *Alpinia galangal*, and *Annona squamosa* on 10 genes of the NF-κB signaling network in HaCaT cells. The investigators found that all of the herbs tested appear to have the capacity to suppress psoriasis by controlling the expression of NF-κB signaling biomarkers, with *C. longa* found to significantly reduce CSF-1, interleukin (IL)-8, NF-κB1, NF-κB2, and RelA expression.[101]

In 2012, Sun et al. found *in vitro* that curcumin reversed the antiapoptotic action of tumor necrosis factor (TNF)-α, thus allowing for the induction of apoptosis in HaCaT cells treated with TNF-α. Their findings, they suggested, provide encouragement for the use of curcumin in psoriasis treatment.[56] The following year, Sun et al. used a mouse model to determine that the topical application of curcumin suppressed imiquimod-induced psoriasis-like inflammation. They deduced that the polyphenol was able to alter the IL-23/IL-17A cytokine axis, which serves a crucial function in psoriasis etiology, by suppressing IL-1β/IL-6 and then obliquely downregulating the synthesis of IL-17A/IL-22. These effects, which were similar to those of clobetasol, reinforced the authors' belief that curcumin will have a role to play in the psoriasis armamentarium.[102]

Antioxidant and Anti-inflammatory Activities of Curcumin

Curcumin is a potent scavenger of various reactive oxygen species (ROS), including superoxide anion radicals, hydroxyl radicals, and nitrogen dioxide radicals at neutral and acidic pH levels.[47,54] It is thought to exhibit 10-fold the potency of vitamin E as an antioxidant [see Chapter 56, Tocopherol (Vitamin E)].[28] The turmeric constituent has manifested particularly high reactivity toward peroxyl radicals.[103] In mouse models, curcumin has been shown to impart antioxidant and anti-inflammatory activity, indicating that curcumin has a beneficial effect against chemo- and photocarcinogenesis. More research is needed to ascertain whether topical applications or oral intake of curcumin can prevent or inhibit skin carcinogenesis in humans.[51,104,105]

Several studies have shown that curcumin displays broad inhibitory action against phospholipase, lipoxygenase, COX-2, leukotrienes, thromboxane, prostaglandins, nitric oxide, collagenase, elastase, hyaluronidase, monocyte chemoattractant protein (MCP)-1, interferon-inducible protein, TNF-α, and IL-12.[16]

A 2001 study on wound healing revealed that the antioxidant effects of curcumin potently inhibited hydrogen peroxide-induced damage in cultured human keratinocytes and fibroblasts.[44]

The anti-inflammatory potency of curcumin was apparent in the results of a 2012 randomized, double-blind trial among 96 male

Iranian veterans with chronic sulphur mustard-induced pruritic skin lesions. Panahi et al. found that curcumin supplementation attenuated inflammation and pruritus in these patients, with significant increases in serum IL-8 and high-sensitivity C-reactive protein, and decreases in calcitonin gene-related peptide; substantial improvements in quality of life were also reported.[106]

In 2013, Thongrakard et al. examined the protective effects on human keratinocytes of extracts of 15 Thai herb species against UVB-induced DNA damage and cytotoxicity. Analysis revealed that the highest antioxidant activity was exhibited by the dichloromethane extract of turmeric. Further, the ethanol extract of turmeric and the dichloromethane extract of ginger demonstrated the maximum UV absorptions and stimulated the production of the antioxidant protein thioredoxin 1, as well as the capacity to protect human keratinocytes from the deleterious effects of UV exposure. The investigators concluded that their findings suggest the viability of incorporating turmeric and ginger extracts into anti-UV cosmetic formulations.[107]

Curcumin, Skin Cancer, and Photoaging

While the anti-inflammatory activity of turmeric and, more recently, curcumin has been the focus of most of its medical applications through the millennia, the preponderance of modern research on curcumin seems to pertain to its anticarcinogenic capacity. In 1988, Huang et al. evaluated the effects of topically applied curcumin as well as caffeic, chlorogenic, and ferulic acids on 12-*O*-tetradecanoylphorbol-13-acetate (TPA)-induced epidermal ornithine decarboxylase (ODC) activity, epidermal DNA synthesis, and skin tumor promotion in female CD-1 mice. Results showed that ODC activity was inhibited by 42 percent in the case of caffeic acid (91 percent by curcumin, 46 percent by ferulic acid, and 25 percent by chlorogenic acid). Curcumin was more successful than the hydroxycinnamic acids in suppressing TPA-promoted DNA synthesis, and more effectively inhibited the number of TPA-induced tumors per mouse after twice weekly topical application with TPA after previous initiation with 7,12-dimethylbenz[a]anthracene (DMBA) (98 percent inhibition by curcumin, 60 percent by chlorogenic acid, 35 percent by ferulic acid, and 28 percent by caffeic acid).[51]

In various animal models, topical application of curcumin has been shown to inhibit initiation and promotion of tumorigenesis. Specifically, curcumin has been shown to block the growth in a broad range of tumors initiated by benzo[a]pyrene (B[a]P) and in TPA-induced or TPA-promoted skin tumors in mice.[34,35] Topical application of curcumin was shown in the early 1990s to exhibit antimutagenic and anticarcinogenic properties, specifically displaying potent inhibitory effects on TPA-induced tumor promotion and DNA synthesis as well as TPA-induced ODC activity and inflammation in mouse skin,[51,104,108] reversing the UVA-enhancing effects of ODC induction.[67] The phytochemical isolate from turmeric has also exhibited significant inhibitory activity against arachidonic acid-induced inflammation *in vivo* in mouse skin and edema of mouse ears, and epidermal lipoxygenase and COX *in vitro*.[34,50,104]

In addition, very low doses of topically applied curcumin have been found to mediate TPA-induced oxidation of DNA bases in the epidermis and tumor promotion in the skin.[109] Pretreatment with curcumin has exhibited the same inhibitory effects on TPA-mediated dermatitis.[67]

An evaluation of four nutraceuticals for their comparative effectiveness against DMBA-initiated and croton oil-promoted skin tumors showed that the topical application of turmeric rhizomes one hour before croton oil exposure resulted in decreases in skin tumor incidence and number of skin tumors, and later onset of skin tumors (30 percent skin tumor incidence, 87.2 percent decrease in skin tumors, and a five-week delay in skin tumor formation) compared with the positive control.[110] Previously, a dose- and time-dependent anticarcinogenic effect of dietary turmeric had been demonstrated on B[a]P-induced forestomach neoplasia and DMBA-induced skin tumorigenesis in female Swiss mice.[111]

Curcumin and its derivatives have been shown in animal models to inhibit the progression of chemically-induced colon and skin cancers. A study of the capacity of curcumin to inhibit the proliferation of primary endothelial cells in the presence and absence of basic fibroblast growth factor (bFGF), and the proliferation of an immortalized endothelial cell line revealed that curcumin imparts direct antiangiogenic activity *in vitro* and *in vivo*, which the researchers believe may account for its cancer-retarding effects in diverse organs.[33]

Other promising findings related to skin cancer include the demonstrated potency of curcumin to potently inhibit the glutathione S-transferase activity towards 1-chloro-2, 4-dinitrobenzene in intact human IGR-39 melanoma cells and its capacity to induce apoptosis in human basal cell carcinoma cells in a dose- and time-dependent manner.[112,113] The molecular mechanisms of action underlying its chemopreventive effects remain undetermined,[114] but in recent research using female ICR mice, investigators found that the topical application of curcumin was associated with the suppression of COX-2 expression by inhibiting ERK activity and NF-κB activation. The researchers believe this may account for the molecular mechanisms that would explain the antitumorigenic effects of curcumin in mouse skin.[114]

In numerous tumor model systems, including skin neoplastic models, curcumin has demonstrated the capacity to inhibit carcinogenesis.[50,111,115] Although its mechanism of action has not been clearly elucidated, curcumin is believed to inhibit cancer initiation, promotion, and progression.[116] In addition, curcumin is known to suppress UVA-induced metallothionein (MT) expression and ODC activity, and to initiate p53-mediated apoptosis, as well as cell membrane-mediated apoptosis through Fas receptor induction and caspase-8 activation.[113,117] Curcumin is also known to be a selective noncompetitive inhibitor of phosphorylase kinase, which fosters photocarcinogenesis in photodamaged skin by activating NF-κB signaling pathways and suppressing apoptosis of photodamaged cells.[56,57]

Recent data suggest a paradoxical aspect to curcumin properties, though. The anticancer activity of the antioxidant has actually promoted the generation of ROS. Chen et al. investigated the antioxidant and anticancer activity of curcumin in human myeloid leukemia (HL-60) cells, finding that the anticancer activity of curcumin was effective in a concentration- and time-dependent manner in lowering the proliferation and viability of leukemia cells, but its effect on ROS depended on concentration. Low concentrations of curcumin reduced ROS generation, but high concentrations yielded the opposite effect. The researchers also found that adding water-soluble antioxidants amplified the antioxidant and anticancer activity of low curcumin concentrations.[118]

In 2009, Sumiyoshi and Kimura examined the effects of a turmeric extract on a cascade of long-term, low-dose UVB exposure in melanin-possessing hairless mice. The researchers found that the polyphenol administered twice daily prevented chronic UVB exposure from enhancing skin thickness and diminishing skin elasticity. Further, the extract thwarted the development of wrinkles and melanin and inhibited the expression of MMP-2.[23]

In a 2010 review article, Heng found that curcumin has shown the capacity to inhibit multiple targets on signaling pathways thus blunting the effects of UV-induced skin aging and carcinogenesis.[48]

Chatterjee and Pandey reported in 2011 that the combination of tamoxifen and curcumin shows potential as chemotherapy. Specifically, they found *in vitro* that chemoresistant melanoma sensitized by tamoxifen to low-dose curcumin resulted in apoptosis and autophagy of melanoma cells while noncancerous cells were unaffected.[1]

Based on experiments in 2011 indicating that curcumin suppressed cutaneous squamous cell carcinoma xenograft growth in SCID mice, Phillips et al., in 2013, performed a randomized experimental study using SKH-1 mice to test the anticancer effects of curcumin.[119] For 14 days, animals were pretreated with oral or topical curcumin or oral or topical control. For 24 weeks, mice were exposed to UVB three times weekly or not at all. No significant differences were observed between groups receiving oral or topical curcumin. Control mice exhibited significantly shorter time to tumor onset and significantly greater tumor formation than the curcumin groups. The researchers concluded that curcumin manifests appreciable chemopreventive potential against skin cancer that warrants investigation in human subjects.[120]

In the previous year, some of the same researchers found that a topical curcumin-based cream was equally effective as dietary curcumin in exerting antiproliferative effects in an aggressive skin cancer cell line tested in a mouse skin cancer model. The investigators, noting that their study was the first to compare topical and oral curcumin, concluded that the turmeric constituent merits use as a chemopreventive agent for cutaneous squamous cell carcinoma particularly when condemned skin is an issue.[121]

Tsai et al. also demonstrated in 2012 that topical application of curcumin to SKH-1 hairless mice delivered significant protective effects against UVB-induced skin tumor formation. Delays in tumor emergence and growth and limited tumor size resulted from the topical application of curcumin before UVB exposure. A significant decline in UVB-induced thymine dimer-positive cells and apoptotic sunburn cells and an increase in p53 and p21/Cip1-positive epidermal cells, among other changes, were generated when curcumin was applied topically before and immediately after a single dose of UVB radiation (180 mJ/cm^2). Curcumin was also found to have significantly suppressed levels of NF-κB, COX-2, prostaglandin E$_2$, and nitric oxide.[122]

In 2013, Hwang et al. found in an *in vitro* investigation using human dermal fibroblast cells that curcumin blocked the UVB-induced expression of MMP-1 and MMP-3 as well as ROS generation, the activation of NF-κB and activator protein-1, and the phosphorylation of p38 and c-Jun N-terminal kinase. The researchers concluded that the potent inhibitory anti-inflammatory activity of curcumin suggests its potential utility in the prevention and treatment of photoaging.[123]

CONCLUSION

The body of research on turmeric and curcumin is increasingly impressive, revealing great potential especially related to its anticarcinogenic and anti-inflammatory activity. Of course, more clinical research is necessary to determine how these promising findings may be applied effectively in the dermatologic armamentarium. The traditional dietary and medical uses of the *C. longa* rhizome provide additional evidence that researchers are moving in the right direction here. Indeed, there appears to be sufficient data to suggest that the potential medical applications of turmeric may certainly prompt some people to pay much more attention to their spice racks.

REFERENCES

1. Chatterjee SJ, Pandey S. Chemo-resistant melanoma sensitized by tamoxifen to low dose curcumin treatment through induction of apoptosis and autophagy. *Cancer Biol Ther*. 2011;11:216.
2. Aggarwal BB, Sundaram C, Malani N, et al. Curcumin: The Indian solid gold. *Adv Exp Med Biol*. 2007;595:1.
3. Jurenka JS. Anti-inflammatory properties of curcumin, a major constituent of Curcuma longa: A review of preclinical and clinical research. *Altern Med Rev*. 2009;14:141.
4. Cohly HH, Taylor A, Angel MF, et al. Effect of turmeric, turmerin and curcumin on H$_2$O$_2$-induced renal epithelial (LLC-PK1) cell injury. *Free Radic Biol Med*. 1998;24:49.
5. Goel A, Kunnumakkara AB, Aggarwal BB. Curcumin as "Curecumin": From kitchen to clinic. *Biochem Pharmacol*. 2008;75:787.
6. Kiuchi F, Goto Y, Sugimoto N, et al. Nematocidal activity of turmeric: Synergistic action of curcuminoids. *Chem Pharm Bull (Tokyo)*. 1993;41:1640.
7. Thornfeldt C. Cosmeceuticals containing herbs: Fact, fiction, and future. *Dermatol Surg*. 2005;31:873.
8. Reddy AC, Lokesh BR. Effect of dietary turmeric (Curcuma longa) on iron-induced lipid peroxidation in the rat liver. *Food Chem Toxicol*. 1994;32:279.
9. Haukvik T, Bruzell E, Kristensen S, et al. Photokilling of bacteria by curcumin in selected polyethylene glycol 400 (PEG 400) preparations. Studies on curcumin and curcuminoids, XLI. *Pharmazie*. 2010;65:600.
10. Strimpakos AS, Sharma RA. Curcumin: Preventive and therapeutic properties in laboratory studies and clinical trials. *Antioxid Redox Signal*. 2008;10:511.
11. Foster S. *An Illustrated Guide to 101 Medicinal Herbs: Their History, Use, Recommended Dosages, and Cautions*. Loveland, CO: Interweave Press; 1998:200–1.
12. Kerr C. Curry ingredient protects skin against radiation. *Lancet Oncol*. 2002;3:713.
13. Rico MJ. Rising drug costs: The impact on dermatology. *Skin Therapy Lett*. 2000;5:1.
14. Aburjai T, Natsheh FM. Plants used in cosmetics. *Phytother Res*. 2003;17:987.
15. Ammon HP, Wahl MA. Pharmacology of Curcuma longa. *Planta Med*. 1991;57:1.
16. Chainani-Wu N. Safety and anti-inflammatory activity of curcumin: A component of tumeric (Curcuma longa). *J Altern Complement Med*. 2003;9:161.
17. *PCT Intl Appl*. 1999;WO9942094:76.
18. Jankasem M, Wuthi-Udomlert M, Gritsanapan W. Antidermatophytic properties of Ar-turmerone, turmeric oil, and Curcuma long preparations. *ISRN Dermatol*. 2013;2013:250597.
19. Singh AG, Kumar A, Tewari DD. An ethnobotanical survey of medicinal plants used in Terai forest of western Nepal. *J Ethnobiol Ethnomed*. 2012;8:19.
20. Saikia AP, Ryakala VK, Sharma P, et al. Ethnobotany of medicinal plants used by Assamese people for various skin ailments and cosmetics. *J Ethnopharmacol*. 2006;106:149.
21. Scartezzini P, Speroni E. Review on some plants of Indian traditional medicine with antioxidant activity. *J Ethnopharmacol*. 2000;71:23.
22. Mills S, Bone K. *Principles and Practice of Phytotherapy*. London: Churchill Livingstone; 2000:569–78.
23. Sumiyoshi M, Kimura Y. Effects of a turmeric extract (Curcuma longa) on chronic ultraviolet B irradiation-induced skin damage in melanin-possessing hairless mice. *Phytomedicine*. 2009;16:1137.
24. Thangapazham RL, Sharad S, Maheshwari RK. Skin regenerative potentials of curcumin. *Biofactors*. 2013;39:141.
25. Hatcher H, Planalp R, Cho J, et al. Curcumin: From ancient medicine to current clinical trials. *Cell Mol Life Sci*. 2008;65:1631.
26. Gupta SC, Patchva S, Koh W, et al. Discovery of curcumin, a component of golden spice, and its miraculous biological activities. *Clin Exp Pharmacol Physiol*. 2012;39:283.
27. Aggarwal BB, Sung B. Pharmacological basis for the role of curcumin in chronic diseases: An age-old spice with modern targets. *Trends Pharmacol Sci*. 2009;30:85.
28. Shishodia S, Sethi G, Aggarwal BB. Curcumin: Getting back to the roots. *Ann N Y Acad Sci*. 2005;1056:206.
29. Schraufstatter E, Bernt H. Antibacterial action of curcumin and related compounds. *Nature*. 1949;164:456.
30. Kuttan R, Bhanumathy P, Nirmala K, et al. Potential anticancer activity of turmeric (Curcuma longa). *Cancer Lett*. 1985;29:197.

31. Singh S, Aggarwal BB. Activation of transcription factor NF-kappaB is suppressed by curcumin (diferuloylmethane). *J Biol Chem*. 1995;270:24995.

32. Ruby J, Kuttan G, Babu KD, et al. Anti-tumor and antioxidant activity of natural curcuminoids. *Cancer Lett*. 1995;94:79.

33. Arbiser JL, Klauber N, Rohan R, et al. Curcumin is an in vivo inhibitor of angiogenesis. *Mol Med*. 1998;4;376.

34. Huang MT, Newmark HL, Frenkel K. Inhibitory effects of curcumin on tumorigenesis in mice. *J Cell Biochem Suppl*. 1997;27:26.

35. Chendil D, Ranga RS, Meigooni D, et al. Curcumin confers radiosensitizing effect in prostate cancer cell line PC-3. *Oncogene*. 2004;23:1599.

36. Jagetia GC, Rajanikant GK. Effect of curcumin on radiation-impaired healing of excisional wounds in mice. *J Wound Care*. 2004;13:107.

37. Cohly HH, Taylor A, Angel MF, et al. Effect of turmeric, turmerin and curcumin on H_2O_2-induced renal epithelial (LLC-PK1) cell injury. *Free Radic Biol Med*. 1998;24:49.

38. Arora RB, Kapoor V, Basu N, et al. Anti-inflammatory studies on Curcuma longa (turmeric). *Indian J Med Res*. 1971;59:1289.

39. Rao TS, Basu N, Siddiqui HH. Anti-inflammatory activity of curcumin analogues. *Indian J Med Res*. 1982;75:574.

40. Basnet P, Skalko-Basnet N. Curcumin: An anti-inflammatory molecule from a curry spice on the path to cancer treatment. *Molecules*. 2011;16:4567.

41. Maheshwari RK, Singh AK, Gaddipati J, et al. Multiple biological activities of curcumin: A short review. *Life Sci*. 2006;78:2081.

42. Sharma OP. Antioxidant activity of curcumin and related compounds. *Biochem Pharmacol*. 1975;25:1811.

43. Surh Y. Molecular mechanisms of chemopreventive effects of selected dietary and medicinal phenolic substances. *Mutat Res*. 1999;428:305.

44. Phan TT, See P, Lee ST, et al. Protective effects of curcumin against oxidative damage on skin cells in vitro: Its implication for wound healing. *J Trauma*. 2001;51:927.

45. Aggarwal BB, Kumar A, Bharti AC. Anticancer potential of curcumin: Preclinical and clinical studies. *Anticancer Res*. 2003;23:363.

46. Surh YJ, Han SS, Keum YS, et al. Inhibitory effects of curcumin and capsaicin on phorbol ester-induced activation of eukaryotic transcription factors, NF-kappaB and AP-1. *Biofactors*. 2000;12:107.

47. Sharma RA, Gescher AJ, Steward WP. Curcumin: The story so far. *Eur J Cancer*. 2005;41:1955.

48. Heng MC. Curcumin targeted signaling pathways: Basis for anti-photoaging and anti-carcinogenic therapy. *Int J Dermatol*. 2010;49:608.

49. Ozaki K, Kawata Y, Amano S, et al. Stimulatory effect of curcumin on osteoclast apoptosis. *Biochem Pharmacol*. 2000;59:1577.

50. Huang MT, Lysz T, Ferraro T, et al. Inhibitory effects of curcumin on in vitro lipoxygenase and cylcooxygenase activities in mouse epidermis. *Cancer Res*. 1991;51:813.

51. Huang MT, Smart RC, Wong CQ, et al. Inhibitory effect of curcumin, chlorogenic acid, caffeic acid, and ferulic acid on tumor promotion in mouse skin by 12-O-tetradecanoylphorbol-13-acetate. *Cancer Res*. 1988;48:5941.

52. Unnikrishnan MK, Rao MN. Inhibition of nitrite induced oxidation of hemoglobin by curcuminoids. *Pharmazie*. 1995;50:490.

53. Mazumder A, Raghavan K, Weinstein J, et al. Inhibition of human immunodeficiency virus type-1 integrase by curcumin. *Biochem Pharmacol*. 1995;49:1165.

54. Kuttan R, Sudheeran PC, Josph CD. Turmeric and curcumin as topical agents in cancer therapy. *Tumori*. 1987;73:29.

55. Srimal RC, Dhawan BN. Pharmacology of diferuloyl methane (curcumin), a non-steroidal anti-inflammatory agent. *J Pharm Pharmacol*. 1973;25:447.

56. Sun J, Han J, Zhao Y, et al. Curcumin induces apoptosis in tumor necrosis factor-alpha-treated HaCaT cells. *Int Immunopharmacol*. 2012;13:170.

57. Heng MC. Signaling pathways targeted by curcumin in acute and chronic injury: Burns and photo-damaged skin. *Int J Dermatol*. 2013;52:531.

58. Srivastava R. Inhibition of neutrophil response by curcumin. *Agents Actions*. 1989;28:298.

59. Srivastava R, Srimal RC. Modification of certain inflammation-induced biochemical changes by curcumin. *Indian J Med Res*. 1985;81:215.

60. Rachmawati H, Edityaningrum CA, Mauludin R. Molecular inclusion complex of curcumin-β-cyclodextrin nanoparticle to enhance

61. curcumin skin permeability from hydrophilic matrix gel. *AAPS PharmSciTech*. 2013;14:1303.

61. Ryan JL, Heckler CE, Ling M, et al. Curcumin for radiation dermatitis: A randomized, double-blind, placebo-controlled clinical trial of thirty breast cancer patients. *Radiat Res*. 2013;180:34.

62. Agrawal R, Kaur IP. Inhibitory effect of encapsulated curcumin on ultraviolet-induced photoaging in mice. *Rejuvenation Res*. 2010;13:397.

63. Aggarwal BB, Harikumar KB. Potential therapeutic effects of curcumin, the anti-inflammatory agent, against neurodegenerative, cardiovascular, pulmonary, metabolic, autoimmune and neoplastic diseases. *Int J Biochem Cell Biol*. 2009;41:40.

64. Saha S, Adhikary A, Bhattacharyya P, et al. Death by design: Where curcumin sensitizes drug-resistant tumours. *Anticancer Res*. 2012;32:2567.

65. Nguyen TA, Friedman AJ. Curcumin: A novel treatment for skin-related disorders. *J Drugs Dermatol*. 2013;12:1131.

66. Shehzad A, Rehman G, Lee YS. Curcumin in inflammatory diseases. *Biofactors*. 2013;39:69.

67. Gupta S, Mukhtar H. Chemoprevention of skin cancer through natural agents. *Skin Pharmacol Appl Skin Physiol*. 2001;14:373.

68. Suwannateep N, Wanichwecharungruang S, Haag SF, et al. Encapsulated curcumin results in prolonged curcumin activity in vitro and radical scavenging activity ex vivo on skin after UVB-irradiation. *Eur J Pharm Biopharm*. 2012;82:485.

69. Esposito E, Ravani L, Mariani P, et al. Effect of nanostructured lipid vehicles on percutaneous absorption of curcumin. *Eur J Pharm Biopharm*. 2013 Dec 20. [Epub ahead of print]

70. Puglia C, Cardile V, Panico AM, et al. Evaluation of monooleine aqueous dispersions as tools for topical administration of curcumin: Characterization, in vitro and ex-vivo studies. *J Pharm Sci*. 2013;102:2349.

71. Gong C, Wu Q, Wang Y, et al. A biodegradable hydrogel system containing curcumin encapsulated in micelles for cutaneous wound healing. *Biomaterials*. 2013;34:6377.

72. Da-Lozzo EJ, Moledo RC, Faraco CD, et al. Curcumin/xanthan-galactomannan hydrogels: Rheological analysis and biocompatibility. *Carbohydr Polym*. 2013;93:279.

73. Mohanty C, Das M, Sahoo SK. Sustained wound healing activity of curcumin loaded oleic acid based polymeric bandage in a rat model. *Mol Pharm*. 2012;9:2801.

74. Kumar K, Rai AK. Proniosomal formulation of curcumin having anti-inflammatory and anti-arthritic activity in different experimental animal models. *Pharmazie*. 2012;67:852.

75. Kaur CD, Saraf S. Topical vesicular formulations of Curcuma longa extract on recuperating the ultraviolet radiation-damaged skin. *J Cosmet Dermatol*. 2011;10:260.

76. Gupta NK, Dixit VK. Development and evaluation of vesicular system for curcumin delivery. *Arch Dermatol Res*. 2011;303:89.

77. Patel NA, Patel NJ, Patel RP. Formulation and evaluation of curcumin gel for topical application. *Pharm Dev Technol*. 2009;14:80.

78. Rungphanichkul N, Nimmannit U, Muangsiri W, et al. Preparation of curcuminoid niosomes for enhancement of skin permeation. *Pharmazie*. 2011;66:570.

79. Lertsutthiwong P, Rojsitthisak P. Chitosan-alginate nanocapsules for encapsulation of turmeric oil. *Pharmazie*. 2011;66:911.

80. Liu CH, Chang FY. Development and characterization of eucalyptol microemulsions for topic delivery of curcumin. *Chem Pharm Bull (Tokyo)*. 2011;59:172.

81. Basnet P, Hussain H, Tho I, et al. Liposomal delivery system enhances anti-inflammatory properties of curcumin. *J Pharm Sci*. 2012;101:598.

82. Liu CH, Huang HY. Antimicrobial activity of curcumin-loaded myristic acid microemulsions against Staphylococcus epidermidis. *Chem Pharm Bull (Tokyo)*. 2012;60:1118.

83. Elad S, Meidan I, Sellam G, et al. Topical curcumin for the prevention of oral mucositis in pediatric patients: Case series. *Altern Ther Health Med*. 2013;19:21.

84. Hsu YC, Chen MJ, Yu YM, et al. Suppression of TGF-β1/SMAD pathway and extracellular matrix production in primary keloid fibroblasts by curcuminoids: Its potential therapeutic use in the chemoprevention of keloid. *Arch Dermatol Res*. 2010;302:717.

85. Dovigo LN, Carmello JC, de Souza Costa CA, et al. Curcumin-mediated photodynamic inactivation of Candida albicans in a murine model of oral candidiasis. *Med Mycol*. 2013;51:243.

86. Takahashi M, Asikin Y, Takara K, et al. Screening of medicinal and edible plants in Okinawa, Japan, for enhanced proliferative

and collagen synthesis activities in NB1RGB human skin fibroblast cells. *Biosci Biotechnol Biochem.* 2012;76:2317.

87. Tu CX, Lin M, Lu SS, et al. Curcumin inhibits melanogenesis in human melanocytes. *Phytother Res.* 2012;26:174.

88. Sidhu GS, Singh AK, Thaloor D, et al. Enhancement of wound healing by curcumin in animals. *Wound Repair Regen.* 1998;6:167.

89. Sidhu GS, Mani H, Gaddipati JP, et al. Curcumin enhances wound healing in streptozotocin induced diabetic rats and genetically diabetic mice. *Wound Rep Regen.* 1999;7:362.

90. Thangapazham RL, Sharma A, Maheshwari RK. Beneficial role of curcumin in skin diseases. *Adv Exp Med Biol.* 2007;595:343.

91. Kundu S, Biswas TK, Das P, et al. Turmeric (Curcuma longa) rhizome paste and honey show similar wound healing potential: A preclinical study in rabbits. *Int J Low Extrem Wounds.* 2005;4:205.

92. Gupta A, Upadhyay NK, Sawhney RC, et al. A poly-herbal formulation accelerates normal and impaired diabetic wound healing. *Wound Repair Regen.* 2008;16:784.

93. Bhagavathula N, Warner RL, DaSilva M, et al. A combination of curcumin and ginger extract improves abrasion wound healing in corticosteroid-impaired hairless rat skin. *Wound Repair Regen.* 2009;17:360.

94. López-Jornet P, Camacho-Alonso F, Jiménez-Torres MJ, et al. Topical curcumin for the healing of carbon dioxide laser skin wounds in mice. *Photomed Laser Surg.* 2011;29:809.

95. Kulac M, Aktas C, Tulubas F, et al. The effects of topical treatment with curcumin on burn wound healing in rats. *J Mol Histol.* 2013;44:83.

96. Chusri S, Settharaksa S, Chokpaisarn J, et al. Thai herbal formulas used for wound treatment: A study of their antibacterial potency, anti-inflammatory, antioxidant, and cytotoxicity effects. *J Altern Complement Med.* 2013;19:671.

97. Chereddy KK, Coco R, Memvanga PB, et al. Combined effect of PLGA and curcumin on wound healing activity. *J Control Release.* 2013;171:208.

98. Kurd SK, Smith N, VanVoorhees A, et al. Oral curcumin in the treatment of moderate to severe psoriasis vulgaris: A prospective clinical trial. *J Am Acad Dermatol.* 2008;58:625.

99. Morelli V, Calmet E, Jhingade V. Alternative therapies for common dermatologic disorders, part 2. *Prim Care.* 2010;37:285.

100. Heng MC, Song MK, Harker J, et al. Drug-induced suppression of phosphorylase kinase activity correlates with the resolution of psoriasis as assessed by clinical, histological and immunohistochemical parameters. *Br J Dermatol.* 2000;143:937.

101. Saelee C, Thongrakard V, Tencomnao T. Effects of Thai medicinal herb extracts with anti-psoriatic activity on the expression on NF-κB signaling biomarkers in HaCaT keratinocytes. *Molecules.* 2011;16:3908.

102. Sun J, Zhao Y, Hu J. Curcumin inhibits imiquimod-induced psoriasis-like inflammation by inhibiting IL-1beta and IL-6 production in mice. *PLoS One.* 2013;8:e67078.

103. Marchiani A, Rozzo C, Fadda A, et al. Curcumin and curcumin-like molecules: From spice to drugs. *Curr Med Chem.* 2014;21:204.

104. Conney AH, Lysz T, Ferraro T, et al. Inhibitory effect of curcumin and some related dietary compounds on tumor promotion and arachidonic acid metabolism in mouse skin. *Adv Enzyme Regul.* 1991;31:385.

105. Nakamura Y, Ohto Y, Murakami A, et al. Inhibitory effects of curcumin and tetrahydrocurcuminoids on the tumor promoter-induced reactive oxygen species generation in leukocytes in vitro and in vivo. *Jpn J Cancer Res.* 1998;89:361.

106. Panahi Y, Sahebkar A, Parvin S, et al. A randomized controlled trial on the anti-inflammatory effects of curcumin in patients with chronic sulphur mustard-induced cutaneous complications. *Ann Clin Biochem.* 2012;49:580.

107. Thongrakard V, Ruangrungsi N, Ekkapongpisit M, et al. Protection from UVB Toxicity in Human Keratinocytes by Thailand Native Herbs Extracts. *Photochem Photobiol.* 2013 Aug 12. [Epub ahead of print]

108. Oguro T, Yoshida T. Effect of ultraviolet A on ornithine decarboxylase and metallothionein gene expression in mouse skin. *Photodermatol Photoimmunol Photomed.* 2001;17:71.

109. Huang MT, Ma W, Yen P, et al. Inhibitory effects of topical application of low doses of curcumin on 12-O-tetradecanoylphorbol-13-acetate-induced tumor promotion and oxidized DNA bases in mouse epidermis. *Carcinogenesis.* 1997;18:83.

110. Villaseñor IM, Simon MK, Villanueva AM. Comparative potencies of nutraceuticals in chemically induced skin tumor prevention. *Nutr Cancer.* 2002;44:66.

111. Azuine MA, Bhide SV. Chemopreventive effect of turmeric against stomach and skin tumors induced by chemical carcinogens in Swiss mice. *Nutr Cancer.* 1992;17:77.

112. Iersel ML, Ploemen JP, Struik I, et al. Inhibition of glutathione S-transferase activity in human melanoma cells by alpha,beta-unsaturated carbonyl derivatives. Effects of acrolein, cinnamaldehyde, citral, crotonaldehyde, curcumin, ethacrynic acid, and trans-2-hexenal. *Chem Biol Interact.* 1996;102:117.

113. Jee SH, Shen SC, Tseng CR, et al. Curcumin induces a p53-dependent apoptosis in human basal cell carcinoma cells. *J Invest Dermatol.* 1998;111:656.

114. Chun KS, Keum YS, Han SS, et al. Curcumin inhibits phorbol ester-induced expression of cyclooxygenase-2 in mouse skin through suppression of extracellular signal-regulated kinase activity and NF-kappB activation. *Carcinogenesis.* 2003;24:1515.

115. Limtrakul P, Lipigorngoson S, Namwong O, et al. Inhibitory effect of dietary curcumin on skin carcinogenesis in mice. *Cancer Lett.* 1997; 116:197.

116. Nagabhushan M, Bhide SV. Curcumin as an inhibitor of cancer. *J Am Coll Nutr.* 1992;11:192.

117. Bush JA, Cheung KJ Jr., Li G. Curcumin induces apoptosis in human melanoma cells through a Fas receptor/caspase-8 pathway independent of p53. *Exp Cell Res.* 2001;271:305.

118. Chen J, Wanming D, Zhang D, et al. Water-soluble antioxidants improve the antioxidant and anticancer activity of low concentrations of curcumin in human leukemia cells. *Pharmazie.* 2005;60:57.

119. Phillips JM, Clark C, Herman-Ferdinandez L, et al. Curcumin inhibits skin squamous cell carcinoma tumor growth in vivo. *Otolaryngol Head Neck Surg.* 2011;145:58.

120. Phillips J, Moore-Medlin T, Sonavane K, et al. Curcumin inhibits UV radiation-induced skin cancer in SKH-1 mice. *Otolaryngol Head Neck Surg.* 2013;148:797.

121. Sonavane K, Phillips J, Ekshyyan O, et al. Topical curcumin-based cream is equivalent to dietary curcumin in a skin cancer model. *J Skin Cancer.* 2012;2012:147863.

122. Tsai KD, Lin JC, Yang SM, et al. Curcumin protects against UVB-induced skin cancers in SKH-1 hairless mouse: Analysis of early molecular markers in carcinogenesis. *Evid Based Complement Alternat Med.* 2012;2012:593952.

123. Hwang BM, Noh EM, Kim JS, et al. Curcumin inhibits UVB-induced matrix metalloproteinase-1/3 expression by suppressing the MAPK-p38/JNK pathways in human dermal fibroblasts. *Exp Dermatol.* 2013;22:371.

CHAPTER 70

Chamomile

Activities:

Anti-inflammatory, antioxidant, analgesic, antimicrobial, antiseptic, antispasmodic, antiulcer, sedative

Important Chemical Components:

Flowers: flavonoids (i.e., apigenin, quercetin, patuletin, luteolin, and their glucosides; isohamnetin), coumarins (herniarin and umbelliferone), mucilages, mono- and oligosaccharides
Essential oil of the flower: the terpenoids (-)-α-bisabolol and its oxides (α-bisabolol A and B), sesquiterpene lactones (anthocotulide), cadinene, farnesene, furfural, spathulenol, spiroethers, the proazulenes matricarin and matricine (also spelled "matricin"), and chamazulene (a transformation product of matricine)[1–4]

Origin Classification:

This ingredient is natural. Organic forms exist.

Personal Care Category:

Anti-inflammatory

Recommended for the following Baumann Skin Types:

DSNT, DSNW, DSPT, DSPW, OSNT, OSNW, OSPT, and OSPW

SOURCE

Topical herbal drugs, including chamomile, have been used for centuries to treat skin conditions.[5] Native to western and southern Europe, western Asia, and India, chamomile (also spelled "camomile") is a sweet-scented flower belonging to the Asteraceae (or Compositae) family, also commonly known as the aster, daisy, or sunflower family. The Compositae family refers to plants in which the flower heads are a composite of individual flowers. They are also given the name Asteraceae because the flower heads are star-shaped (*aster* is Greek for star). Chamomile has been used as a medicinal herb worldwide for thousands of years.[6,7] It remains one of the most widely used medicinal herbs as well as one of the most frequently studied plants.[8]

The generic designation "chamomile" is rooted in the Greek expressions *khamai* or *chamos* (on the ground, or ground) and *melon* (apple).[9,10] There are two primary types of chamomile: *Chamaemelum nobile* (Roman chamomile, sometimes referred to as English chamomile) and *Matricaria recutita*, also known as *Chamomilla recutita* or *Matricaria chamomilla* (German chamomile, sometimes referred to as Hungarian chamomile, mayweed, sweet false chamomile, true chamomile, or wild chamomile).[1,3,11–13] Roman chamomile is a low-growing perennial that emits an apple-like aroma when trod upon. German chamomile is a robust, self-seeding annual plant.

TABLE 70-1
Pros and Cons of Chamomile

PROS	CONS
Long history of traditional use	Paucity of clinical trials
Strong evidence of anti-inflammatory activity seen *in vitro* and in animal studies	Individuals with allergies to members of the Asteraceae (Compositae) family are susceptible to allergic reactions
Fair empirical evidence of efficacy in humans	Source of the plant determines the amount of beneficial components in the extracts used
One of the most frequently studied plants	No studies evaluating use in rosacea
Inexpensive and readily available	

Both plants have been used for medicinal purposes, with Roman chamomile considered therapeutic for burns, bruises, boils, as well as small cuts and reputed to foster the natural healing of acne, dermatitis, and athlete's foot. Compared to Roman chamomile, German chamomile contains a higher concentration of key active ingredients that have shown anti-inflammatory activity *in vivo*, namely the terpenoids chamazulene and α-bisabolol (also known as levomenol)[4,14]; therefore, German chamomile is the focus of this chapter. In Germany, chamomile is referred to as *alles zutraut* ("capable of anything").[15] Its traditional medical uses include inflammatory conditions such as eczema, gout, neuralgia, and rheumatic discomfort.[1,12,16] Despite a long history of traditional use (Table 70-1), chamomile has only been subjected to the rigors of the scientific method during the past 40 years.

HISTORY

Chamomile has long been used in folk medicine and aromatherapy, systemically and topically, to treat inflammation disorders, primarily gastrointestinal and cutaneous.[17] Through human migration, this sweet-scented plant has also become abundant throughout North America, growing freely throughout much of the continent. The earliest recorded uses of chamomile date back 2,500 years to the time of Hippocrates (circa 500 BCE), who is believed to have recognized therapeutic properties in the herb.[18] Later recorded writings on chamomile were also attributed to the Greek-speaking Roman physician Galen as well as Dioscorides.[3,10] Ancient Egyptians, Greeks, and Romans used crushed chamomile flowers for medicinal purposes, such as treating erythema and dry skin brought on by harsh, dry weather.[10,19] Chamomile tea has also been used as a folk remedy in eye washing to treat conjunctivitis and other superficial ocular conditions.[20] Decoctions of chamomile in cold wet packs have been used traditionally to treat acute, exudative eczema.[21] In 1951, α-bisabolol, one of the primary active ingredients of chamomile, was isolated and is now included in many cosmetic skin care products to prevent and treat inflammation.[22]

A recent ethnobotanical survey in southwestern Serbia revealed that chamomile was one of the most highly valued medicinal plants used in local folk medicine, primarily for curing minor gastrointestinal, respiratory, and cutaneous conditions.[23] Chamomile is also widely used for wound care in Europe.[21] Currently, chamomile is one of the seven most common herbs used for medical purposes.[19] A large body of research conducted over the last 40 years has buttressed the traditional uses of the herb,[10] and it is now listed as a drug in the official pharmacopoeias of 26 nations (including Belgium, France, Germany, and the United Kingdom).[10,15]

CHEMISTRY

Chamazulene, flavonoids (which are known to have antioxidant properties), coumarins, mucilages, and mono- and oligosaccharides are the primary active components of *M. recutita* deemed medically important among the 120 identified compounds in chamomile flowers.[1,24] Chamazulene is a transformation product of matricine and both of these constituents of chamomile extracts have shown anti-inflammatory and antipyretic activity *in vivo*.[4,25] Chamazulene, but not matricine, is thought to be involved in exerting anti-inflammatory activity in chamomile by suppressing leukotriene production.[24]

Levomenol, or α-bisabolol, is another key anti-inflammatory component found in great abundance in German chamomile, and comprises nearly half of its essential oil.[22] It is believed to confer significant effects on skin, such as soothing inflammation and diminishing pruritus (itching). The combined effects of levomenol, a natural moisturizer, and chamazulene are said to soothe skin exhibiting inflammation due to eczema, allergy, and sunburn.

In addition to reports of anti-inflammatory effects, chamomile is believed, based on chemical assays, to possess some antioxidant properties.[26] These characteristics are mainly associated with the terpenoid matricine as well as the flavonoids apigenin, luteolin, and quercetin, with the flavonoids recognized for strongly inhibiting histamine release and the infiltration of leukocytes, and for possessing antioxidant properties.[24,27] As a result of its various beneficial properties, chamomile is now included in many cosmetic products intended to improve skin appearance. Of note, chamomile has been reported to cause allergic contact dermatitis in susceptible types,[28] such as those with known allergies to the Compositae family (e.g., ragweed and feverfew) (see Chapter 66, Feverfew).

Chamomile is notably versatile in the medicinal realm, with the dried flowers of *M. recutita* exhibiting sedative and antispasmodic properties.[29] Chamomile also acts as an antiallergenic and antibacterial. The traditional indications for chamomile and its various teas and topical formulations range from stomach cramping and pains, menstrual cramping, and diarrhea, to inflammatory skin and eye problems, mood disorders, and even the flu.

In a 2006 review by McKay and Blumberg, chamomile was found to deliver moderate *in vitro* antioxidant and antimicrobial as well as significant antiplatelet activities. Strong anti-inflammatory as well as mild antimutagenic and cholesterol-reducing activities have been displayed by the herb in animal experiments, they noted, in addition to some antispasmodic and anxiolytic effects, but data from human studies are limited.[1]

A key active ingredient in German chamomile that is believed to deliver anti-inflammatory and soothing activity is α-bisabolol (matricine), as well as α-bisabolol oxide A and B. These are known to exhibit anti-inflammatory activity due to inhibition of cyclooxygenase (COX) and lipoxygenase (see Chapter 64, Anti-inflammatory Agents).[30] For this reason, α-bisabolol is commonly included in various personal care products, including moisturizing creams and ointments, lotions, cleansers, sunscreens, antiperspirants, and makeup.[22]

ORAL USES

Globally, chamomile is one of the most popular medicinal plants and is extensively consumed as a beverage in herbal teas (or tisanes) brewed from dried flower heads.[1,31] In fact, as of 2006, it was estimated that chamomile is consumed in more than a million cups per day around the world.[32,33] As an infusion, chamomile has also been traditionally used to ease colic and teething in babies, and to calm restless children. In addition, this bittersweet herb has been shown to be effective in relieving acid indigestion, intestinal gas, constipation, and peptic ulcers. Importantly, chamomile herbal tea is not just for drinking. The use of chamomile tea as an eye wash for conjunctivitis and other external ocular symptoms is a traditional remedy.[20] Oral uses of chamomile are extensive and a detailed description is beyond the scope of this chapter.

TOPICAL USES

Topically applied chamomile oil is used to soothe cutaneous inflammation and is well tolerated. Chamomile is thought to diminish photodamage and pruritus,[18] and it is believed to act as a natural moisturizer.[18,34,35] It is a common home remedy to treat inflammation of various causes including sunburn, insect bites, and rashes.

Atopic Dermatitis

In a 1985 study of 161 patients with eczema on their hands, forearms, and lower legs, Aertgeerts et al. compared the effects of a chamomile-containing cream (Kamillosan®) with 0.25 percent hydrocortisone, 0.75 percent fluocortin butyl ester, and 5 percent bufexamac as maintenance therapy over three to four weeks. In this bilateral comparative study, they found that the herbal cream was equally effective as hydrocortisone and achieved better results than the nonsteroidal anti-inflammatory drug (NSAID) bufexamac and the glucocorticoid aging fluocortin butyl ester.[36]

In 2000, Patzelt-Wenczler and Ponce-Pöschl performed a two-week, partially double-blind, randomized half-side comparison of Kamillosan® cream (which contains chamomile extract) and 0.5 percent hydrocortisone cream and placebo in patients with moderate atopic eczema. This proof of efficacy revealed that the chamomile formulation was marginally better than hydrocortisone and placebo in diminishing symptoms of atopic eczema.[37] Previously, clinical studies demonstrated that the chamomile-containing patented Camocare® cream was efficacious and safe as a maintenance therapy after corticosteroid treatment for severe inflammatory conditions and as single therapy for milder cutaneous inflammatory issues.[10]

In 2010, Lee et al. induced atopic dermatitis in mice using 1 percent 2,4-dinitrochlorobenzene (DNCB) to sensitize and then challenge the animals. Subsequently, the researchers daily applied 3 percent German chamomile oil on the dorsal skin for four weeks or a saline or jojoba oil in controls (see Chapter 12, Jojoba Oil). Significantly lower histamine levels were recorded in the chamomile group compared to controls after two weeks, and scratching was displayed much less frequently by the mice treated with chamomile. The investigators reported that this was the first study to show the immunoregulatory potential of chamomile to ease atopic dermatitis by affecting the activation of Th2 cells.[38]

Anti-inflammatory Activity

In 1984, Tubaro et al. induced ear edema in male albino Swiss mice using croton oil to assess the anti-inflammatory activity of topically applied chamomile. They found that the herbal extract was as effective as a reference NSAID in reducing inflammation.[39]

In an animal study in which inflammation was induced via the injection of carrageenan and prostaglandin E_1, German chamomile was found to inhibit the inflammatory effect as well as leukocyte infiltration.[40] Specifically, chamazulene decreases the inflammatory process by inhibiting leukotriene synthesis.[4]

In an *in vitro* model, Srivastava et al. showed in 2009 that aqueous extracts of chamomile inhibited COX-2 enzyme activity, hindering the release of lipopolysaccharide (LPS)-induced prostaglandin E_2 and limiting LPS-induced COX-2 mRNA and protein expression, without altering COX-1 expression. The investigators found that chamomile acted similarly to NSAIDs in this context and suggested that their findings may have implications regarding the prevention and management of inflammatory and neoplastic disorders.[33]

In 2010, Bhaskaran et al. showed that chamomile suppresses LPS-induced nitric oxide production and inducible nitric oxide synthase gene expression, thus implying its viability as an anti-inflammatory agent.[12]

In 2013, Drummond et al. investigated the potential use as anti-inflammatory agents of chamomile, meadowsweet (*Filipendula ulmaria*), and willow bark (*Salix alba*), based on their traditional uses. The researchers isolated polyphenols from each herb (apigenin, quercetin, and salicylic acid, respectively) and, along with aqueous herbal extracts, incubated the compounds with THP1 macrophages. Both apigenin and quercetin significantly lowered interleukin (IL)-6 and tumor necrosis factor (TNF)-α. Overall, willow bark exerted the greatest anti-inflammatory activity and chamomile, the least. The authors noted that this was the first study to reveal that these herbal extracts display positive anti-inflammatory activity in human macrophages, suggesting that *in vivo* study is warranted.[41]

In a small skin penetration study with nine healthy female volunteers, Merfort et al. showed in 1994 that the chamomile flavones apigenin, luteolin, and apigenin 7-O-β-glucoside were adsorbed at the skin surface and also penetrated into deeper skin layers, suggesting suitability as anti-inflammatory agents.[42]

Wound Healing

In 2009, Martins et al. conducted *in vitro* as well as *in vivo* studies in male rats that indicated that chamomile facilitated significantly faster wound healing as compared to corticosteroids.[13]

Using 30 male albino Wistar rats with linear incisional wounds on the back in a 2010 study, Jarrahi et al. randomized the animals into control, olive oil, and chamomile treatment groups (see Chapter 14, Olive Oil). No drug or cold cream was administered to the control group. Topical olive oil was administered to the olive oil group once daily until wounds were completely healed. *M. chamomilla* extract dissolved in olive oil was used topically on the chamomile group. Statistically significant differences were observed on most days between the olive oil and treatment groups. The investigators concluded that topically applied chamomile exhibits potential as a wound-healing agent, supporting findings by Jarrahi in a similar experiment two years earlier.[43,44]

Cutaneous benefits of chamomile have been demonstrated in various ways. A 2011 controlled clinical study of 72 colostomy patients revealed that a German chamomile solution was effective in alleviating pruritus and inflammation associated with peristomal skin lesions. Twice daily application of the chamomile solution promoted healing and was more effective than hydrocortisone 1 percent ointment.[45]

In a literature review intended to identify the potential uses of complementary and alternative therapies in relation to dermatologic surgery, Reddy et al. found citations for numerous natural ingredients that can be used perioperatively, including chamomile, as well as other ingredients discussed in this text such as honey, propolis, vitamin C, aloe vera gel, turmeric, calendula, and lavender oil [see Chapter 55, Ascorbic Acid (Vitamin C), Chapter 60, Honey/Propolis/Royal Jelly, Chapter 65, Aloe Vera, Chapter 69, Turmeric, Chapter 71, Calendula, and Chapter 73, Lavandula]. Specifically, they found that chamomile was conducive to wound healing, decreasing edema and purpura, and delivering anti-inflammatory effects in animals.[46]

SAFETY ISSUES

The use of chamomile in any form is considered by the United States Food and Drug Administration as generally recognized as safe (GRAS) with few side effects. There have been some reports of contact dermatitis as well as contact urticaria and angioedema following the topical application of chamomile products. Allergic conjunctivitis has also been reported in patients who manifested positive skin prick reactions to chamomile tea extract, *M. chamomilla* pollen, and *Artemisia vulgaris* (mugwort) pollen extracts.[20,47] Overall, reactions to chamomile tend to be mild-to-moderate, and occur in individuals with sensitivities to members of the Compositae family (see Table 70-2).[48] *M. recutita* is known as a weak sensitizer.[7,49,50] De la Torre et al. have identified significant *in vivo* cross-reactivity between *A. vulgaris* and chamomile.[51] In addition, there have been reports of adverse reactions to topically applied chamomile or chamomile orally consumed in individuals allergic to other plants in the daisy family.[1] Specifically, sensitization has been linked to the use of various chamomile creams, ointments, and lotions, and, to a lesser degree, chamomile oil and tea. Chamomile, comfrey, and tea tree oil are considered the ingredients in cosmeceutical formulations at highest risk of eliciting a reaction (see Chapter 77, Tea Tree Oil).[52]

In 2004, Jovanovic´ et al. found an overall prevalence of 30 percent Compositae-sensitivity among patients with extrinsic or allergic atopic dermatitis who were patch tested with

TABLE 70-2

Some Members of the Compositae (Asteraceae) Family of Plants

Burdock

Chamomile

Chrysanthemum

Daisy

Dandelion

Echinacea

Edelweiss

Feverfew

Marigold

Ragweed

Sunflower

Yarrow

Compositae mix, including its individual ingredients, extracts of arnica (*Arnica montana*), chamomile (*C. recutita*), tansy (*Tanacetum vulgare*), feverfew (*Tanacetum parthenium*), and yarrow (*Achillea millefolium*); sesquiterpene lactone mix; and specific series for atopic dermatitis patients (see Chapter 66, Feverfew). Five patients were specifically sensitive to chamomile. The researchers concluded that atopic dermatitis is a risk factor for Compositae allergy.[53]

Type-IV allergic reactions to chamomile manifesting as allergic contact dermatitis are not uncommon. Andres et al. suggested, based on a case study of an anaphylactic response to chamomile tea, that the incidence and risk of type-I allergic responses may be underestimated.[54] In addition, Paulsen et al. advised caution to Compositae-sensitive patients regarding the topical use of cosmetics or remedies containing Compositae ingredients.[28]

Certainly the risk of allergy depends upon the compounds in the herb and these can vary by geographic origin. For instance, chamomile from Argentina has been found to contain higher levels of the potent allergen anthocotulide, perhaps due to contamination with the morphologically comparable *Anthemis cotula* (dog fennel).[7,35] Up to 7.3 percent anthocotulide is found in dog fennel; the sesquiterpene lactone is found in only trace amounts in chamomile of European origin.[7] In the commercial production of the chamomile product Kamillosan®, the final product is filtered to eliminate allergens.[7]

Chamomile is one among the several herbs that can interact with warfarin, elevating the risk of bleeding or other adverse effects for a patient on warfarin therapy.[55] Herniarin (7-methoxycoumarin), the main coumarin found in the plant, is responsible for the antiplatelet activity and has been identified as one of the non-sesquiterpene lactone sensitizers in German chamomile.[2] NSAIDs, particularly aspirin, have the potential to interact with herbal supplements that contain coumarin, such as chamomile, augmenting the risk of bleeding and bruising.[56]

The German Commission E approved of chamomile for internal use to treat gastrointestinal spasms and inflammatory disorders, and as an inhalant for respiratory inflammation; for external use, for the treatment of mucocutaneous disorders as well as wounds and burns, genital inflammation, and bacterial skin disorders, including the oral cavity and gums.[10,52] Chamomile is one of the most commonly used herbs for treating morning sickness, but there is contradictory evidence amid an overall dearth of data on whether use of chamomile is safe during pregnancy.[57]

Bisabolol

Ogata et al. showed in a study using rats, that α-bisabolol oxide A is essentially safe in the conventional use of German chamomile.[58] However, α-bisabolol has been linked to cases of periorbital swelling and contact cheilitis from lipstick.[22,59,60] In 2010, Russell and Jacob recommended, based on reports in Europe of contact dermatitis from bisabolol, that patch testing with α-bisabolol or α-bisabolol-containing products be included in the work-up of patients with presumptive allergic contact dermatitis or aggravated atopic dermatitis.[22]

ENVIRONMENTAL IMPACT

The environmental impact from the cultivation and commercial use of German chamomile is not well reported; however, it is a naturally occurring plant and organically grown crops are available.

FORMULATION CONSIDERATIONS

Chamomile is included in a wide array of cosmetic products to provide anti-inflammatory and soothing activity for sensitive skin. Various processes are used to isolate the active compounds from the plants, and the formulation considerations depend upon which processes are used.

USAGE CONSIDERATIONS

Chamomile is available in several forms including alcohol extracts, tea infusions, and oil.[50,52] It is often formulated in cleansers, lotions, creams, and serums.[50]

SIGNIFICANT BACKGROUND

In a 2005 survey of English-language medical journals and symposia, Thornfeldt identified German chamomile as one of the top dozen important botanicals used in cosmeceutical products.[52] A 2007 ethnobotanical survey on the highest mountain in Central Serbia identified 83 wild species, with *M. chamomilla* found to be one of the most frequently used for health purposes; skin injuries and issues were second only to gastrointestinal illnesses as the main indication.[61] Recent studies appear to suggest a wider range of biologic activity than first thought, such as antioxidant, antiparasitic, hypocholesterolemic, antiaging, and anticancer properties.[12] Nevertheless, despite increasing popular use of herbal products, and those including chamomile in particular, clinical evidence substantiating the cutaneous effects of chamomile remains sparse, according to the 2010 findings of a systematic review by Rügge et al.[62]

In 1996, Ramos et al. performed preliminary experiments toward incorporating plant extracts as sun-protective agents, finding that liquid and dry extracts of *M. recutita*, *Hamamelis virginiana* (witch hazel), *Aesculus hippocastanum* (horse chestnut), *Rhamnus purshiana*, and *Cinnamomum zeylanicum* amplified the solar protection factors (SPF) of a 2 percent solution of the synthetic sunscreen octylmethoxycinnamate (see Chapter 74, Horse Chestnut). They concluded that such herbal extracts could intensify SPF values when included in commercial sunscreens, while also enhancing the emollient activity of the product.[63]

Anticancer Activity

Chamomile is incorporated along with six other standardized botanical extracts (*Panax ginseng*, cranberry, green tea, grape skin, grape seed, and *Ganoderma lucidum*) in a proprietary botanical agent, Traditional Botanical Supplement-101 (TBS-101), demonstrated by Evans et al. in 2009 to have a good safety profile and significant anticancer activities (see Chapter 47, Green Tea). The botanical agent dose-dependently inhibited cell growth and induced apoptosis of PC-3 cells in a xenograft mouse model and, according to the investigators, merits consideration as a treatment for aggressive prostate cancer. They ascribed the contributions of chamomile to its constituent apigenin, which has been found to suppress cell proliferation and induce apoptosis.[64,65]

In 2013, Mamalis et al. investigated the antioxidant activity of key constituents of chamomile, silymarin, and halophilic bacteria (α-bisabolol, silymarin, and ectoin, respectively) finding that each substance hindered the *in vitro* upregulation of H_2O_2-induced free radicals in human skin fibroblasts. The researchers concluded that the antioxidant capacities of these herbs deserve additional study in clinical trials to ascertain their antiaging and anticancer potential.[66]

Later that year, Kogiannou et al. analyzed the phenolic profile of six herbal infusions and investigated potential anticarcinogenic properties, identifying chamomile as rich in genistein, a potent isoflavone (see Chapter 45, Soy). They found that the molecular target for chamomile in epithelial colon cancer appears to be nuclear factor-κB, and it, along with the other herbal infusions, displayed antiradical activity in relation to total phenolic content.[67]

Antiviral Activity

Koch et al. screened the essential oils of several plants, including chamomile, in 2008, to ascertain inhibitory activity against herpes simplex virus type 2 (HSV-2). All of the essential oils (which also included anise, hyssop, thyme, ginger, and sandalwood), displayed a dose-dependent virucidal capacity against HSV-2 (see Chapter 59, Ginger). The researchers noted a high selectivity index for chamomile, suggesting that it was especially promising among the herbs tested for topical therapeutic use for genital herpes.[68]

Oral Mucositis

In 2013, Curra et al. examined the effects of topical chamomile and corticosteroid treatment on IL-1β and TNF-α levels in 5-fluorouracil-induced oral mucositis in hamsters, with 36 animals randomized into control, chamomile, and corticosteroid groups. They found that topically applied chamomile was associated with lower scores for both proinflammatory cytokines, indicating the anti-inflammatory activity of the herb in treating oral mucositis.[8]

In an earlier experiment with 105 hamsters with oral mucositis induced by 5-fluorouracil, Pavesi et al. randomized animals into control, topical chamomile, and corticosteroid groups. The group treated with chamomile exhibited milder clinical symptoms throughout the study and had a 12-fold greater chance of being clear of mucositis than the control group. Histopathological results showed that chamomile-treated hamsters displayed milder symptoms of mucositis than the other groups throughout the evaluation period.[35]

Notably, a mouthwash containing German chamomile was found to be effective in resolving oral mucositis arising from methotrexate therapy in a patient with rheumatoid arthritis.[69]

CONCLUSION

Although the health benefits of chamomile might be most often associated with its tea preparation in the popular consciousness, there is a long history of effective, therapeutic application of various types of chamomile extracts to the skin. The body of clinical research on chamomile is relatively slim, but does support its use as a natural anti-inflammatory ingredient. Caution must be taken when used in individuals with a history of allergy to plants in the Compositae family. Double-blind, placebo-controlled trials are necessary to establish the range of therapeutic potential of this herb and to compare its efficacy with other natural anti-inflammatory ingredients such as willow bark, argan oil, and feverfew.

REFERENCES

1. McKay DL, Blumberg JB. A review of the bioactivity and potential health benefits of chamomile tea (Matricaria recutita L.). *Phytother Res*. 2006;20:519.
2. Paulsen E, Otkjaer A, Andersen KE. The coumarin herniarin as a sensitizer in German chamomile [Chamomilla recutita (L.) Rauschert, Compositate]. *Contact Dermatitis*. 2010;62:338.
3. No authors listed. Matricaria chamomilla (German chamomile). Monograph. *Altern Med Rev*. 2008;13:58.
4. Safayhi H, Sabieraj J, Sailer ER, et al. Chamazulene: An antioxidant-type inhibitor of leukotriene B4 formation. *Planta Med*. 1994;60:410.
5. Hörmann HP, Korting HC. Evidence for the efficacy and safety of topical herbal drugs in dermatology: Part I: Anti-inflammatory agents. *Phytomedicine*. 1994;1:161.
6. O'Hara M, Kiefer D, Farrell K, et al. A review of 12 commonly used medicinal herbs. *Arch Fam Med*. 1998;7:523.
7. Paulsen E. Contact sensitization from Compositae-containing herbal remedies and cosmetics. *Contact Dermatitis*. 2002;47:189.
8. Curra M, Martins MA, Lauxen IS, et al. Effect of topical chamomile on immunohistochemical levels of IL-1β and TNF-α in 5-fluoouracil-induced oral mucositis in hamsters. *Cancer Chemother Pharmacol*. 2013;71:293.
9. Grieve M. A Modern Herbal (Vol. I). New York: Dover Publications; 1971:185.
10. Ross SM. An integrative approach to eczema (atopic dermatitis). *Holist Nurs Pract*. 2003;17:56.
11. Wu J. Anti-inflammatory ingredients. *J Drugs Dermatol*. 2008;7:s13.
12. Bhaskaran N, Shukla S, Srivastava JK, et al. Chamomile: An anti-inflammatory agent inhibits inducible nitric oxide synthase expression by blocking RelA/p65 activity. *Int J Mol Med*. 2010;26:935.
13. Martins MD, Marques MM, Bussadori SK, et al. Comparative analysis between Chamomilla recutita and corticosteroids on wound healing. An in vitro and in vivo study. *Phytother Res*. 2009;23:274.
14. Barene I, Daberte I, Zvirgzdina L, et al. The complex technology on products of German chamomile. *Medicina (Kaunas)*. 2003;39(Suppl 2):127.
15. Foster S. An Illustrated Guide to 101 Medicinal Herbs: Their History, Use, Recommended Dosages, and Cautions. Loveland, CO: Interweave Press; 1998:54-55.
16. Srivastava JK, Gupta S. Antiproliferative and apoptotic effects of chamomile extract in various human cancer cells. *J Agric Food Chem*. 2007;55:9470.
17. Dohil MA. Natural ingredients in atopic dermatitis and other inflammatory skin disease. *J Drugs Dermatol*. 2013;12:s128.
18. Baumann LS. Less-known botanical cosmeceuticals. *Dermatol Ther*. 2007;20:330.
19. Dockrell TR, Leever JS. An overview of herbal medications with implications for the school nurse. *J Sch Nurs*. 2000;16:53.
20. Subiza J, Subiza JL, Alonso M, et al. Allergic conjunctivitis to chamomile tea. *Ann Allergy*. 1990;65:127.
21. Reuter J, Merfort I, Schempp CM. Botanicals in dermatology: An evidence-based review. *Am J Clin Dermatol*. 2010;11:247.
22. Russell K, Jacob SE. Bisabolol. *Dermatitis*. 2010;21:57.
23. Savikin K, Zdunić G, Menković N, et al. Ethnobotanical study on traditional use of medicinal plants in South-Western Serbia, Zlatibor district. *J Ethnopharmacol*. 2013;146:803.
24. Máday E, Szöke E, Muskáth Z, et al. A study of the production of essential oils in chamomile hairy root cultures. *Eur J Drug Metab Pharmacokinet*. 1999;24:303.
25. Hoffmann D. Medical Herbalism: The Science and Practice of Herbal Medicine. Rochester, VT: Healing Arts Press; 2003:68.
26. Lee KG, Shibamoto T. Determination of antioxidant potential of volatile extracts isolated from various herbs and spices. *J Agric Food Chem*. 2002;50:4947.
27. Reszko AE, Berson D, Lupo MP. Cosmeceuticals: Practical applications. *Dermatol Clin*. 2009;27:401.
28. Paulsen E, Christensen LP, Andersen KE. Cosmetics and herbal remedies with Compositae plant extracts - are they tolerated by Compositae-allergic patients? *Contact Dermatitis*. 2008;58:15.
29. Avallone R, Zanoli P, Puia G, et al. Pharmacological profile of apigenin, a flavonoid isolated from Matricaria chamomilla. *Biochem Pharmacol*. 2000;59:1387.
30. Wu J. Skin care update: The role of natural products in clinical practice. Introduction. *J Drugs Dermatol*. 2008;7:s1.
31. Chandrashekhar VM, Halagali KS, Nidavani RB, et al. Anti-allergic activity of German chamomile (Matricaria recutita L.) in mast cell mediated allergy model. *J Ethnopharmacol*. 2011;137:336.
32. Speisky H, Rocco C, Carrasco C, et al. Antioxidant screening of medicinal herbal teas. *Phytother Res*. 2006;20:462.

33. Srivastava JK, Pandey M, Gupta S. Chamomile, a novel and selective COX-2 inhibitor with anti-inflammatory activity. *Life Sci.* 2009;85:663.

34. Gardiner P. Complementary, holistic, and integrative medicine: Chamomile. *Pediatr Rev.* 2007;28:e16.

35. Pavesi VC, Lopez TC, Martins MA, et al. Healing action of topical chamomile on 5-fluoracil induced oral mucositis in hamster. *Support Care Cancer.* 2011;19:639.

36. Aertgeerts P, Albring M, Klaschka F, et al. Comparative testing of Kamillosan cream and steroidal (0.25% hydrocortisone, 0.75% fluocortin butyl ester) and non-steroidal (5% bufexamac) dermatologic agents in maintenance therapy of eczematous diseases. *Z Hautkr.* 1985;60:270.

37. Patzelt-Wenczler R, Ponce-Pöschl E. Proof of efficacy of Kamillosan® cream in atopic eczema. *Eur J Med Res.* 2000;5:171.

38. Lee SH, Heo Y, Kim YC. Effect of German chamomile oil application on alleviating atopic dermatitis-like immune alterations in mice. *J Vet Sci.* 2010;11:35.

39. Tubaro A, Zilli C, Redaelli C, et al. Evaluation of anti-inflammatory activity of a chamomile extract after topical application. *Planta Med.* 1984;50:359.

40. Shipochliev T, Dimitrov A, Aleksandrova E. Anti-inflammatory action of a group of plant extracts. *Vet Med Nauki.* 1981;18:87.

41. Drummond EM, Harbourne N, Marete E, et al. Inhibition of pro-inflammatory biomarkers in THP1 macrophages by polyphenols derived from chamomile, meadowsweet and willow bark. *Phytother Res.* 2013;27:588.

42. Merfort I, Heilmann J, Hagedorn-Leweke U, et al. In vivo skin penetration studies of chamomile flavones. *Pharmazie.* 1994;49:509.

43. Jarrahi M, Vafaei AA, Taherian AA, et al. Evaluation of topical Matricaria chamomilla extract activity on linear incisional wound healing in albino rats. *Nat Prod Res.* 2010;24:697.

44. Jarrahi M. An experimental study of the effects of Matricaria chamomilla extract on cutaneous burn wound healing in albino rats. *Nat Prod Res.* 2008;22:422.

45. Charousaei F, Dabirian A, Mojab F. Using chamomile solution or a 1% topical hydrocortisone ointment in the management of peristomal skin lesions in colostomy patients: Results of a controlled clinical study. *Ostomy Wound Manage.* 2011;57:28.

46. Reddy KK, Grossman L, Rogers GS. Common complementary and alternative therapies with potential use in dermatologic surgery: Risks and benefits. *J Am Acad Dermatol.* 2013;68:e127.

47. Foti C, Nettis E, Panebianco R, et al. Contact urticaris from Matricaria chamomile. *Contact Dermatitis.* 2000;42:360.

48. Compositae Allergy. http://www.dermnetnz.org/dermatitis/compositae-allergy.html. Accessed March 16, 2014.

49. Paulsen E, Andersen KE. Patch testing with constituents of Compositae mixes. *Contact Dermatitis.* 2012;66:241.

50. Aburjai T, Natsheh FM. Plants used in cosmetics. *Phytother Res.* 2003;17:987.

51. de la Torre Morín F, Sánchez Machín I, García Robaina JC, et al. Clinical cross-reactivity between Artemisia vulgaris and Matricaria chamomilla (chamomile). *J Investig Allergol Clin Immunol.* 2001;11:118.

52. Thornfeldt C. Cosmeceuticals containing herbs: Fact, fiction, and future. *Dermatol Surg.* 2005;31:873.

53. Jovanović M, Poljacki M, Duran V, et al. Contact allergy to Compositae plants in patients with atopic dermatitis. *Med Pregl.* 2004;57:209.

54. Andres C, Chen WC, Ollert M, et al. Anaphylactic reaction to chamomile tea. *Allergol Int.* 2009;58:135.

55. Heck AM, De Witt BA, Lukes AL. Potential interactions between alternative therapies and warfarin. *Am J Health Syst Pharm.* 2000;57:1221.

56. Abebe W. Herbal medication: Potential for adverse interactions with analgesic drugs. *J Clin Pharm Ther.* 2002;27:391.

57. Wilkinson JM. What do we know about herbal morning sickness treatments? A literature survey. *Midwifery.* 2000;16:224.

58. Ogata I, Kawanai T, Hashimoto E, et al. Bisabololoxide A, one of the main constituents in German chamomile extract, induces apoptosis in rat thymocytes. *Arch Toxicol.* 2010;84:45.

59. Wilkinson SM, Hausen BM, Beck MH. Allergic contact dermatitis from plant extracts in a cosmetic. *Contact Dermatitis.* 1995;33:58.

60. Pastor N, Silvestre JF, Mataix J, et al. Contact cheilitis from bisabolol and polyvinylpyrrolidone/hexadecane copolymer in lipstick. *Contact Dermatitis.* 2008;58:178.

61. Jarić S, Popović Z, Macukanović-Jocić M, et al. An ethnobotanical study on the usage of wild medicinal herbs from Kopaonik Mountain (Central Serbia). *J Ethnopharmacol.* 2007;111:160.

62. Rügge SD, Nielsen M, Jacobsen AS, et al. Evidence of dermatological effects of chamomile. *Ugeskr Laeger.* 2010;172:3492.

63. Ramos MF, Santos EP, Bizarri CH, et al. Preliminary studies towards utilization of various plant extracts as antisolar agents. *Int J Cosmet Sci.* 1996;18:87.

64. Evans S, Dizeyi N, Abrahamsson PA, et al. The effect of a novel botanical agent TBS-101 on invasive prostate cancer in animal models. *Anticancer Res.* 2009;29:3917.

65. Shukla S, Gupta S. Apigenin suppresses insulin-like growth factor I receptor signaling in human prostate cancer: An in vitro and in vivo study. *Mol Carcinog.* 2009;48:243.

66. Mamalis A, Nguyen DH, Brody N, et al. The active natural antioxidant properties of chamomile, milk thistle, and halophilic bacterial components in human skin in vitro. *J Drugs Dermatol.* 2013;12:780.

67. Kogiannou DA, Kalogeropoulos N, Kefalas P, et al. Herbal infusions; their phenolic profile, antioxidant and anti-inflammatory effects in HT29 and PC3 cells. *Food Chem Toxicol.* 2013;61:152.

68. Koch C, Reichling J, Schneele J, et al. Inhibitory effect of essential oils against herpes simplex virus type 2. *Phytomedicine.* 2008;15:71.

69. Mazokopakis EE, Vrentzos GE, Papadakis JA, et al. Wild chamomile (Matricaria recutita L.) mouthwashes in methotrexate-induced oral mucositis. *Phytomedicine.* 2005;12:25.

CHAPTER 71

Calendula

Activities:

Anti-inflammatory, antioxidant, antimicrobial, antiseptic, immunomodulatory, photoprotective

Important Chemical Components:

Triterpenoids (i.e., sesquiterpene lactones, faradiol, taraxasterol), flavonoids (i.e., quercetin, rutin, isorhamnetin, kaempferol, narcissin), phenolic acids, ubiquinone (CoQ_{10}) and other quinines (including polyprenylquinones), mucilages, saponins, carotenoids (i.e., β-carotene, lutein, lycopene, xanthophylls), essential oils (1,8-cineole, α-pinene, α-thujene, dihydrotagetone, T-muurolol), resins, sterins, sugars, sterins, sterols, tocopherols [1–7]

Origin Classification:

This ingredient is natural. Organic forms exist.

Personal Care Category:

Analgesic, anti-inflammatory

Recommended for the following Baumann Skin Types:

DSNT, DSNW, DSPT, DSPW, OSNT, OSNW, OSPT, and OSPW

SOURCE

Popularly known as pot marigold, garden marigold, holligold/holigold, marigold, marybud, common marigold, maravilla, ruddles, and goldbloom, *Calendula officinalis* is a bright, flowering annual herb native to Asia, central and southern Europe, northern Africa, and the Mediterranean region.[2,8] Despite one of its appellations, it is not related to the garden marigolds of the *Tagetes* genus, also within the Asteraceae (or Compositae) family.[9] Like many other members of the Asteraceae family, which includes daisies, arnica, feverfew, chamomile, edelweiss, and yarrow, calendula is now cultivated throughout the world (see Chapter 70, Chamomile, and Chapter 72, Edelweiss). Like many other popular herbs, calendula is valued for its culinary and medicinal uses and is cultivated for ornamental purposes. Through traditional use, calendula has long been considered a soothing herb that, more

TABLE 71-1
Pros and Cons of Calendula

PROS	CONS
Considered to have potent anti-inflammatory properties	Limited clinical data
Broad naturopathic uses	Risk of allergy
	Efficacy greatly depends upon the source of the herb and the formulation

recently, has been found to possess anti-inflammatory, antibacterial, and antioxidant properties.[6,7,10] Today, its primary indications are cutaneous and inflammatory conditions, scalds, bruises, boils, rashes, and first-degree burns, including sunburns[8,11] (Table 71-1).

HISTORY

In ancient Rome, calendula was regarded for its properties in breaking fevers. It was used as a topical anti-inflammatory agent prior to the 12th century in medieval Europe,[12] where its use further spread in the 13th century,[13] when it was grown in monastery gardens and used for wound healing. Calendula has continued to serve as a staple among topical and systemic homeopathic remedies through the succeeding centuries.[1,11] In the 1860s, it was used to treat battle wounds during the United States Civil War. Essentially, the antiseptic properties were seen to prevent gangrene and clean and repair wounds. Further, calendula has been used traditionally for treating an array of burns, bruises, skin tumors, cutaneous lesions, gastric ulcers and other stomach ailments, dysmenorrhea, edema, jaundice, and nervous disorders.[3,9] In Bulgarian folk medicine, it has been used as an anti-inflammatory, antipyretic, and antitumorigenic agent.[14] In Ayurvedic and Unani medicine, *C. officinalis* has been noted for conferring anti-inflammatory, antipyretic, antiepileptic, and antimicrobial activity.[3] Currently, calendula is broadly accepted in Europe for mild burns, sunburn, and slow-healing wounds; it is approved in Germany and other European countries specifically for leg ulcers and slow-healing wounds.[9]

CHEMISTRY

The mechanism of action is not fully understood, but the constituents in calendula that likely play a role in the chemical activity of the herb include saponins, carotenoids, essential oil, sterols, flavonoids, and mucilage. Triterpenoids, though, appear to be the most significant anti-inflammatory components of the flower.[15] The anti-inflammatory activity of calendula seems to be supported by emerging scientific evidence. A study with mice showed significant anti-inflammatory evidence by several members of the Compositae family, including calendula.[16] As is the case with all members of the Compositae family, calendula can cause contact dermatitis and it seems to be the sesquiterpene lactones most responsible for eliciting these allergic reactions.[17]

Research has shown that the butanolic fraction of *C. officinalis* displays antioxidant, free radical-scavenging activity.[18] The concentrations of flavonoids and carotenoids in calendula are sufficiently high that calendula flowers have been used as natural orange-yellow dyes. More importantly, such components are quite possibly responsible for yielding the reputed antioxidant effect. In fact, calendula flowers contain the potent antioxidant carotenoids β-carotene, lutein, and lycopene. This may at least partially account for the anti-inflammatory, antiseptic, antihemorrhagic, antiulcerogenic, and immunostimulating characteristics that have been attributed to calendula. Recent research indeed continues to bear out the viability of producing formulations with biological activity using the extracts of C. officinalis, given the prevalence of saponins, triterpenes, and flavonols.[5]

ORAL USES

Naturopathic healers ascribe antispasmodic, antimicrobial, and antiviral activity to calendula. As such, these practitioners consider calendula indicated systemically for digestive problems and as a gargle for oral/dental problems such as sores and toothaches.

Notably, orally administered C. officinalis extract has been shown to accelerate wound healing in rats with burn injury, with collagen-hydroxyproline and hexosamine levels significantly elevated in treated animals and lipid peroxidation significantly reduced compared to untreated controls.[19]

TOPICAL USES

Calendula is a popular antiseptic component in the armamentarium for the treatment of scrapes, cuts, burns, and wounds. Naturopathic healers also recommend its use for treating eczema, and note that the nontoxic herb acts topically as an anti-inflammatory and systemically to promote blood clotting. Topically applied calendula formulations have been found to be effective in treating diaper rash and for nipples tender from breastfeeding. Nearly 200 cosmetic creams, lotions, and shampoos are thought to contain C. officinalis extract.[2,3] The myriad topical uses by naturopathic practitioners include as an external wash, for ocular inflammations, abscesses, acne, bee stings, boils, eczema, and varicose veins.

Among homeopathic practitioners, calendula is considered a suitable home remedy for treating scrapes and burns.[20] Western medicine has also incorporated calendula as an antiseptic and anti-inflammatory agent, treating some skin disorders and pain.[18] Like the expansive range of calendula products, the number of potential indications is wide and growing. In vitro anti-HIV activity has been discerned in organic C. officinalis extract, which has prompted research into possible therapeutic applications, especially given the known antiviral properties of the flavonoid components of the plant.[14] In addition, several calendula cream formulations have also been demonstrated, in healthy volunteers, to protect against irritant contact dermatitis provoked by sodium lauryl sulfate.[21] In cosmetic or personal care products, it is used for skin conditioning in concentrations ranging from 0.1 to 1 percent.[8]

Diaper Dermatitis

A postmarketing surveillance study performed in Italy in 2007 comparing the efficacy and safety of two baby creams in 82 infants with diaper dermatitis revealed that the calendula-based cream was rated slightly safer and equally efficacious as a zinc oxide-based cream. Both creams were well tolerated and rated, with approximately 80 percent of physicians labeling the creams as "very good" or "good"; in 78 percent of cases, the doctor would prescribe the calendula cream and in 65.9 percent, the zinc oxide cream.[22]

Panahi et al. conducted a randomized, double-blind trial to compare the effects of calendula ointment and aloe vera cream on the frequency and severity of diaper dermatitis in 66 infants treated three times daily for 10 days (see Chapter 65, Aloe Vera). No adverse reactions were reported for either group. Symptoms

were mitigated in both groups, but the calendula group experienced significantly fewer rash sites. The researchers concluded that both botanicals, but especially topical calendula, offer safe and effective treatment options for diaper dermatitis.[23]

Radiation Dermatitis

In 2004, Pommier et al. performed a Phase III randomized trial to compare the effects of calendula and trolamine in 254 patients treated in a regional cancer center in France for the prevention of acute radiation dermatitis after breast cancer surgery. They found that acute dermatitis of grade 2 or higher occurred significantly less often in the calendula group (41 percent vs. 63 percent), with fewer interruptions in radiotherapy and less radiation-induced pain in patients treated with calendula. Although calendula was deemed more difficult to apply than trolamine, patient self-assessment revealed that calendula treatment was more satisfying. The investigators concluded that calendula is extremely effective in preventing acute dermatitis of grade 2 or higher and is a worthy option for patients undergoing postoperative radiotherapy for breast cancer.[24]

Five years later, Kassab et al. conducted a database review of randomized controlled trials (RCTs) of homeopathic medicines used to treat the adverse effects associated with cancer treatments. Eight controlled trials met inclusion criteria, with the Pommier and colleagues study cited above indicating that topical calendula was more effective than topical trolamine in preventing radiation dermatitis, and a small study with 32 subjects showing the superiority of Traumeel S® (a proprietary homeopathic formulation that includes calendula along with 11 other natural ingredients) over placebo as a mouthwash in treating chemotherapy-induced stomatitis.[25]

A 2010 systematic literature review of skin toxicity management during radiation therapy in Australia and New Zealand by Kumar et al. identified only seven articles, of 29 meeting search criteria, citing statistically significant side-effect management outcomes. Calendula was one of the topical therapies associated with such results.[26]

In a 2011 clinical update covering the previous four years of publications on evidence-based skin care management in radiation therapy, McQuestion highlighted the Pommier report on calendula cream as having the potential to lower the incidence of grade 2 or 3 cutaneous reactions in women with breast cancer, with the Radiodermatitis Putting Evidence into Practice (PEP) Resource consequently categorizing the herb as "likely to be effective."[27,28]

However, in 2013, an international interdisciplinary study group of experts convened to develop RCT-based guidelines on radiation dermatitis prevention and treatment was less impressed. Following an extensive literature review, they determined that while some evidence supported the use of silver sulfadiazine cream to lower dermatitis score, insufficient evidence had been compiled to support the use of numerous topical treatments, including calendula (see Chapter 80, Silver). For that reason, the panel recommended against the use of such interventions.[29]

SAFETY ISSUES

In terms of oral safety, the United States Food and Drug Administration (FDA), in 1997, labeled the dried flower of calendula used in spices and other natural seasonings and flavorings as generally recognized as safe (GRAS).[2,8]

Calendula has been associated with cases of contact dermatitis and can cause allergy in those allergic to ragweed and other members of the Compositae family (see Table 70-2). Reider et al.

tested 443 consecutive patients with Compositae mix, sesquiterpene lactone mix, arnica, calendula, and propolis, along with the European standard and other series, in a 2001 contact sensitization study. Nine patients (approximately 2.03 percent) reacted to calendula, of whom four were among the total of 18 subjects who reacted to Compositae mix. The researchers observed that calendula and arnica sensitization was often correlated with colophonium, fragrance mix, Myroxylon Pereirae resin, and propolis reactions (see Chapter 60, Honey/Propolis/Royal Jelly). They concluded that testing calendula and arnica sensitivity only with Compositae or sesquiterpene mix alone is insufficient and that Compositae allergy is a significant contributor to the prevalence of contact dermatitis. Further, they suggested that given the pervasive use of extracts of such plants in cosmetic and occupational products, patch testing should be adapted accordingly, with additional plant extracts or additions to the commercial Compositae mix.[30]

Some authors believe that the increasing use of herbal medicine and herb-based cosmetics may lead to an increase in contact dermatitis as some of the more popular herbs (e.g., arnica, chamomile, marigold, and echinacea) are members of the Compositae family. It is not yet known what the relative risks of provoking contact dermatitis are from the use of products containing herbs of the Compositae family.[17] In addition, despite a growing body of research on the use of calendula, current data are not sufficient to establish a scientific standard of safety for *C. officinalis* extract in cosmetic formulations.[2]

The results of a prospective, multicenter, observational study of adverse drug reactions to Asteraceae extracts in German primary care between September 2004 to September 2006 indicated that calendula was the second most prescribed agent, and that the use of these agents (including chamomile and arnica) was not linked to a high risk of adverse reactions (see Chapter 70, Chamomile).[31]

According to a report by the Cosmetic Ingredient Review (CIR) Expert Panel in 2010, *C. officinalis* ingredients (extract, flower, flower extract, flower oil, and seed oil) are safe for use in cosmetic formulations for the uses and concentrations considered. Though some of the ingredients may act as mild ocular irritants, they were not found to be sensitizing, photosensitizing, or otherwise irritating in animal or clinical testing.[32]

ENVIRONMENTAL IMPACT

The significance of the environmental impact from the cultivation and commercial use of *C. officinalis* is not well reported. The herb is known to grow rapidly and for being easy to germinate and tend.[33]

FORMULATION CONSIDERATIONS

A 2010 *in vivo* experiment in rats conducted by Vargas et al. indicated that hyperbranched polyglycerol electrospun nanofibers containing *C. officinalis* may be an effective bioactive wound dressing in the clinical setting.[34] The researchers noted the challenges of producing bioactive preparations of the herb due to poor solubility and decreased uptake of pharmaceutical ingredients.[34]

Kassab et al. suggest that formulation adjustments for the calendula ointment used successfully in the study by Pommier et al. in acute radiation dermatitis should be considered given that 30 percent of the participants complained that it was difficult to apply.[25]

With all herbal extracts, the source of the herb greatly affects the amount of active constituents in the preparation. Assays that look at the final product help determine efficacy. Bernatoniene et al. describe the preparation of a hydrophilic calendula-containing cream in a 2011 published study.[35] Calendula can be prepared as a tea, oil, cream, serum, or lotion.

USAGE CONSIDERATIONS

In Germany, calendula is prescribed for dermatitis and eczema as well as several non-dermatologic indications, such as upper respiratory conditions, conjunctival disorders, middle ear and mastoid ailments, and arthropathies.[31] Absorption rates of the preparation and interactions with other ingredients depend on the type of preparation used and the presence of other ingredients.

SIGNIFICANT BACKGROUND

The German Commission E, European Scientific Co-operative on Phytotherapy, British Herbal Pharmacopoeia, and World Health Organization monographs acknowledge *C. officinalis* for wound-healing and anti-inflammatory properties.[3] Calendula has, indeed, long been used as a topical agent for its anti-inflammatory activity. In recent years, the presence of several active ingredients, including flavonoids and phenolic acids, has fueled research into potential antioxidant activity.

Wound Healing

In 2009, Preethi and Kuttan found that oral administration and topical application of *C. officinalis* exhibited potent wound-healing activity in a rat model. Wound closure was found to be 90 percent in the extract-treated group and 51.1 percent in the control group after eight days. Reepithelialization took 17.7 days for the control group, but 14 days in animals receiving a 20 mg/kg/wt. dose and 13 days for animals administered 100 mg/kg/wt. Compared to control rats, significant increases in hydroxyl proline and hexosamine content were recorded in the animals treated with calendula.[36]

The next year, Parente et al. used a rat model to demonstrate that the healing activity associated with calendula, particularly its constituent triterpenes and steroids, can be partly attributed to the positive influence the herb exerts on angiogenesis, as indicated by the promotion of neovascularization.[13]

Photoprotection and Antiaging Activity

Fonseca et al. conducted an investigation in 2010 into the potential of orally administered *C. officinalis* extract to prevent ultraviolet (UV) B-induced oxidative stress in the skin of hairless mice. They found that doses of 150 and 300 mg/kg maintained glutathione levels nearly to the level of nonexposed control mice. The investigators acknowledged this photoprotective effect but suggested that more research is necessary to fully elucidate the protective activity delivered to the skin by calendula.[11]

The next year, the same team studied the possible preventive effects of topical *C. officinalis* extracts against UVB-induced skin damage. Using hairless mice, the researchers found that although all of the tested formulations were physically and functionally stable, the gel formulation was the most effective for topical delivery. The gel maintained diminished glutathione levels approximating those of nonirradiated mice, but did not alter the UVB-enhanced activities of gelatinase-9 or myeloperoxidase. Histologic examination revealed that the calendula gel attenuated UVB-induced effects that manifest as changes to collagen fibrils. The authors attributed the observed photoprotective effect from topically applied calendula to the effect of the gel in potentially enhancing collagen production in the connective tissue of the hairless mice.[37]

Using the Cutometer 580 MPA on 21 healthy human volunteers over eight weeks earlier in 2011, Akhtar et al. determined that a topically applied calendula formulation was effective in rendering significant improvements in skin hydration and firmness.[38]

In 2012, Mishra et al. assessed the effects of a cream containing *C. officinalis* essential oil on the skin of albino rats exposed to UVB. In comparison to untreated controls, animals exposed to one month of daily UVB exposure and treatment with 4 or 5 percent calendula cream experienced significant reductions in malondialdehyde levels and significant increases in catalase, glutathione, superoxide dismutase, ascorbic acid, and total protein levels. The investigators concluded that topically applied calendula essential oil cream prevents UVB-induced changes in cutaneous antioxidant levels.[4] Previously, Mishra et al. showed, *in vitro*, that a calendula oil in cream formulation displayed an appreciable sun protection factor (SPF) and has potential to exert photoprotective effects in sunscreen creams.[33]

Anticancer Activity

In 2013, Ali et al. used the two-stage skin carcinogenesis model in mice to evaluate the chemopreventive effects of the methanolic extracts of three medicinal herbs (*Trigonella foenum-graecum*, *Eclipta alba*, and *C. officinalis*) over 32 weeks. All three extracts were effective in suppressing proliferation by boosting endogenous antioxidant defense, hindering nuclear factor-κB, diminishing inflammation, augmenting immunosurveillance of the genetically mutated cells, and silencing cell cycle progression signals. The investigators noted that the herbal extracts also engendered the stable cytoplasmic expression of p53-mediated apoptosis, resulting in fewer and regressed tumors.[39] *C. officinalis* is also considered among herbalists and naturopathic practitioners to be among the herbs useful in supporting a holistic approach to cancer treatment.[6]

Chronic Venous Leg Ulcer Treatment

Thirty-four patients with venous leg ulcers were clinically examined by Duran et al. in 2005 after 21 were treated with a topical *C. offinalis* ointment and 13, a control ointment, for three weeks. Total surface area of the ulcers declined by 41.71 percent in the experimental group, with complete epithelialization achieved in seven patients. A reduction of 14.52 percent was recorded in the control group, with four patients achieving epithelialization. While the investigators viewed their results as preliminary, they acknowledged the statistically significant acceleration of wound healing in patients using the calendula ointment, suggesting its viability in venous ulcer epithelialization.[40]

In 2012, Kundaković et al. conducted a seven-week prospective nonrandomized pilot study of the effects of Herbadermal® ointment, which combines calendula, garlic, and St. John's wort, on the epithelialization and microbial flora of 25 patients (15 women, 10 men) with venous ulcers. Epithelialization was measured as 99.1 percent after seven weeks, with no significant impact on microbial flora identified. The investigators found this topical botanical formulation effective in delivering antierythematous, antiedematous, epithelializing activity.[41]

Other Uses

In 2012, Saini et al. investigated the effects of calendula on human gingival fibroblast-mediated collagen degradation and matrix metalloproteinase (MMP) activity based on the prominent role of quercetin among components of the flower. They found that calendula 2 to 3 percent completely inhibited MMP-2 activity and fibroblast-mediated collagen degradation as did various doxycycline and quercetin doses, but calendula was more effective than the corresponding concentrations of pure quercetin, which the researchers ascribed to other key constituents of the herb. Given these findings, they speculated that calendula has the potential to arrest periodontal disease progression.[1]

CONCLUSION

There is a long history of traditional medical use of calendula and compelling anecdotal evidence of its efficacy for certain dermatologic conditions. As is also the case with most herbs and herbal ingredients in cosmeceuticals, there is a paucity of randomized, double-blind, placebo-controlled studies establishing incontrovertible evidence of efficacy. Products containing calendula do appear to be safe but there is potential for products of the Compositae family to elicit allergic reactions. Additional research is necessary to assess the relative safety of these products and to determine if such herbal cocktails, with calendula as a leading active ingredient, can impart the same or similar benefits as those reported from traditional use of the less dilute form of the herb.

REFERENCES

1. Saini P, Al-Shibani N, Sun J, et al. Effects of Calendula officinalis on human gingival fibroblasts. *Homeopathy*. 2012;101:92.
2. Anonymous. Final report on the safety assessment of Calendual officinalis extract and Calendula officinalis. *Int J Toxicol*. 2001;20(Suppl 2):13.
3. Arora D, Rani A, Sharma A. A review on phytochemistry and ethnopharmacological aspects of genus Calendula. *Pharmacogn Rev*. 2013;7:179.
4. Mishra AK, Mishra A, Verma A, et al. Effects of calendula essential oil-based cream on biochemical parameters of skin of albino rats against ultraviolet B radiation. *Sci Pharm*. 2012;80:669.
5. Pérez-Carreón JI, Cruz-Jiménez G, Licea-Vega JA, et al. Genotoxic and anti-genotoxic properties of Calendula officinalis extracts in rat liver cell cultures treated with diethylnitrosamine. *Toxicol In Vitro*. 2002;16:253.
6. Hoffmann D. *Medical Herbalism: The Science and Practice of Herbal Medicine*. Rochester, VT: Healing Arts Press; 2003:458, 488, 491, 535.
7. Preethi KC, Kuttan G, Kuttan R. Anti-inflammatory activity of flower extract of Calendula officinalis Linn. And its possible mechanism of action. *Indian J Exp Biol*. 2009;47:113.
8. Re TA, Mooney D, Antignac E, et al. Application of the threshold of toxicological concern approach for the safety evaluation of calendula flower (Calendula officinalis) petals and extracts used in cosmetic and personal care products. *Food Chem Toxicol*. 2009;47:1246.
9. Foster S. *An Illustrated Guide to 101 Medicinal Herbs: Their History, Use, Recommended Dosages, and Cautions*. Loveland, CO: Interweave Press; 1998:44-45.
10. Mills S, Bone K. *Principles and Practice of Phytotherapy: Modern Herbal Medicine*. London: Churchill Livingstone; 2000:133.
11. Fonseca YM, Catini CD, Vicentini FT, et al. Protective effect of Calendula officinalis extract UVB-induced oxidative stress in skin: Evaluation of reduced glutathione levels and matrix metalloproteinase secretion. *J Ethnopharmacol*. 2010;127:596.
12. Basch E, Bent S, Foppa I, et al. Marigold (Calendula officinalis L.): An evidence-based systematic review by the Natural Standard Research Collaboration. *J Herb Pharmacother*. 2006;6:135.
13. Parente LM, Andrade MA, Brito LA, et al. Angiogenic activity of Calendula officinalis flowers L. in rats. *Acta Cir Bras*. 2011;26:19.
14. Kalvatchev Z, Walder R, Garzaro D. Anti-HIV activity of extracts from Calendula officinalis flowers. *Biomed Pharmacother*. 1997;51:176.

15. Della Loggia R, Tubaro A, Sosa S, et al. The role of triterpenoids in the topical anti-inflammatory activity of Calendula officinalis flowers. *Planta Med.* 1994;60:516.

16. Akihisa T, Yasukawa K, Oinuma H, et al. Triterpene alcohols from the flowers of compositae and their anti-inflammatory effects. *Phytochemistry.* 1996;43:1255.

17. Paulsen E. Contact sensitization from Compositae-containing herbal remedies and cosmetics. *Contact Dermatitis.* 2002;47:189.

18. Cordova CA, Siqueira IR, Netto CA, et al. Protective properties of butanolic extract of the Calendula officinalis L. (marigold) against lipid peroxidation of rat liver microsomes and action as free radical scavenger. *Redox Rep.* 2002;7:95.

19. Chandran PK, Kuttan R. Effect of Calendula officinalis flower extract on acute phase proteins, antioxidant defense mechanism and granuloma formation during thermal burns. *J Clin Biochem Nutr.* 2008;43:58.

20. Kaplan B. Homeopathy: 3. Everyday uses for all the family. *Prof Care Mother Child.* 1994;4:212.

21. Fuchs SM, Schliemann-Willers S, Fischer TW, et al. Protective effects of different marigold (Calendula officinalis L.) and rosemary cream preparations against sodium-lauryl-sulfate-induced irritant contact dermatitis. *Skin Pharmacol Physiol.* 2005;18:195.

22. Guala A, Oberle D, Ramos M. Efficacy and safety of two baby creams in children with diaper dermatitis: Results of a postmarketing surveillance study. *J Altern Complement Med.* 2007;13:16.

23. Panahi Y, Sharif MR, Sharif A, et al. A randomized comparative trial on the therapeutic efficacy of topical aloe vera and Calendula officinalis on diaper dermatitis in children. *Scientific WorldJournal.* 2012;2012:810234.

24. Pommier P, Gomez F, Sunyach MP, et al. Phase III randomized trial of Calendula officinalis compared with trolamine for the prevention of acute dermatitis during irradiation for breast cancer. *J Clin Oncol.* 2004;22:1447.

25. Kassab S, Cummings M, Berkovitz S, et al. Homeopathic medicines for adverse effects of cancer treatments. *Cochrane Database Syst Rev.* 2009;2:CD004845.

26. Kumar S, Juresic E, Barton M, et al. Management of skin toxicity during radiation therapy: A review of the evidence. *J Med Imaging Radiat Oncol.* 2010;54:264.

27. McQuestion M. Evidence-based skin care management in radiation therapy: Clinical update. *Semin Oncol Nurs.* 2011;27:e1.

28. Feight D, Baney T, Bruse S, et al. Putting evidence into practice. *Clin J Oncol Nurs.* 2011;15:481.

29. Wong RK, Bensadoun RJ, Boers-Doets CB, et al. Clinical practice guidelines for the prevention and treatment of acute and late radiation reactions from the MASCC Skin Toxicity Study Group. *Support Care Cancer.* 2013;21:2933.

30. Reider N, Komericki P, Hausen BM, et al. The seamy side of natural medicines: Contact sensitization to arnica (Arnica montana L.) and marigold (Calendula officinalis L.). *Contact Dermatitis.* 2001;45:269.

31. Jeschke E, Ostermann T, Lüke C, et al. Remedies containing Asteraceae extracts: A prospective observational study of prescribing patterns and adverse drug reactions in German primary care. *Drug Saf.* 2009;32:691.

32. Andersen FA, Bergfeld WF, Belsito DV, et al. Final report of the Cosmetic Ingredient Review Expert Panel amended safety assessment of Calendula officinalis-derived cosmetic ingredients. *Int J Toxicol.* 2010;29:221S.

33. Mishra A, Mishra A, Chattopadhyay P. Assessment of in vitro sun protection factor of Calendula officinalis L. (Asteraceae) essential oil formulation. *J Young Pharm.* 2012;4:17.

34. Vargas EA, do Vale Baracho NC, de Brito J, et al. Hyperbranched polyglycerol electrospun nanofibers for wound dressing applications. *Acta Biomater.* 2010;6:1069.

35. Bernatoniene J, Masteikova R, Davalgiene J, et al. Topical application of Calendula officinalis (L.): Formulation and evaluation of hydrophilic cream with antioxidant activity. *J Med Plants Res.* 2011;5:868.

36. Preethi KC, Kuttan R. Wound healing activity of flower extract of Calendula officinalis. *J Basic Clin Physiol Pharmacol.* 2009;20:73.

37. Fonseca YM, Catini CD, Vicentini FT, et al. Efficacy of marigold extract-loaded formulations against UV-induced oxidative stress. *J Pharm Sci.* 2011;100:2182.

38. Akhtar N, Zaman SU, Khan BA, et al. Calendula extract: Effects on mechanical parameters of human skin. *Acta Pol Pharm.* 2011;68:693.

39. Ali F, Khan R, Khan AQ, et al. Assessment of augmented immune surveillance and tumor cell death by cytoplasmic stabilization of p53 as a chemopreventive strategy of 3 promising medicinal herbs in murine 2-stage skin carcinogenesis. *Integr Cancer Ther.* 2013 Dec 19. [Epub ahead of print]

40. Duran V, Matic M, Jovanović M, et al. Results of the clinical examination of an ointment with marigold (Calendula officinalis) extract in the treatment of venous leg ulcers. *Int J Tissue React.* 2005;27:101.

41. Kundakovic T, Milenković M, Zlatković S, et al. Treatment of venous ulcers with the herbal-based ointment Herbadermal®: A prospective non-randomized pilot study. *Forsch Komplementmed.* 2012;19:26.

CHAPTER 72

Edelweiss

Activities:

Anti-inflammatory, antimicrobial, antioxidant, analgesic, DNA-protective[1]

Important Chemical Components:

Polyphenols, including quercetin-3-*O*-β-D-glucoside, luteolin-7-*O*-β-D-glucoside, luteolin-3'-*O*-β-D-glucoside, luteolin-4'-*O*-β-D-glucoside, apigenin-7-*O*-β-D-glucoside, 6-hydroxy-luteolin-7-*O*-β-D-glucoside, luteolin-7,4'-di-*O*-β-D-glucoside, chrysoeriol-7-*O*-β-D-glucoside, leontopodic acid and 3,5-dicaffeolyquinic acid; sesquiterpenes, such as isocomene, 14-acetoxy-isocomene, silphiperfolene acetate, silphinene, and bisabolane derivatives [2]; lignans, including leoligin [(2S,3R,4R)-4-(3,4-dimethoxybenzyl)-2-(3,4-dimethoxyphenyl)tetrahydrofuran-3-yl]methyl (2Z)-2-methylbut-2-enoat; β-sitosterol; coumarins; benzofurans[3,4]

Origin Classification:

This ingredient is natural. Organic forms exist.

Personal Care Category:

Anti-inflammatory, skin protective, conditioning

Recommended for the following Baumann Skin Types:

DSNT, DSPT, DSNW, DSPW, OSNT, OSPT, OSNW, and OSPW

SOURCE

Leontopodium alpinum, better known as edelweiss (German for "noble whiteness" and understood as "noble purity"; the scientific name "leontopodium" is a Latin adaptation of the Greek *leontopódion* for "lion's paw"), is a European mountain flower found in the Alps, Pyrenees, and Carpathians, as well as the Balkan Peninsula.[5] Edelweiss is a member of the sunflower (Asteraceae, or less commonly known as Compositae) family long used ornamentally and honored symbolically in national currency, badges, song (perhaps most famously in the Rodgers and Hammerstein musical *The Sound of Music*), and other forms of national pride, including as the national flower of Switzerland.[5] Of medical interest, the plant has been used in traditional alpine folk medicine to treat abdominal disorders, angina, bronchitis, cancer, colitis, diarrhea, dysentery, fever, rheumatoid arthritis, and tonsillitis (Table 72-1).[2,6,7]

HISTORY

Folk medicine uses of edelweiss were founded on the anti-inflammatory qualities of the herb.[1,7,8] Diarrhea and dysentery were listed as indications in 1582, as was breast cancer, which was treated with a compress infused with the boiled extract.[1,5,6] The use of *L. alpinum* in Polish traditional medicine to treat tumors was reported in the 1960s and cardioprotective benefits of the herb were cited in 1975.[6] Recent phytochemical and pharmacologic investigations of the aerial and root portions of the plant have uncovered constituents exhibiting anti-inflammatory, antimicrobial, and leukotriene-inhibiting properties.[2]

CHEMISTRY

In 2006, Schwaiger et al. identified and measured the major phenolic constituents of edelweiss. They compared retention times, ultraviolet (UV) and mass spectra of nearly all separated constituents to commercially available reference compounds or those isolated from the plant using column chromatography. Among the constituent compounds of edelweiss were found several known polyphenolic antioxidants, including quercetin-3-*O*-β-D-glucoside, luteolin-7-*O*-β-D-glucoside, luteolin-3'-*O*-β-D-glucoside, luteolin-4'-*O*-β-D-glucoside, apigenin-7-*O*-β-D-glucoside, 6-hydroxy-luteolin-7-*O*-β-D-glucoside, luteolin-7,4'-di-*O*-β-D-glucoside, chrysoeriol-7-*O*-β-D-glucoside, leontopodic acid, and 3,5-dicaffeolyquinic acid. A new natural product [3,4,5-tri-(E)-caffeoly-D-glucaric acid] was also discovered in the process and named leontopodic acid B.[9] Various secondary active metabolites have also been detected, including highly bioactive sesquiterpenes, diterpenes, lignans, and benzofurans, as well as the aforementioned polyphenols.[1]

Leoligin has been identified as the major lignan, and key active component, found in the roots of edelweiss.[3,10] In fact, it has been shown to act as a safe and effective cholesteryl ester transfer protein agonist, demonstrating potential for influencing high-density lipoprotein metabolism.[10] In addition, the isocomene and related compounds found in the plant are thought to show promise as antidementia agents.[2] Overall, substantial antioxidant, antibacterial, and anti-inflammatory properties associated with edelweiss extracts have been confirmed in several pharmacologic studies.[11]

ORAL USES

In traditional alpine medicine, edelweiss has been boiled with milk and honey to alleviate stomach aches, in humans and livestock.[4,6] The herb was boiled in wine and mixed with milk to treat oral conditions.[6] Other indications treated with edelweiss tea include bronchitis, diarrhea, and dysentery.[4,6]

TABLE 72-1
Pros and Cons of Edelweiss

Pros	Cons
Used as an anti-inflammatory agent in folk medicine	Few clinical or basic science findings available
Several bioactive constituents identified and found to exhibit potent antioxidant and anti-inflammatory activity	Activities of the extract depend upon plant sourcing and methods of extraction used

In 2006, Speroni et al. gauged the anti-inflammatory and analgesic effects of the dichloromethane, methanolic, and carbon dioxide extracts of the aerial parts and roots of edelweiss after oral administration to rats and mice. In pretreated specimens, histological examination revealed significant decreases in carrageenan-induced rat paw inflammation. In the rat paw edema assay, the most activity was seen in the lipophilic extracts of the aerial plant parts, with swelling diminished by 80 percent from the dichloromethane extract and 72 percent from the carbon dioxide extract. The presence in high concentrations of linoleic and linolenic acids, known to inhibit the arachidonic acid cascade, in the aerial parts of the plant is thought to at least partially account for the greater anti-inflammatory effectiveness from this area. Analgesic effects were more salient in association with treatment from the root extracts as compared to the aerial parts, which the authors suggested was indicative of varying mechanisms of action. Also, they evaluated the antioxidant properties of some of the extracts to ascertain any correlations with the observed anti-inflammatory characteristics. The investigators speculated that flavonoid glycosides in the aerial parts contributed to antioxidant strength, whereas terpenes, lignans, coumarins, and benzofurans were deemed active root constituents.[4]

TOPICAL USES

Edelweiss has been incorporated into several topical preparations, primarily touted for antiaging activity. There is little published literature or clinical evidence to support such inclusion. The anti-inflammatory and antioxidant properties identified in the aerial parts of the cultivated plant have been recently exploited in various cosmetic formulations, particularly sunscreens, intended to provide cutaneous protection against UV-induced chronic inflammation, photoaging, and cancer.[7,9]

In 2004, Dobner et al. conducted a study using *L. alpinum* that offered dermatologic implications. Specifically, they examined the aerial (i.e., capitula, inflorescence leaves, stems, stem leaves, and leaves of the basal rosette)[9] parts of edelweiss for their *in vivo* topical anti-inflammatory effects on croton oil-induced ear dermatitis in mice. They found that dichloromethane extract dose-dependently reduced edema, with the extract conferring greater activity than methanol and 70 percent aqueous methanol extracts. Dichloromethane extracts from the aerial parts of the plant were also found to be more active than dichloromethane root extracts. The investigators noted that fatty acids contribute significantly to the antiedema effect of the aerial dichloromethane extract while the anti-inflammatory activity of the root extract could be attributed to bisabolane sesquiterpenes, tricyclic sesquiterpenes, coumarins, and lignans.[8]

SAFETY ISSUES

There are no reports of adverse side effects associated with *L. alpinum* usage; however, it is a member of the Compositae family (see Table 70.2) and therefore may cause allergic contact dermatitis in those allergic to ragweed, feverfew, chamomile, and marigold.

ENVIRONMENTAL IMPACT

L. alpinum grows sparsely in several European mountain ranges. It is a protected species in various countries and, in 1886, became the first protected plant in Austria.[7,8] Given perceived public concerns about the potential overexploitation of a wild protected species for medicinal and cosmetic purposes, Switzerland created plantations of edelweiss for cultivation in 2004.[7] In 2012, Daniela et al. found that the production of callus/tissue cultures established at these plantations may be an ideal venue for the biotechnological production of complex molecules suitable for medical and cosmetic application. Specifically, they found that a concentrated ethanolic extract of leontopodic acid-laden culture exhibited significant anti-inflammatory activity in primary human keratinocytes and endotheliocytes exposed to UVA and UVB, lipopolysaccharide, oxidized low-density lipoprotein, and various proinflammatory cytokines. The investigators concluded that edelweiss cell cultures are viable environmentally- and species-sensitive sources of anti-inflammatory agents potentially suitable for treating chronic inflammatory skin and other conditions.[7]

FORMULATION CONSIDERATIONS

Various processes are used to isolate the active compounds from edelweiss plants, and the formulation considerations depend upon which processes are used. The soil in which the plants are raised, the geographic location, and the climate can all affect the type and amount of components in plant extracts; therefore, efficacy can vary depending on the source of the plants.

USAGE CONSIDERATIONS

No interactions with other ingredients are known by the author.

SIGNIFICANT BACKGROUND

Lignans, polyphenolic plant metabolites derived from phenylalanine, are thought to exhibit antioxidant, anti-inflammatory, antihypertensive, antithrombotic, and lipid-lowering activity.[3] In 2009, Reisinger et al. found that leoligin, the primary lignan active in edelweiss, strongly suppressed intimal hyperplasia as well as vascular smooth muscle cell proliferation, by inducing G_1-phase cell cycle arrest, suggesting its viability as a nontoxic, nonthrombogenic treatment option for vein graft disease.[3]

It is thought that the constituents of edelweiss that have provided protection in a harsh environment, particularly its exposure to and absorption of UV radiation, may in turn have the potential to be harnessed to confer protection to human skin.[12,13] In addition, the significant polyphenolic and flavonoid content in edelweiss is thought to imbue the plant with substantial radical-scavenging, antioxidant, and photoprotective properties, with components such as β-sitosterol, luteolin-4'-O-β-D-glucoside, and bisabolane derivatives believed to impart soothing effects to its extracts.[11,12] The leontopodic acid found in *L. alpinum* is also thought to deliver antioxidant as well as DNA-protecting qualities, and to inhibit elastase, which may yield an antiaging effect.[14]

The white filamentary hair covering edelweiss bracts is thought to play an important protective role against dehydration as well as cold and UV exposure, absorbing rather than reflecting UV radiation.[13] Better understanding this UV screening process may lead to innovations in various products, including UV-protective sunscreen ingredients in cosmetic formulations.[13]

In Vitro Studies

In 2003, Dobner et al. evaluated the antimicrobial activity of extracts and several individual components of edelweiss. Using agar diffusion assays and the microbroth dilution method to ascertain minimum inhibitory concentrations, they noted significant antimicrobial activities displayed against *Enterococcus faecium*, *Escherichia coli*, *Pseudomonas aeruginosa*, *Staphylococcus aureus*, *Streptococcus pneumoniae*, and *Streptococcus pyogenes* strains. The researchers concluded that their findings buttress the previously observed traditional folk medicine uses of edelweiss to treat abdominal and respiratory conditions.[6]

In 2009, some of the same investigators, led by Costa, assessed the chemopreventive effects of the antioxidant leontopodic acid isolated from *L. alpinum*. After pretreatment with leontopodic acid, they evaluated various mycotoxins in two different cell lines, aflatoxin B_1 on HepG$_2$ cells and deoxynivalenol on U937 cells. Leontopodic acid was demonstrated to have protected U937 cells from deoxynivalenol-induced cell damage, though it did not protect HepG$_2$ cells from aflatoxin B_1 toxicity. The investigators also found that the edelweiss isolate enhanced glutathione peroxidase activity in U937; it had no such effect on glutathione S-transferase activity in HepG$_2$. They concluded that the primary mechanism of the potent antioxidant-associated chemopreventive activity delivered by leontopodic acid is the elevation of detoxifying enzymes, with the edelweiss constituent acting as a potent antioxidant.[15]

CONCLUSION

Edelweiss has been used in traditional medicine and continues to be used for some health issues in contemporary times. However, there is a conspicuous dearth of research to support the claims of effectiveness for edelweiss in topical formulations. For edelweiss to be established as a genuinely useful ingredient in skin care, like numerous other botanical sources of medication, much more research and clinical investigation is necessary. The scant data available suggest that such work is warranted.

REFERENCES

1. Safer S, Cicek SS, Pieri V, et al. Metabolic fingerprinting of Leontopodium species (Asteraceae) by means of ¹H NMR and HPLC-ESI-MS. *Phytochemistry*. 2011;72:1379.
2. Hornick A, Schwaiger S, Rollinger JM, et al. Extracts and constituents of Leontopodium alpinum enhance cholinergic transmission: Brain ACh increasing and memory improving properties. *Biochem Pharmacol*. 2008;76:236.
3. Reisinger U, Schwaiger S, Zeller I, et al. Leoligin, the major lignin from Edelweiss, inhibits intimal hyperplasia of venous bypass grafts. *Cardiovasc Res*. 2009;82:542.
4. Speroni E, Schwaiger S, Egger P, et al. In vivo efficacy of different extracts of Edelweiss (Leontopodium alpinum Cass.) in animal models. *J Ethnopharmacol*. 2006;105:421.
5. Safer S, Tremetsberger K, Guo YP, et al. Phylogenetic relationships in the genus Leontopodium (Asteraceae: Gnaphalieae) based on AFLP data. *Bot J Linn Soc*. 2011;165:364.
6. Dobner MJ, Schwaiger S, Jenewein IH, et al. Antibacterial activity of Leontopodium alpinum (Edelweis). *J Ethnopharmacol*. 2003;89:301.
7. Daniela L, Alla P, Maurelli R, et al. Anti-inflammatory effects of concentrated ethanol extracts of Edelweiss (Leontopodium alpinum Cass.) callus cultures towards human keratinocytes and endothelial cells. *Mediators Inflamm*. 2012;2012:498373.
8. Dobner MJ, Sosa S, Schwaiger S, et al. Anti-inflammatory activity of Leontopodium alpinum and its constituents. *Planta Med*. 2004;70:502.
9. Schwaiger S, Seger C, Wiesbauer B, et al. Development of an HPLC-PAD-MS assay for the identification and quantification of major phenolic edelweiss (Leontopodium alpinum Cass.) constituents. *Phytochem Anal*. 2006;17:291.
10. Duwensee K, Schwaiger S, Tancevski I, et al. Leoligin, the major lignin from Edelweiss, activates cholesteryl ester transfer protein. *Atherosclerosis*. 2011;219:109.
11. Ganzera M, Greifeneder V, Schwaiger S, et al. Chemical profiling of Edelweiss (Leontopodium alpinum Cass.) extracts by micellar electrokinetic capillary chromatography. *Fitoterapia*. 2012;83:1680.
12. Wenzel AF. Edelweiss (Leontopodium alpinum): Monograph on the biological effects of extracts of L. alpinum used in cosmetics, medical devices and medicinal products. *PSST*. 17 December, 2012.
13. Vigneron JP, Rassart M, Vértesy Z, et al. Optical structure and function of the white filamentary hair covering the edelweiss bracts. *Phys Rev E Stat Nonlin Soft Matter Phys*. 2005;71:011906.
14. Schwaiger S, Cervellati R, Seger C, et al. Leontopodic acid – A novel highly substituted glucaric acid derivative from edelweiss (Leontopodium alpinum Cass.) and its antioxidative and DNA protecting properties. *Tetrahedron*. 2005;61:4621.
15. Costa S, Schwaiger S, Cervellati R, et al. In vitro evaluation of the chemoprotective action mechanisms of leontopodic acid against aflatoxin B1 and deoxynivalenol-induced cell damage. *J Appl Toxicol*. 2009;29:7.

CHAPTER 73

Lavandula

Activities:

Anti-inflammatory, antimicrobial, antiseptic, anticolic, antispasmodic, antidepressant, sedative[1,2]

Important Chemical Components:

Tannins, coumarins (e.g., coumarin, umbelliferone), flavonoids (e.g., luteolin), triterpenes (e.g., ursolic acid), essential oil (i.e., linalyl acetate, linalool, 1,8-cineole, β-ocimene, limonene, lavandulyl acetate, terpinen-4-ol, borneol, β-caryophyllene, camphor, carvacrol, nerolidol, fenchone, perillyl alcohol)[3–8]

Origin Classification:

This ingredient is natural. Many organic options exit.

Personal Care Category:

Soothing, sedating, anti-inflammatory, analgesic

Recommended for the following Baumann Skin Types:

DSNT, DSPT, DSNW, DSPW, OSNT, OSNW, OSPT, and OSPW

SOURCE

Widely cultivated in southern Europe, the United States, the United Kingdom, and Australia for its essential oil, *Lavandula angustifolia*, better known as lavender, is a fragrant, hardy perennial shrub belonging to the Labiatae (Lamiaceae), or mint, family.[9,10] Native to the Mediterranean region, seeds of the shrub were transported to England and France through migration several hundred years ago. Many species of lavender have been used for therapeutic, cosmetic, culinary, and commercial purposes for much longer, on the order of thousands of years. *L. angustifolia*, also known as English lavender, or true lavender, is a commercially important species in the lucrative perfume industry. Though all 28 lavender species are believed to impart some therapeutic benefits to varying degrees, *L. angustifolia* (previously known as *L. officinalis*) is the species included most often in medicinal formulations and is known to exhibit anti-inflammatory qualities.[6] *L. latifolia*, *L. stoechas* (known as French lavender in Europe and Spanish lavender in the United States),[2] and *L. intermedia* (a sterile hybrid of *L. angustifolia* and *L. latifolia* and also known as lavandin) are also popular for cosmetic and therapeutic uses.[2,7,11,12] Topical application of lavender essential oil, extracted by steam distillation from the freshly cut aerial parts of the plant, is thought to alleviate the discomfort characteristic of rheumatism.[6] Indeed, traditional uses of lavender oil include relaxation, wound healing, and improving circulation to the skin.[4,9]

HISTORY

Lavender was used in ancient societies for perfumery as well as medical purposes (Table 73-1). Derived from the Latin word *lavare* ("to wash"), the plant was named for its practical antiseptic and disinfectant applications in ancient Arabia, Greece, and Rome.[9,10] Lavender blossoms, believed to be from *L. stoechas*, were used by ancient Greeks and Romans to scent bath water, bathe wounds, and prevent infections at communal baths. Its activity as an antiseptic formed the foundation of its earliest traditional uses:[13] Lavender oil was used in ancient Egypt in the mummification process.[9,10] In Iranian medicine, *L. angustifolia* has been used for several centuries to treat inflammatory conditions, with its roots dating back to ancient Persia when the herb (*ostokhoddous* in Persian) was cited by the physician/polymaths Muhammad ibn Zakariya al-Razi (Latinized as Rhazes or Rasis) in his *Continens* circa 900 CE and, about 100 years later, Ibn Sina (Latinized as Avicenna) in his *The Canon of Medicine*.[9,11,14] It was used to treat psychiatric conditions in ancient Indian and Tibetan medicine.[9] The Ayurvedic pharmacopoeia currently includes *L. angustifolia* for multiple indications, including depressive and digestive disorders.[9]

Traditionally, lavender was hung in the home to repel mosquitoes, flies, fleas, and lice, and placed in linen closets to repel moths.[12] Its disinfectant and fumigant properties were also useful for sanitizing floors. Other folk claims made regarding the uses of lavender oil include activity as an analgesic, anticonvulsive, antidepressant, antibacterial, antifungal, antirheumatic, antispasmodic, diuretic, and sedative agent.[2,9,14] It was also used to treat headaches, particularly those resulting from tension or stress.[15] In addition, the essential oil distillate was and is used to treat wounds, bites, burns (including sunburns), lacerations, and even acne, psoriasis, fungal conditions, and herpes. Despite a long history of various applications, modern scientific research into the reputed benefits of lavender has largely been conducted only in the last 20 years, though the modern use of lavender in aromatherapy can be traced to 1932, when French perfumer René Gattefossé directly applied the essential oil to severe burns and published his accounts of healing.[9] While many of the biologic activities attributed to the herb have not been substantiated, recent scientific and clinical findings appear to support the traditional applications of lavender.[2]

TABLE 73-1
Pros and Cons of Lavandula

Pros	Cons
Used for thousands of years for therapeutic purposes	Scant clinical evidence of dermatologic efficacy
Wide range of reputed biologic activities	Limited scientific evidence to support many of its purported health benefits
Well regarded for aromatherapy	

CHEMISTRY

The active chemical components that provide lavender with its reputed medicinal properties include tannins, coumarins, flavonoids, triterpenoids, and essential oil components, themselves an intricate mix of mono- and sesquiterpenoid alcohols, esters, ketones, and oxides.[5] Linalool (3,7-dimethylocta-1,6-dien-3-ol) is the most important phytochemical constituent of the essential oil of lavender and is considered its primary active component, though it is present in lower concentration than its parent compound linalyl acetate (3,7-dimethyl-1,6-octadien-3yl acetate), another key active substance in the essential oil.[3,4,16,17] In animals and humans, lavender has been shown to exhibit sedative activity upon inhalation.[3] Lavender oil is believed to be one of the mildest of the known essential oils.[4]

In 2003, Hajhashemi et al. studied the effects of the hydroalcoholic extract, polyphenolic fraction, and essential oil of *L. angustifolia* in formalin- and acetic acid-exposed mice. Results from these tests along with a carageenan test in rats buttressed the traditional uses of lavender for anti-inflammatory and analgesic indications.[14]

ORAL USES

Lavender essential oil should not be taken internally, but the dry herb can be consumed as an infusion and is endorsed by the German Commission E.[6]

A 2009 randomized, between-subject, double-blind study to measure the effects of orally administered lavender essential oil on responses to watching anxiety-provoking film clips revealed that lavender exerts an anxiolytic effect in humans under low-anxiety conditions, but such effects many not hold in high-anxiety conditions.[18]

TOPICAL USES

Lavender is included in a wide variety of skin care products including soaps, moisturizers, lotions, bath gels, lip balms, hand creams, shampoos, and hair conditioners.[19] Current data on the uses of lavender bear out many of its traditional uses. Researchers have demonstrated the sedative qualities of *L. angustifolia* in humans and animals.[3] Positive effects on human skin have been demonstrated. Investigators studying perineal pain among women who had recently given birth found an association between use of lavender oil in baths and reduced discomfort.[20] Lavender has been reported to be of use in many different areas of medicine; in fact, there is a report in the literature of lavender oil (among several other essential oils) being used with moderate success for alopecia areata. In a randomized, double-blind, controlled trial lasting seven months, 86 patients received daily scalp massage treatments with either essential oil in a mixture of carrier oils or carrier oil only. Six of 41 in the control group showed improvement whereas 19 of 43 patients in the treatment group exhibited significant improvement.[21]

A 2005 report by Sosa et al. indicated that another lavender species, *L. multifada*, used in Moroccan traditional medicine, has also exhibited topical anti-inflammatory activity. In this study in mice, ethanol and aqueous extracts from the aerial parts of the plant dose-dependently suppressed croton oil-induced ear edema.[22]

Head Lice

In 2010, Barker and Altman led a randomized, assessor-blind, parallel-group, comparative efficacy trial in 123 patients with live head lice to evaluate three topical treatments, including a "suffocation" product, a formulation containing pyrethrins and piperonyl butoxide, and a tea tree oil and lavender oil combination (see Chapter 77, Tea Tree Oil). The herbal combination and the suffocation product were equally efficacious, with 97.6 percent in each group presenting as free of lice one day after the last treatment, as opposed to 25 percent in the pyrethrins-based product. The investigators suggested that the herbal as well as suffocation products appear to be viable alternatives to those based on pyrethrins.[23]

Episiotomy/Perineal Pain Treatment

Lavender oil may be prescribed to alleviate the pain associated with episiotomy due to its antiseptic and soothing activity. In 2012, Sheikhan et al. conducted a randomized controlled clinical trial with 60 primiparous women admitted for labor in Karaj, Iran. Patients were randomized into a treatment group using lavender oil and a control group, matching the standard hospital protocol. A statistically significant difference was recorded in pain intensity between the groups after four hours and five days following episiotomy, though such differences were not significant at 12 hours after surgery. Five days after episiotomy, the average redness, edema, ecchymosis, drainage, approximation (REEDA) score was significantly lower in the lavender group. The investigators concluded that lavender essential oil is an effective analgesic agent for diminishing perineal pain after episiotomy and may be a suitable option over povidone-iodine.[24] These results support the findings of a larger clinical trial conducted in 120 primiparous women in Iran in 2011 with lavender essential oil derived from *L. stoechas*.[25]

Prior to the publication of these studies, Jones reviewed the evidence on use of lavender oil on perineal trauma, particularly in light of increasing anecdotal reports of effectiveness. She found negligible support for the notion that lavender oil accelerated healing, but acknowledged the benefits of lavender in aromatherapy. Further, she cautioned that women applying lavender oil directly to the perineum should use highly diluted forms.[26]

Aphthous Ulceration

In 2012, Altaei conducted laboratory and clinical assessments of the efficacy of lavender oil to treat recurrent aphthous ulceration. Initially, rabbits with induced ulcers were tested in a randomized, double-blind, placebo-controlled study, with animals treated with lavender oil manifesting significantly diminished ulcer size, accelerated mucosal repair, and faster healing than controls. Lavender oil also demonstrated broad antibacterial activity against all strains tested. In the clinical study, 115 patients were divided into topical lavender and placebo groups. Significant declines in inflammation, ulcer size, healing time, and pain were experienced by the subjects treated with lavender oil compared to baseline and the placebo group, with no adverse effects noted.[27] However, the next year, Baccaglini commented in response to this study, suggesting that the data undergirding topical lavender oil as a palliative treatment for recurrent aphthous stomatitis (RAS) are actually limited, the Altaei animal data were essentially irrelevant because mucosal injuries in rabbits differ from RAS in humans, and the human study was beset with multiple design flaws.[28]

Hirsutism

In 2013, Tirabassi et al. conducted a prospective, open-label, placebo-controlled, randomized study with 24 young women with mild idiopathic hirsutism to compare the potential efficacy of lavender and tea tree oils. Subjects received oil spray containing lavender and tea tree oil or placebo twice daily for three months in affected areas. Investigators reported a statistically significant reduction in hair diameter and hirsutism total score in the herbal group and no such difference in the placebo group. They concluded that the topical application of lavender and tea tree oils is effective in diminishing mild idiopathic hirsutism (see Chapter 77, Tea Tree Oil).[29]

SAFETY ISSUES

There are no reports of significant adverse effects from the use of lavender for therapeutic or cosmetic purposes. Similarly, there are no reports of drug interactions with lavender.[6] Mild contact dermatitis has been identified, though, from the use of dried lavender flowers used in items such as pillows and to disinfect ambient air.[30] Conversely, researchers have shown, *in vivo* and *in vitro*, that lavender oil has the capacity to mediate sudden allergic reactions by inhibiting mast cell degranulation.[31] However, there are caveats and contraindications.

In 2004, Prashar et al. showed that lavender oil was cytotoxic to human skin (endothelial cells and fibroblasts) *in vitro* at a concentration of 0.25 percent (v/v). Individual assays revealed that the activity of linalool corresponded to that of the whole oil, while linalyl acetate cytotoxicity was higher, indicating that linalool may be the active component with linalyl acetate activity hampered by an unknown factor in the oil.[4]

In addition, researchers have shown that linalool and linalyl acetate, the primary components of lavender oil, undergo auto-oxidation on air exposure, forming allergenic oxidation products, with linalool acting as a stronger sensitizing agent implicated in allergic contact dermatitis.[32] The same investigators subsequently demonstrated that lavender oil is devoid of natural protection against auto-oxidation, meaning that lavender oil exposed to air can lead to the development of potent contact allergenic hydroperoxides.[33] Nevertheless, linalool and linalyl acetate are rarely reported to be the sources of contact allergy.[4,32] Although the genotoxic profile of lavender oil has been deemed difficult to delineate, linalool, in particular, is thought to be safe.[17] That said, in 2003, the 7th Amendment to the European Cosmetic Directive mandated that cosmetic products incorporating any of 26 identified natural ingredients, including linalool, be labeled as possibly allergenic.[5]

Contact allergy to lavender oil is reportedly highest in Japan, where its frequency of use has been known to be prevalent.[30] It is advised that lavender oil and its constituents be used cautiously and in dilute forms, particularly in topical application.[4] Lavender oil in ketoprofen has also been implicated in photoallergic contact dermatitis.[34,35]

A small 2007 study with three prepubertal boys presenting with gynecomastia is also noteworthy. Henley et al. discerned that the patients were healthy otherwise with normal endogenous steroid levels. Gynecomastia emerged in each case through the topical use of products containing lavender and tea tree oils (see Chapter 77, Tea Tree Oil). Discontinuation of the product spurred resolution of the condition. The investigators also examined the natural oils in human cell lines and observed estrogenic and antiandrogenic properties. They concluded that chronic exposure to these oils likely accounted for the development of gynecomastia.[36]

ENVIRONMENTAL IMPACT

Cultivation in hot, dry climates at medium altitudes is necessary for optimal yields of *L. angustifolia* essential oils, which are produced in relatively low quantities.[5] Lavender species can endure intense heat, wind, and occasional frost.[5] Most commercial supplies are produced in France, where *L. angustifolia* is sometimes intermixed with *L. latifolia* and *L. intermedia*.[9]

FORMULATION CONSIDERATIONS

In 2006, Francis et al. found that degassing water facilitated the dispersion of natural, water-immiscible oils, particularly lavender, tea tree, and eucalyptus (see Chapter 77, Tea tree Oil). The process yields micron-sized droplets without the need for additives, with these natural oils in pure water left well suited for use in skin care formulations and oral sprays, according to the authors.[37] Lavender should be packaged in airless pumps to prevent oxidation.

USAGE CONSIDERATIONS

Lavender oil is now primarily used as a carminative, relaxant, and sedating agent in aromatherapy, and is one of the more popular of the 40 major essential oils.[13,38] Pharmaceutical grade lavender oil is typically composed of 0.8 to 3 percent volatile oil.[9] Both of the main constituents of lavender essential oil, linalool and linalyl acetate, are readily absorbed into the skin, usually within five minutes of topical application.[9]

SIGNIFICANT BACKGROUND

Research into the potential applications of lavender, particularly lavender essential oil, in medicine and dermatology, specifically, is ongoing but not especially extensive.

Antibacterial Activity

Roller et al. conducted a study in 2009 using four different lavender species to compare their antimicrobial efficacy singly and in combination on methicillin-sensitive and -resistant *Staphylococcus aureus* (MSSA and MRSA , respectively). They found that lavender oils from *L. angustifolia*, *L. latifolia*, *L. stoechas,* and *L. luisieri* suppressed MSSA and MRSA growth by direct contact except in the vapor phase. Two combinations (*L. luisieri* and *L. stoechas*; *L. luisieri* and *L. angustifolia*) of several binary combinations tested resulted in larger inhibition zones than those achieved by using individual oil. The researchers suggested that lavender oils might warrant more serious consideration for inclusion in antibacterial formulations.[7]

Also that year, Warnke et al. found that lavender oil was among several essential oils shown *in vitro* to evince strong efficacy against several common and hospital-acquired bacterial and yeast isolates (six *Staphylococcus* strains including MRSA, four *Streptococcus* strains, and three *Candida* strains including *Candida krusei*), suggesting potential viability as inexpensive and effective antiseptic topical treatment options even for antibiotic-resistant bacterial strains and antimycotic-resistant *Candida* species.[39]

Anticancer Activity

Work is scant in this area, but lavender may have a role to play in acting against mutations and, more relevant to current patients, alleviating some of the related stress.

Evandri et al. performed bacterial reverse mutation assays in 2005 and ascertained that lavender oil displayed potent anti-mutagenic activity, concentration-dependently shrinking mutant colonies in the *Salmonella typhimurium* TA98 strain exposed to the direct mutagen 2-nitrofluorene. In addition, lavender oil exhibited moderate antimutagenic properties against the same strain exposed to the direct mutagen 1-nitropyrene. The researchers concluded that these findings suggest a wide array of potential medical applications of lavender oil.[13] *In vitro* investigations into prospective anticancer properties of lavender oil have indicated that trace compounds, such as perillyl alcohol, do manifest such activity, including angiogenesis inhibition.[5,40,41]

In 2012, Boehm et al. conducted a systematic review of preclinical and clinical trial evidence on the benefits and safety of aromatherapy for cancer patients. Regarding lavender essential oil, they noted that patients with estrogen-dependent tumors should exercise caution in using topical lavender because of findings that it has contributed to engendering reversible prepubertal gynecomastia (see Safety section). They added, though, that lavender aromatherapy may have a beneficial effect for patients by reducing levels of the stress hormone cortisol.[38]

Aromatherapy

The use of lavender in aromatherapy is supported by anecdotal reports as well as recent data. Indeed, the essential oil of lavender is reputed to confer sedative, antispasmodic, and tranquilizing effects and, thus, has become a staple ingredient in aromatherapy. Such characteristics have been central, understandably, in research regarding mood and cognitive effects. In 2000, Saeki performed a randomized, crossover, controlled study using essential oil of lavender in a hot foot bath, finding that small but distinct changes in autonomic activity indicated relaxation in subjects.[42]

In a single-blind, randomized controlled trial of depression in 80 women, negative responses were reduced in the group treated with 80 percent grapeseed oil/20 percent lavender oil baths as opposed to 100 percent grapeseed oil baths for two weeks.[43] In a placebo-controlled trial with blinded observer, lavender oil administered via aroma stream resulted in slight improvement of agitated behavior among patients with severe dementia.[44]

A study of the olfactory effects of essential oils of lavender and rosemary on mood and cognitive performance offered disparate but telling results. Lavender was associated with a significant drop in performance of working memory and reduced attention span, suggesting a sedative effect.[45] The rosemary group was much more alert than the lavender and control groups. In a subjective evaluation of relative mood, the control group was significantly less content than the lavender and rosemary groups. Mood enhancement through treatment with lavender has been seen elsewhere.

In a one-month, double-blind, randomized trial, researchers studying depression found that a tincture of *L. angustifolia* may have therapeutic benefits as an adjunct to other treatments for moderate depression, thus warranting further investigation.[15]

In 2008, Xu et al. investigated the pharmaco-physio-psychologic effect of Ayurvedic oil-dripping treatment [Shirodhara, which combines the Sanskrit words *shiro* (head) and *dhhara* (flow)] using *L. angustifolia* essential oil in 16 healthy females. Shirodhara usually entails using medicated herbal sesame oils. Subjects were assigned randomly to robotic arm oil-dripping with either plain sesame oil (plain Shirodhara), sesame oil with lavender essential oil, or the control supine position. The researchers observed that lavender Shirodhara acted as a strong anxiolytic and induced or promoted an altered state of consciousness, also yielding the greatest climb in foot skin temperature of the interventions. The well-established relaxing effect of *L. angustifolia* essential oils was thought to partially account for these findings, as well as the pharmacologic action of sesame oil or lavender essential oil absorbed via the skin or mucosa.[46]

Although lavender aroma is reputed to exert a substantial relaxation effect, much of the supportive evidence is anecdotal. Howard and Hughes conducted a double-blind, mixed factorial, placebo-controlled trial in 96 healthy undergraduate women in 2008 to gauge the effects of lavender aromatherapy. Participants were exposed to lavender, placebo, or no scent while evaluated physiologically following a stimulating cognitive task. An instructional procedure, upon the introduction of an aroma, manipulated the expectations of the participants regarding the likely effects of the aroma on their ability to relax. The investigators found that while galvanic skin response was unaffected by the aroma, the instructional prompt did influence relaxation patterns, with subjects relaxing more when expecting to be hindered by the aroma and relaxing less when expecting to be calmed by the aroma. The authors concluded that their results suggest the potential of expectancy biases, which they claimed could be easily manipulated, influencing prior reports of lavender aroma facilitating relaxation.[47]

A more recent study by Grunebaum and colleagues (including the author of this text) randomized 30 subjects with no prior experience with cosmetic facial injections to exposure to lavender essential oil aroma or placebo during elective Botox injections to correct glabellar wrinkles. Participants exposed to lavender oil aroma experienced a significant decrease in heart rate after injection compared to their heart rate prior to injection. No such differences were seen in patients exposed to placebo. The investigators found that lavender did not influence pain perception, but the lavender aroma did elevate subjects' parasympathetic activity. They concluded that lavender aromatherapy appears to have the capacity to reduce anxiety for those undergoing minimally invasive cosmetic procedures.[48]

In 2011, Hongratanaworakit showed that the blended essential oils of lavender and bergamot topically applied to 40 healthy volunteers synergistically interacted to impart a relaxing effect. Specifically, the formulation applied to the abdomen yielded significant reductions in pulse rate, as well as systolic and diastolic blood pressure, as compared to those taking placebo, revealing diminished autonomic arousal in the treatment group. A comparative reduction in subjective behavioral arousal was also noted between the groups. The author suggested that the lavender/bergamot blend may be suitable in the clinical setting for treating anxiety or depression.[49]

CONCLUSION

Topical products that contain lavender appear to be safe, with mild allergic reactions as the most likely adverse responses. Research has established a scientific and clinical foundation for the traditional uses of lavender. It remains to be seen if double-blind, randomized, placebo-controlled trials will establish the use of lavender for dermatologic purposes. While it is unlikely that commercially available topical formulations including lavender are harmful, it appears just as unlikely that such products impart clinically significant benefits. Linking a well-regarded plant known for soothing qualities to potentially therapeutic activity is an effective marketing strategy that manufacturers employ with lavender among several other herbal ingredients.

REFERENCES

1. Mills S, Bone K. *Principles and Practice of Phytotherapy: Modern Herbal Medicine*. London: Churchill Livingstone; 2000:29–30.
2. Cavanagh HM, Wilkinson JM. Biological activities of lavender essential oil. *Phytother Res*. 2002;16:301.
3. Lis-Balchin M, Hart S. Studies on the mode of action of the essential oil of lavender (Lavandula angustifolia P. Miller). *Phytother Res*. 1999;13:540.
4. Prashar A, Locke IC, Evans CS. Cytotoxicity of lavender oil and its major components to human skin cells. *Cell Prolif*. 2004;37:221.
5. Woronuk G, Demissie Z, Rheault M, et al. Biosynthesis and therapeutic properties of Lavandula essential oil constituents. *Planta Med*. 2011;77:7.
6. Hoffmann D. *Medical Herbalism: The Science and Practice of Herbal Medicine*. Rochester, VT: Healing Arts Press; 2003:489, 561–2.
7. Roller S, Ernest N, Buckle J. The antimicrobial activity of high-necrodane and other lavender oils on methicillin-sensitive and –resistant Staphylococcus aureus (MSSA and MRSA). *J Altern Complement Med*. 2009;15:275.
8. Ben Salah M, Abderraba M, Tarhouni MR, et al. Effects of ultraviolet radiation on the kinetics of in vitro percutaneous absorption of lavender oil. *Int J Pharm*. 2009;382:33.
9. Denner SS. Lavandula angustifolia Miller: English lavender. *Holist Nurs Pract*. 2009;23:57.
10. Basch E, Foppa I, Liebowitz R, et al. Lavender (Lavandula angustifolia Miller). *J Herb Pharmacother*. 2004;4:63.
11. Wu J. Treatment of rosacea with herbal ingredients. *J Drugs Dermatol*. 2006;5:29.
12. Aburjai T, Natsheh FM. Plants used in cosmetics. *Phytother Res*. 2003;17:987.
13. Evandri MG, Battinelli L, Daniele C, et al. The antimutagenic activity of Lavandula angustifolia (lavender) essential oil in the bacterial reverse mutation assay. *Food Chem Toxicol*. 2005;43:1381.
14. Hajhashemi V, Ghannadi A, Sharif B. Anti-inflammatory and analgesic properties of the leaf extracts and essential oil of Lavandula angustifolia Mill. *J Ethnopharmacol*. 2003;89:67.
15. Akhondzadeh S, Kashani L, Fotouhi A, et al. Comparison of Lavandula angustifolia Mill. Tincture and imipramine in the treatment of mild to moderate depression: A double-blind, randomized trial. *Prog Neuropsychopharmacol Biol Psychiatry*. 2003;27:123.
16. Bickers D, Calow P, Greim H, et al. A toxicologic and dermatologic assessment of linalool and related esters when used as fragrance ingredients. *Food Chem Toxicol*. 2003;41:919.
17. Di Sotto A, Mazzanti G, Carbone F. Genotoxicity of lavender oil, linalyl acetate, and linalool on human lymphocytes in vitro. *Environ Mol Mutagen*. 2011;52:69.
18. Bradley BF, Brown SL, Chu S, et al. Effects of orally administered lavender essential oil on responses to anxiety-provoking film clips. *Hum Psychopharmacol*. 2009;24:319.
19. Baumann LS. Less-known botanical cosmeceuticals. *Dermatol Ther*. 2007;20:330.
20. Cornwell S, Dale A. Lavender oil and perineal repair. *Mod Midwife*. 1995;5:31.
21. Hay IC, Jamieson M, Ormerod AD. Randomized trial of aromatherapy. Successful treatment for alopecia areata. *Arch Dermatol*. 1998;134:1349.
22. Sosa S, Altinier G, Politi M, et al. Extracts and constituents of Lavandula multifada with topical anti-inflammatory activity. *Phytomedicine*. 2005;12:271.
23. Barker SC, Altman PM. A randomized, assessor blind, parallel group comparative efficacy trial of three products for the treatment of head lice in children – Melaleuca oil and lavender oil, pyrethrins and piperonyl butoxide, and a "suffocation" product. *BMC Dermatol*. 2010;10:6.
24. Sheikhan F, Jahdi F, Khoei EM, et al. Episiotomy pain relief: Use of Lavender oil essence in primiparous Iranian women. *Complement Ther Clin Pract*. 2012;18:66.
25. Vakilian K, Atarha M, Bekradi R, et al. Healing advantages of lavender essential oil during episiotomy recovery: A clinical trial. *Complement Ther Clin Pract*. 2011;17:50.
26. Jones C. The efficacy of lavender oil on perineal trauma: A review of the evidence. *Complement Ther Clin Pract*. 2011;17:215.
27. Altaei DT. Topical lavender oil for the treatment of recurrent aphthous ulceration. *Am J Dent*. 2012;25:39.
28. Baccaglini L. There is limited evidence that topical lavender oil is effective for palliative treatment of recurrent aphthous stomatitis. *J Evid Based Dent Pract*. 2013;13:47.
29. Tirabassi G, Giovannini L, Paggi F, et al. Possible efficacy of lavender and tea tree oils in the treatment of young women affected by mild idiopathic hirsutism. *J Endocrinol Invest*. 2013;36:50.
30. Sugiura M, Hayakawa R, Kato Y, et al. Results of patch testing with lavender oil in Japan. *Contact Dermatitis*. 2000;43:157.
31. Kim HM, Cho SH. Lavender oil inhibits immediate-type allergic reaction in mice and rats. *J Pharm Pharmacol*. 1999;51:221.
32. Sköld M, Hagvall L, Karlberg AT. Autoxidation of linalyl acetate, the main component of lavender oil, creates potent contact allergens. *Contact Dermatitis*. 2008;58:9.
33. Hagvall L, Sköld M, Bråred-Christensson J, et al. Lavender oil lacks natural protection against autoxidation, forming strong contact allergens on air exposure. *Contact Dermatitis*. 2008;59:143.
34. Goiriz R, Delgado-Jiménez Y, Sánchez-Pérez J, et al. Photoallergic contact dermatitis from lavender oil in topical ketoprofen. *Contact Dermatitis*. 2007;57:381.
35. Matthieu L, Meuleman L, Van Hecke E, et al. Contact and photo-contact allergy to ketoprofen. The Belgian experience. *Contact Dermatitis*. 2004;50:238.
36. Henley DV, Lipson N, Korach KS, et al. Prepubertal gynecomastia linked to lavender and tea tree oils. *N Engl J Med*. 2007;356:479.
37. Francis MJ, Gulati N, Pashley RM. The dispersion of natural oils in de-gassed water. *J Colloid Interface Sci*. 2006;299:673.
38. Boehm K, Büssing A, Ostermann T. Aromatherapy as an adjuvant treatment in cancer care – a descriptive systematic review. *Afr J Tradit Complement Altern Med*. 2012;9:503.
39. Warnke PH, Becker ST, Podschun R, et al. The battle against multi-resistant strains: Renaissance of antimicrobial essential oils as a promising force to fight hospital-acquired infections. *J Craniomaxillofac Surg*. 2009;37:392.
40. Zhang Z, Chen H, Chan KK, et al. Gas chromatographic-mass spectrometric analysis of perillyl alcohol and metabolites in plasma. *J Chromatogr B Biomed Sci Appl*. 1999;728:85.
41. Loutrari H, Hatziapostolou M, Skouridou V, et al. Perillyl alcohol is an angiogenesis inhibitor. *J Pharmacol Exp Ther*. 2004;311:568.
42. Saeki Y. The effect of foot-bath with or without the essential oil of lavender on the autonomic nervous system: A randomized trial. *Complement Ther Med*. 2000;8:2.
43. Morris N. The effects of lavender (Lavendula angustifolium) baths on psychological well-being: Two exploratory randomized control trials. *Complement Ther Med*. 2002;10:223.
44. Holmes C, Hopkins V, Hensford C, et al. Lavender oil as a treatment for agitated behavior in severe dementia: A placebo controlled study. *Int J Geriatr Psychiatry*. 2002;17:305.
45. Moss M, Cook J, Wesnes K, et al. Aromas of rosemary and lavender essential oils differentially affect cognition and mood in healthy adults. *Int J Neurosci*. 2003;113:15.
46. Xu F, Uebaba K, Ogawa H, et al. Pharmaco-physio-psychologic effect of Ayurvedic oil-dripping treatment using an essential oil from Lavandula angustifolia. *J Altern Complement Med*. 2008;14:947.
47. Howard S, Hughes BM. Expectancies, not aroma, explain impact of lavender aromatherapy on psychophysiological indices of relaxation in young healthy women. *Br J Health Psychol*. 2008;13:603.
48. Grunebaum LD, Murdock J, Castanedo-Tardan MP, et al. Effects of lavender olfactory input on cosmetic procedures. *J Cosmet Dermatol*. 2011;10:89.
49. Hongratanaworakit T. Aroma-therapeutic effects of massage blended essential oils on humans. *Nat Prod Commun*. 2011;6:1199.

CHAPTER 74

Horse Chestnut

Activities:

Anti-inflammatory, antioxidant, antiedematous, vasoconstrictive, venotonic

Important Chemical Components:

Saponins (particularly aescin, found in horse chestnut seeds), hydroxycoumarins (i.e., aesculin, fraxin, and scopolin, found in the bark), flavonoids (i.e., quercetin and kampferol, and their glycoside derivatives astragalin, isoquercitrin, and rutin), tannins (i.e., leucocyanidin, proanthocyanidin A$_2$), sterols, polysaccharides and oligosaccharides, and essential oils (e.g., oleic and linoleic acids, found in the leaves and flowers)[1–4]

Origin Classification:

This ingredient is natural. Organic forms exist.

Personal Care Category:

Chronic venous insufficiency, hemorrhoids, edema

Recommended for the following Baumann Skin Types:

DRNT, DRNW, DRPT, DRPW, DSNT, DSNW, DSPT, DSPW, ORNT, ORNW, ORPT, ORPW, OSNT, OSNW, OSPT, and OSPW

TABLE 74-1
Pros and Cons of Horse Chestnut

Pros	Con
Long history of traditional medical use	Appropriateness for broader, particularly antiaging, dermatologic indications is not well established
Shown in several randomized controlled trials to be an effective short-term treatment for mild-to-moderate CVI	
Effective orally and topically for edema and related cutaneous issues	

SOURCE

There are 15 known species of horse chestnut, which is found as both a tree and a shrub in all the temperate regions of Europe, Asia, and North America. Believed to have originated in the northern Greece/Balkan region of southeast Europe,[3] the European horse chestnut, *Aesculus hippocastanum*, which belongs to the Hippocastanaceae family, is the species of horse chestnut most often used in medical applications, traditionally for bronchitis, dysentery, hemorrhoids, and venous issues.[5] It is not known whether other species of horse chestnut have been thoroughly evaluated for their potential medicinal value. The European horse chestnut is not related to the more familiar sweet chestnut (*Castanea vesca*).[3] Its common name is believed to be based on the appearance of the seeds and the horseshoe-shaped mark that remains on the twig after autumnal leaf shedding.[3]

HISTORY

Traditional uses of *A. hippocastanum* are traced to the region of its provenance. For instance, *A. hippocastanum* is one of 227 plants identified in an ethnopharmacologic study found to be used traditionally for health purposes in Bosnia and Herzegovina.[6] The species was introduced into Western Europe around 1576 (Table 74-1).[7] As early as that century, nuts of the *A. hippocastanum* tree were used for medical applications ranging from persistent fever, with the first written record appearing in 1720,[3,8] to use on hemorrhoids as early as 1886,[8] and later varicose veins in the legs, phlebitis, and petechiae.[9,10] Early traditional uses also included rheumatism, leg cramps, gastrointestinal and bladder conditions, and rectal issues.[3,10,11] The bark was used in folk medicine to treat diarrhea and hemorrhoids.[7] In North America, Native Americans are said to have harnessed the toxic qualities of the seeds to stun fish.[7] The use of topically applied horse chestnut in cosmetic formulations emerged in 1980, with descriptions of applications to the face, scalp, oral cavity, body, hands, feet, and legs, as well as for foot and bodily hygiene and hemorrhoids.[1] Horse chestnut is now widely used in the pharmaceutical and cosmetics industries.[2] Antiaging or antiwrinkling uses have also been suggested, as Masaki et al. discovered in 1995 that *A. hippocastanum* extracts strongly scavenge active oxygen.[12]

CHEMISTRY

Most of the aerial sections of the European horse chestnut tree, such as the seeds, leaves, and bark, were traditionally utilized in medical treatments. Modern horse chestnut formulations are derived from extracts from the seeds, which are high in the active component aescin (also spelled as "escin"). In 1960, Lorenz and Marek found that β-aescin was the constituent of the saponin mixture in *A. hippocastanum* responsible for conferring antiedematous and vasoprotective activity.[3,13] The selective vascular permeabilization of aescin allows a higher sensitivity (e.g., of calcium channels) to molecular ions leading to increased venous contractile activity.[8]

The seeds contain hydroxycoumarins, flavonoids, tannins, sterols, saponins, the antioxidant proanthocyanidin A$_2$, and glycosides. "Aescin" is actually the collective name for the alkylated triterpene glycosides, or saponins, that represent 3 to between 6 and 10 percent of the active constituents of the seeds.[5,10,14] Aescin is present in α and β forms, the latter of which is composed of more than 30 triterpenoid derivatives of protoaescigenin and barrintogenol C and found in horse chestnut seed extract (HCSE) pharmaceuticals used for venous insufficiency.[1,3,8] Saponins are strong anti-inflammatory substances with a gentle, soapy texture.

Several flavonoids have been identified in horse chestnut seeds, with di- and triglycosides of quercetin and kaempferol shown to be dominant forms. Kapusta et al. observed that glycosides of these flavonoids can be obtained from industrial horse chestnut wastewater to be used in cosmetics, nutraceuticals, and food supplements.[2] In 1999, Wilkinson and Brown noted that an HCSE rich in quercetin and kaempferol derivatives displayed greater oxygen-scavenging capacity than 65 other tested plant extracts as well as antioxidant potency exceeding that of vitamin E, with cell-protective effects associated with the antiaging characteristics of antioxidants.[1]

The mechanism of action is not fully understood, but it is speculated that HCSE may work by inhibiting leukocyte activation.[15] Aescin, the major active ingredient of HCSE,[8] is believed to inhibit enzymes that attack vein interiors and thus fosters normal, healthy tone in vein walls and enhances circulation.[16] Specifically, aescin in HCSE facilitates the contraction of elastic fibers in capillary walls thereby increasing the contractility of the vessels and increasing venous tone.[17,18] Aescin has been found to hinder elastase and hyaluronidase *in vitro*. Both enzymes are involved in the degradation of proteoglycans, an important element in the extravascular matrix and component of endothelium. Researchers speculate that the aescin in horse chestnut alters the equilibrium between proteoglycans synthesis and degradation resulting in the prevention of vascular leakage.[5,15] Proanthocyanidin A_2 is also said to inhibit hyaluronidase activity.[1] Interestingly, extracts of *A. hippocastanum* were shown to be more effective than aescin alone in accounting for the potent venotonic activity associated with the plant, suggesting that the suppression of other enzymes (i.e., collagenase, elastase, and β-glucuronidase) is involved.[1,19]

Aescin is also associated with the release of prostaglandin F $2α$ ($PGF_{2α}$) from veins, antagonism to 5-hydroxytryptamine (5-HT, or better known as serotonin) and histamine, and decreased catabolism of tissue mucopolysaccharides.[8]

Rutin, which is believed to strengthen fragile capillaries, is another active ingredient in horse chestnut seeds. Several European investigators claim that aescin and rutin work synergistically with other active components to enhance circulation and ease inflammation and discomfort. The leaves of the horse chestnut tree purportedly have antioxidant properties that may slow skin wrinkling, though such claims have not been confirmed through controlled clinical trials. The amassed evidence clearly shows that horse chestnut ameliorates circulatory vein function.

ORAL USES

The oral administration of standardized HCSE is well established as an effective treatment primarily for chronic venous insufficiency (CVI) and edema, as well as diarrhea, fever, hemorrhoids, neuralgia, phlebitis, prostate enlargement, rectal issues, and rheumatism.[1,11] CVI is characterized by edema, enlarged veins near the skin surface, and leg fatigue. Indeed, there is copious, strong evidence, as Ernst et al. identified in a systematic review of randomized controlled trials (RCTs), for the effectiveness of oral HCSE for treatment of CVI.[20] The same researchers previously conducted a comprehensive review of placebo-controlled studies finding that

HCSE was superior to placebo in all cases.[15] They also noted reductions in lower-leg volume, leg circumference at the calf and ankle, and improvement in symptoms such as leg pain, pruritus, fatigue, and tension with only mild adverse reactions occurring rarely. The same study found equivalence between horse chestnut and O-(β-hydroxyethyl)-rutosides against the reference medication and equivalence between horse chestnut and compression therapy.[15]

In a 2012 literature search of six placebo-controlled trials assessing leg pain, Pittler and Ernst reported a significant reduction of leg pain in the groups treated with HCSE as compared to the placebo groups or reference treatments, with only mild and infrequent side effects. They concluded that horse chestnut is safe and effective for short-term CVI therapy, but more rigorous RCTs are necessary to evaluate overall, long-term efficacy.[21]

In a 12-week, randomized, partially-blinded, placebo-controlled parallel study of 240 patients, significant and equivalent reduction of edema resulted from horse chestnut and compression therapy as compared to placebo; both effective therapies were well tolerated with no adverse side effects.[18]

Another study, in which 5,000 patients with CVI were treated with standardized HCSE, showed improvement or clearing of all of the investigated symptoms (i.e., discomfort, fatigue, tension and edema in the leg, and pruritus).[22]

In 2013, Sipos et al., having earlier found that aescin suppresses allergic dermatitis in murine models, used a new porcine model to further test safe and novel alternatives to glucocorticoids and antihistamines. Orally administered pretreatment of animals with aescin potently and dose-dependently blocked allergic skin responses induced by the compound 48/80. The investigators concluded that their findings suggest the use of oral aescin as a new antiallergic agent.[23]

In addition, *A. hippocastanum*, as supplemented orally in the diet, is considered one of the several botanical extracts that may alleviate the symptoms of hemorrhoids and varicose veins.[24,25] The recommended dose for CVI in the United States is one 50-mg capsule taken twice daily for 2 to 16 weeks, though 50 to 75 mg is not uncommon.[25,26] The German Commission E suggests a total daily dose of 100 mg.[14]

TOPICAL USES

There are various uses for this herbal product in traditional Chinese medicine (TCM). Known as *tien shi li*, horse chestnut is used as an astringent, an anti-inflammatory, a diuretic, and an expectorant and for a wide range of conditions including circulatory problems and viruses. Western medicine uses HCSE as an astringent and an anti-inflammatory. Horse chestnut is a common ingredient in lotions, creams, massage oils, and other skin care products, often in combination with other herbal ingredients. Most such topical products tout the capacity of horse chestnut to combat varicose veins, swelling, and water retention, but some of the newer products ascribe antioxidant potency to horse chestnut and purport to combat wrinkling. The extract is also effective when used in a sitz bath for the treatment of hemorrhoids.

The topical application of standardized HCSE balm with 2 percent aescin supports healthy skin, blood vessels, and muscles,[9,27,28] particularly in the legs and hemorrhoidal plexus.[27] One double-blind, randomized, single-dose study assessing the effectiveness of a topically-applied standardized HCSE balm (2 percent aescin) for localized swelling and blood accumulation showed that the product containing aescin significantly reduced tenderness in the affected area as compared to placebo.[9] Indeed, aescin has demonstrated clinically significant activity in the treatment of hemorrhoids, CVI, and postoperative edema.[8]

SAFETY ISSUES

The crude form of *A. hippocastanum* (e.g., bark, leaves, and seeds) is toxic; only processed extracts should be used for medicinal purposes.[7] Horse chestnut is contraindicated for patients who have bleeding disorders or who take anticoagulant drugs, such as warfarin, because the herb reduces blood coagulation, or clotting. Nonsteroidal anti-inflammatory drugs (NSAIDs), particularly aspirin, as well as the analgesic acetaminophen/paracetamol potentially interact with coumarin-containing herbal supplements (such as horse chestnut), increasing the risk of bleeding.[14,29] Notably, though, aesculin, the primary coumarin present in *A. hippocastanum*, is found in the bark but not the seeds.[3] Due to lack of clinical data, oral HCSE is contraindicated in pregnant or nursing women.[3] An adverse reaction rate of 0.9 to 3.0 percent has been reported in association with the oral use of HCSE for CVI, with dizziness, headache, pruritus, and gastrointestinal disturbances more common.[5,8]

Topical horse chestnut has been associated, in a few instances, with allergic skin reactions. Overall, though, horse chestnut is generally thought to be safe as used in recommended doses. It should not be applied to ulcerated or broken skin.[10]

ENVIRONMENTAL IMPACT

There is no significant environmental impact of commercial horse chestnut production known by the author. In the United States, *A. hipposcastanum* is usually grown as a shade tree.[7] The modern medical supply of horse chestnut is cultivated and produced primarily in Poland.[7]

FORMULATION CONSIDERATIONS

Typically applied three to four times per day, topical HSCE formulations usually contain 2 percent aescin (1–3 percent is recommended).[3,30] A wide array of personal care products now include extracts of horse chestnuts, including creams and lotions, bath and shower foams, shampoos, and toothpastes.[1]

USAGE CONSIDERATIONS

HCSE is used both internally and externally to treat CVI and the related conditions such as varicose veins, leg cramps, phlebitis, and hemorrhoids (varicose veins of the anus and rectum). In topical form, horse chestnut is also used for wound healing and treating sprains and strains. Topical application of gels or creams containing 2 percent aescin, three or four times per day, is popular in Europe for eliminating hemorrhoids, skin ulcers, and varicose veins and healing bruises, sports injuries, and similar traumas. It is the most widely prescribed treatment for edema with venous insufficiency in Germany, where standardized HCSE has been approved by the Commission E for the treatment of pathological conditions of the veins of the legs, including pruritus, edema, nocturnal cramping in the calves, discomfort and a sensation of heaviness, as well as varicose and spider veins.[4,7]

There are some claims that horse chestnut may even be effective in the treatment of wrinkles, dark circles under the eyes, hair loss, cellulite, backache, and arthritis, but there is no reliable evidence in the literature to substantiate these claims. As an ingredient in facial creams and shaving products, it is intended for sensitive skin.

SIGNIFICANT BACKGROUND

While some have noted the adequacy of horse chestnut in the early phases of CVI as a result of its capacity to close venular endothelial gaps, compression therapy remains indicated for later stages (though horse chestnut may have the potential to act at later stages of CVI).[31] Various authors note that poor compliance is associated with the relatively uncomfortable compression therapy, rendering an oral and, perhaps, topical therapy such as horse chestnut more preferable. The sooner such therapy is initiated, the better the chance of avoiding painful compression therapy.

Both topical and systemic HCSEs are popular in Europe for the treatment of CVI and varicose veins. The aescin in HCSEs clearly possesses anti-inflammatory properties and has been demonstrated to ease edema after trauma, especially following head and sports injury, and surgery.[9,16] A topical aescin preparation is also popular for use during sporting events in Europe for treatment of acute sprains.

Chronic Venous Insufficiency

The inhibitory effect exerted on the catalytic degradation of capillary wall proteoglycans is thought to account for the efficacy associated with HCSE formulations.[5] Several RCTs show that *A. hippocastanum* is effective in reducing edema associated with CVI.[32] However, in a 2002 four-week open, controlled, comparative study of HCSE (Venostasin) and Pycnogenol used to treat 40 patients with CVI, Koch found that while both medications were well tolerated, Venostasin only moderately improved symptoms whereas Pycnogenol significantly diminished lower limb circumference as well as cholesterol and low-density lipoprotein values (see Chapter 49, Pycnogenol).[33]

Aesculaforce®, a fresh plant HCSE, was found in five clinical trials (four on CVI, one on varicose veins) as a topical gel, oral tincture, or tablet, to decrease objective measures of lower leg edema and, subjectively, relieve patients of pruritus, leg pain, and heaviness associated with CVI and varicose veins. The fresh plant HCSE formulation was safe and well tolerated, and, according to a 2006 review by Suter et al., suitable for patients with mild-to-moderate venous insufficiency.[5] In addition, an Australian study that year suggested that the use of HCSE may be more cost-effective than conventional therapy for the treatment of venous leg ulcers.[34]

Rathbun and Kirkpatrick note that multiple RCTs have shown that the use of HCSE has achieved short-term improvement in CVI signs and symptoms, though caution is necessary when considering herbal supplements insofar as they are not regulated or licensed by the United States Food and Drug Administration.[26] Pittler and Ernst, in their 2012 database review, echoed the conclusion that HCSE provides efficacious short-term relief from CVI, while calling for larger RCTs to verify the efficacy of the herbal treatment.[21]

Photoprotection and Antiaging Activity

In 1996, Ramos et al. assessed liquid and dry extracts of *A. hippocastanum*, *Hamamelis virginiana* (witch hazel), *Matricaria recutita* (chamomile), *Rhamnus purshiana* (cascara), and

Cinnamomum zeylanicum (cinnamon) to determine their viability as antisolar agents. After incorporation into an octylmethoxycinnamate synthetic sunscreen, the researchers noted that the solar protection factors (SPFs) intensified (see Chapter 70, Chamomile). They concluded that inclusion in sunscreens of such plant extracts, which can also deliver emollient qualities to the formulation, may allow for providing greater SPF and, thus, skin protection from UV exposure.[35]

Noting that contraction forces generated by nonmuscle cells, such as fibroblasts, contribute to wound healing and vasoconstriction, Fujimura et al. set out in 2006 to identify plant extracts (among 100 of those listed in the Japanese cosmetic ingredients codex) capable of creating such forces in fibroblast-populated collagen gels. Finding that an extract of horse chestnut met such parameters, they conducted a nine-week clinical trial with 40 healthy female volunteers, who applied the 3 percent extract gel around the eyes three times daily. At six weeks, significant reductions in wrinkle scores for the corners of the eye and lower eyelid were noted in comparison with scores for the control group, with similar differences seen at nine weeks. The investigators concluded that horse chestnut appears to be a considerable antiaging agent *in vivo*, though more research is necessary, including comparisons to other agents.[36]

CONCLUSION

The use of horse chestnut in chronic venous insufficiency and other venous disorders has some support by randomized controlled trials due to the effects of aescin on venous tone. Like many other such herbs, the potential efficacy of its inclusion in modern topical products remains questionable, though the evidence for topical use for edema is well established. Many products targeted for eye puffiness or dark circles under the eyes contain horse chestnut due to the purported effects on blood flow and circulation around the eyes. These claims remain unproven. Much more research with topical horse chestnut is needed to support some of the more recent assertions regarding efficacy in providing photoprotection, treating wrinkles, dark circles under the eyes, spider veins, and hair loss (Table 74-1).

REFERENCES

1. Wilkinson JA, Brown AM. Horse chestnut – Aesculus hippocastanum: Potential applications in cosmetic skin-care products. *Int J Cosmet Sci.* 1999;21:437.
2. Kapusta I, Janda B, Szajway B, et al. Flavonoids in horse chestnut (Aesculus hippocastanum) seeds and powdered waste water byproducts. *J Agric Food Chem.* 2007;55:8485.
3. No authors listed. Aesculus hippocastanum (Horse chestnut). Monograph. *Altern Med Rev.* 2009;14:278.
4. Thornfeldt C. Cosmeceuticals containing herbs: Fact, fiction, and future. *Dermatol Surg.* 2005;31:873.
5. Suter A, Bommer S, Rechner J. Treatment of patients with venous insufficiency with fresh plant horse chestnut seed extract: A review of 5 clinical studies. *Adv Ther.* 2006;23:179.
6. Redzić SS. The ecological aspect of ethnobotany and ethnopharmacology of population in Bosnia and Herzegovina. *Coll Antropol.* 2007;31:869.
7. Foster S. *An Illustrated Guide to 101 Medicinal Herbs: Their History, Use, Recommended Dosages, and Cautions.* Loveland, CO: Interweave Press; 1998:116–7.
8. Sirtori CR. Aescin: Pharmacology, pharmacokinetics and therapeutic profile. *Pharmacol Res.* 2001;44:183.
9. Calabrese C, Preston P. Report of the results of a double-blind, randomized, single-dose trial of a topical 2% escin gel versus placebo in the acute treatment of experimentally-induced hematoma in volunteers. *Planta Med.* 1993;59:394.
10. Mills S, Bone K. *Principles and Practice of Phytotherapy: Modern Herbal Medicine.* London: Churchill Livingstone; 2000:448–455.
11. Grieve M. *A Modern Herbal* (Vol. II). New York: Dover Publications; 1971:192–193.
12. Masaki H, Sakaki S, Atsumi T, et al. Active-oxygen scavenging activity of plant extracts. *Biol Pharm Bull.* 1995;18:162.
13. Lorenz D, Marek ML. The active therapeutic principle of horse chestnut (Aesculus hippocastanum). Part I. Classification of the active substance. *Arzneimittelforschung.* 1960;10:263.
14. Hoffmann D. *Medical Herbalism: The Science and Practice of Herbal Medicine.* Rochester, VT: Healing Arts Press; 2003:524.
15. Pittler MH, Ernst E. Horse-chestnut seed extract for chronic venous insufficiency. A criteria-based systematic review. *Arch Dermatol.* 1998;134:1356.
16. Guillaume M, Padioleau F. Veinotonic effect, vascular protection, anti-inflammatory and free radical scavenging properties of horse chestnut extract. *Arzneimittelforschung.* 1994;44:25.
17. Bisler H, Pfeifer R, Klüken N, et al. Effects of horse-chestnut see extract on transcapillary filtration in chronic venous insufficiency. *Dtsch Med Wochenschr.* 1986;111:1321.
18. Diehm C, Trampisch HJ, Lange S, et al. Comparison of leg compression stocking and oral horse-chestnut seed extract therapy in patients with chronic venous insufficiency. *Lancet.* 1996;347:292.
19. Facino RM, Carini M, Stefani R, et al. Anti-elastase and anti-hyaluronidase activities of saponins and sapogenins from Hedera helix, Aesculus hippocastanum, and Ruscus aculeatus: Factors contributing to their efficacy in the treatment of venous insufficiency. *Arch Pharm (Weinheim).* 1995;328:720.
20. Ernst E, Pittler MH, Stevinson C. Complementary/alternative medicine in dermatology: Evidence-assessed efficacy of two diseases and two treatments. *Am J Clin Dermatol.* 2002;3:341.
21. Pittler MH, Ernst E. Horse chestnut seed extract for chronic venous insufficiency. *Cochrane Database Syst Rev.* 2012;11:CD003230.
22. Greeske K, Pohlmann BK. Horse chestnut seed extract – an effective therapy principle in general practice. Drug therapy of chronic venous insufficiency. *Fortschr Med.* 1996;114:196.
23. Sipos W, Reutterer B, Frank M, et al. Escin inhibits type I allergic dermatitis in a novel porcine model. *Int Arch Allergy Immunol.* 2013;161:44.
24. MacKay D. Hemorrhoids and varicose veins: A review of treatment options. *Altern Med Rev.* 2001;6:126.
25. Dattner AM. From medical herbalism to phytotherapy in dermatology: Back to the future. *Dermatol Ther.* 2003;16:106.
26. Rathbun SW, Kirkpatrick AC. Treatment of chronic venous insufficiency. *Curr Treat Options Cardiovasc Med.* 2007;9:115.
27. Tozzi E, Scatena M, Castellacci E. Anti-inflammatory local frigotherapy with a combination of escin, heparin and polyunsaturated phosphatidylcholine (EPL). *Clin Ter.* 1981;98:517.
28. Desogus AI, D'Alia G. Venotropic therapy: Results of clinical experimentation. *Clin Ter.* 1986;118:339.
29. Abebe W. Herbal medication: Potential for adverse interactions with analgesic drugs. *J Clin Pharm Ther.* 2002;27:391.
30. Hexsel D, Orlandi C, Zechmeister do Prado D. Botanical extracts used in the treatment of cellulite. *Dermatol Surg.* 2005;31:866.
31. Ottillinger B, Greeske K. Rational therapy of chronic venous insufficiency—chances and limits of the therapeutic use of horse-chestnut seeds extract. *BMC Cardiovasc Disord.* 2001;1:5.
32. Reuter J, Wölfle U, Korting HC, et al. Which plant for which skin disease? Part 2: Dermatophytes, chronic venous insufficiency, photoprotection, actinic keratoses, vitiligo, hair loss, cosmetic indications. *J Dtsch Dermatol Ges.* 2010;8:866.
33. Koch R. Comparative study of Venostasin and Pycnogenol in chronic venous insufficiency. *Phytother Res.* 2002;16 (Suppl 1):S1.
34. Leach MJ, Pincombe J, Foster G. Using horse chestnut seed extract in the treatment of venous leg ulcers: A cost-benefit analysis. *Ostomy Wound Manage.* 2006;52:68.
35. Ramos MF, Santos EP, Bizarri CH, et al. Preliminary studies towards utilization of various plant extracts as antisolar agents. *Int J Cosmet Sci.* 1996;18:87.
36. Fujimura T, Tsukahara K, Moriwaki S, et al. A horse chestnut extract, which induces contraction forces in fibroblasts, is a potent anti-aging ingredient. *J Cosmet Sci.* 2006;57:369.

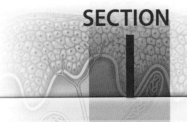

CHAPTER 75

Overview of Acne

Four main etiologic factors have been implicated in the pathophysiology of acne: sebaceous gland hyperactivity, inflammation, abundance of *Propionibacterium acnes*, and dysfunction of the desquamation of the hair follicle (see Chapter 64, Anti-inflammatory Agents). These causal elements work interdependently and are mediated by such important influences as diet, stress, heredity, and hormonal activity.

SEBACEOUS GLAND HYPERACTIVITY

Sebum, composed of lipids, is continuously synthesized by the sebaceous glands and secreted to the skin surface through the hair follicle pore. The sebaceous glands are located all over the body but are largest and most numerous in the face, back, chest, and shoulders. These glands become more active during puberty because of the increase in androgens, particularly testosterone, which spurs sebum production. Oral drugs that inhibit sebaceous gland activity, such as antiandrogens, estrogens, and retinoids, are important treatment modalities in the successful control of acne. At this time, there are no topical ingredients that can reduce sebum secretion, most likely because the sebaceous gland is deep in the hair follicle and unreachable by most topical agents.

FOLLICULAR KERATINIZATION

The keratinocytes that line the hair follicle undergo the maturation process known as keratinization. Once they mature into stratum corneum cells, they desquamate into the hair follicle. In acne patients, these keratinocytes have a tendency to stick together due to the effects of positive and negative charges, the actions of the enzyme transglutaminase, and the viscosity of sebum. The clumped keratinocytes block the pore/follicle, creating a blackhead if the pore is open ("open comedone") or a whitehead if it is closed ("closed comedone"). The clogged pore is a great nutritional source for *P. acnes* bacteria.

THE INFLUENCE OF BACTERIA

P. acnes has been cited as a key component in the etiologic pathway of acne, a *sine qua non* feature, because it is typically present in higher concentrations in teenagers with acne than in controls without acne.[1] When *P. acnes* is present, immune system cells are activated to initiate an inflammatory immune response. In addition, *P. acnes* itself releases inflammatory mediators when it ingests sebum. This inflammation leads to the red pus-filled bump known as a "pimple."

Corynebacterium acnes is another bacteria associated with the pathophysiologic pathway of acne. Antibiotic resistance to *P. acnes* bacteria is estimated to be as high as 60 percent in some patient populations.[2] Erythromycin, methicillin, and clindamycin are the most common antibiotics to which bacteria have been reportedly found to be resistant.[3] For this reason, erythromycin and clindamycin should no longer be used as monotherapy for acne. Benzoyl peroxide (BPO), lauric acid, triclosan, and colloidal silver display antibacterial properties that make them attractive as antiacne agents that should not lead to bacterial resistance.[4-6] Combining BPO with erythromycin or clindamycin has been proven to prevent the emergence of resistant strains of *P. acnes*;[3,7,8], therefore, the current clinical acne recommendation is to include BPO in topical antiacne regimens that employ antibiotics.[9] Triclosan is a known allergen, so it is not used for acne. Lauric acid and silver are still under investigation, but their utility in the treatment of acne is promising.

Acne is characterized by clogged pores, open and closed comedones, red papules, pustules, and cysts. Treatments include anti-inflammatories, antimicrobials, exfoliants to prevent clogged follicles, and retinoids. Blue light is effective to reduce *P. acnes* levels and red light can be used to decrease inflammation. Most acne treatments are by prescription. This section will cover over-the-counter (OTC) acne ingredients.

The best way to treat acne is through combination therapy using an exfoliant, an antimicrobial, a retinoid, and anti-inflammatory ingredients. This section will focus on BPO, as an antimicrobial, salicylic acid, for its dual role as an exfoliant and an anti-inflammatory, and retinoids, as the mainstay of acne treatment, as well as alternatives such as tea tree oil and silver. Although retinoids are usually prescription medications, retinol and other retinoids are available over the counter. It is important to realize that many ingredients can cause acne (see Table 75-1). One of the frequent culprits is isopropyl myristate, which is common in skin and hair care products.

The etiologic pathway of acne is convoluted and its treatment variable, multistep, and most effective when individualized to the patient. An extensive exploration of this most common of dermatologic conditions, particularly the cases resistant to treatment, will not be pursued in this section. Instead, the focus is on basic OTC ingredients for patients with mild-to-moderate acne. Note that there are many drugs approved by the United States Food and Drug Administration (FDA) for acne, including tretinoin, adapalene, and tazarotene, that are beyond the scope

TABLE 75-1
List of Potential Acne-Causing Ingredients Found in Cosmetic Products

Anhydrous Lanolin	Crisco	Isopropyl Palmitate	PG Dicaprylate/Caprate
Apricot Kernel Oil	D & C Red # 3	Isostearyl Isostearate	PG Dipelargonate
Arachidic Acid	D & C Red # 4	Isostearyl Neopentanoate	Polyethylene Glycol (PEG 400)
Ascorbyl Palmitate	D & C Red # 6	Jojoba Oil	Polyethylene Glycol 300
Avocado Oil	D & C Red # 7	Lanolin Alcohol	Polyglyceryl-3-Diisostearate
Azulene	D & C Red # 9	Lanolin Oil	Potassium Chloride
BHA	D & C Red # 17	Lanolin Wax	Propylene Glycol Monostearate
Beeswax	D & C Red # 19	Laureth 23	Red Algae
Benzaldehyde	D & C Red # 21	Laureth 4	Sandalwood Seed Oil
Benzoic Acid	D & C Red # 27	Lithium Stearate	Sesame Oil
β-Carotene	D & C Red # 30	Magnesium Stearate	Shark Liver Oil
Bubussa Oil	D & C Red # 33	Menthyl Anthranilate	Simethicone
Butyl Stearate	D & C Red # 36	Mink Oil	Sodium Chloride (Salt)
Butylated Hydroxyanisole (BHA)	D & C Red # 40	Myristic Acid	Sodium Laureth Sulfate
Butylene Glycol	Decyl Oleate	Myristyl Lactate	Sodium Lauryl Sulfate
Cajeput Oil	Dimethicone	Myristyl Myristate	Solulan 16
Calendula	Dioctyl Succinate	Octyl Palmitate	Sorbitan Laurate
Camphor	Disodium Oleamido	Octyl Stearate	Sorbitan Oleate
Candelilla Wax	PEG 2-Sulfosuccinate	Oleth-3	Soybean Oil
Capric Acid	Emulsifying Wax NF	Oleth-10	Squalane
Caprylic Acid	Ethoxylated Lanolin	Oleyl Alcohol	Steareth 10
Carbomer 940	Ethylhexyl Palmitate	Olive Oil	Steareth 2
Carnuba Wax	Evening Primrose Oil	PEG 100 Distearate	Steareth 20
Carotene	Glyceryl Stearate NSE	PEG 100 Stearate	Stearic Acid
Carrageenan	Glyceryl Stearate SE	PEG 150 Distearate	Stearic Acid Tea
Castor Oil	Glyceryl Tricapylo/Caprate	PEG 16 Lanolin	Stearyl Alcohol
Cetearyl Alcohol	Glyceryl-3-Diisostearate	PEG 20 Stearate	Stearyl Heptanoate
Cetyl Alcohol	Hexadecyl Alcohol	PEG 200 Dilaurate	Sulfated Castor Oil
Chamomile	Hexylene Glycol	PEG 8 Stearate	Sulfated Jojoba Oil
Chaulmoogra Oil	Hydrogenated Castor Oil	PG Caprylate/Caprate	Stearyl Heptanoate
Cocoa Butter	Hydrogenated Vegetable Oil	PG Dipelargonate	Talc
Coconut Butter	Hydroxypropylcellulose	PG Monostearate	Triethanolamine
Coconut Oil	Isocetyl Stearate	PPG 2 Myristyl Propionate	Vitamin A Palmitate
Colloidal Sulfur	Isodecyl Oleate	Palmitic Acid	Wheat Germ Glyceride/Oil
Corn Oil	Isopropyl Isostearate	Peanut Oil	Xylene
Cotton Seed Oil	Isopropyl Myristate	Pentarythrital Tetra Isostearate	Zinc Oxide

of this book because they are prescription products. These acne drugs must undergo a formal clinical research process (Phase I to Phase III research trials) in order to prove safety and efficacy and to receive FDA drug approval. After hundreds of millions of dollars and at least three years of effort, the acne drug may receive approval from the FDA, which dictates and strictly enforces the manufacturing processes, labeling, and marketing claims. OTC medications claimed by manufacturers to improve acne do not require FDA drug approval but they must contain ingredients that have been ruled as "safe" and "effective for acne" by the FDA. Their use is governed by an official ruling known as a "monograph." See Table 75-2 for a set of

TABLE 75-2
Summary of Warnings and Directions Required for OTC Acne Medications[10]

WARNINGS

For external use only
When using this product
- Skin irritation and dryness is more likely to occur if you use another topical acne medication at the same time. If irritation occurs, only use one topical acne medication at a time.

DIRECTIONS
- Clean the skin thoroughly before applying this product
- Cover the entire affected area with a thin layer one to three times daily
- Because excessive drying of the skin may occur, start with one application daily, then gradually increase to two or three times daily if needed or as directed by a doctor
- If bothersome dryness or peeling occurs, reduce application to once a day or every other day.

Products, such as soaps and masks, which are applied and removed, should include appropriate directions in addition to the directions set forth above. For example, the second bullet of the standard directions listed above may be revised to read "cover the entire affected area with a thin layer and rinse thoroughly one to three times daily."

In addition to the required directions, all OTC topical acne products marketed under the monograph may contain the following optional direction:

"*Sensitivity Test for a New User.* Apply product sparingly to one or two small affected areas during the first 3 days. If no discomfort occurs, follow the directions stated (select one of the following: 'elsewhere on this label,' 'above,' or 'below')."

TABLE 75-3
OTC Acne Monograph (21 CFR part 333, subpart D)[11]

SUBPART D – TOPICAL ACNE DRUG PRODUCTS

Sec. 333.301 Scope

a. An over-the-counter acne drug product in a form suitable for topical application is generally recognized as safe and effective and is not misbranded if it meets each of the conditions in this subpart and each general condition established in 330.1 of this chapter

b. References in this subpart to regulatory sections of the Code of Federal Regulations are to chapter I of title 21 unless otherwise noted

Sec. 333.303 Definitions

As used in this subpart:

a. *Acne.* A disease involving the oil glands and hair follicles of the skin which is manifested by blackheads, whiteheads, acne pimples, and acne blemishes

b. *Acne blemish.* A flaw in the skin resulting from acne

c. *Acne drug product.* A drug product used to reduce the number of acne blemishes, acne pimples, blackheads, and whiteheads

d. *Acne pimple.* A small, prominent, inflamed elevation of the skin resulting from acne

e. *Blackhead.* A condition of the skin that occurs in acne and is characterized by a black tip

f. *Whitehead.* A condition of the skin that occurs in acne and is characterized by a small, firm, whitish elevation of the skin

Sec. 333.310 Acne active ingredients

The active ingredient of the product consists of any of the following:

a. Benzoyl peroxide, 2.5 to 10 percent

b. Resorcinol, 2 percent, when combined with sulfur in accordance with 333.320(a)

c. Resorcinol monoacetate, 3 percent, when combined with sulfur in accordance with 333.320(b)

d. Salicylic acid, 0.5 to 2 percent

e. Sulfur, 3 to 10 percent

f. Sulfur, 3 to 8 percent, when combined with resorcinol or resorcinol monoacetate in accordance with 333.320

[75 FR 9776, Mar. 4, 2010]

Sec. 333.320 Permitted combinations of active ingredients

a. Resorcinol identified in 333.310(b) may be combined with sulfur identified in 333.310(f)

b. Resorcinol monoacetate identified in 333.310(c) may be combined with sulfur identified in 333.310(f)

[75 FR 9776, Mar. 4, 2010]

Sec. 333.350 Labeling of acne drug products

a. *Statement of identity.* The labeling of the product contains the established name of the drug, if any, and identifies the product as an "acne medication," "acne treatment," "acne medication" (insert dosage form, e.g., "cream," "gel," "lotion," or "ointment"), or "acne treatment" (insert dosage form, e.g., "cream," "gel," "lotion," or "ointment")

b. *Indications.* The labeling of the product states, under the heading "Indications," the phrase listed in paragraph (b)(1) of this section and may contain any of the additional phrases listed in paragraph (b)(2) of this section. Other truthful and nonmisleading statements, describing only the indications for use that have been established and listed in paragraph (b) of this section, may also be used, as provided in 330.1(c)(2) of this chapter, subject to the provisions of section 502 of the Federal Food, Drug, and Cosmetic Act (the act) relating to misbranding and the prohibition in section 301(d) of the act against the introduction or delivery for introduction into interstate commerce of unapproved new drugs in violation of section 505(a) of the act

1. "For the" (select one of the following: "management" or "treatment") "of acne"

2. In addition to the information identified in paragraph (b)(1) of this section, the labeling of the product may contain any one or more of the following statements:

    i.   (Select one of the following: "clears," "clears up," "clears up most," "dries," "dries up," "dries and clears," "helps clear," "helps clear up," "reduces the number of," or "reduces the severity of") (select one or more of the following: "acne blemishes," "acne pimples," "blackheads," or "whiteheads") which may be followed by "and allows skin to heal"

    ii. "Penetrates pores to" (select one of the following: "eliminate most," "control," "clear most," or "reduce the number of") (select one or more of the following: "acne blemishes," "acne pimples," "blackheads," or "whiteheads")

    iii. "Helps keep skin clear of new" (select one or more of the following: "acne blemishes," "acne pimples," "blackheads," or "whiteheads")

    iv. "Helps prevent new" (select one or more of the following: "acne blemishes," "acne pimples," "blackheads," or "whiteheads") which may be followed by "from forming."

    v.   "Helps prevent the development of new" (select one or more of the following: "acne blemishes," "acne pimples," "blackheads," or "whiteheads")

c. *Warnings.* The labeling of the product contains the following warnings under the heading "Warnings":

1. *For products containing any ingredients identified in 330.310*

    i.   The labeling states "For external use only"

    ii. The labeling states "When using this product ● skin irritation and dryness is more likely to occur if you use another topical acne medication at the same time. If irritation occurs, only use one topical acne medication at a time"

2. *For products containing sulfur identified in 333.310(e) and (f)*

    i.   The labeling states "Do not use on ● broken skin ● large areas of the skin"

    ii. The labeling states "When using this product ● apply only to areas with acne"

3. *For products containing any combination identified in 333.320.* (i) The labeling states "When using this product ● rinse right away with water if it gets in eyes"

    i.   The labeling states "Stop use and ask a doctor ● if skin irritation occurs or gets worse"

4. *For products containing benzoyl peroxide identified in 333.310(a)*

    i.   The labeling states "Do not use if you ● have very sensitive skin ● are sensitive to benzoyl peroxide"

    ii. The labeling states "When using this product ● avoid unnecessary sun exposure and use a sunscreen ● avoid contact with the eyes, lips, and mouth ● avoid contact with hair and dyed fabrics, which may be bleached by this product ● skin irritation may occur, characterized by redness, burning, itching, peeling, or possibly swelling. Irritation may be reduced by using the product less frequently or in a lower concentration"

    iii. The labeling states "Stop use and ask a doctor if ● irritation becomes severe"

d. *Directions.* The labeling of the product contains the following information under the heading "Directions":

1. *For products applied containing any ingredient identified in 333.310.* The labeling states " ● clean the skin thoroughly before applying this product ● cover the entire affected area with a thin layer one to three times daily ● because excessive drying of the skin may occur, start with one application daily, then gradually increase to two or three times daily if needed or as directed by a doctor ● if bothersome dryness or peeling occurs, reduce application to once a day or every other day"

2. *For products applied and left on the skin containing benzoyl peroxide identified in 333.310(a)*

    i.   The labeling states the directions in paragraph (d)(1) of this section

    ii. The labeling states " ● if going outside, apply sunscreen after using this product. If irritation or sensitivity develops, stop use of both products and ask a doctor"

3. *For products applied and removed from the skin containing any ingredient identified in 333.310.* Products, such as soaps and masks, may be applied and removed and should include appropriate directions. All products containing benzoyl peroxide should include the directions in paragraph (d)(2)(ii) of this section

4. *Optional directions.* In addition to the required directions in paragraphs (d)(1) and (d)(2) of this section, the product may contain the following optional labeling: "Sensitivity Test for a New User. Apply product sparingly to one or two small affected areas during the first 3 days. If no discomfort occurs, follow the directions stated (select one of the following: 'elsewhere on this label,' 'above,' or 'below')"

[56 FR 41019, Aug. 16, 1991, as amended at 75 FR 9776, Mar. 4, 2010]

FDA required warnings on the label of OTC acne products containing BPO or salicylic acid as per FDA OTC regulations 21 CFR 333, subpart D. Some ingredients such as BPO are found in both prescription and OTC acne products (see Table 75-3).

REFERENCES

1. Zaenglein AL, Graber EM. Thiboutot DM. Acne vulgaris and acneiform eruptions. In: Goldsmith LA, Katz SI, Gilchrest B, et al. eds. *Fitzpatrick's Dermatology in General Medicine.* 8th ed. New York: McGraw-Hill; 2012:900.

2. Nishijima S, Akamatsu H, Akamatsu M, et al. The antibiotic susceptibility of Propionibacterium acnes and Staphylococcus epidermidis isolated from acne. *J Dermatol*. 1994;21:166.

3. Kircik LH. The role of benzoyl peroxide in the new treatment paradigm for acne. *J Drugs Dermatol*. 2013;12:s73.

4. Nakatsuji T, Kao MC, Fang JY, et al. Antimicrobial property of lauric acid against Propionibacterium acnes: Its therapeutic potential for inflammatory acne vulgaris. *J Invest Dermatol*. 2009;129:2480.

5. Domínguez-Delgado CL, Rodríguez-Cruz IM, Escobar-Chávez JJ, et al. Preparation and characterization of triclosan nanoparticles intended to be used for the treatment of acne. *Eur J Pharm Biopharm*. 2011;79:102.

6. Lansdown AB. Silver. I: Its antibacterial properties and mechanism of action. *J Wound Care*. 2002;11:125.

7. Eady EA, Farmery MR, Ross JI, et al. Effects of benzoyl peroxide and erythromycin alone and in combination against antibiotic-sensitive and -resistant skin bacteria from acne patients. *Br J Dermatol*. 1994;131:331.

8. Leyden J, Levy S. The development of antibiotic resistance in Propionibacterium acnes. *Cutis*. 2001;67:21.

9. Thiboutot D, Gollnick H, Bettoli V, et al. New insights into the management of acne: An update from the Global Alliance to Improve Outcomes in Acne group. *J Am Acad Dermatol*. 2009;60:S1.

10. U.S. Department of Health and Human Services, Food and Drug Administration, Center for Drug Evaluation and Research (CDER). Guidance for Industry Topical Acne Drug Products for Over-the-Counter Human Use–Revision of Labeling and Classification of Benzoyl Peroxide as Safe and Effective Small Entity Compliance Guide. Posted June 2011. http://www.fda.gov/downloads/Drugs/GuidanceCompliance RegulatoryInformation/Guidances/UCM259744.pdf. Accessed August 11, 2013.

11. CFR–Code of Federal Regulations Title 21 – Food and Drugs Chapter I, Subchapter D, Drugs for Human Use, Part 333 Topical Antimicrobial Drug Products for Over-the-Counter Human Use, Subpart D, Topical Acne Drug Products, Food and Drug Administration. http://www.accessdata.fda.gov/scripts/cdrh/cfdocs/cfcfr/CFRSearch.cfm?CFRPart=333&showFR=1&subpart Node=21:5.0.1.1.12.4. Accessed August 11, 2013.

CHAPTER 76

Benzoyl Peroxide

Activities:

Anti-inflammatory, antibacterial, keratolytic, wound healing

Important Chemical Components:

Benzoyl peroxide, an organic compound in the peroxide family, is metabolized to benzoic acid within the skin.

Origin Classification:

Synthesized in the laboratory

Personal Care Category:

Acne therapy

Recommended for the following Baumann Skin Types:

OSNT, OSNW, OSPT, OSPW (but only by those with the Type 1 subtype, S_1, of the four BST sensitive skin types). Should be avoided by very dry types and S_4 sensitive skin allergic types because they often have an impaired barrier and are irritated by benzoyl peroxide.

TABLE 76-1
Pros and Cons of Benzoyl Peroxide

Pros	Cons
Strong antibacterial activity with no risk of bacterial resistance	Risk of irritation especially in dry skin types
Works quicker than most acne ingredients	Produces free radicals that may age skin
Comedolytic	
Inexpensive	
Many forms available	
Safe	
Covered by an FDA monograph	

SOURCE

Benzoyl peroxide (BPO) is one of the two most common ingredients in over-the-counter (OTC) acne treatments.[1] It is also found in many prescription drug acne therapies. Both OTC and prescription versions have been shown to be effective in the treatment of acne.[2] BPO was originally derived from chlorhydroxyquinoline, a component of coal tar.[3] Currently, BPO is usually prepared by treating hydrogen peroxide with benzoyl chloride.

HISTORY

BPO is used for many purposes including bleaching flour and as a catalyst for chemical production of resins.[4] There are conflicting reports about the history of the medical use of BPO but Merker provides a thorough historical review in his 2002 article in the *International Journal of Dermatology*.[5] BPO seems to have first been used as a topical agent in the management of various skin lesions, especially burns, by Loevenhart in 1905.[5] The first description of BPO in the treatment of acneiform eruptions dates back to 1934 and, in 1958, Fishman was credited as the first to suggest BPO as a viable treatment for acne.[6] In the 1960s, it was used as a treatment for leg ulcers and decubitus ulcers, and its regular use in acne therapy dates back to 1979.[1] But Pace is credited for publishing his results using BPO, identifying it as the main active ingredient in a chlorhydroxyquinoline ointment, for acne in 1965, and developing a commercially available product with Werner Stiefel.[7,8] This began a flurry of patents to improve BPO for use in acne. Richard DeVillez found that BPO would dissolve in dimethyl isosorbide and remain stable with increased skin penetration.[9] Won and colleagues developed a porous styrene-divinylbenzene polymer structure, which is now known as microsponge technology.[3,10] In 1980, Fulton patented the use of BPO and glycerin to treat acne.[11] In 1983, Klein and Fox (Dermik Laboratories) improved the stability of BPO by adding dioctyl sodium sulfosuccinate.[12] In 1985, Flynn and colleagues patented the use of the combination of BPO and silica to remove excess skin oils found around acne lesions, which was launched in the Oxy acne product line.[13] In 1985, Klein filed the first patent for BPO in combination with erythromycin, an antibiotic (Benzamycin, Dermik Laboratories).[3] In the last few decades many advances have been achieved in the formulations of BPO and there are hundreds of variations on the market. The inclusion of BPO in an OTC product for acne is covered in the Food and Drug Administration (FDA) monograph 21 CFR 333, subpart D (Table 76-1).

CHEMISTRY

The structural formula of BPO is $[C_6H_5C(O)]_2O_2$. It consists of two benzoyl groups bridged by a peroxide link (Figure 76-1).

ORAL USES

BPO is used to whiten teeth but is not used orally for skin care reasons.

TOPICAL USES

BPO is one of the most common ingredients used topically to treat acne. It can be used alone or combined with other ingredients, including antibiotics and retinoids. When using

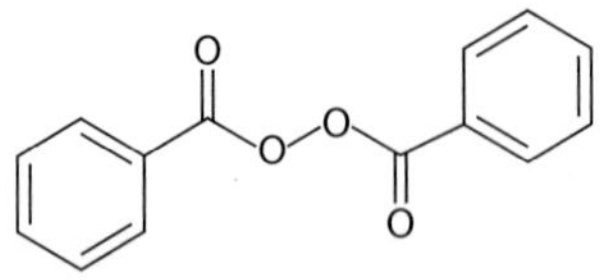

▲ **FIGURE 76-1** Chemical structure of benzoyl peroxide.

oral antibiotics, the concurrent use of BPO can minimize the emergence of bacterial resistance.[14,15]

BPO is known to penetrate into the skin and absorb unchanged into the stratum corneum (SC). In the epidermis or dermis it is metabolized to benzoic acid. It is absorbed as benzoate and excreted in the urine.[15] BPO is not degraded in the liver. Nacht et al. demonstrated that in an eight-hour time period, 4.5 percent of BPO is absorbed into the skin when applied topically.[16] Yeung et al. showed that BPO had an *in vitro* flux of 0.6 µg/cm² through human skin independent of the drug concentration.[17]

BPO is safe and effective in the treatment of acne but is tolerated better by people with oily skin types as opposed to dry skin types. This is due to the fact that BPO can be an irritant and individuals with an impaired skin barrier, such as S_4 Baumann Skin Types and dry skin types, have impaired barrier function, which allows increased BPO penetration. BPO is also a weak allergen but most reactions to it are due to its potential as an irritant, which more commonly occurs at higher concentrations. The delivery systems and the vehicles used and the choice of other ingredients and products in the skin care regimen play an important role in BPO sensitivity. Some studies have shown that if irritant-type sensitivity develops, BPO can be stopped for four days and restarted with less irritation.

Antibacterial Uses

BPO exerts its bactericidal activity by releasing highly reactive oxygen able to oxidize proteins in bacterial cell membranes. It has been shown to have bactericidal effects against *Propionibacterium acnes* and *Corynebacterium acnes*, the bacteria known to cause acne.[18] It has also been shown to kill *Staphylococcus capitis*, *S. epidermis*, *S. hominis*, *P. avidum*, *P. granulosum*, and the yeast *Pityrosporum ovale*.[19] BPO does not seem to leave any residual subpopulations of bacteria; therefore, overgrowth of other organisms is not expected to occur with the use of BPO.

Antibiotic resistance is of great interest in medicine right now, including the acne realm where *P. acnes* resistance rates are estimated to be as high as 60 percent in some patient populations.[20] Erythromycin, methicillin, and clindamycin are the most common antibiotics to which bacteria have reportedly developed resistance.[21] Combining BPO with erythromycin or clindamycin has been proven to prevent the emergence of resistant strains of *P. acnes*;[21–23] therefore, the current clinical acne recommendation is to include BPO in topical antiacne regimens that utilize antibiotics.[24] In more than 45 years of use in acne management, bacterial resistance to BPO has not been reported.[25]

Keratolytic Activity

BPO tends to clear acne lesions and comedones faster than other acne therapies. Its keratotic activity (i.e., ability to increase desquamation) may be one reason that the acne lesions clear more rapidly. Waller and colleagues performed a study quantifying the amount of SC removed after tape stripping. They compared BPO, salicylic acid (SA) 2 percent, and retinoic acid (RA) 0.05 percent.[26] After three hours, BPO was significantly more effective in disrupting SC cohesion than SA and RA, but after six hours all three agents showed similar keratolytic activity. The authors noted that the ability of BPO to disrupt the SC barrier may increase penetration of drugs that are coadministered; however, this would depend on the formulation of the BPO.[3]

Keratolytic refers to the separation of the SC keratinocytes allowing increased desquamation of the skin cells.

Desquamation is the process of skin cells separating from each other and flaking off of the surface of the skin. Exfoliation is the process by which a chemical or mechanical force is used to encourage desquamation. Therefore, BPO can be considered an exfoliant.

Acne

Many studies have shown that BPO is an effective agent for the topical treatment of acne.[27] It seems to increase efficacy of other topically applied antimicrobials. There are several mechanisms by which BPO is thought to improve acne. BPO is a highly lipophilic molecule able to penetrate through the sebum and into the pilosebaceous unit. Its bactericidal activity has been well demonstrated. In addition, BP exhibits keratolytic and anti-inflammatory activity.[26]

BPO may help increase the efficacy of other antiacne antimicrobials by preventing bacterial resistance and by facilitating penetration into the sebum, keratin, and polysaccharides to reach the target bacteria. The predominant organism that causes acne, *P. acnes*, is capable of secreting biofilm polysaccharides, which hinder antimicrobials from reaching *P. acnes*.[28,29] BPO, by virtue of its oxidative properties, may destroy this biofilm, thereby expediting the delivery of topical antibiotics and other agents to the targeted bacteria.

Several studies have demonstrated that the combination of BPO with antimicrobials such as clindamycin is more effective than using either topical BPO or clindamycin alone. One study showed that the combination of clindamycin and BPO resulted in a 61 percent reduction of inflammatory lesions after three months as compared with 39 percent and 35 percent, respectively, when the agents were used alone.[30] BPO is also often combined with SA.[31]

BPO tends to more rapidly yield improvement of acne as compared to retinoids and other acne therapies.[3,32] One study showed that after two days of treatment with BPO 5 percent, an almost 2 $\log_{10}$ decrease in *P. acnes* counts was observed.[33] In 2011, a systematic review of the acne study literature revealed that that at 2 to 4 weeks, a 5 percent BPO + SA combination was most effective at reducing inflammatory and noninflammatory acne lesions. However, at later time points (10–12 weeks), 5 percent BPO + SA was similar to BPO + clindamycin. Therefore, it appears that BPO can engender a more rapid improvement of acne, which may contribute to greater compliance. However, the dryness and irritation associated with its use may undermine compliance. For these reasons, the formulation of BPO and the combinations of other ingredients in the regimen is crucial. Several studies have demonstrated that BPO is effective in cleanser form and may be less irritating.[31]

SAFETY ISSUES

Photocarcinogenicity

In 1992 the FDA formed an advisory committee that reviewed the safety of BPO because there were a few reports that suggested that BPO would predispose mice to skin cancer, especially when combined with sun exposure.[34–41]

The following statement was issued by the FDA:

"During the 1992 Advisory Committee meeting, industry representatives stated that published studies in mice showed no evidence of benzoyl peroxide being photocarcinogenic. However, the Committee concluded that the studies were insufficient to determine whether benzoyl peroxide is carcinogenic. The Committee indicated that the studies were inconclusive because none of the studies used sufficient numbers of mice and the mice should have been observed over their entire lifespan. Therefore, the Committee unanimously agreed that a new photocarcinogenicity study should be conducted."[34,42]

The FDA advisory committee recommended that:

- New photocarcinogenicity studies on BPO should be conducted.
- Current animal safety data regarding BPO should be conveyed in labeling.
- Acne drug products containing BPO should stay on the market while new studies are being performed.

During the period of 1992 to 2011 new safety studies were conducted. In 2011 the FDA published a new ruling that changed the classification of BPO to Category I and stated:

"We now conclude that benzoyl peroxide, in concentrations of 2.5 to 10 percent, is GRASE (GRASE = Generally Recognized As Safe and Effective) for the OTC topical treatment of acne. This conclusion is based on safety data that we received and evaluated since publication of the 1995 proposed rule that proposed classifying benzoyl peroxide as Category III. As recommended by the Committee, these new data include studies examining the carcinogenic and photocarcinogenic potential of benzoyl peroxide. In addition to discussing these new studies in this section of the document, we provide a summary of earlier studies discussed in previous OTC acne drug product rulemakings. We believe the combined results of the earlier and new studies support the GRASE finding for benzoyl peroxide."[42] (See Table 76-2 for additional warnings and directions issued by the FDA in 2011 for the use of OTC benzoyl peroxide.)

TABLE 76-2

Additional Required Warnings and Directions for OTC Topical Acne Products Containing Benzoyl Peroxide or a Combination of Active Ingredients (the FDA recommended labeling language for benzoyl peroxide in addition to the labeling requirements presented in Chapter 80, Overview of Acne, Table 76-2)[62]

ADDITIONAL REQUIRED WARNINGS	ADDITIONAL REQUIRED DIRECTIONS
Do not use if you - have very sensitive skin - are sensitive to benzoyl peroxide	- If going outside, apply sunscreen after using this product. If irritation or sensitivity develops, stop use of both products and ask a doctor.
When using this product - avoid unnecessary sun exposure and use a sunscreen - avoid contact with the eyes, lips, and mouth - avoid contact with hair and dyed fabrics, which may be bleached by this product - skin irritation may occur, characterized by redness, burning, itching, peeling, or possibly swelling. Irritation may be reduced by using the product less frequently or in a lower concentration.	
Stop use and ask a doctor if - irritation becomes severe	

Safety in Pregnancy

Many patients develop acne in pregnancy. Although no specific safety studies using BPO in pregnant patients have been performed, several publications contend that only about 5 percent of topically applied BPO is absorbed systemically, suggesting that BPO is a safe option during pregnancy.[15,43–45]

Irritation

BPO causes skin irritation, either as contact dermatitis or irritant dermatitis, in approximately 1 percent of patients.[46,47] Agents that increase penetration would increase the susceptibility to irritation while lower strengths of BPO would be less likely to cause irritation. Using barrier repair moisturizers may decrease incidence of irritation but this has not been studied or proven.

Skin Aging

When BPO breaks down into benzoic acid in the skin, benzoyloxy, a free radical, forms as an intermediate.[48] Benzoyloxy can decarboxylate into a phenyl radical.[49] It has been shown that BPO depletes membrane and cytosolic antioxidants.[50] These free radicals produce oxidative stress, which may cause DNA strand breaks in keratinocytes or harm proteins or lipids.[50–52] A study by Ibbotson et al. showed that topically applied BPO induced photodamage in mouse skin that resembled that of UVB.[48]

◼ ENVIRONMENTAL IMPACT

BPO is used for many different indications including bleaching flour used in food and is rated as GRASE by the FDA. It is synthesized in laboratories for widespread use in the cosmeceutical world and should not exert an appreciable impact on the environment.

◼ FORMULATION CONSIDERATIONS

BPO consists of white crystal agglomerates that are insoluble in water but soluble in organic solvents.[3,53] BPO is stable at room temperature but flammable and explosive when heated greater than 100°C. In 1974, Fulton et al. showed that the vehicle for BPO delivery is critical. Alcohol gels increase efficacy because once the alcohol evaporates, residual BPO is left on the skin.[54] Water-based preparations are less irritating than alcohol-based preparations,[55] likely because less BPO is deposited on the skin. Irritation potential may be reduced through micronizing the BPO particle or making it softer and less abrasive. Urea, glycerin, and the emollient dimethicone also improve tolerability. Encapsulating the BPO or placing it in a microsponge may slow delivery of BPO, reducing the risk of irritation.[3]

◼ USAGE CONSIDERATIONS

The use of BPO in acne therapies is associated with a decrease in antibiotic resistance.[21] Therefore, it is often combined with other acne therapies. Because BPO kills bacteria by generating reactive oxygen species (ROS) in the sebaceous follicle, the chemical compatibility of BPO with other agents should be considered.[16] BPO, as a strong oxidizer, could oxidize other agents such as tretinoin and hydroquinone, thus reducing the efficacy of these agents.[56] One study demonstrated that BPO tends to degrade tretinoin to about 80 percent of initial content and this effect is dramatically increased in the presence of indoor light. Adapalene is not degraded by BPO even in the presence of light.[56]

When BPO is used in body washes, studies have shown that greater efficacy is realized when the product is left on for five minutes before rinsing.[57,58] The efficacy associated with BPO in cleansing products equals that seen in leave-on products but with less irritation provoked by the cleansers.[55,59]

The order of products used is important when BPO is incorporated in the regimen because it can inactivate other ingredients. For example, when applied simultaneously with topical tretinoin, BPO can denature the tretinoin and reduce its effectiveness.[56]

SIGNIFICANT BACKGROUND

BPO has been used for over 45 years for acne treatment. It is available as a prescription medication alone or combined with tretinoin, adapalene, or clindamycin. The FDA monograph also allows it to be sold without a prescription as long as the label includes the information covered in the FDA monograph. BPO is being studied for use in rosacea, seborrheic dermatitis, and in other skin diseases, but is currently only approved for use in acne. Its use is limited by the fact that it causes irritation in some skin types and generates ROS. Carefully selecting a treatment regimen that uses the proper ingredients in the proper sequence can help mitigate these pitfalls of BPO.

CONCLUSION

BPO has a colorful history in dermatology. It is very effective as an acne medication and is one of the few acne medications that is available both over the counter and by prescription in the United States. In some other countries, BPO is available only by prescription. It is an important medication because it helps prevent antibiotic resistance to erythromycin and clindamycin. Bacterial resistance is a serious problem in the United States and the treatment of acne with erythromycin and clindamycin is thought to contribute to this problem. However, the use of BPO is limited in dry skin with an impaired barrier because of the risk of irritation. It reacts with other ingredients such as tretinoin, thereby reducing tretinoin's efficacy. Most importantly, BPO is a source of free radicals to the skin, which may contribute to glycation, mitochondrial damage, and skin aging.[60,61] Combined use with antioxidants is suggested to minimize skin damage.

REFERENCES

1. Bowe WP, Shalita AR. Effective over-the-counter acne treatments. *Semin Cutan Med Surg.* 2008;27:170.
2. Green L, Kircik LH, Gwazdauskas J. Randomized, controlled, evaluator-blinded studies conducted to compare the efficacy and tolerability of 3 over-the-counter acne regimens in subjects with mild or moderate acne. *J Drugs Dermatol.* 2013;12:180.
3. Tanghetti EA, Popp KF. A current review of topical benzoyl peroxide: New perspectives on formulation and utilization. *Dermatol Clin.* 2009;27:17.
4. Kraus AL, Munro IC, Orr JC, et al. Benzoyl peroxide: An integrated human safety assessment for carcinogenicity. *Regul Toxicol Pharmacol.* 1995;21:87.
5. Merker PC. Benzoyl peroxide: A history of early research and researchers. *Int J Dermatol.* 2002;41:185.
6. Fishman IM. Benzoyl peroxide in acne: Reply. *J Am Acad Dermatol.* 1989;20:518.
7. Pace WE. A benzoyl peroxide-sulfur cream for acne vulgaris. *Can Med Assoc J.* 1965;93:252.
8. Cox RM, Ciufo LR, inventors; Stiefel Laboratories, Inc, assignee. Stable benzoyl peroxide composition. US patent 3 535 422. October 20, 1970.
9. DeVillez RL, inventor; Board of Regents, The University of Texas System, assignee. Therapeutic compositions containing benzoyl peroxide. US patent 4 923 900. May 8, 1990.
10. Won R, inventor; Advanced Polymer Systems, Inc, assignee. Method for delivery an active ingredient by controlled release utilizing a novel delivery vehicle which can be prepared by a process utilizing the active ingredient as a porogen. US patent 4 690 825. September 1, 1985.
11. Fulton JE Jr, inventor; AHC Pharmacal, Inc, assignee. Composition and method for the treatment of acne. US patent 4 189 501. February 19, 1980.
12. Klein RW, Foxx ME, inventors; Dermik Laboratories, Inc, assignee. Stable benzoyl peroxide composition. US patent 4 387 107. June 7, 1983.
13. Flynn RG, Pitkin CG, Hileman GA, inventors; Norcliff Thayer, Inc, assignee. Use of fumed silica for treating oily skin and acne. US patent 4 536 399. August 20, 1985.
14. Mays RM, Gordon RA, Wilson JM, et al. New antibiotic therapies for acne and rosacea. *Dermatol Ther.* 2012;25:23.
15. Pugashetti R, Shinkai K. Treatment of acne vulgaris in pregnant patients. *Dermatol Ther.* 2013;26:302.
16. Nacht S, Yeung D, Beasley JN Jr, et al. Benzoyl peroxide: Percutaneous penetration and metabolic disposition. *J Am Acad Dermatol.* 1981;4:31.
17. Yeung D, Nacht S, Bucks D, et al. Benzoyl peroxide: Percutaneous penetration and metabolic disposition. II. Effect of concentration. *J Am Acad Dermatol.* 1983;9:920.
18. Drucker CR. Update on topical antibiotics in dermatology. *Dermatol Ther.* 2012;25:6.
19. Cove JH, Holland KT. The effect of benzoyl peroxide on cutaneous micro-organisms in vitro. *J Appl Bacteriol.* 1983;54:379.
20. Nishijima S, Akamatsu H, Akamatsu M, et al. The antibiotic susceptibility of Propionibacterium acnes and Staphylococcus epidermidis isolated from acne. *J Dermatol.* 1994;21:166.
21. Kircik LH. The role of benzoyl peroxide in the new treatment paradigm for acne. *J Drugs Dermatol.* 2013;12:s73.
22. Eady EA, Farmery MR, Ross JI, et al. Effects of benzoyl peroxide and erythromycin alone and in combination against antibiotic-sensitive and -resistant skin bacteria from acne patients. *Br J Dermatol.* 1994;131:331.
23. Leyden J, Levy S. The development of antibiotic resistance in Propionibacterium acnes. *Cutis.* 2001;67:21.
24. Thiboutot D, Gollnick H, Bettoli V, et al. New insights into the management of acne: An update from the Global Alliance to Improve Outcomes in Acne group. *J Am Acad Dermatol.* 2009;60:S1.
25. Gollnick H, Cunliffe W, Berson D, et al. Management of acne: A report from a Global Alliance to Improve Outcomes in Acne. *J Am Acad Dermatol.* 2003;49:S1.
26. Waller JM, Dreher F, Behnam S, et al. 'Keratolytic' properties of benzoyl peroxide and retinoic acid resemble salicylic acid in man. *Skin Pharmacol Physiol.* 2006;19:283.
27. Sagransky M, Yentzer BA, Feldman SR. Benzoyl peroxide: A review of its current use in the treatment of acne vulgaris. *Expert Opin Pharmacother.* 2009;10:2555.
28. Burkhart CN, Burkhart CG. Genome sequence of Propionibacterium acnes reveals immunogenic and surface-associated genes confirming existence of the acne biofilm. *Int J Dermatol.* 2006;45:872.
29. Burkhart CN, Burkhart CG. Microbiology's principle of biofilms as a major factor in the pathogenesis of acne vulgaris. *Int J Dermatol.* 2003;42:925.
30. Lookingbill DP, Chalker DK, Lindholm JS, et al. Treatment of acne with a combination clindamycin/benzoyl peroxide gel compared with clindamycin gel, benzoyl peroxide gel and vehicle gel: Combined results of two double-blind investigations. *J Am Acad Dermatol.* 1997;37:590.
31. Simpson RC, Grindlay DJ, Williams HC. What's new in acne? An analysis of systematic reviews and clinically significant trials published in 2010–11. *Clin Exp Dermatol.* 2011;36:840.
32. do Nascimento LV, Guedes AC, Magalhães GM, et al. Single-blind and comparative clinical study of the efficacy and safety of benzoyl peroxide 4% gel (BID) and adapalene 0.1% gel (QD) in the treatment of acne vulgaris. *J Dermatolog Treat.* 2003;14:166.
33. Bojar RA, Cunliffe WJ, Holland KT. The short-term treatment of acne vulgaris with benzoyl peroxide: Effects on the surface and follicular cutaneous microflora. *Br J Dermatol.* 1995;132:204.

34. Food and Drug Administration. Classification of Benzoyl Peroxide as Safe and Effective and Revision of Labeling to Drug Facts Format; Topical Acne Drug Products for Over-the-Counter Human Use; Final Rule. Posted March 4, 2010. http://www.regulations.gov/#!documentDetail;D=FDA-1981-N-0114-0001. Accessed August 24, 2013.

35. Hazlewood C, Davies MJ. Benzoyl peroxide-induced damage to DNA and its components: Direct evidence for the generation of base adducts, sugar radicals, and strand breaks. *Arch Biochem Biophys*. 1996;332:79.

36. Slaga TJ, Klein-Szanto AJ, Triplett LL, et al. Skin tumor-promoting activity of benzoyl-peroxide, a widely used free radical-generating compound. *Science*. 1981;213:1023.

37. Reiners JJ Jr, Nesnow S, Slaga TJ. Murine susceptibility to two-stage skin carcinogenesis is influenced by the agent used for promotion. *Carcinogenesis*. 1984;5:301.

38. O'Connell JF, Klein-Szanto AJ, DiGiovanni DM, et al. Enhanced malignant progression of mouse skin tumors by the free-radical generator benzoyl peroxide. *Cancer Res*. 1986;46:2863.

39. Iversen OH. Carcinogenesis studies with benzoyl peroxide (Panoxyl gel 5%). *J Invest Dermatol*. 1986;86:442.

40. Iversen OH. Skin tumorigenesis and carcinogenesis studies with 7,12-dimethylbenz[a]anthracene, ultraviolet light, benzoyl peroxide (Panoxyl gel 5%) and ointment gel. *Carcinogenesis*. 1988;9:803.

41. Athar M, Raza H, Bickers DR, et al. Inhibition of benzoyl peroxide-mediated tumor promotion in 7,12-dimethylbenz[a] anthracene-initiated skin of Sencar mice by antioxidants nordihydroguaiaretic acid and diallyl sulfide. *J Invest Dermatol*. 1990;94:162.

42. Food and Drug Administration, HHS. Classification of benzoyl peroxide as safe and effective and revision of labeling to drug facts format; topical acne drug products for over-the-counter human use, final rule. *Fed Regist*. 2010;75:9767.

43. Hale EK, Pomeranz MK. Dermatologic agents during pregnancy and lactation: An update and clinical review. *Int J Dermatol*. 2002;41:197.

44. Bozzo P, Chua-Gocheco A, Einarson A. Safety of skin care products during pregnancy. *Can Fam Physician*. 2011;57:665.

45. Kong YL, Tey HL. Treatment of acne vulgaris during pregnancy and lactation. *Drugs*. 2013;73:779.

46. Greiner D, Weber J, Kaufmann R, et al. Benzoyl peroxide as a contact allergen in adhesive tape. *Contact Dermatitis*. 1999;41:233.

47. Balato N, Lembo G, Cuccurullo FM, et al. Acne and allergic contact dermatitis. *Contact Dermatitis*. 1996;34:68.

48. Ibbotson SH, Moran MN, Nash JF, et al. The effects of radicals compared with UVB as initiating species for the induction of chronic cutaneous photodamage. *J Invest Dermatol*. 1999;112:933.

49. Binder RL, Aardema MJ, Thompson ED. Benzoyl peroxide: Review of experimental carcinogenesis and human safety data. *Prog Clin Biol Res*. 1995;391:245.

50. Valacchi G, Rimbach G, Saliou C, et al. Effect of benzoyl peroxide on antioxidant status, NF-kappaB activity and interleukin-1alpha gene expression in human keratinocytes. *Toxicology*. 2001;165:225.

51. Akman SA, Doroshow JH, Kensler TW. Copper-dependent site-specific mutagenesis by benzoyl peroxide in the supF gene of the mutation reporter plasmid pS189. *Carcinogenesis*. 1992;13:1783.

52. Saladino AJ, Willey JC, Lechner JF, et al. Effects of formaldehyde, acetaldehyde, benzoyl peroxide, and hydrogen peroxide on cultured normal human bronchial epithelial cells. *Cancer Res*. 1985;45:2522.

53. Cotterill JA. Benzoyl peroxide. *Acta Derm Venereol Suppl (Stockh)*. 1980;Suppl 89:57.

54. Fulton JE Jr, Farzad-Bakshandeh A, Bradley S. Studies on the mechanism of action to topical benzoyl peroxide and vitamin A acid in acne vulgaris. *J Cutan Pathol*. 1974;1:191.

55. Fakhouri T, Yentzer BA, Feldman SR. Advancement in benzoyl peroxide-based acne treatment: Methods to increase both efficacy and tolerability. *J Drugs Dermatol*. 2009;8:657.

56. Martin B, Meunier C, Montels D, et al. Chemical stability of adapalene and tretinoin when combined with benzoyl peroxide in presence and in absence of visible light and ultraviolet radiation. *Br J Dermatol*. 1998;139(Suppl 52):8.

57. Leyden JJ. Efficacy of benzoyl peroxide (5.3%) emollient foam and benzoyl peroxide (8%) wash in reducing Propionibacterium acnes on the back. *J Drugs Dermatol*. 2010;9:622.

58. Bikowski J. A review of the safety and efficacy of benzoyl peroxide (5.3%) emollient foam in the management of truncal acne vulgaris. *J Clin Aesthet Dermatol*. 2010;3:26.

59. Burkhart CG, Scheinfeld NS. Benzoyl peroxide skin washes: Basis, logic, effectiveness and tolerance. *Skinmed*. 2005;4:370.

60. Babizhayev MA, Deyev AI, Savel'yeva EL, et al. Skin beautification with oral non-hydrolized versions of carnosine and carcinine: Effective therapeutic management and cosmetic skincare solutions against oxidative glycation and free-radical production as a causal mechanism of diabetic complications and skin aging. *J Dermatolog Treat*. 2012;23:345.

61. Cadenas E, Davies KJ. Mitochondrial free radical generation, oxidative stress, and aging. *Free Radic Biol Med*. 2000;29:222.

62. U.S. Department of Health and Human Services, Food and Drug Administration, Center for Drug Evaluation and Research (CDER). Guidance for Industry Topical Acne Drug Products for Over-the-Counter Human Use – Revision of Labeling and Classification of Benzoyl Peroxide as Safe and Effective Small Entity Compliance Guide. Posted June 2011. http://www.fda.gov/downloads/Drugs/GuidanceComplianceRegulatoryInformation/Guidances/UCM259744.pdf. Accessed August 24, 2013.

CHAPTER 77

Tea Tree Oil

Activities:

Analgesic, anti-inflammatory, antibacterial, antifungal, antimicrobial, antipruritic, antiseptic, insecticidal, anti-skin cancer[1-4]

Important Chemical Components:

Terpinen-4-ol, γ-terpinene, α-terpinene, α-terpineol, terpinolene, α-pinene, and cineole are primary constituents. Tea tree oil contains more than 100 chemical compounds, mainly terpenes and alcohols, including D-limonene.[5,6]

Origin Classification:

This ingredient is considered natural. As an ingredient used for dermatologic purposes, it is laboratory made.

Personal Care Category:

Antiacne, analgesic, antifungal

Recommended for the following Baumann Skin Types:

DSNT, DSPT, DSNW, DSPW, OSNT, OSPT, OSNW, and OSPW

SOURCE

Melaleuca alternifolia, a member of the Myrtaceae family and the source of tea tree oil (TTO), is a small tree native to Australia. Although there are three different species of coniferous Myrtaceae growing in Australia, New Zealand, and Southeast Asia known as tea trees, only the essential oil derived from the needles or leaves of the Australian *M. alternifolia* is used in medical and cosmetic products. Aromatherapists do use the essential oils of all three species, but only *M. alternifolia* has been extensively tested for toxicity, and its antimicrobial activity evaluated.[7] A clear liquid that ranges from colorless to faint yellow but with a sharp, camphoraceous aroma, TTO contains over 100 natural compounds.

Steam distillation is used to extract the oil from the leaves. A menthol-like cooling sensation is yielded by the essential oil.[6] Its common name is based on the brewing of the leaves for tea by early settlers in Australia.[8] It is also known by the Maori and Samoan expression "ti tree oil."[1,9]

Recent data support its use to treat acne vulgaris, seborrheic dermatitis, and chronic gingivitis as well as to promote wound healing.[4] In addition, TTO has been shown to display anti-skin cancer activity.[4]

HISTORY

An essential oil of the *M. alternifolia* tree or shrub, TTO is thought to have been used for thousands of years by Australian natives for healing purposes,[10] and has been used for nearly a century, at least, by the Bundjalung indigenous tribe in Australia as an herbal medicine to treat upper respiratory tract infections.[1,6] Australian aborigines also use TTO to treat bruises and skin infections, and the essential oil is now thought to be a suitable alternative option in the acne armamentarium.[11] The antiseptic and disinfectant properties of TTO were reported by Penfold and Grant in the 1920s, with the finding that it exhibited 13 times more antiseptic activity than carbolic acid, leading to the investigation and usage of the essential oil.[12,13] Further studies in the 1930s established TTO in Australia as an effective topical antiseptic and broad-spectrum antimicrobial agent, particularly against *Candida albicans*, *Escherichia coli*, *Staphylococcus aureus*, *S. epidermidis*, and *Propionibacterium acnes*.[3,12,14] In fact, the broad-spectrum antibacterial activity of TTO forms the basis for its use in acne therapy.[4,15]

CHEMISTRY

TTO is obtained through the steam distillation of the leaves and terminal branchlets of the *M. alternifolia* tree.[16] Terpinene-4-ol constitutes up to 60 percent of the oil. Australian standards set a minimum content of 30 percent terpinene-4-ol.[14]

ORAL USES

TTO is considered toxic when consumed orally. Reported adverse effects from consuming TTO include nausea, diarrhea, vomiting, drowsiness, confusion, hallucinations, weakness, and coma.[6,10,17]

TOPICAL USES

Acne, psoriasis, fungal infections, vaginal infections, tinea, lice, rashes, cold sores, cuts, scratches, and various burns are among the indications for topical TTO. Accordingly, the botanical is found in a wide range of over-the-counter (OTC) personal care, hair, skin cream, and cosmetic formulations.[8,18]

Antiacne Activity

In a seminal study of topically applied TTO in 1990, Bassett et al. conducted a single-blind, randomized clinical trial in 124 patients with mild-to-moderate acne to assess efficacy and skin tolerance. Subjects were treated with either 5 percent TTO gel or 5 percent benzoyl peroxide. Both treatments demonstrated significant effects in improving acne by lowering the number of inflamed lesions, both open and closed comedones. Although TTO oil took longer to exert its effects, patients using TTO exhibited fewer side effects. Investigators concluded that using a higher concentration of TTO might have yielded faster yet still effective action.[3]

In a literature review conducted in 2000, Ernst and Huntley analyzed data from six electronic databases to identify randomized clinical trials using TTO. They were able to find only four trials. Evidence indicated that the botanical appeared to be an effective treatment for acne and fungal infections, with any side effects, typically allergic reactions, found to be mild and short-lived.[19]

A 2007 randomized, double-blind clinical trial in 60 patients with mild-to-moderate acne revealed the efficacy of 5 percent TTO gel. Patients, randomly assigned to one of two groups (30 each), were treated with TTO or placebo and followed every 15 days over a 45-day period. Investigators found that the TTO gel was 3.55 times more effective than placebo in reducing total acne lesion counts and 5.75 times more effective than placebo in lowering the acne severity index. Side effects were similarly mild and tolerable in both groups.[15] Topical application of TTO three or four times daily is a recommended regimen to treat acne.[14]

Anticancer Activity

In 2012, Ireland et al. reported that topically applied TTO in a dilute (10 percent) dimethyl sulfoxide formulation quickly leads to a direct anticancer effect in subcutaneous tumor-bearing mice. The *in vivo* cytotoxicity of TTO was linked to its penetration, according to the researchers. They suggested that future investigations should focus on enhancing skin penetration to increase *in situ* terpene concentration.[20] Previously, Greay et al. reported that topically applied TTO had shown *in vivo* antitumor activity in fully immune-competent subcutaneous tumor-bearing mice.[21] Also that year, the same team of investigators found that TTO and terpinen-4-ol exhibited significant antiproliferative activity–inducing necrosis and cell cycle arrest–against two murine tumor cell lines.[22]

Antibacterial, Antifungal, and Antiviral Activity

TTO is well known to have displayed antibacterial and antifungal activity.[2,5] A 2001 *in vitro* study by D'Auria et al. revealed the effectiveness of lipophilic TTO in blocking the conversion of *C. albicans* (and other yeasts, including *Schizosaccharomyces pombe* and *Debaryomyces hansenii*) from the yeast to the pathogenic mycelial form. The investigators concluded that such inhibitory activity positions TTO as a potentially suitable agent for treating fungal mucosal and cutaneous infections.[2] According to a 2000 study by Zhang et al., TTO also may have the capacity to attack many of the microbes typically associated with otitis externa and otitis media, though some ototoxicity is feared.[23] Since then, though, the risks have been shown to be minimal, with broad-spectrum activity being increasingly attributed to the herbal agent.

In a 2008 case report, Millar and Moore documented their successful treatment of a pediatric patient with warts on her right middle finger through the once-daily topical application of TTO for 12 days. They concluded that this shows the potential of TTO to treat warts caused by the human papilloma virus.[24]

Based on a recent uncontrolled, open-label case series that began with 19 patients and ended with 11, Edmondson et al. reported that TTO, while it failed to decolonize methicillin-resistant *S. aureus* (MRSA) (the primary aim of the study), did not inhibit wound healing and was associated with a reduction in wound size.[25] More recently, in a 2013 study by Thomsen et al. to ascertain the antimicrobial susceptibility of *Staphylococcus* spp. after acclimation to low levels of topical TTO, the investigators habituated methicillin-susceptible *S. aureus* (MSSA), MRSA, and coagulase-negative staphylococci (CoNS) to 0.075 percent TTO for three days. They uncovered no evidence that TTO

contributes to resistance to antimicrobial agents (i.e., fusidic acid, mupirocin, chloramphenicol, linezolid, and vancomycin).[18]

Seborrheic Dermatitis and Other Indications

Seborrheic dermatitis may also be alleviated by TTO.[26] In a 2002 randomized trial of 126 patients with dandruff conducted by Satchell et al., subjects using 5 percent TTO shampoo experienced a 41 percent improvement whereas patients using a placebo showed only an 11 percent improvement in the quadrant area severity score.[27] That same year, Satchell et al. also conducted a randomized, controlled, double-blind, four-week study of 158 patients with interdigital tinea pedis that demonstrated the efficacy and safety of 25 and 50 percent TTO for the treatment of the dermatophyte. An appreciable clinical response was noted by the investigators, with 68 percent of the 50 percent TTO group and 72 percent of the 25 percent TTO group improving, compared to 39 percent in the placebo group.[28]

In 2010, Barker and Altman conducted a randomized, assessor-blind, parallel-group, comparative efficacy trial in 123 subjects to evaluate three treatments for head lice in children. A pediculicide containing TTO and lavender oil was found to be equally effective as a head lice "suffocation" product and significantly more effective than the product containing pyrethrins and piperonyl butoxide (41 of 42 patients were louse-free one day after the last treatment with tea tree and lavender oils compared to 10 of 40 patients using the pyrethrins and piperonyl butoxide).[29] In addition, TTO has been used successfully to treat blepharitis secondary to ocular demodicosis.[30]

In 2013, Sakr et al. formulated a multimodal microemulsion composed of minoxidil, diclofenac, and TTO and conducted a pilot study in 32 women (from 18 to 30 years old) with androgenetic alopecia who were randomized to apply 1 mL of the microemulsion, minoxidil alone, or placebo twice daily for 32 weeks. The combination treatment was associated with significantly better mean hair counts, mean hair weight, and mean hair thickness. In fact, the stability, safety, and efficacy of the microemulsion containing TTO were far superior to minoxidil alone or placebo.[31]

The combination of TTO and lavender oil was also evaluated more recently by Tirabassi et al. in a prospective, open-label, placebo-controlled, randomized study in 24 women with mild idiopathic hirsutism. Twelve women were randomized to use an oil spray containing the botanicals twice daily for three months in the affected areas and the remaining 12 women used a placebo spray. Statistically significant reductions were noted in hirsutism total score and hair diameter in the group using TTO and lavender, unlike the placebo group. The researchers concluded that the topical application of TTO and lavender is a safe and practical approach to treating mild idiopathic hirsutism.[32]

In addition, TTO, through its main active constituent terpinen-4-ol, may also deliver an antipsoriatic effect.[16]

■ SAFETY ISSUES

In a recent multicenter Italian study on the use of topical botanically-derived products, Corazza et al. reported that of 2,661 patients surveyed, 1,274 (48 percent) claimed to have used such products of whom 139 (11 percent) experienced adverse cutaneous reactions. Propolis, Compositae extracts, and TTO were the three most frequently cited allergens.[33]

Terpinen-4-ol, the primary constituent of TTO, has been implicated in mild allergic contact reactions, such as allergic contact dermatitis (ACD) (see Table 77-1). Photooxidation

TABLE 77-1
Pros and Cons of Tea Tree Oil

Pros	Cons
Appears to have potential as a versatile agent in the dermatologic armamentarium	Implicated in causing mild allergic reactions
Evidence suggests suitability for the treatment of mild-to-moderate acne	Dearth of randomized, controlled, double-blind, placebo-controlled clinical trials for acne treatment

within a few days to several months of exposure leads to the synthesis of peroxides, epoxides, and endoperoxides, such as ascaridol and 1,2,4-trihydroxymethane, which are likely responsible in cases of ACD.[34] The increase in use of TTO over the last 15 years is expected to contribute to a higher incidence of reports of contact dermatitis and eczema, according to some authors.[35,36]

Contact sensitization and ACD have been associated with the use of topical TTO, but in low numbers. The most recent prevalence rates indicate that 1.4 percent of patients referred for patch testing experienced a positive reaction to TTO, which was added to the North American Contact Dermatitis Group screening panel in 1999.[6] However, some components of TTO may actually alleviate hypersensitivity reactions and TTO is considered safe and effective for use by most patients.

Studies on mice conducted by Brand et al. in 2002 suggest that some constituents of TTO may actually diminish hypersensitivity reactions. In one study, two components of topical TTO, terpinen-4-ol and α-terpineol, were found to regulate the edema associated with the efferent phase of a contact hypersensitivity reaction.[37] In a separate study, terpninen-4-ol was also found to be effective in controlling the histamine-induced edema often correlated with type I allergic reactions.[38]

Adverse reactions in humans can be mitigated through correct storage; not using the neat oil; limiting exposure to aged, oxidized oil; and using more dilute preparations.[1,9,20,39–41] The track record for safe usage is approximately 90 years.[1] There is a report of gynecomastia occurring in three prepubertal boys in association with the topical application of lavender and tea tree oils. The condition subsided in each patient soon after cessation of product usage and each patient had been found to be otherwise healthy with normal serum concentrations of endogenous steroids.[42]

ENVIRONMENTAL IMPACT

TTO is harvested throughout the year. *M. alternifolia* are robust, sturdy plants native to New South Wales, Australia that recover quickly from harvesting and live for up to a decade.

FORMULATION CONSIDERATIONS

Optimal TTO solubility in the base and optimal TTO delivery to targeted skin in proper concentrations are important considerations.[12] The presence of preservatives or surfactants may or may not amplify the antimicrobial effects of TTO. Australian standards require a minimum content of 30 percent terpinene-4-ol in TTO products.[14]

USAGE CONSIDERATIONS

TTO is available in liquid and semisolid formulations. TTO should be stored in a cool, dark, dry area in a container with little air as oil stability can be affected by heat, light, moisture, and air exposure.[1]

SIGNIFICANT BACKGROUND

With increasing frequency, TTO, usually in concentrations of 5 to 10 percent, is found as an ingredient in several cosmetic products, including shampoos, massage oils, skin and nail creams, as well as household products such as laundry detergents (for eliminating mites).[6] TTO has long been regarded as an effective topical antiseptic and broad-spectrum antimicrobial agent.[12] In recent years, a more expansive demographic has come to use this essential oil for a wide range of indications including acne, psoriasis, fungal infections (e.g., oral candidiasis), vaginal infections, tinea, lice, rashes, cold sores, cuts, scratches, various burns (including sunburns), and for dental applications.[1,39,43] It is also being studied for potential effectiveness against recurrent herpes labialis.[44] Given its reputation and anecdotal reports of effectiveness, TTO has been incorporated into antifungal soaps and shampoos, dental products (e.g., mouthwashes and toothpastes), veterinary products (to protect against fleas and ticks), and several household and industrial disinfectants. An antioxidant application of TTO in skin care formulations has been proposed, though one study from 2000 suggests that TTO lacks antioxidant properties.[7] Importantly, in terms of its antiacne activity, TTO exhibits anti-inflammatory properties by lowering histamine-induced cutaneous inflammation.[45]

Contradictory Findings

Despite numerous favorable reports on its varied beneficial effects, the amount of valid research showing the positive effects of TTO on dermatologic conditions is relatively small. In one study of complementary and alternative medicine (CAM) comparing the effectiveness of *Aloe vera* gel and TTO in treating two selected conditions (atopic dermatitis and chronic venous insufficiency), neither product was found to be effective.[46] In a review of four randomized clinical trials, researchers acknowledged that TTO might be effective in treating acne and fungal infections, but declared that there is no compelling evidence showing that TTO is truly effective in treating any dermatologic condition.[19] Since then, however, more favorable findings have emerged. In fact, TTO is thought to have potential as a standard acne therapy,[11] and is included in OTC products designed to treat acne.[47]

CONCLUSION

Tea tree oil has been recently touted for a wide range of dermatologic conditions and, accordingly, become an extremely popular ingredient in skin care products. While anecdotal reports may hold some sway, it is important to consider the relative paucity of clinical evidence on tea tree oil. That is, much more research, particularly randomized, double-blind, controlled trials, are needed to establish the efficacy of products with tea tree oil as the main active ingredient. Nevertheless, the evidence, derived mostly from *in vitro* work, that has emerged does seem to support the reputed broad range of activity.

In particular, the antimicrobial and anti-inflammatory effects of the essential oil of *Melaleuca alternifolia* have been well established and the data on its use as an acne adjuvant are particularly promising.

REFERENCES

1. Carson CF, Hammer KA, Riley TV. Melaleuca alternifolia (Tea Tree) oil: A review of antimicrobial and other medicinal properties. *Clin Microbiol Rev.* 2006;19:50.
2. D'Auria FD, Laino L, Strippoli V, et al. In vitro activity of tea tree oil against Candida albicans mycelia conversion and other pathogenic fungi. *J Chemother.* 2001;13:377.
3. Bassett IB, Pannowitz DL, Barnetson RS. A comparative study of tea-tree oil versus benzoylperoxide in the treatment of acne. *Med J Aust.* 1990;153:455.
4. Pazyar N, Yaghoobi R, Bagherani N, et al. A review of applications of tea tree oil in dermatology. *Int J Dermatol.* 2013;52:784.
5. Morelli V, Calmet E, Jhingade V. Alternative therapies for common dermatologic disorders, part 2. *Prim Care.* 2010;37:285.
6. Larson D, Jacob SE. Tea tree oil. *Dermatitis.* 2012;23:48.
7. Lis-Balchin M, Hart SL, Deans SG. Pharmacological and antimicrobial studies on different tea-tree oils (Melaleuca alternifolia, Leptospermum scoparium or Manuka and Kunzea ericoides or Kanuka), originating in Australia and New Zealand. *Phytother Res.* 2000;14:623.
8. Aburjai T, Natsheh FM. Plants used in cosmetics. *Phythother Res.* 2003;17:987.
9. Carson CF, Riley TV. Safety, efficacy and provenance of tea tree (Melaleuca alternifolia) oil. *Contact Dermatitis.* 2001;45:65.
10. American Cancer Society. Tea tree oil. http://www.cancer.org/Treatment/TreatmentsandSideEffects/ComplementaryandAlternativeMedicine/HerbsVitaminsandMinerals/tea-tree-oil. Accessed October 8, 2013.
11. Reuter J, Merfort I, Schempp CM. Botanicals in dermatology: An evidence-based review. *Am J Clin Dermatol.* 2010;11:247.
12. Thomsen PS, Jensen TM, Hammer KA, et al. Survey of the antimicrobial activity of commercially available Australian tea tree (Melaleuca alternifolia) essential oil products in vitro. *J Altern Complement Med.* 2011;17:835.
13. Foster S. *An Illustrated Guide to 101 Medicinal Herbs: Their History, Use, Recommended Dosages, and Cautions.* Loveland, CO: Interweave Press; 1998:196-197.
14. Hoffmann D. *Medical herbalism: The science and practice of herbal medicine.* Rochester, VT: Healing Arts Press; 2003:439.
15. Enshaieh S, Jooya A, Siadat AH, et al. The efficacy of 5% topical tea tree oil gel in mild to moderate acne vulgaris: A randomized, double-blind placebo-controlled study. *Indian J Dermatol Venereol Leprol.* 2007;73:22.
16. Pazyar N, Yaghoobi R. Tea tree oil as a novel antipsoriasis weapon. *Skin Pharmacol Physiol.* 2012;25:162.
17. Crawford GH, Sciacca JR, James WD. Tea tree oil: Cutaneous effects of the extracted oil of Melaleuca alternifolia. *Dermatitis.* 2004;15:59.
18. Thomsen NA, Hammer KA, Riley TV, et al. Effect of habituation to tea tree (Melaleuca alternifolia) oil on the subsequent susceptibility of Staphylococcus spp. to antimicrobials, triclosan, tea tree oil, terpinen-4-ol and carvacrol. *Int J Antimicrob Agents.* 2013;41:343.
19. Ernst E, Huntley A. Tea tree oil: A systematic review of randomized clinical trials. *Forsch Komplementarmed Klass Naturheilkd.* 2000;7:17.
20. Ireland DJ, Greay SJ, Hooper CM, et al. Topically applied Melaleuca alternifolia (tea tree) oil causes direct anti-cancer cytotoxicity in subcutaneous tumour bearing mice. *J Dermatol Sci.* 2012;67:120.
21. Greay SJ, Ireland DJ, Kissick HT, et al. Inhibition of established subcutaneous murine tumour growth with topical Melaleuca alternifolia (tea tree) oil. *Cancer Chemother Pharmacol.* 2010;66:1095.
22. Greay SJ, Ireland DJ, Kissick HT, et al. Induction of necrosis and cell cycle arrest in murine cancer cell lines by Melaleuca alternifolia (tea tree) oil and terpinen-4-ol. *Cancer Chemother Pharmacol.* 2010;65:877.
23. Zhang SY, Robertson D. A study of tea tree oil ototoxicity. *Audiol Neurootol.* 2000;5:64.
24. Millar BC, Moore JE. Successful topical treatment of hand warts in a paediatric patient with tea tree oil (Melaleuca alternifolia). *Complement Ther Clin Pract.* 2008;14:225.
25. Edmondson M, Newall N, Carville K, et al. Uncontrolled, open-label, pilot study of tea tree (Melaleuca alternifolia) oil solution in the decolonisation of methicillin-resistant Staphylococcus aureus positive wounds and its influence on wound healing. *Int Wound J.* 2011;8:375.
26. Morelli V, Calmet E, Jhingade V. Alternative therapies for common dermatologic disorders, part I. *Prim Care.* 2010;37:269.
27. Satchell AC, Saurajen A, Bell C, et al. Treatment of dandruff with 5% tea tree oil shampoo. *J Am Acad Dermatol.* 2002;47:852.
28. Satchell AC, Saurajen A, Bell C, et al. Treatment of interdigital tinea pedis with 25% and 50% tea tree oil solution: A randomized, placebo-controlled, blinded study. *Australas J Dermatol.* 2002;43:175.
29. Barker SC, Altman PM. A randomized, assessor blind, parallel group comparative efficacy trial of three products for the treatment of head lice in children – Melaleuca oil and lavender oil, pyrethrins and piperonyl butoxide, and a "suffocation" product. *BMC Dermatol.* 2010;10:6.
30. Patel KG, Raju VK. Ocular demodicosis. *W V Med J.* 2013;109:16.
31. Sakr FM, Gado AM, Mohammed HR, et al. Preparation and evaluation of a multimodal minoxidil microemulsion versus minoxidil alone in the treatment of androgenetic alopecia of mixed etiology: A pilot study. *Drug Des Devel Ther.* 2013;7:413.
32. Tirabassi G, Giovannini L, Paggi F, et al. Possible efficacy of Lavender and Tea tree oils in the treatment of young women affected by mild idiopathic hirsutism. *J Endocrinol Invest.* 2013;36:50.
33. Corazza M, Borghi A, Gallo R, et al. Topical botanically derived products: use, skin reactions, and usefulness of patch tests. A multicentre Italian study. *Contact Dermatitis.* 2014;70:90.
34. Hausen BM, Reichling J, Harkenthal M. Degradation products of monoterpenes are the sensitizing agents in tea tree oil. *Am J Contact Dermat.* 1999;10:68.
35. Khanna M, Qasem K, Sasseville D. Allergic contact dermatitis to tea tree oil with erythema multiforme-like id reaction. *Am J Contact Dermat.* 2000;11:238.
36. Knight TE, Hausen BM. Melaleuca oil (tea tree oil) dermatitis. *J Am Acad Dermatol.* 1994;30:423.
37. Brand C, Grimbaldeston MA, Gamble JR, et al. Tea tree oil reduces the swelling associated with the efferent phase of a contact hypersensitivity response. *Inflamm Res.* 2002;51:236.
38. Brand C, Townley SL, Finlay-Jones JJ, et al. Tea tree oil reduces histamine-induced oedema in murine ears. *Inflamm Res.* 2002;51:283.
39. Hammer KA, Carson CF, Riley TV. Effects of Melaleuca alternifolia (tea tree) essential oil and the major monoterpene component terpinen-4-ol on the development of single- and multistep antibiotic resistance and antimicrobial susceptibility. *Antimicrob Agents Chemother.* 2012;56:909.
40. Hammer KA, Carson CF, Riley TV, et al. A review of the toxicity of Melaleuca alternifolia (tea tree) oil. *Food Chem Toxicol.* 2006;44:616.
41. Rutherford T, Nixon R, Tam M, et al. Allergy to tea tree oil: Retrospective review of 41 cases with positive patch tests over 4.5 years. *Australas J Dermatol.* 2007;48:83.
42. Henley DV, Lipson N, Korach KS, et al. Prepubertal gynecomastia linked to lavender and tea tree oils. *N Engl J Med.* 2007;356:479.
43. Baumann L. Botanical ingredients in cosmeceuticals. *J Drugs Dermatol.* 2007;6:1084.
44. Carson CF, Ashton L, Dry L, et al. Melaleuca alternifolia (tea tree) oil gel (6%) for the treatment of recurrent herpes labialis. *J Antimicrob Chemother.* 2001;48:450.
45. Koh KJ, Pearce AL, Marshman G, et al. Tea tree oil reduces histamine-induced skin inflammation. *Br J Dermatol.* 2002;147:1212.
46. Ernst E, Pittler MH, Stevinson C. Complementary/alternative medicine in dermatology: Evidence-assessed efficacy of two diseases and two treatments. *Am J Clin Dermatol.* 2002;3:341.
47. Bowe WP, Shalita AR. Effective over-the-counter acne treatments. *Semin Cutan Med Surg.* 2008;27:170.

CHAPTER 78

Salicylic Acid

Activities:

Anti-inflammatory, pore cleansing

Important Chemical Components:

Also known as 2-hydroxybenzoic acid, the chemical formula of salicylic acid is $C_6H_4(OH)COOH$. Its molecular formula is $C_7H_6O_3$.

Origin Classification:

Natural and organic forms are derived from willow bark, wintergreen leaves, and sweet birch. Most salicylic acid is laboratory made.

Personal Care Category:

Cleansing, antiacne, pore minimizing, exfoliating

Recommended for the following Baumann Skin Types:

DSNT, DSNW, DSPT, DSPW, OSNT, OSNW, OSPT, and OSPW. Salicylic acid may cause stinging in type 3 (S_3) sensitive skin (stinging subtype), but it is beneficial for S_1 (acne) and S_2 (rosacea) sensitive skin.

SOURCE

Salicylic acid (SA) is derived primarily from willow bark, but has also been extracted from wintergreen leaves, sweet birch, myrtle, and meadow sweet flowers.[1] Additional natural sources of SA include almonds, water chestnuts, peanuts, mushrooms, and various unripe fruits and vegetables, including blackberries, blueberries, cantaloupes, dates, raisins, kiwi, guavas, apricots, broccoli, green peppers, olives, tomatoes, as well as radishes and chicory, among others.[2]

SA is known to exhibit anti-inflammatory and comedolytic properties, which accounts for its inclusion in the dynamic antiacne arsenal (Table 78-1). This aromatic acid is also used as a denaturant, hair-conditioning agent, and skin-conditioning ingredient in cosmetic formulations.[3]

TABLE 78-1
Pros and Cons of Salicylic Acid

Pros	Cons
Anti-inflammatory	May cause stinging
Inexpensive	May thin the stratum corneum, leading to increased risk of photodamage
Covered for acne use by FDA monograph	
Long history of traditional anti-inflammatory and antipyretic use	

HISTORY

In antiquity, the willow bark (*Salix alba*) was considered a medicine by the Greek physicians Hippocrates and Dioscorides as well as the Roman naturalist, philosopher, and author Pliny the Elder.[4] Derivatives of the willow species *S. alba* were traditionally used as an analgesic for head and other aches, rheumatism, and gout; it was also used to treat fever.[5–7] Indigenous peoples in North America are believed to have used willow species for medical purposes for 2,000 years, with the Houma employing black willow root as a blood thinner and the Creek using willow root tea as an anti-inflammatory and antipyretic.[8]

The modern history of SA is traced back to 1763 when England's Reverend Edward Stone found that willow bark extract was effective in treating malarial fever.[4,5,9] In Italy in 1824, Bartolomeo Rigatelli therapeutically used an extract of willow bark and Francesco Fontana characterized the compound, labeling it "salicina" (based on the Latin expression for white willow, *Salix alba*).[9] However, the German chemist Johann Andreas Buchner was given credit for naming the active ingredient of white willow bark after he isolated salicin in 1826.[10] French pharmacist Henri Leroux isolated a larger amount in 1828 or 1829.[4,10] In 1838, Raffaele Piria, an Italian chemist working in Paris, became the first to synthesize SA from salicin,[1,4,9,10] as well as name the product "salicylic acid,"[11] and Hermann Kolbe is credited with using sodium phenate and carbon dioxide to generate SA.[4] These mid-1800s developments and the discovery that salicylates were the active constituents of willow species paved the way for the development of acetylsalicylic acid (aspirin), first prepared from carbolic acid in 1853 by Charles Gerhardt, who was unable to identify its structure.[4,8,12] With its structure discovered, aspirin was first synthesized, from willow bark, in 1897 by Arthur Eichengrün, Felix Hoffmann, and Heinrich Dreser working at Friedrich Bayer Company, which recorded acetylsalicylic acid under the name "Aspirin" in 1899.[4–6,13] This acetylated salicylic acid became the world's first truly blockbuster drug.

The use of SA in the treatment of acne began appearing in the medical literature in the 1960s and has since become a mainstay of topical acne therapy, particularly in over-the-counter (OTC) products.

Many companies, in the attempt to capitalize upon the popularity of α-hydroxy acids (AHAs) such as glycolic acid, have marketed SA as a "β-hydroxy acid" (BHA). However, because SA is an aromatic compound, it is actually incorrect to refer to it as a β-hydroxy acid. Nevertheless, "β-hydroxy acid" or "BHA" is a popular component in many OTC cosmetic products.

CHEMISTRY

SA is the best known simple phenol, with well-established antipyretic and anti-inflammatory activity.[14] It is the only member of the BHA family, so named because the aromatic carboxylic acid has a hydroxy group in the β position (Figure 78-1).

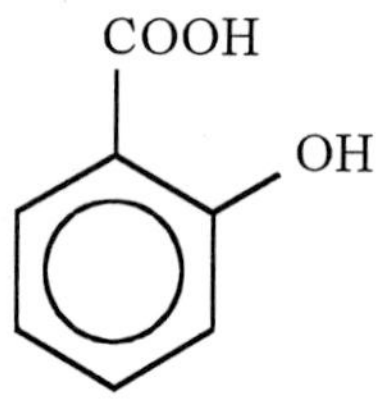

▲ **FIGURE 78-1** Chemical structure of salicylic acid.

This is actually a misnomer because the carbons of aromatic compounds are traditionally given Arabic numerals (1, 2, etc.) rather than the Greek letter designations typical for nonaromatic structures. As a member of the salicylate family, like aspirin, SA contains anti-inflammatory capabilities due to its effects on the arachidonic acid cascade.[15]

Product labels will state the percentage of SA in a formula; however, the most important aspect is the amount of available free acid in the formulation. The amount of free acid itself is affected by the following: concentration of the SA (percent SA), the pKa of the acid preparation, the pH of the solution (which is also affected by the type of vehicle used), and whether or not the formula is buffered. Because of this complex interplay of factors, it is difficult to compare one brand of SA to another. For example, a 20 percent SA peel from one company is not necessarily the same strength as a 20 percent SA peel from another company. The acid percentage is only a small part of the story. It is necessary to consider the pH, the amount of free acid, the additive ingredients, and whether or not the peel is buffered in order to make a truly useful comparison between different SA brands.

Significance of the pKa

In order to use SA properly, one must understand the pKa as well as how the pH of a formula impacts its efficacy. The pKa of a compound measures its capacity to donate protons. The pKa is the pH at which the level of free acid equals the level of the salt form of the acid. When the pH is lower than the pKa, the free acid form, which is responsible for exfoliation of the skin, predominates; when the pH is higher than the pKa, the salt form predominates. The acid form is the "active form" in the preparation because it spurs exfoliation. To create an efficacious peel that provokes minimal irritation, having the proper balance of salt and acid forms is necessary. The pKa for SA is 2.97, whereas it is 3.83 for AHAs.[16] Because of this significant disparity in pKa, it is difficult to formulate a combination product containing both a BHA and an AHA that reaches an optimal pH. For example, in a combination AHA-BHA product with a pH of 3.5, the AHA acid form but BHA salt form would predominate. Consequently, the effects of BHA would be undermined or rendered suboptimal. For this reason, products containing SA alone are preferable to products that contain both AHA and SA.[17]

Significance of the pH

The higher the pH, the more alkaline or basic the solution is; the lower the pH, the more acidic the solution. The irritation engendered by a product is often directly related to how low its pH is, with a lower pH causing increased irritation, but greater efficacy.

Buffered Solutions

Some SA formulations are "buffered," which numerous companies claim enhances the tolerability of these agents. A solution is buffered by the addition of a base compound such as sodium bicarbonate or sodium hydroxide. This yields an increased amount of the salt form, less free acid, and a higher pH. In addition, buffered solutions are resistant to fluctuations in pH upon the addition of a salt or an acid to the preparation. Fewer side effects are associated with buffered solutions because of the lower pH and reduced amount of free acid, but a decrease in efficacy may also be seen. These formulations are safer, but less effective.

Forms of Salicylic Acid

SA is found in various forms in cosmetic preparations. The salt forms of SA used as preservatives include magnesium salicylate, MEA-salicylate (SA compounded with 2-aminoethanol), sodium salicylate, and calcium salicylate. The TEA salt of SA is used as an ultraviolet (UV) light absorber.[3] Ethylhexyl salicylate (formerly known as octyl salicylate) is used as a fragrance ingredient, sunscreen agent, and UV light absorber and methyl salicylate is used as a denaturant and flavoring agent.

ORAL USES

SA is not used orally because it induces gastrointestinal irritation. The uses of aspirin and other oral forms of salicylates are beyond the scope of this chapter.

TOPICAL USES

The penetration of SA into the skin is regulated by the barrier function of the skin. One study demonstrated that impairing the skin barrier with acetone, tape stripping, or detergent (sodium lauryl sulfate) led to increased penetration of SA. The penetration of SA significantly correlated with the measurements of barrier perturbation by transepidermal water loss ($P = 0.01$) and erythema ($P = 0.02$) for each individual.[18] As a keratolytic agent, SA is used in concentrations of 3 to 6 percent to treat ichthyoses, keratosis pilaris, palmoplantar keratosis, pityriasis rubra pilaris, and psoriasis.[19] It is also used for removal of warts and corns in concentrations of 5 to 40 percent.[19]

Acne

Comedolytics, such as SA and AHAs, are used to loosen the keratinocytes and "unclog" the pores. BHA is more effective in reducing the number of comedones than are AHAs.

SA is one of the most effective and frequently used therapies for acne. In fact, SA is well established as an effective treatment, along with benzoyl peroxide (BPO), and low-dose retinoids, for mild acne.[20] It is covered in the United States Food and Drug Administration (FDA) monograph for acne for 0.05 to 2 percent strengths in OTC products and is considered effective for acne in 3 percent concentration in prescription medications, as stipulated by the FDA.[21,22] At-home cleansers, blemish treatments and toners, gels, and moisturizers contain SA in addition to at-home chemical peels or in-office chemical peels.

Lee and Kim investigated the efficacy and safety of a 30 percent SA peel in 35 Korean patients with facial acne. They found that inflammatory as well as noninflammatory lesion counts declined proportionately with increased treatment time. The investigators also reported that all patients were satisfied with the results and side effects were generally tolerable. They concluded that SA peels are an effective and safe therapy for Asian patients with facial acne.[23]

In 2008, Kessler et al. conducted a split-face, double-blind, randomized, controlled study with 20 patients with mild-to-moderately severe facial acne to compare the efficacy of AHAs and BHA. The AHA glycolic acid (30 percent) was applied to one side and 30 percent SA was applied on the other side every two weeks for six treatments overall. Both peels were significantly and equally effective after two treatments, with sustained effectiveness and fewer side effects associated with SA.[24]

A 2010 meta-analysis compared studies of BPO, clindamycin, BPO and SA, and BPO/clindamycin and found that the combination of BPO and SA was most effective in acne treatment.[25] SA plays a role in acne because of its keratolytic effects, ability to decrease the number of comedones, and its anti-inflammatory characteristics.

In 2011, Babayeva et al. conducted a 12-week, prospective, single-blind, randomized, comparative clinical study comparing the efficacy and tolerability of a 3 percent alcohol-based SA preparation combined with clindamycin and tretinoin 0.05 percent cream combined with clindamycin in 46 patients (between 18 and 35 years old) with mild-to-moderate facial acne. Ultimately, both regimens were found to be equally efficacious in lowering total lesion, inflammatory, and non-inflammatory lesion counts. Lesion counts did decline faster in the tretinoin group. Neither formulation was found to influence stratum corneum (SC) hydration, but skin sebum values did fall in the SA group.[26] Previously, NilFroushzadeh et al. had shown in a single-blinded, randomized clinical trial with 42 female patients (between the ages of 15 and 25 years) that a 1 percent clindamycin and 2 percent SA lotion used twice daily for 12 weeks was significantly more efficacious than 1 percent clindamycin alone in terms of total lesion count and Acne Severity Index score. No significant differences were seen, though, between the clindamyc/ SA group and a group treated once nightly with 1 percent clindamycin and 0.025 percent tretinoin lotion.[27]

In an open, baseline-controlled clinical study with 20 patients (18 females and 2 males between the ages of 19 and 32 years) with mild-to-moderate facial acne conducted in 2013, Zheng et al. assessed the safety and efficacy of an antioxidant optimized topical SA 1.5 percent cream containing natural skin penetration enhancers. Patients were instructed to apply the formulation twice daily for four weeks. No side effects were noted and 95 percent of the subjects improved (complete clearing in 20 percent, significant improvement in 30 percent, moderate improvement in 15 percent, mild improvement in 30 percent).[22]

Also that year, Raone et al. conducted a prospective, observational, multicenter, open-label, postmarketing Phase IV study to assess the efficacy and tolerability of a 30 percent SA, triethyl citrate, and ethyl linoleate peel combined with a home therapy with three topical agents (triethyl citrate, ethyl linoleate, and SA 0.5 percent cream) for the treatment of moderate facial acne. The average Global Acne Grading System score fell 49 percent for the 53 patients as the investigators concluded that the therapy was effective and universally well tolerated.[28] The authors noted that SA peels also enhance the penetration of other topical ingredients used to treat acne.[28]

Although SA has been used steadily for several years to treat acne, the number of well designed, controlled clinical trials to test its safety and efficacy is relatively small.

Anti-inflammatory Uses

Unlike AHAs, BHA affects the arachidonic acid cascade and, therefore, exhibits anti-inflammatory capabilities. In addition, salicylates inhibit nuclear factor-κB and suppress cytokine gene expression in activated monocytes and macrophages.[29] These properties may allow SA peels to be effective while inducing less irritation than AHA peels. The lower incidence of perceived irritation of SA compared to AHA was confirmed in a 1997 double-blind consumer-perception study of neurosensory discomfort after three weeks of use. In this study, 20 percent of the patients treated with an in-office AHA peel reported subjective adverse reactions versus only 4 to 7 percent of the SA group.[30] The anti-inflammatory effects of SA may also make it a useful adjuvant in the treatment of rosacea.[17]

Antimicrobial

SA in 5 percent concentrations has shown activity against Gram-positive and Gram-negative bacteria, yeast, and fungi. The pH must be within a range of 2 to 5 to exert this activity.

Pore Minimizing

Comedolytics, such as BHA and AHAs, are used to loosen the keratinocytes and "unclog" the pores. BHA is more effective in reducing the number of comedones than are AHAs. A study by Kligman demonstrated that biopsy specimens from patients treated with SA displayed fewer comedones when compared to those treated with AHAs. This is due to the fact that AHAs are not lipid soluble.[30] The lipophilicity of SA enables it to penetrate the sebaceous material in the hair follicle and exfoliate the pores.[31,32] However, AHAs, which are water soluble, do not have this comedolytic property.[33]

Photoaging

AHAs and BHA are naturally-occurring organic acids used in at-home as well as in-office products to assist in exfoliation and accelerating the cell cycle. They impact corneocyte cohesiveness in the lower levels of the SC,[34] where they alter its pH, thus affecting the skin.[35] The topical application of AHAs and BHA in high concentrations causes the detachment of keratinocytes and epidermolysis; application at lower concentrations diminishes intercorneocyte cohesion directly above the granular layer, promoting desquamation and SC thinning.[35] The two main effects, then, are accelerating the cell cycle, which slows with age, and augmenting desquamation, which helps reduce hyperpigmentation and smoothes the skin surface.

Although glycolic acid is the most commonly used acid in the antiaging armamentarium, SA is frequently found in products used to treat photoaged skin. SA functions as an exfoliant and accelerates the cell cycle (thus cell renewal) in the same way that AHAs have been shown to do. A study examining the antiaging benefits of topically applied SA up to concentrations of 30 percent showed fading of pigment spots, decreased surface roughness, reduction of fine lines, and improvement of seborrheic keratosis.[17,36,37] In 1992, Swinehart found that using a buffered 50 percent SA ointment peel, after pretreatment with topical tretinoin and localized 20 percent trichloroacetic acid, on the hands and forearms of patients exhibiting actinically-induced pigmentary changes was very effective in eliminating lentigines, pigmented keratoses, and actinic damage.[37]

■ SAFETY ISSUES

In February 2000, the Cosmetic Ingredients Review (CIR) Expert Panel published an opinion that the use of SA-related substances in cosmetics is "safe as used when formulated to avoid irritation and when formulated to avoid increased sun sensitivity."[3] It is advised that all patients treated with SA-containing products should use a broad-spectrum sunscreen as part of their daily skin care regimen.

Salicylates are absorbed percutaneously. Around 10 percent of applied salicylates can remain in the skin.[3] Little acute toxicity (LD$_{50}$ in rats >2 g/kg) via a dermal exposure route is seen for SA, methyl salicylate, tridecyl salicylate, and butyloctyl salicylate.

SA is neither phototoxic nor a photosensitizer.[3] In fact, SA and ethylhexyl salicylate act as low-level photoprotective agents.[3] Because these ingredients are often used as exfoliating agents, concern has emerged that repeated use may effectively increase exposure of the dermis and epidermis to UV radiation by reducing SC thickness. Daily use of sun protection is emphasized for this reason.

Although SA is relatively safe, its use is associated with risks. The most common risk is burning of the skin, which can occur if the skin is prepared too vigorously, if the patient's SC is thin from exfoliation or concomitant retinoid use, or if the skin barrier is impaired as seen with the use of foaming cleansers and soap. Toxic levels of salicylates have not been reported in association with the concentrations currently used for SA peels.[38] However, there have been case reports of children with multiple excoriations and elderly patients with ichthyosis who developed salicylism after being treated with topical products containing SA.[39] The CIR panel found that an oral dose of baby aspirin (81 mg) by a 58 kg female would result in a salicylate exposure of 1.4 mg/kg/day, which would not be expected to pose any reproductive risk.[3] They concluded that the risk of using a cosmetic product with SA could result in an exposure of 0.4 to 0.5 mg/kg/day of SA, which is significantly less than with a baby aspirin. To minimize the risk of toxicity, patients that are taking aspirin should be cautioned to avoid using topical SA products.

Because of the risk of salicylism, it is unwise to peel large surface areas of the body in the same office visit. The signs of salicylism include nausea, disorientation, and tinnitus. SA use, if it is improper or too frequent or in high concentrations, can cause redness, itching, peeling, increased skin sensitivity, and blisters. There are no reported cases of salicylism from SA acne products.[19] SA is contraindicated in patients who are pregnant, breast-feeding, or allergic to aspirin. Nevertheless, safety data are lacking for pregnant patients, and SA is considered among the safe and effective topical treatments for mild-to-moderate acne in this population.[40] While animal data do support the practice of pregnant women avoiding the use of many topical agents, including SA,[19] the systemic absorption of SA through the skin is sufficiently minimal to warrant confidence that topical SA would pose no risk to the developing fetus.[40,41] SA peels should not be used during pregnancy, however.

ENVIRONMENTAL IMPACT

SA has been synthesized in the laboratory for the last century. While numerous plants contain this organic acid, few if any are targeted specifically for SA on a large-scale, industrial basis; therefore, the likely environmental impact is minimal.

FORMULATION CONSIDERATIONS

SA-containing formulations are available in OTC at-home products that have lower concentrations of acids (usually 0.5–2 percent),[21] and medical strength to be used in the dermatologist's office (usually 20–35 percent). The CIR panel report did not establish a limit on concentration of SA or identify the minimum pH of formulations containing SA.[3] SA seems to absorb well in skin. The absorption of 5 percent SA in human skin was measured and it was found that vehicles containing an aqueous base allowed more penetration of SA into human skin as compared to a Vaseline base.[3] The effects of pH on penetration were measured and a pH of 2 was found to be associated with the highest level of penetration. Studies suggest that the SC is the largest barrier of penetration to SA. Application of large amounts of SA to the body of psoriatic patients does result in increased serum levels of SA and urinary excretion of SA. The amount of SA absorbed depends on the pH, the vehicle, and the condition of the skin's permeability barrier (i.e., SC).[3] Ethanol-containing vehicles were linked to the highest penetration followed by aqueous vehicles while lipophilic vehicles displayed the least penetration.

USAGE CONSIDERATIONS

SA is popular as an in-office chemical peeling method because of its efficacy and ease of use. It is unique among peeling agents insofar as it forms a white precipitate once the peel is complete. Any area that has been inadequately peeled can be easily identified and treated by applying the SA solution in the areas that were missed. In addition, timing and neutralizing the peel is unnecessary. Once the vehicle becomes volatile, which occurs in approximately two minutes, there is very little penetration of the active agent; this makes timing and neutralizing the peel unnecessary. Therefore, SA is much easier to use on areas that are difficult to easily rinse such as the back and the arms.

SA peels may exert a whitening effect in patients with darker skin types. In a 2006 study by Ahn and Kim of 24 Asian women with acne who were treated with biweekly facial peeling with 30 percent SA in absolute ethanol for three months, subjects exhibited some skin lightening.[31] However, such peels can also result in postinflammatory hyperpigmentation. Practitioners should explain to patients with darker skin types the risks of skin lightening or darkening from using SA peels. The key is to use a peel that is strong enough to exert the desired effect but not strong enough to induce inflammation. If in doubt, start with a lower-strength peel and titrate to stronger peels in later treatments.

SA reportedly enhances percutaneous penetration of vitamin A and triamcinolone acetonide but not hydrocortisone, methyl nicotinate, or cyclosporine.[3] Studies have shown that it does not increase sensitivity to other agents and in fact may reduce the erythema seen with sensitizing agents.[3]

SIGNIFICANT BACKGROUND

In a literature review including Ovid, MEDLINE, EMBASE, and Cochrane Database Library searches, Gamble et al. found multiple controlled trials showing BPO, topical antibiotics, and topical retinoids used in combination as the therapies offering optimal efficacy and safety for mild-to-moderate acne, but acknowledged SA as one of several alternatives not extensively studied that have proven efficacious and safe when combined with traditional treatment options.[42] SA is often the treatment of choice for patients that find a topical retinoid too irritating.[43]

There is no one therapeutic option that addresses each of the etiologic factors in acne vulgaris. Only SA, BPO, and steroids treat lesions already visible on the skin.

CONCLUSION

Salicylic acid is a versatile component in the antiacne armamentarium. Importantly, it is safe and reduces inflammation. It is also inexpensive. Because it has a low pH, salicylic acid may provoke stinging, particularly in individuals with S_3 sensitive skin. More research is necessary to ascertain the role of salicylic acid in other inflammatory skin diseases, but its use as a topical therapy, particularly in combination, for mild-to-moderate acne is well researched and substantiated.

REFERENCES

1. Mahdi JG, Mahdi AJ, Mahdi AJ, et al. The historical analysis of aspirin discovery, its relation to the willow tree and antiproliferative and anticancer potential. *Cell Prolif.* 2006;39:147.
2. Duthie GG, Wood AD. Natural saliyclates: Foods, functions and disease prevention. *Food Funct.* 2011;2:515.
3. Cosmetic Ingredient Review Expert Panel. Safety assessment of Salicylic Acid, Butyloctyl Salicylate, Calcium Salicylate, C12-15 Alkyl Salicylate, Capryloyl Salicylic Acid, Hexyldodecyl Salicylate, Isocetyl Salicylate, Isodecyl Salicylate, Magnesium Salicylate, MEA-Salicylate, Ethylhexyl Salicylate, Potassium Salicylate, Methyl Salicylate, Myristyl Salicylate, Sodium Salicylate, TEA-Salicylate, and Tridecyl Salicylate. *Int J Toxicol.* 2003;22(Suppl 3):1.
4. Lafont O. From the willow to aspirin. *Rev Hist Pharm (Paris).* 2007;55:209.
5. Pasero G, Marson P. A short history of anti-rheumatic therapy. II. Aspirin. *Reumatismo.* 2010;62:148.
6. Rishton GM. Natural products as a robust source of new drugs and drug leads: Past successes and present day issues. *Am J Cardiol.* 2008;101:43D.
7. Hoffmann D. *Medical Herbalism: The Science and Practice of Herbal Medicine.* Rochester, VT: Healing Arts Press; 2003:579.
8. Foster S. *101 Medicinal Herbs: An Illustrated Guide.* Loveland, CO: Interweave Press; 1998:210–211.
9. Marson P, Pasero G. The Italian contributions to the history of salicylates. *Reumatismo.* 2006;58:66.
10. Jeffreys D. *Aspirin: The remarkable story of a wonder drug.* New York: Bloomsbury; 2005:38–40.
11. Fuster V, Sweeny JM. Aspirin: A historical and contemporary therapeutic overview. *Circulation.* 2011;123:768.
12. Rainsford KD. Anti-inflammatory drugs in the 21st century. *Subcell Biochem.* 2007;42:3.
13. Schmidt B, Ribnicky DM, Poulev A, et al. A natural history of botanical therapeutics. *Metabolism.* 2008;57:S3.
14. Mills S, Bone K. *Principles and Practice of Phytotherapy: Modern Herbal Medicine.* London: Churchill Livingstone; 2000:23–25, 61.
15. Weirich EG, Longauer JK, Kirkwood AH. Dermatopharmacology of salicylic acid. III. Topical contra-inflammatory effect of salicylic acid and other drugs in animal experiments. *Dermatologica.* 1976;152:87.
16. Clark CP 3rd. Alpha hydroxyl acids in skin care. *Clin Plast Surg.* 1996;23:49.
17. Baumann L, Saghari S. Chemical peels. In: Baumann L, Saghari S, Weisberg E, eds. *Cosmetic Dermatology: Principles and Practice.* 2nd ed. New York: McGraw-Hill; 2009:148–162.
18. Benfeldt E, Serup J, Menné T. Effect of barrier perturbation on cutaneous salicylic acid penetration in human skin: In vivo pharmacokinetics using microdialysis and non-invasive quantification of barrier function. *Br J Dermatol.* 1999;140:739.
19. Akhavan A, Bershad S. Topical acne drugs: Review of clinical properties, systemic exposure, and safety. *Am J Clin Dermatol.* 2003;4:473.
20. Whitney KM, Ditre CM. Management strategies for acne vulgaris. *Clin Cosmet Investig Dermatol.* 2011;4:41.
21. Kaminsky A. Less common methods to treat acne. *Dermatology.* 2003;206:68.
22. Zheng Y, Wang M, Chen H, et al. Clinical evidence on the efficacy and safety of an antioxidant optimized 1.5% salicylic acid (SA) cream in the treatment of facial acne: An open, baseline-controlled clinical study. *Skin Res Technol.* 2013;19:125.
23. Lee HS, Kim IH. Salicylic acid peels for the treatment of acne vulgaris in Asian patients. *Dermatol Surg.* 2003;29:1196.
24. Kessler E, Flanagan K, Chia C, et al. Comparison of alpha- and beta-hydroxy acid chemical peels in the treatment of mild to moderately severe facial acne vulgaris. *Dermatol Surg.* 2008;34:45.
25. Seidler EM, Kimball AB. Meta-analysis comparing efficacy of benzoyl peroxide, clindamycin, benzoyl peroxide with salicylic acid, and combination benzoyl peroxide/clindamycin in acne. *J Am Acad Dermatol.* 2010;63:52.
26. Babayeva L, Akarsu S, Fetil E, et al. Comparison of tretinoin 0.05% cream and 3% alcohol-based salicylic acid preparation in the treatment of acne vulgaris. *J Eur Acad Dermatol Venereol.* 2011;25:328.
27. NilFroushzadeh MA, Siadat AH, Baradaran EH, et al. Clindamycin lotion alone versus combination lotion of clindamycin phosphate plus tretinoin versus combination lotion of clindamycin phosphate plus salicylic acid in the topical treatment of mild to moderate acne vulgaris: A randomized control trial. *Indian J Dermatol Venereol Leprol.* 2009;75:279.
28. Raone B, Veraldi S, Raboni R, et al. Salicylic acid peel incorporating triethyl citrate and ethyl linoleate in the treatment of moderate acne: A new therapeutic approach. *Dermatol Surg.* 2013;39:1243.
29. Stevenson MA, Zhao MJ, Asea A, et al. Salicylic acid and aspirin inhibit the activity of RSK2 kinase and repress RSK2-dependent transcription of cyclic AMP response element binding protein- and NF-kappaB-responsive genes. *J Immunol.* 1999;163:5608.
30. Kligman AM. A comparative evaluation of a novel low-strength salicylic acid cream and glycolic acid products on human skin. *Cosmet Dermatol.* 1997;10:S11.
31. Ahn HH, Kim IH. Whitening effect of salicylic acid peels in Asian patients. *Dermatol Surg.* 2006;32:372.
32. Bowe WP, Shalita AR. Effective over-the-counter acne treatments. *Semin Cutan Med Surg.* 2008;27:170.
33. Davies M, Marks R. Studies on the effect of salicylic acid on normal skin. *Br J Dermatol.* 1976;95:187.
34. Van Scott EJ, Yu RJ. Hyperkeratinization, corneocyte cohesion, and alpha hydroxy acids. *J Am Acad Dermatol.* 1984;11:867.
35. Berardesca E, Distante F, Vignoli GP, et al. Alpha hydroxyacids modulate stratum corneum barrier function. *Br J Dermatol.* 1997;137:934.
36. Kligman D, Kligman AM. Salicylic acid peels for the treatment of photoaging. *Dermatol Surg.* 1998;24:325.
37. Swinehart JM. Salicylic acid ointment peeling of the hands and forearms. Effective nonsurgical removal of pigmented lesions and actinic damage. *J Dermatol Surg Oncol.* 1992;18:495.
38. Rubin MG. Salicylic acid peels. In: *Manual of Chemical Peels: Superficial and Medium Depth.* Philadelphia, PA: Lippincott Williams & Wilkins; 1995:19–20.
39. Brubacher JR, Hoffman RS. Salicylism from topical salicylates: Review of the literature. *J Toxicol Clin Toxicol.* 1996;34:431.
40. Pugashetti R, Shinkai K. Treatment of acne vulgaris in pregnant patients. *Dermatol Ther.* 2013;26:302.
41. Bozzo P, Chua-Gocheco A, Einarson A. Safety of skin care products during pregnancy. *Can Fam Physician.* 2011;57:665.
42. Gamble R, Dunn J, Dawson A, et al. Topical antimicrobial treatment of acne vulgaris: An evidence-based review. *Am J Clin Dermatol.* 2012;13:141.
43. Strauss JS, Krowchuk DP, Leyden JJ, et al. Guidelines of care for acne vulgaris management. *J Am Acad Dermatol.* 2007;56:651.

CHAPTER 79

Retinol, Retinyl Esters, and Retinoic Acid

Activities:

Anti-inflammatory

Important Chemical Components:

Retinol: A form of vitamin A also known as (2E,4E,6E,8E)-3,7-dimethyl-9-(2,6,6-trimethylcyclohex-1-enyl)nona-2,4,6,8-tetraen-1-ol. Its molecular formula is $C_{20}H_{30}O$.

Retinoic acid: A metabolite of vitamin A also known as all-*trans* retinoic acid and (2E,4E,6E,8E)-3,7-dimethyl-9-(2,6,6-trimethylcyclohexen-1-yl)nona-2,4,6,8-tetraenoic acid. Its molecular formula is $C_{20}H_{28}O_2$.

Retinyl palmitate: Also known as retinol palmitate, vitamin A palmitate and [(2E,4E,6E,8E)-3,7-Dimethyl-9-(2,6,6-trimethyl-1-cyclohexenyl)nona-2,4,6,8-tetraenyl] hexadecanoate. Its molecular formula is $C_{36}H_{60}O_2$.

Origin Classification:

Retinol occurs in nature as vitamin A, but the retinol found in personal care products is laboratory made.

Personal Care Category:

Antiacne, photoprotection

BST Treatable with this Ingredient:

DRPW, DRNW, DSNT, DSPT, DSNW, DSPW, ORNW, ORPW, OSNT, OSNW, OSPT, and OSPW. These are the preferred ingredients for subtype S_1 sensitive skin (acne).

SOURCE

All of the natural and synthetic derivatives of vitamin A are included in a family of compounds known as the retinoids. Many prescription retinoids, including tretinoin, adapalene, and tazarotene, have been approved by the United States Food and Drug Administration (FDA) for use in treating acne. While retinol is not FDA approved for use in acne and is not included in the FDA monograph ingredients that can be used for the disorder it certainly exerts antiacne effects. Although vitamin A is naturally occurring and is found in foods that contain carotenoids such as carrots, the retinols used in over-the-counter (OTC) skin care products are laboratory made. Putting carrots, carrot extract, or β-carotene on the skin would not be sufficient because of the lack of skin penetration of the ingredients. For this reason, effective skin care products use retinoic acid (tretinoin), retinol, adapalene, or tazarotene as the form of retinoid. Some skin care products use retinyl esters such as retinyl palmitate (RP), but the efficacy is questionable because penetration rates are minimal. Carotenoids, a large family of secondary metabolic products that provide pigment to the many fruits and vegetables in which they are found, are precursors to vitamin A. Although some carotenoids (such as β-carotene, lycopene, lutein, astaxanthin, and zeaxanthin)

are known to confer antioxidant activity and photoprotective effects,[1,2] a discussion of these compounds is beyond the scope of this text.

HISTORY

In 1937, the Nobel Prize was awarded to Karrer et al. for determining the structure of retinol.[3] Retinol was successfully synthesized in 1943 and soon thereafter became commercially available. Since that time, the number of retinoid formulations has proliferated, now numbering over 2,500 products including prescription and nonprescription preparations. Prescription topical retinoids, including tretinoin (Retin A), tazarotene (Tazorac), and adapalene (Differin), have been widely used for decades to treat moderate acne based on their efficacy in reducing comedogenesis,[4,5] and normalizing keratinization.[6-9] The two most common retinoids found in OTC products are retinol and RP. Due to their "cosmetic" status under FDA regulations, retinol and RP are commonly listed as "inactive" ingredients in OTC skin care products. Although early reviews of retinol deemed the ingredient ineffective, it was later determined that this was due to the molecule's photoinstability (Table 79-1). With light exposure, retinol degrades to a biologically inactive molecule. This breakdown can be avoided with the addition of an antioxidant or incorporation into a vehicle that resists oxidation. Retinol is now known to induce the same effects on the retinoic acid receptor as tretinoin and prescription retinoids.

CHEMISTRY

Vitamin A is found in several forms that convert to each other through the actions of various enzymes (see Figure 79-1).

Retinoids

Initially, a "retinoid" was defined as a compound the structure and action of which resembled the parent compound retinol. Through the last several decades, chemists have made extensive modifications to the naturally-occurring molecule that have resulted in the development of many forms of retinoids. The vitamin A or "retinoid" family now includes retinyl esters, retinol, tretinoin (retinoic acid), adapalene, tazarotene, and oral isotretinoin (Accutane) in addition to four carotenoids including β-carotene.

TABLE 79-1
Pros and Cons of Retinol

Pros	Cons
Many brand options	Can cause redness and flaking
Strong scientific justification for use	Stability affected by other ingredients
Has effects on wrinkles as well as acne	Unstable when exposed to light
	Insufficient number of studies on retinol
	Retinyl esters are not well absorbed

Retinyl ester ← → Retinol ← → Retinal → Retinoic acid

▲ **FIGURE 79-1** Conversion flow of retinoids.

The retinoids exhibit many important biologic activities, which include regulating growth and differentiation in epithelial cells, inhibiting tumor promotion during experimental carcinogenesis, diminishing malignant cell growth, reducing inflammation, and bolstering the immune system.[10] At the molecular level, retinoids confer such effects by regulating gene transcription and influencing cellular differentiation and proliferation. Retinoids can act directly, by inducing transcription from genes with promoter regions that contain retinoid response elements, or indirectly, by blocking the transcription of particular genes.[11]

RETINOID RECEPTORS Retinoid-binding proteins were discovered in the 1970s.[12] In 1987, the identification of retinoic acid receptors paved the way to understanding that tretinoin functions as a hormone.[13,14] Much research has since been conducted to ascertain the mechanisms of these binding proteins and receptors. The biologic effects of retinoic acid are now known to be mediated by various biological systems: binding proteins such as cellular retinoic acid-binding proteins I and II (CRABP I and II); cellular retinol-binding protein (CRBP)[15]; and nuclear receptors divided into two categories, retinoic acid receptors (RARs) and retinoid X receptors (RXRs).[16] All of these nuclear receptors belong to a large family called nuclear hormone superfamily receptors, of which the receptors for vitamin D, estradiol, glucocorticoids, and thyroid hormone are members.[17]

RARs heterodimerize specifically with RXRs in order to interact with their retinoic acid response elements (RAREs) and mediate classic retinoid activity and toxicity. RXRs are more promiscuous, heterodimerizing with multiple members of the steroid receptor superfamily, including peroxisome proliferator-activated receptors (PPARs), vitamin D receptors, thyroid hormone receptors, and several orphan receptors, such as liver X receptors (LXRs), pregnane X receptors (PXRs), and farnesoid X receptors (FXRs).[18] More research is needed to elucidate the interaction of retinoid agents with other hormones.

ORAL USES

Retinoids are used orally in the form of isotretinoin (Accutane). A discussion of oral compounds is beyond the scope of this text.

TOPICAL USES

Many studies have looked at the efficacy of retinoids in treating acne and have resulted in FDA approval of many tretinoin-, adapalene-, and tazarotene-containing acne medications. The discussions in this book are limited to the OTC ingredients retinol and RP and their use in acne. There are no published studies examining the efficacy of retinol and RP in acne; however, they are frequently used in dermatology practices for this indication. The discussion will concentrate on the reasons why it is believed that retinol may play a role in the treatment of acne, although its efficacy has not been proven. RP is not likely to have a role in acne therapy because of its limited absorption. However, new types of retinoids are being synthesized, which should lead to more options in the near future. RP is the main retinyl ester occurring in the diet, stored in the body, and incorporated in topical preparations.[19]

Retinoids by definition all bind an RAR, leading to a predictable response. The primary distinguishing characteristics among retinoid types are the amount of absorption of the molecule, on which enzymes act to convert it to retinoic acid, and the amount of irritation caused. In 1997, Duell et al. showed that unoccluded retinol is more effective at penetrating human skin *in vivo* than RP or retinoic acid.[20] In this study, retinol at 0.25 percent was found to induce the cellular and molecular changes observed with the application of 0.025 percent retinoic acid, without the irritation usually seen with retinoic acid. Conversely, RP is considered a storage form of vitamin A, accounting for approximately 70 percent of the total vitamin A present in human skin.[19,21] RP requires cutaneous cleavage of its ester bond in order to be transformed into retinol, which then requires conversion into retinoic acid in order to impart benefits when topically applied.

Mechanism in Acne

COMEDOLYTIC Retinoids help remove comedones (blackheads and whiteheads) through desquamation,[22] affecting cell adhesion, and regulating keratinization.[23] Using retinoids helps prevent and treat comedones. The comedolytic properties of retinoids are similar to those associated with benzoyl peroxide and salicylic acid.[24] Retinoids should be considered a first-line therapy for acne because the elimination of keratinocyte accretion in the hair follicle facilitates the penetration of antibiotics and other acne medications. Comedolytic properties are also important because improvement in comedones helps the patient see progress faster and increases compliance with acne therapy. Receding of the papules and pustules of acne can take 8 to 12 weeks, while comedones may start to subside within days of initial treatment.

EFFECTS ON TOLL-LIKE RECEPTOR 2 The transmembrane proteins known as Toll-like receptors (TLRs) are thought to play a key role in the pathogenesis of acne. TLR-2 is activated by ligands, such as bacterial components, and modulates the expression of various immune response genes involved in acne development.[25] Evidence suggests that *Propionibacterium acnes*, the bacteria implicated in acne etiology, can induce TLR-2 expression through secreted proinflammatory compounds. Retinoids downregulate TLR-2 expression, resulting in acne symptom improvement.[26] The mechanism of action of TLR-2 in acne development is not known but one study showed that TLR-2 activation yielded increases in interleukin (IL)-1α.[27]

EFFECTS ON INFLAMMATORY CYTOKINES In 2005, Kang et al. demonstrated that transcription factors nuclear factor-κB and activator protein-1 are activated in acne lesions, ultimately resulting in increased expression of inflammatory cytokines and matrix metalloproteinases (MMPs).[28,29] Others have since shown that several inflammatory cytokines are involved in acne. For example, IL-1α, induced by TLR-2, is known to influence comedone development.[30] In 2013, Agak et al. reported that IL-17 is induced by *P. acnes* but suppressed by retinoids.[31]

Proinflammatory cytokine production promoted by *P. acnes* has been shown to decline with the addition of retinoids to culture media.[26] MMPs have recently gained attention for playing a role in acne pathogenesis. Notably, investigators have observed significant increases in MMP-1, MMP-3, and MMP-9 in lesional skin in comparison to donor-matched normal skin.[28,32] The scarring associated with many cases of moderate-to-severe acne may be attributable, in part, to the overexpression of these MMPs. Retinoids may target this MMP expression as part of its therapeutic mechanism of action.

EFFECTS ON SEBUM PRODUCTION Patients with cystic acne, or those who are unresponsive to all other regimens, can be treated with oral retinoids such as isotretinoin. This oral medication has been shown to alter sebaceous gland function, and a marked decrease in sebum production occurs within two weeks of the start of therapy.[33] Topical retinoids have not yet been shown to affect sebaceous gland function. This is likely due to the fact that sebaceous glands are located at a level in the hair follicle beyond which topical retinoids have been demonstrated to penetrate.

SAFETY ISSUES

In 2010, a controversial report by the Environmental Working Group (EWG) warned of possible photocarcinogenicity associated with RP-containing sunscreens. This warning was based in part on a 2006 report by Xia et al. that demonstrated that ultraviolet (UV) A and UVB exposure led to the formation of photodecomposition products, synthesis of reactive oxygen species (ROS), and lipid peroxidation induction.[34] Reacting to the EWG report, Wang et al. acknowledged that of the eight *in vitro* studies published by the FDA from 2002 to 2009, four revealed that RP generated ROS after UVA exposure.[34–39] However, Wang contended that the National Toxicology Program (NTP) study on which the EWG based its report failed to prove that the combination of RP and UV results in photocarcinogenesis and, in fact, was rife with reasons for skepticism.[35,36] The EWG offered its own counter arguments and stood by its report. This heated debate was covered by the *Journal of the American Academy of Dermatology*.[35] It is important to note that the RP studies did not consider RP products that contain sun protection factor (SPF) protection; therefore, it is not known if these effects could be mitigated by concomitant use of SPF.

ENVIRONMENTAL IMPACT

There is no environmental impact of commercial topical retinoid formulation manufacture known by the author.

FORMULATION CONSIDERATIONS

Retinol-containing products must be manufactured and packaged in special low-light conditions to ensure stability, as retinol is degraded immediately upon exposure to light. Other ingredients such as benzoyl peroxide can affect the stability of retinoids, especially upon exposure to light.[40] Some products include selected antioxidants added to maintain stability. Most OTC products contain 0.04 to 0.1 percent retinol.

USAGE CONSIDERATIONS

Skin irritation, desquamation, and redness are the most frequent side effects associated with topical retinoid use. Dry skin, likely due to an increase in transepidermal water loss (TEWL) characteristic of topical retinoid use, is also a common complaint of patients treated with retinoids. The

increase in TEWL is believed to be linked to a perturbation of the stratum corneum (SC) water barrier function.[41,42] Although retinoids augment cell proliferation, this yields a short-term decline in ceramide biosynthesis. This reduction in the production of ceramides, a key constituent of the water barrier of the SC, may partly account for the xerosis observed with retinoid use.[43]

Typically within four days of starting retinoid therapy, the side effects commonly associated with these agents become apparent. These side effects can usually be alleviated by directing the patient to apply small amounts of the retinoid at less frequent intervals. Applying the retinoid along with a barrier repair moisturizer (see Chapter 19, Barrier Repair Ingredients), or on top of a moisturizer or oil-containing product reduces retinoid absorption and eases side effects. At the beginning of retinoid therapy, it is advisable to suggest that a patient use the product once and wait four days to gauge any skin irritation. If excessive redness, flaking, or stinging occurs, then the retinol product should be used every three to four days for the first two weeks. The patient can then begin to apply the retinoid every other night for two weeks. After tolerating the retinoid for two weeks every other night, the patient can switch to nightly use. The lowest available dose should be started initially. Once the patient is nightly applying the retinol on a consistent basis, the strength of the agent used can be increased. The irritation seen with retinoids at the beginning of therapy is the reason for poor patient compliance with this ingredient. Consequently, patients should be given clear instructions on how to begin product usage. It is important to remember that the entire skin care regimen and order of products applied greatly affects the tolerability and efficacy of retinoids.

Retinoids possess neither phototoxic nor photosensitizing activity; therefore, they can be used even by people getting sun exposure. Retinoids should not be used by women who are pregnant or breastfeeding.

SIGNIFICANT BACKGROUND

An increasing compilation of clinical data suggests that the topical application of retinoids can mitigate and even somewhat reverse mild-to-moderate symptoms of photoaging.[44–47] [Please see Chapter 83, Retinoids (Retinol), for a discussion of such effects delivered by topical retinoids.] This is an important area of continuing clinical study of these agents. Oral retinoids are already being used to treat photodamage.

Types of OTC Retinoids

RETINOL Retinol is a fat-soluble diterpenoid that belongs to the vitamin A or "retinoid" family of molecules (Figure 79-2). Retinol is synthesized from the breakdown of β-carotene. It is a prodrug that can be converted to all-*trans* retinoic acid in the skin. This change to retinoic acid within the keratinocytes is essential for retinol to be active.[48] Although it is a precursor to retinoic acid, retinol is classified as a cosmetic rather than a drug; therefore, it is used in numerous OTC formulations.[49] Further, because cosmetic companies cannot claim that their retinol products exert a biologic action, retinol is listed on many cosmetic products as an "inactive ingredient." There is no FDA monograph for retinol supporting claims that it ameliorates acne or photodamaged skin. This regulatory loophole has only enhanced the views of some, based on the instability and fleeting shelf life of early forms of retinol, that retinol

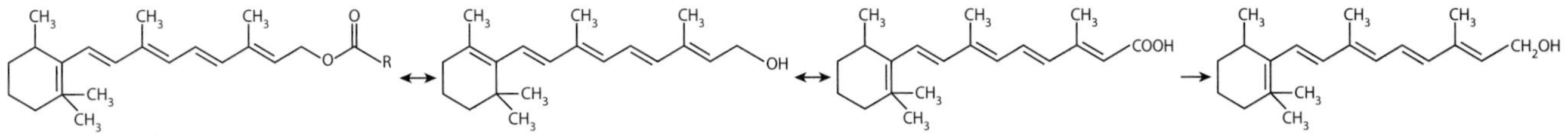

▲ **FIGURE 79-2** Chemical formulas for retinol and other retinoids.

exhibits minimal, if any, biologic activity. Notably, though, retinol-containing products may have only minute amounts of retinol, may be manufactured and packaged incorrectly, or may be formulated with ingredients that undermine stability. As a result, not all retinol-containing products are efficacious. Nevertheless, retinol has been shown to display significant biologic action and efficacy at the proper doses. Retinol must be distinguished from retinoid esters such as RP and retinyl linoleate. Many companies claim that their product contains "retinol" when, in fact, the product contains these esters, which are less effective than, and do not penetrate into the skin as well as, retinol.

RETINOL ESTERS RP is a storage form of retinol and the main form of vitamin A found naturally in the skin (Figure 79-2).[21] It was also the subject of a controversial EWG report in the summer of 2010 that warned of possible photocarcinogenicity associated with RP-containing sunscreens (see the Safety Issues section above). In 2005, Yan et al. investigated the phototoxicity of RP, anhydroretinol (AR), and 5,6-epoxyretinyl palmitate (5,6-epoxy-RP) in human skin Jurkat T-cells with and without light irradiation. Little damage occurred from irradiation of cells in the absence of a retinoid, but the presence of RP, 5,6-epoxy-RP or AR (50, 100, 150, and 200 μM) led to DNA fragmentation, with apoptosis occurring at retinoid concentrations of at least 100 μM. The researchers concluded that DNA damage and cytotoxicity are engendered by RP and its photodecomposition products in conjunction with exposure to UVA and visible light. In addition, they found that UVA irradiation of these retinoid products yielded free radicals that promote DNA strand cleavage.[21]

Based on the observation that exogenous RP builds up from topically applied cosmetic and skin care formulations, Yan et al., in 2006, studied the time course for the accumulation and disappearance of RP and retinol in the stratified layers of female SKH-1 mice skin singly or repeatedly dosed with topical creams containing 0.5 or 2 percent RP. The investigators noted that within 24 hours of application, RP quickly diffused into the SC and epidermal skin layers. RP and retinol levels were highest in the epidermis, lowest in the dermis, highest in the epidermis, lowest in the dermis, and intermediate in the SC. In separated skin layers and intact skin, RP and retinol levels decreased over time, but RP levels were higher than controls for 18 days. The researchers concluded that topically applied RP altered the normal physiological levels of RP and retinol in mouse skin.[50]

CONCLUSION

Prescription retinoids have convincingly been shown to be effective for acne treatment. Although retinol has not been studied in acne, it is reasonable to assume that it will exhibit similar effects because it is converted to retinoic acid in the skin. Retinol is unstable, so not all formulations are efficacious. It is impossible to ascertain by reading the label which products

are manufactured and packaged properly; therefore, using reputable brands is the best approach. Retinol products are most efficacious when used at night, when degradation by light is minimal. With respect to the controversy swirling around RP, the author advises patients to avoid daytime use of products with RP unless they use a concomitant SPF. The order of ingredients placed on the skin is important when retinoids are used because other ingredients can affect the absorption and stability of retinoids.

REFERENCES

1. Eichler O, Sies H, Stahl W. Divergent optimum levels of lycopene, beta-carotene and lutein protecting against UVB irradiatioin in human fibroblasts. *Photochem Photobiol.* 2002;75:503.
2. Dinkova-Kostova AT. Phytochemicals as protectors against ultraviolet radiation: Versatility of effects and mechanisms. *Planta Med.* 2008;74:1548.
3. Karrer P, Morf R, Schopp K. Zur kenntnis des vitamin-a aus fischtranin. *Helv Chim Acta.* 1931;14:1036.
4. Thielitz A, Abdel-Naser MB, Fluhr JW, et al. Topical retinoids in acne – An evidence-based overview. *Dtsch Dermatol Ges.* 2008;6:1023.
5. Thiboutot D, Gollnick H, Bettoli V, et al. New insights into the management of acne: An update from the Global Alliance to Improve Outcomes in Acne group. *J Am Acad Dermatol.* 2009;60:S1.
6. Alexis AF. Clinical considerations on the use of concomitant therapy in the treatment of acne. *J Dermatolog Treat.* 2008;19:199.
7. Amichai B, Shemer A, Grunwald MH. Low-dose isotretinoin in the treatment of acne vulgaris. *J Am Acad Dermatol.* 2006;54:644.
8. Akhavan A, Bershad S. Topical acne drugs: Review of clinical properties, systemic exposure, and safety. *Am J Clin Dermatol.* 2003;4:473.
9. Fluhr JW, Vienne MP, Lauze C, et al. Tolerance profile of retinol, retinaldehyde and retinoic acid under maximized and long-term clinical conditions. *Dermatology.* 1999;199(Suppl 1):57.
10. Keller KL, Fenske NA. Uses of vitamins A, C, and E and related compounds in dermatology: A review. *J Am Acad Dermatol.* 1998;39:611.
11. Chandraratna RA. Tazarotene – First of a new generation of receptor-selective retinoids. *Br J Dermatol.* 1996;135(Suppl 49):18.
12. Chytil F, Ong D. Cellular retinoid-binding proteins. In: Sporn MB, Roberts A, Goodman D, eds. *The Retinoids.* Vol. 2. Orlando: Academic Press; 1984:89–123.
13. Giguere V, Ong ES, Segui P, et al. Identification of a receptor for the morphogen retinoic acid. *Nature.* 1987;330:624.
14. Petkovich M, Brand NJ, Krust A, et al. A human retinoic acid receptor which belongs to the family of nuclear receptors. *Nature.* 1987;330:444.
15. Kligman L, Kligman AM. Photoaging – Retinoids, alpha hydroxy acids, and antioxidants. In: Gabard B, Elsner P, Surber C, Treffel P, eds. *Dermatopharmacology of Topical Preparations.* New York: Springer; 2000:383.
16. Pfahl M. The molecular mechanism of retinoid action. Retinoids today and tomorrow. *Retinoids Dermatol.* 1996;44:2.
17. Petkovich M. Regulation of gene expression by vitamin A: The role of nuclear retinoic acid receptors. *Annu Rev Nutr.* 1992;12:443.
18. Lippman SM, Lotan R. Advances in the development of retinoids as chemopreventive agents. *J Nutr.* 2000;130:479S.
19. Fu, PP, Xia Q, Boudreau MD, et al. Physiological role of retinyl palmitate in the skin. *Vitam Horm.* 2007;75:223.
20. Duell EA, Kang S, Voorhees JJ. Unoccluded retinol penetrates human skin in vivo more effectively than unoccluded retinyl palmitate or retinoic acid. *J Invest Dermatol.* 1997;109:301.

21. Yan J, Xia Q, Cherng SH, et al. Photo-induced DNA damage and photocytotoxicity of retinyl palmitate and its photodecomposition products. *Toxicol Ind Health*. 2005;21:167.

22. Bikowski JB. Mechanisms of the comedolytic and anti-inflammatory properties of topical retinoids. *J Drugs Dermatol*. 2005;4:41.

23. Varani J, Nickoloff BJ, Dixit VM, et al. All-trans retinoic acid stimulates growth of adult human keratinocytes cultured in growth factor-deficient medium, inhibits production of thrombospondin and fibronectin, and reduces adhesion. *J Invest Dermatol*. 1989;93:449.

24. Waller JM, Dreher F, Behnam S, et al. 'Keratolytic' properties of benzoyl peroxide and retinoic acid resemble salicylic acid in man. *Skin Pharmacol Physiol*. 2006;19:283.

25. Heymann WR. Toll-like receptors in acne vulgaris. *J Am Acad Dermatol*. 2006;55:691.

26. Liu PT, Krutzik SR, Kim J, et al. Cutting edge: All-trans retinoic acid down-regulates TLR2 expression and function. *J Immunol*. 2005;174:2467.

27. Selway JL, Kurczab T, Kealey T, et al. Toll-like receptor 2 activation and comedogenesis: Implications for the pathogenesis of acne. *BMC Dermatol*. 2013;13:10.

28. Kang S, Cho S, Chung JH, et al. Inflammation and extracellular matrix degradation mediated by activated transcription factors nuclear factor-kappaB and activator protein-1 in inflammatory acne lesions in vivo. *Am J Pathol*. 2005;166:1691.

29. Emanuele E, Bertona M, Altabas K, et al. Anti-inflammatory effects of a topical preparation containing nicotinamide, retinol, and 7-dehydrocholesterol in patients with acne: A gene expression study. *Clin Cosmet Investig Dermatol*. 2012;5:33.

30. Downie MM, Sanders DA, Kealey T. Modelling the remission of individual acne lesions in vitro. *Br J Dermatol*. 2002;147:869.

31. Agak GW, Qin M, Nobe J, et al. Propionibacterium acnes induces an IL-17 response in acne vulgaris that is regulated by vitamin A and vitamin D. *J Invest Dermatol*. 2013 Aug 7. [Epub ahead of print]

32. Trivedi NR, Gilliland KL, Zhao W, et al. Gene array expression profiling in acne lesions reveals marked upregulation of genes involved in inflammation and matrix remodeling. *J Invest Dermatol*. 2006;126:1071.

33. Farrell LN, Strauss JS, Stranieri AM. The treatment of severe cystic acne with 13-cis-retinoic acid. Evaluation of sebum production and the clinical response in a multiple-dose trial. *J Am Acad Dermatol*. 1980;3:602.

34. Xia Q, Yin JJ, Wamer WG, et al. Photoirradiation of retinyl palmitate in ethanol with ultraviolet light – Formation of photodecomposition products, reactive oxygen species, and lipid peroxides. *Int J Environ Res Public Health*. 2006;3:185.

35. Wang SQ, Dusza SW, Lim HW. Safety of retinyl palmitate in sunscreens: A critical analysis. *J Am Acad Dermatol*. 2010;63:903.

36. Burnett ME, Wang SQ. Current sunscreen controversies: A critical review. *Photodermatol Photoimmunol Photomed*. 2011;27:58.

37. Yin JJ, Xia Q, Fu PP. UVA photoirradiation of anhydroretinol – Formation of singlet oxygen and superoxide. *Toxicol Ind Health*. 2007;23:625.

38. Xia Q, Yin JJ, Cherng SH, et al. UVA photoirradiation of retinyl palmitate – Formation of singlet oxygen and superoxide, and their role in induction of lipid peroxidation. *Toxicol Lett*. 2006;163:30.

39. Cherng SH, Xia Q, Blankenship LR, et al. Photodecomposition of retinyl palmitate in ethanol by UVA light-formation of photodecomposition products, reactive oxygen species, and lipid peroxides. *Chem Res Toxicol*. 2005;18:129.

40. Martin B, Meunier C, Montels D, et al. Chemical stability of adapalene and tretinoin when combined with benzoyl peroxide in presence and in absence of visible light and ultraviolet radiation. *Br J Dermatol*. 1998;139(Suppl 52):8.

41. Tagami H, Tadaki T, Obata M, et al. Functional assessment of the stratum corneum under the influence of oral aromatic retinoid (etretinate) in guinea-pigs and humans. Comparison with topical retinoic acid treatment. *Br J Dermatol*. 1992; 127:470.

42. Effendy I, Kwangsukstith C, Lee LY, et al. Functional changes in human stratum corneum induced by topical glycolic acid: Comparison with all-trans retinoic acid. *Acta Derm Venereol*. 1995;75:455.

43. Griffiths CE, Voorhees JJ. Human in vivo pharmacology of topical retinoids. *Arch Dermatol Res*. 1994;287:53.

44. Rawlings AV, Stephens TJ, Herndon JH, et al. The effect of a vitamin A palmitate and antioxidant-containing oil-based moisturizer on photodamaged skin of several body sites. *J Cosmet Dermatol*. 2013;12:25.

45. Tucker-Samaras S, Zedayko T, Cole C, et al. A stabilized 0.1% retinol facial moisturizer improves the appearance of photodamaged skin in an eight-week, double-blind, vehicle-controlled study. *J Drugs Dermatol*. 2009;8:932.

46. Kikuchi K, Suetake T, Kumasaka N, et al. Improvement of photoaged facial skin in middle-aged Japanese females by topical retinol (vitamin A alcohol): A vehicle-controlled, double-blind study. *J Dermatolog Treat*. 2009;20:276.

47. Antoniou C, Kosmadaki MG, Stratigos AJ, et al. Photoaging: Prevention and topical treatments. *Am J Clin Dermatol*. 2010;11:95.

48. Kurlandsky SB, Xiao JH, Duell EA, et al. Biological activity of all-trans retinol requires metabolic conversion to all-trans retinoic acid and is mediated through activation of nuclear retinoid receptors in human keratinocytes. *J Biol Chem*. 1994;269:32821.

49. Baumann L, Saghari S. Retinoids. In: Baumann L, Saghari S, Weisberg E. eds. *Cosmetic Dermatology: Principles and Practice*. 2nd ed. New York: McGraw-Hill; 2009:256–62.

50. Yan J, Wamer WG, Howard PC, et al. Levels of retinyl palmitate and retinol in the stratum corneum, epidermis, and dermis of female SKH-1 mice topically treated with retinyl palmitate. *Toxicol Ind Health*. 2006;22:181.

CHAPTER 80

Silver

Activities:

Anti-inflammatory, antibacterial, antifungal, antiviral, wound healing, antitumorigenic

Important Chemical Components:

Silver ion Ag$^+$

Origin Classification:

Natural element

Personal Care Category:

Acne therapy, antimicrobial

Recommended for the following Baumann Skin Types:

DSNT, DSPT, DSNW, DSPW, OSNT, OSNW, OSPT, and OSPW. This is the treatment of choice for dry acne-prone skin.

SOURCE

Silver is a naturally occurring chemical element on our planet (with the chemical symbol Ag). It is obtained by mining. Nanoparticles are produced in the laboratory and are designed to be a particular size and shape. Silver salts are formed by combining silver with other agents. This can occur spontaneously or in the laboratory setting.

HISTORY

The medicinal use of silver dates back at least to the time of ancient Greek historian Herodotus, who lived in the 5th century BCE and stated that when the King of Persia went to war, he would take boiled water stored in flagons of silver to treat wounds.[1,2] But the awareness of metallic silver dates back further to 4,000 BCE.[2] The Phoenicians were known to store water and other liquids in silver vats to prevent them from spoiling. Although the metallic silver in the vats was not soluble in water and therefore would not have antimicrobial properties, the beneficial properties noted by the Romans and Phoenicians can be explained by the fact that leeching of silver ions into water occurred when the water was stored for long periods of time.[3] Silver nitrate was cited in a Roman pharmacopeia published in 69 BCE (Table 80-1).[2] Over three hundred years earlier, Hippocrates, the father of medicine, documented the beneficial healing and disease-modifying properties of silver.[4] Avicenna is reported to have used silver as a blood purifier circa 980 CE and Paracelsus used silver systemically, and topically applied silver nitrate to wounds in the early 1500s, a practice that has continued into modern times.[2]

In 1869, Raulin observed that the fungus *Aspergillus niger* could not grow in silver vessels.[5] The Swiss botanist von Nägeli was

TABLE 80-1
Pros and Cons of Silver

PROS	CONS
Strong antibacterial activity with minimal risk of bacterial resistance	Theoretical risk of contact dermatitis
Works quicker than most acne ingredients	Not FDA approved for acne
No risk of irritation especially in dry skin types	Not covered by an FDA monograph
Inexpensive	More clinical studies needed
Anti-inflammatory	Not FDA approved for nail and foot fungus
Long history of use	Oral use associated with argyria
Does not impair barrier	
Can be used before and after procedures, including facials	
Antifungal and antiviral activity	

studying silver when he devised the term "oligodynamic" to describe any metal that exhibits bactericidal properties at minute concentrations (*oligos*, small + *dynamis*, power). Silver nitrate was introduced by Credé in 1884 for the prevention of ophthalmia neonatorum, an infection in the eyes of newborn babies also known as gonorrheal ophthalmia.[2,6]

In 1901, Philadelphia doctor Albert Barnes and German chemist Hermann Hille developed Argyrol, a mild vacuum-dried silver nitrate precipitate of the protein vitellin (derived from wheat), which they marketed in 1902 to treat gonorrhea and gonorrheal neonatal blindness. Argyrol contained up to 30 percent silver and was also indicated for catarrhal conjunctivitis and follicular conjunctivitis in addition to ophthalmia neonatorum.[7] Barnes convinced Hille not to patent the product, but vigorously defended it against imitators. They marketed directly to physicians. Barnes bought out Hille and was a millionaire by 1907. He sold the enterprise in 1928, subsequently amassing a world famous art collection, including works by, among others, Cézanne, Matisse, Picasso, Modigliani, Renoir, van Gogh, Degas, Seurat, and Rousseau, now housed in the Barnes Foundation in Philadelphia.[7] Not long after Barnes sold his business, antibiotics were discovered and displaced the silver-based Argyrol.

In the early 1900s, people often deposited silver dollars in milk bottles to prolong the milk's freshness. Before the advent of penicillin, clinicians placed silver wafers on contaminated wounds during World War I to help prevent infection. In fact, before antibiotics were introduced, silver was the most important antimicrobial agent and a major component in wound healing.[2] Moyer is credited with resurrecting interest in silver (in the form of silver nitrate) in the 1960s,[8] but newer delivery technologies fuel the more recent interest in the medical applications of the element.

Indeed, silver compounds, in metallic, nanocrystalline, and ionic preparations, have exhibited broad antibacterial activity and have garnered recent interest for topical antiseptic use in wound dressings.[9] Nanocrystalline silver dressings were introduced commercially as antimicrobial dressings in 1998.[10]

Today silver is used in dressings, catheters, cleansers, ophthalmic ointments, and many other medical products. It is so popular that it has been estimated that 15 metric tons of silver were incorporated into medical products worldwide in 2010 alone.[11] Silver is also being used in personal care products, textiles, and water purification devices.

CHEMISTRY

Silver is element number 47 on the periodic table and is designated as Ag, which comes from the Latin word *argentum* (árgyros in Greek), derived from the Indo-European root "arg-," meaning "shining," "white," or "gray." It has the highest electrical conductivity of all metals and is classified as a noble metal. Noble metals resist corrosion and oxidation in moist environments and are usually valuable due to their limited amounts. Other noble metals include ruthenium, rhodium, palladium, osmium, iridium, platinum, and gold. Silver is stable in pure air and water, but tarnishes when it is exposed to air or water containing ozone or hydrogen sulfide.

Metallic silver is insoluble in water; however, it is highly reactive and easily converts to salt forms such as Ag^+, Ag^{2+}, Ag^{3+}, and Ag^0. These salt forms render silver compounds such as silver nitrate ($AgNO_3$) and silver chloride ($AgCl$) soluble in water. Silver is present in these four oxidation states. Ag^0 and Ag^+ are the most abundant. The most common oxidation state of silver is +1 of which $AgNO_3$ is an example. Less common are the +2 compounds (e.g., silver(II) fluoride, AgF_2), and the even less common +3 and +4 compounds.[12] Single-charged silver Ag^+ is the most biologically active form. In the environment, silver is often naturally complexed with sulfide, sulfate, bicarbonate, or chlorides.[13]

There are several designations used when describing the type of silver used in topical skin formulations:

1. *Colloidal silver:* This term describes a suspension of silver particles in an aqueous base.
2. *Nanosilver:* Ag nanoparticles can be produced in various sizes and shapes.[3] Nanoparticles range from 1 to 100 nm in at least one dimension.

Silver exhibits many activities that account for its various effects on infectious organisms. Silver ions are known to react with nucleophilic amino acid residues in proteins, and attach to membrane or enzyme proteins leading to protein denaturation. Silver is also known to inhibit a number of oxidative enzymes such as yeast alcohol dehydrogenase, the uptake of succinate by membrane vesicles, and the respiratory chain of bacteria, as well as causing metabolite efflux, interfering with DNA replication, and affecting the NaC-translocating NADH: ubiquinone oxidoreductase system.[14,15]

ORAL USES

Several online businesses enthusiastically promote oral colloidal silver products as supplements and for prevention and treatment of many diseases. The US Food and Drug Administration (FDA) stated in Sec. 310.548 of a 2012 ruling that "there is a lack of adequate data to establish general recognition of the safety and effectiveness of colloidal silver ingredients or silver salts for over-the-counter (OTC) use in the treatment or prevention of any disease."[16] This ruling was in response to the indiscriminate use of oral silver products, some of which led to toxicity such as argyria.[17] Oral use of silver-containing products is not advised until well-designed research trials demonstrate safety and efficacy.

TOPICAL USES

There are many silver-containing topical formulations on the market, some containing silver ions and some with nanoparticles. The topical absorption of silver into the skin depends on several factors including the vehicle used, concentration, charge, particle size, particle shape, whether it is a silver salt or a nanoparticle, and the coating (in the case of nanoparticles). As expected, smaller nanometer particles (15 nm in rat skin and 6 nm in human skin) penetrate better than larger particles (102 nm and 198 nm, respectively).[18]

Colloidal silver is the most common preparation found in OTC silver-containing preparations, and the efficacy varies based on the vehicle, concentration of silver in parts per million, the pH, and the length of time of exposure. Nanosilver behaves very differently than colloidal silver preparations because the small size yields different characteristics, primarily due to its high surface-area-to-volume ratio. This renders the molecules more reactive in some cases. The most common form of silver used topically is silver sulfadiazine 1 percent cream, which has a long record of successful use as a safe and effective treatment to reduce *Pseudomonas* infection in wounds. Silver sulfadiazine 1 percent cream contains a sulfa antibiotic, so it cannot be used by individuals allergic to sulfa-containing medications. It is important to note that sulfa and sulphur are different compounds. Sulfur smells like rotten eggs and is often found in acne medications. Sulfa is found in the antibiotic known as Bactrim and an allergy to it can be life threatening.

Antibacterial Uses

Many healthcare products contain silver, including silver-coated catheters, wound dressings, and pre-procedure cleansers.[15] Silver has been shown to deliver antimicrobial effects against bacteria, viruses, and fungi and to inhibit the formation of bacterial biofilms.[15,19] Despite the long-standing and increasing use of silver ions and nanoparticles, its antibacterial mode of action remains unclear but most data suggest that the bactericidal effect is due to damage to the bacterial membrane. Silver exerts its bactericidal activity by acting on the bacteria at several levels including the cell membrane, enzymes, uncoupling of the respiratory chain from oxidative phosphorylation,[11] actions on DNA, and induction of proton leakage through the bacterial membrane, resulting in complete de-energization and, ultimately, cell death.[20]

Antibiotic resistance is of great interest in public health and medicine right now, including the acne realm where *Propionibacterium acnes* resistance rates are estimated to be as high as 60 percent in some patient populations.[21] Erythromycin, methicillin, and clindamycin are the most common antibiotics to which bacteria have reportedly developed resistance.[22] Combining benzoyl peroxide (BPO) with erythromycin or clindamycin has been proven to prevent the emergence of resistant strains of *P. acnes*;[22–25] therefore, the current clinical acne recommendation is to include BPO in topical antiacne regimens that utilize antibiotics (see Chapter 76, Benzoyl Peroxide).[25] However, BPO kills bacteria by producing free radicals, which may increase skin aging and inflammation, so another option to prevent antibiotic-resistant *P. acnes* is needed. Silver may be the solution to antibacterial resistance in acne patients. Although silver-resistant bacteria have been reported since 1975,[26–36] lack of standardized methodology for assessing bacterial susceptibility to Ag^+, small sample sizes, and differing overall methodologies make it difficult to draw firm conclusions about the true incidence of antibiotic resistance to silver.[37–39]

Examples of silver-resistant bacterial strains that have been isolated include *Escherichia coli*, *Enterobacter cloacae*, *Klebsiella pneumoniae*, *Acinetobacter baumannii*, *Salmonella typhimurium*, and *Pseudomonas stutzeri*, but resistant *P. acnes* has not been reported.[15,26,36,40] Unlike antibiotics, resistance to antiseptics such as silver is rare and sporadic. However, it is important to note that bacteria have been exposed to subinhibitory levels of silver for over four billion years and no widespread resistance has been evident to date, whereas widespread antibiotic resistance has developed within the last 60 years.

Anti-inflammatory Uses

Noble metals, including silver, have been shown for years to have anti-inflammatory capabilities.[41–45] These effects seem to be mediated by the impact that silver exerts on the cytokine system. Silver nanoparticles suppress the activity of interleukin (IL)-6 and tumor necrosis factor (TNF)-α, IL-12, and IL-1β. The effects on the cytokine system account for why silver has been demonstrated to relieve rheumatoid arthritis symptoms.[10]

A study by Nadworny demonstrated that nanocrystalline silver treatments decreased dinitrochlorobenzene (DNCB)-induced erythema and edema, increased apoptosis (programmed cell death) in dermal cells, and decreased matrix metalloproteinase (MMP) and proinflammatory cytokine expression.[10] She postulated that the decreased TNF-α seen in the silver-treated animals resulted from the elimination of inflammatory cells by apoptosis. In 2005, Bhol and Schechter showed that nanocrystalline silver inhibited allergic contact dermatitis in mice, suppressed the expression of TNF-α and IL-12, and induced apoptosis of inflammatory cells.[46] The previous year, Bhol et al. used DNCB to induce allergic contact dermatitis in a guinea pig model and found that topical nanocrystalline silver cream was comparably effective as topical steroids and immunosuppressants in dose-dependently reducing erythema.[47]

Anticancer Activity

Silver complexes containing various types of ligands such as carboxylic acids, amino acids, nitrogen, phosphorus, or sulfur donor ligands have shown significant antiproliferative effects. Although the mechanism is not known, it is thought to be due in part to the interactions of silver with DNA and proteins.[48] Silver causes apoptosis when combined with other agents (ligands). These silver-ligand complexes have been shown to exert greater cytotoxicity than the chemotherapeutic agent cisplatin on certain cancer cells. Studies using silver complexes have revealed efficacy in the treatment of breast cancer.[48]

Wound Healing

Silver sulfadiazine cream (Silvadeen™) was the earliest commercially available silver-containing preparation to treat wounds. It was developed in the 1960s for the treatment of burns. It is known that *P. acnes*, the bacteria that causes acne and forms biofilms, is a major cause of wound infections, especially after shoulder surgery, and could play a role in the development of granulomas and skin infections (due to biofilms) seen after dermal filler injections.[19] For this reason, silver-containing cleansers such as Theraworx™ are used to cleanse skin prior to surgery and other invasive procedures such as urinary catheterization without the skin barrier damage caused by other pre-surgical cleansing products such as chlorhexidine or Hibiclens™. Pre-procedure skin cleansers such as GCP Skincare have been developed to cleanse skin prior to dermal filler injections (e.g., Juvéderm, Voluma, and Restylane), chemical peels, botulinum toxin (i.e., Botox and Dysport) injections, facials, and other cosmetic procedures. The other pre-procedure cleansing options, chlorhexidine and Hibiclens, are contraindicated for use on the face. In addition, chlorhexidine and Hibiclens cannot be used before chemical peels because they impair the skin barrier,[49] which could lead to increased depth of the chemical peel resulting in burning, postinflammatory hyperpigmentation, and possible scarring. These colloidal silver-containing cleansers are safe to use on wounded skin, including after surgery, laser treatments, and chemical peels. In addition to silver-containing cleansers, a recent trend toward the use of wound cover dressings that contain silver has resulted in a large selection of commercially available foam, film, hydrocolloid, gauze, and dressings with hydrofiber technology impregnated with silver.[15]

Burns

$AgNO_3$ has been used in burns but the reduction of AG^+ to Ag^0 that occurs leaves the wound blackened. For this reason, silver sulfadiazine, a topical antibiotic cream used for decades to prevent secondary skin infections in wounds, is a more popular option and the wound healing ointment of choice of many medical professionals. Another formulation marketed as Silvazine in the United States is a topical cream that contains 1 percent silver sulfadiazine plus 0.2 percent chlorhexidine digluconate in a water-immiscible cream base. It also exhibits antibacterial activity but the chlorhexidine can impair the skin barrier and cause an allergic reaction, so silver sulfadiazine alone is preferable.[49]

There are numerous studies in the literature showing the efficacy of silver-impregnated dressings for wounds. In some cases, direct current electricity was used to accelerate the release of Ag^+ from the bandage into the damaged tissue.[50,51]

In addition to colloidal silver and silver-impregnated dressings, nanoparticle silver in various forms has been used to treat burns. Treatment of murine infected burns with silver nanoparticles has increased the rate of healing and decreased scarring in comparison with silver sulfadiazine.[52] This was accompanied by increased expression of IL-10, vascular endothelial growth factor, and interferon-γ, with reduced IL-6 expression. The literature includes more studies of silver products in burns and wounds that are beyond the scope of this chapter.

Acne

Acne is caused by the presence of the bacteria *P. acnes*, which leads to an inflammatory response in the skin. Silver functions as a bactericidal and anti-inflammatory agent, without the production of free radicals seen with BPO. For this reason it is a good option for acne treatment. Silver is not approved by the FDA for use in acne, and has not been proven safe or efficacious for this condition. (Acne medications with the exception of salicylic acid and BPO must undergo a formal FDA drug approval process.) Despite the fact that formal acne studies have not been performed, silver sulfadiazine has been used "off-label" for this purpose for years. The use of silver sulfadiazine for acne is limited by the risk of sulfa allergy and the thick white pasty consistency of the preparation. Silver-containing cleansers and textiles are other options for acne treatment.

Textiles

Textiles coated with silver have been shown to reduce skin bacteria counts. Silver is incorporated into textiles by integrating silver nanoparticles into the polymer used to form yarn or by coating the yarn with silver.[53] Some textiles have every strand coated while others coat every 5th or 6th strand. There does not seem to be a difference in efficacy between the textiles with every strand coated versus every 5th strand coated; however, the textiles with every 5th strand coated are softer. The loss of silver during washing varies between textile technologies. Fabrics that lose a negligible amount of silver during washings and that are comfortable are preferable. These textiles can be used to manufacture pillowcases, face masks, and shirts to treat acne. Textiles containing silver have been used in other skin disorders such as atopic dermatitis but no formal studies in acne have been conducted.

Atopic Dermatitis

One study in patients with atopic dermatitis showed that silver-coated textiles were able to reduce *Staphylococcus aureus* density significantly after two days of wearing, lasting until the end of treatment (day 7) and even one week after removal of the textiles.[54] The silver-coated textiles, compared to cotton, were able to improve objective and subjective symptoms of atopic dermatitis significantly within two weeks without measurable side effects. One technology known as Padycare® incorporates silver into micromesh material (82 percent polyamide, 18 percent lycra) for clothing and bedding.[55] Textiles have the added benefit of preventing scratching and providing protection from irritating substances and allergens. The amount of silver lost from textiles during washing can vary from 100 percent loss after four washings to less than one percent loss.[56] Concerns have been raised about the silver leaking from the textiles into the water supply, killing beneficial bacteria used to treat the water.

SAFETY ISSUES

Humans are exposed to silver on a daily basis, most commonly by ingestion in the diet via water and food.[13] Other sources of silver are inhalation of silver dust, contact with jewelry, acupuncture needles, dental amalgams, cleaning products, and creams used to treat burns.[13] Silver in any form is not carcinogenic and is not thought to be toxic to the immune, cardiovascular, nervous, or reproductive systems.[13]

Colloidal silver preparations are much less likely to penetrate into the skin because of the large size of the silver ion. Recent concern about the safety of nanoparticles has emerged because of the ability of nanoparticles to enter the skin and possibly the circulatory system. Silver nanoparticles usually consist of 20 to 15,000 silver atoms and are smaller than the required 100 nm or less to be called a "nanoparticle."[13] Of more than 800 consumer products that contain nanomaterial, 30 percent are claimed to contain silver particles.[13] Studies have shown that nanosilver can penetrate into the skin, but this ability depends on the size, shape, and vehicle used as well as the length of exposure. In 2009, it was demonstrated for the first time that silver applied as nanoparticles coated with polyvinylpirrolidone was able to permeate skin and enter the stratum corneum and upper epidermis. The silver nanoparticle absorption through intact and damaged skin was very low but detectable.[57] In 2013, topically applied nanocrystalline silver dressings were applied to intact human skin destined to be removed via surgery to determine if the silver ions were absorbed into skin and subsequently into the circulation. The skin was surgically excised and then analyzed by tissue mass spectrometry, light microscopy, scanning electron microscopy (SEM), and X-ray diffusion spectrography (XRD). Silver clusters as large as 750 nm could be discerned in the dermis. Pre- and post-dressing serum silver levels were compared and there was no rise in silver in serum samples. This study shows that nanoparticles of silver can be absorbed into the dermis but do not enter the circulatory system.[58]

Silver does not pose the toxic threat to humans that other heavy metals do. It is taken up in the intestine and passed through the blood, liver, and bone marrow, and, ultimately, is excreted in urine.

Argyria

Argyria is typically an irreversible blue-gray coloring of the skin, eyes, and mucous membranes caused by deposits of silver granules in regions around hair follicles and sweat ducts.[59] The condition is rare and the vast majority of cases are due to oral exposure to silver. Argyria occurs when silver is absorbed into the circulatory system and precipitates in the dermis, usually in the form of silver sulfide. Although this condition does not harm an individual's health, it is disfiguring and usually permanent. This condition is one of the reasons the FDA prohibited the use of oral silver to treat medical conditions. There are a few reports in the literature of lasers being used to treat the blue-gray color characteristic of argyria.

ENVIRONMENTAL IMPACT

Silver naturally occurs in our environment, but rarely. Concentrations can be elevated by activities such as coal combustion, manufacturing of electronic goods, and disposal of photographic supplies. It is released into the air and water naturally by rain and rock erosion. The general population is exposed to silver in drinking water and food. Dietary intake of silver is estimated at 70 to 90 μg per day.[13]

It has been shown that nanosilver in textiles washes out and enters the water supply. However, silver has been used for years in water treatment plants and is often used in washing machines.[13] Farmers are concerned that the antimicrobial effects of nanosilver will affect beneficial bacteria in the soil.[60] A review by Wijnhoven et al. discussed the environmental impact of silver and concluded that because there are many different forms of silver it is difficult to accurately predict the effects on the environment and to know which forms of silver are the safest.[13] Nanosilver may have various effects because of its size, shape, and different properties. Little is known about the effects of nanosilver on the environment and if it should prompt increased concern compared to naturally occurring silver ions.

FORMULATION CONSIDERATIONS

Silver metal easily dissolves in nitric acid yielding $AgNO_3$, an inorganic, transparent, photosensitive, crystalline solid that is readily water soluble.[61,62] Colloidal silver formulations are usually comprised of silver ions suspended in an aqueous solution.

Given the propensity of silver to complex with so many molecules, it is obviously important to consider what interactions may occur between silver and other cosmeceutical ingredients. Silver reacts with proteins and amino acids and, therefore, would not be a good option to combine with peptides, growth factors, or stem cell ingredients.

Silver sulfadiazine is highly insoluble in water, which accounts for its thick white pasty consistency when formulated into a topical cream.[63]

USAGE CONSIDERATIONS

Silver reacts strongly with proteins. This should be taken into account when applying along with growth factor-, collagen-, or peptide-containing ingredients and the regimens should be adjusted to minimize contact between these ingredients.

SIGNIFICANT BACKGROUND

The antifungal effects of spherical silver nanoparticles (nano-Ag) on fungal pathogens of the skin have been investigated. Nano-Ag showed potent activity against strains of *Trichophyton mentagrophytes* and *Candida* species. The activity of nano-Ag was comparable to that of amphotericin B, but superior to that of fluconazole.[64] Silver has also been shown to have strong antiviral effects. Studies have not been conducted but it is likely that topical silver formulations can play a role in the treatment of nail fungus, foot fungus, and herpes simplex viral infections.

CONCLUSION

Silver has been used as a medicinal therapy for centuries but is not currently FDA approved to treat any medical conditions including acne. Its antimicrobial and anti-inflammatory activities, its gentleness to the skin barrier, and its usability on the face make it popular for pre- and post-procedure application, especially in relation to dermal fillers, botulinum toxin injections, and chemical peels. It is used off-label for many purposes but safety and efficacy trials are lacking. Silver may be a good adjuvant for acne therapy because of the low risk of bacterial resistance, the lack of irritation, and the preservation of the skin barrier as contrasted to other acne medications such as retinoids, antibiotics, and BPO. However, further studies are necessary.

REFERENCES

1. Blakeney EH, ed. *The History of Herodotus* [Rawlinson G, trans.]. London: Dent & Sons, 1945:188.
2. Alexander JW. History of the medical use of silver. *Surg Infect (Larchmt)*. 2009;10:289.
3. Jones VE. Nanocrystalline Silver: Use in wound care. In: Slevin M, ed. *Current Advances in the Medical Application of Nanotechnology*. Manchester, UK: Bentham Books, 2012:25–31.
4. Salcido RS. Silver: An old wine in a new bottle. *Adv Skin Wound Care*. 2006;19:472.
5. Raulin J. *Sci Nat*. 1869;11:93. Berk (3) Abstr 1.
6. Novak JM. Current status of Credé prophylaxis. *Am J Optom Physiol Opt*. 1984;61:340.
7. Hodson TJ, Gillies WE. Argyrol, argyrosis and the acquisition of art. *Aust N Z J Ophthalmol*. 1985;13:391.
8. Moyer CA, Brentano L, Gravens DL, et al. Treatment of large human burns with 0.5 percent silver nitrate solution. *Arch Surg*. 1965;90:812.
9. Lipsky BA, Hoey C. Topical antimicrobial therapy for treating chronic wounds. *Clin Infect Dis*. 2009;49:1541.
10. Nadworny PL, Wang J, Tredget EE, et al. Anti-inflammatory activity of nanocrystalline silver in a porcine contact dermatitis model. *Nanomedicine*. 2008;4:241.
11. Randall CP, Oyama LB, Bostock JM, et al. The silver cation (Ag⁺): Antistaphylococcal activity, mode of action and resistance studies. *J Antimicrob Chemother*. 2013;68:131.
12. Riedel S, Kaupp M. The highest oxidation states of the transition metal elements. *Coord Chem Rev*. 2009;253:606.
13. Wijnhoven SWP, Peijnenburg WJGM, Herberts CA, et al. Nano-silver – A review of available data and knowledge gaps in human and environmental risk assessment. *Nanotoxicology*. 2009;3:109.
14. Hostýnek JJ, Hinz RS, Lorence CR, et al. Metals and the skin. *Crit Rev Toxicol*. 1993;23:171.
15. Percival SL, Bowler PG, Russell D. Bacterial resistance to silver in wound care. *J Hosp Infect*. 2005;60:1.
16. U.S. Food and Drug Administration. Code of Federal Regulations Title 21, Subchapter D – Drugs for Human Use. http://www.accessdata.fda.gov/scripts/cdrh/cfdocs/cfcfr/cfrsearch.cfm?fr=310.548. Accessed October 19, 2013.
17. Fung MC, Bowen DL. Silver products for medical indications: Risk-benefit assessment. *J Toxicol Clin Toxicol*. 1996;34:119.
18. Labouta HI, Schneider M. Interaction of inorganic nanoparticles with the skin barrier: Current status and critical review. *Nanomedicine*. 2013;9:39.
19. Percival SL, Bowler PG, Dolman J. Antimicrobial activity of silver-containing dressings on wound microorganisms using an in vitro biofilm model. *Int Wound J*. 2007;4:186.
20. Dibrov P, Dzioba J, Gosink KK, et al. Chemiosmotic mechanism of antimicrobial activity of Ag(+) in Vibrio cholerae. *Antimicrob Agents Chemother*. 2002;46:2668.
21. Nishijima S, Akamatsu H, Akamatsu M, et al. The antibiotic susceptibility of Propionibacterium acnes and Staphylococcus epidermidis isolated from acne. *J Dermatol*. 1996;21:166.
22. Kircik LH. The role of benzoyl peroxide in the new treatment paradigm for acne. *J Drugs Dermatol*. 2013;12:s73.
23. Eady EA, Farmery MR, Ross JI, et al. Effects of benzoyl peroxide and erythromycin alone and in combination against antibiotic-sensitive and -resistant skin bacteria from acne patients. *Br J Dermatol*. 1994;131:331.
24. Leyden J, Levy S. The development of antibiotic resistance in Propionibacterium acnes. *Cutis*. 2001;67:21.
25. Thiboutot D, Gollnick H, Bettoli V, et al. New insights into the management of acne: An update from the Global Alliance to Improve Outcomes in Acne group. *J Am Acad Dermatol*. 2009;60:S1.
26. McHugh GL, Moellering RC, Hopkins CC, et al. Salmonella typhimurium resistance to silver nitrate, chloramphenicol, and ampicillin. *Lancet*. 1975;1:235.
27. Annear DI, Mee BJ, Bailey M. Instability and linkage of silver resistance, lactose fermentation, and colony structure in Enterobacter cloacae from burn wounds. *J Clin Pathol*. 1976;29:441.
28. Hendry AT, Stewart IO. Silver-resistant Enterobacteriaceae from hospital patients. *Can J Microbiol*. 1979;25:915.
29. Bridges K, Kidson A, Lowbury EJ, et al. Gentamicin- and silver-resistant pseudomonas in a burns unit. *Br Med J*. 1979;1:446.
30. Belly RT, Kydd GC. Silver resistance in microorganisms. *Dev Ind Microbiol*. 1982;23:567.
31. Haefeli C, Franklin C, Hardy K. Plasmid-determined silver resistance in Pseudomonas stutzeri isolated from a silver mine. *J Bacteriol*. 1984;158:389.
32. Kaur P, Saxena M, Vadehra DV. Plasmid mediated resistance to silver ions in Escherichia coli. *Indian J Med Res*. 1985;82:122.
33. Kaur P, Vadehra DV. Mechanism of resistance to silver ions in Klebsiella pneumoniae. *Antimicrob Agents Chemother*. 1986;29:165.
34. Starodub ME, Trevors JT. Mobilization of Escherichia coli R1 silver-resistance plasmid pJT1 by Tn5-Mob into Escherichia coli C600. *Biol Met*. 1990;3:24.
35. Deshpande LM, Chopade BA. Plasmid mediated silver resistance in Acinetobacter baumannii. *Biometals*. 1994;7:49.
36. Silver S. Bacterial silver resistance: Molecular biology and uses and misuses of silver compounds. *FEMS Microbiol Rev*. 2003;27:341.
37. Ip M, Lui SL, Chau SS, et al. The prevalence of resistance to silver in a burns unit. *J Hosp Infect*. 2006;63:342.
38. Maple PA, Hamilton-Miller JM, Brumfitt W. Comparison of the in-vitro activities of the topical antimicrobials azelaic acid, nitrofurazone, silver sulphadiazine and mupirocin against methicillin-resistant Staphylococcus aureus. *J Antimicrob Chemother*. 1992;29:661.
39. Ug A, Ceylan O. Occurrence of resistance to antibiotics, metals, and plasmids in clinical strains of Staphylococcus spp. *Arch Med Res*. 2003;34:130.
40. Silver S, Phung le T, Silver G. Silver as biocides in burn and wound dressings and bacterial resistance to silver compounds. *J Ind Microbiol Biotechnol*. 2006;33:627.

41. Mizushima Y, Okumura H, Kasukawa R. Effects of gold and platinum on necrotizing factor, skin sensitizing antibody, and complement. *Jpn J Pharmacol.* 1965;15:131.
42. Suzuki S, Okubo M, Kaise S, et al. Gold sodium thiomalate selectivity inhibits interleukin-5-mediated eosinophil survival. *J Allergy Clin Immunol.* 1995;96:251.
43. Eisler R. Chrysotherapy: A synoptic review. *Inflamm Res.* 2003;52:487.
44. Abraham GE, Himmel PB. Management of rheumatoid arthritis: Rationale for the use of colloidal metallic gold. *J Nutr Env Med.* 1997;7:295.
45. Handel ML, Nguyen LQ, Lehmann TP. Inhibition of transcription factors by anti-inflammatory and anti-rheumatic drugs: Can variability in response be overcome? *Clin Exp Pharmacol Physiol.* 2000;27:139.
46. Bhol KC, Schechter PJ. Topical nanocrystalline silver cream suppresses inflammatory cytokines and induces apoptosis of inflammatory cells in a murine model of allergic contact dermatitis. *Br J Dermatol.* 2005;152:1235.
47. Bhol KC, Alroy J, Schechter PJ. Anti-inflammatory effect of topical nanocrystalline silver cream on allergic contact dermatitis in a guinea pig model. *Clin Exp Dermatol.* 2004;29:282.
48. Banti CN, Hadjikakou SK. Anti-proliferative and anti-tumor activity of silver(I) compounds. *Metallomics.* 2013;5:569.
49. Silvestri DL, McEnery-Stonelake M. Chlorhexidine: Uses and adverse reactions. *Dermatitis.* 2013;24:112.
50. Matylevich NP, Chu CS, McManus AT, et al. Direct current reduces plasma protein extravasation after partial-thickness burn injury in rats. *J Trauma.* 1996;41:424.
51. Chu CS, Matylevich NP, McManus AT, et al. Accelerated healing with a mesh autograft/allodermal composite skin graft treated with silver nylon dressings with and without direct current in rats. *J Trauma.* 2000;49:115.
52. Tian J, Wong KK, Ho CM, et al. Topical delivery of silver nanoparticles promotes wound healing. *ChemMedChem.* 2007;2:129.
53. Lansdown ABG. *Silver in Healthcare: Its Antimicrobial Efficacy and Safety in Use.* Anderson D, ed. London: Royal Society of Chemistry, 2010:159.
54. Gauger A. Silver-coated textiles in the therapy of atopic eczema. *Curr Probl Dermatol.* 2006;33:152.
55. Gauger A, Fischer S, Mempel M, et al. Efficacy and functionality of silver-coated textiles in patients with atopic eczema. *J Eur Acad Dermat`ol Venereol.* 2006;20:534.
56. Benn TM, Westerhoff P. Nanoparticle silver released into water from commercially available sock fabrics. *Environ Sci Technol.* 2008;42:4133.
57. Larese FF, D'Agostin F, Crosera M, et al. Human skin penetration of silver nanoparticles through intact and damaged skin. *Toxicology.* 2009;255:33.
58. George R, Merten S, Wang TT, et al. In vivo analysis of dermal and systemic absorption of silver nanoparticles through healthy human skin. *Australas J Dermatol.* 2013 Sep 5. [Epub ahead of print]
59. Bouts BA. Images in clinical medicine. Argyria. *N Engl J Med.* 1999;340:1554.
60. Murata T, Kanao-Koshikawa M, Takamatsu T. Effects of Pb, Cu, Sb, In and Ag contamination on the proliferation of soil bacterial colonies, soil dehydrogenase activity, and phospholipid fatty acid profiles of soil microbial communities. *Water Air Soil Pollut.* 2005;164:103.
61. Asaad K, Mashhadi S. Topical application of silver nitrate. *Int J Low Extrem Wounds.* 2013;12:324.
62. Klasen HJ. A historical review of the use of silver in the treatment of burns. II. Renewed interest for silver. *Burns.* 2000;26:131.
63. Clement JL, Jarrett PS. Antibacterial silver. *Metal Based Drugs.* 1994;1:467.
64. Kim KJ, Sung WS, Moon SK, et al. Antifungal effect of silver nanoparticles on dermatophytes. *J Microbiol Biotechnol.* 2008;18:1482.

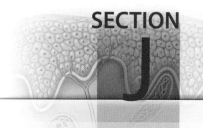

Antiaging Ingredients

C H A P T E R   8 1

Overview of Aging

CLINICAL SIGNS OF AGING

There are two main processes of skin aging, intrinsic and extrinsic.[1] Intrinsic aging is controlled by genes. The genes that contribute to skin aging have not yet been elucidated although some are thought to play a role in aging. Extrinsic aging is caused by external factors such as smoking, excessive use of alcohol, poor nutrition, and sun exposure, which in many cases can be reduced with effort. It is believed that as much as 80 percent of facial aging can be ascribed to sun exposure (extrinsic aging).[2] It is also speculated that some factors implicated in extrinsic cutaneous aging may impact the intrinsic aging process.[3]

Extrinsic aging accounts for most facial aging. Extrinsically aged skin appears predominantly in exposed areas such as the face, chest, and extensor surfaces of the arms. It is a result of the cumulative effects of a lifetime of exposure to ultraviolet radiation (UVR) and other insults such as pollution. Clinical findings of photoaged skin include fragility, thinning, wrinkles, dryness, rough texture, poor light reflection, sallowness, pigmented lesions such as lentigines (dark patches), sagging, diminished elasticity, and decreased hysteresis (ability to resume shape after deformation).

SCIENCE OF AGING SKIN

The clinical signs of aged skin are primarily thought to be caused by a loss of or dysfunction in collagen, elastin, and/or the glycosaminoglycans hyaluronic acid (HA). The goal of antiaging skin care products is to prevent the loss of collagen, elastin, and HA as well as increase the production of collagen and HA. At this time, no procedures or products have been developed to increase the production of functional elastin. Matrix metalloproteinases (MMPs), glycation, dysfunction of organelles such as mitochondria and lysosomes, telomere shortening, sirtuin expression, stem cell function, accumulation of senescent cells, and DNA damage also play a role in skin aging.

Matrix Metalloproteinases

The mechanism of action of UVR induction of collagen damage has been well characterized in the last decade. It is now known that UVR exposure dramatically upregulates the production of enzymes known as MMPs. This occurs by the following mechanism: UV exposure causes an increase in the amount of the transcription factor c-Jun; c-Fos is abundant without UV exposure. When UV exposure occurs, these two transcription factors, c-Jun and c-Fos, combine to produce activator protein (AP)-1, which activates the MMP genes resulting in production of MMPs including collagenase, gelatinase, and stromelysin. It has been demonstrated in humans that MMPs, specifically collagenase and gelatinase, are induced within hours of UVB exposure.[4] Fisher et al. showed that multiple exposures to UVB yield a sustained induction of MMPs.[5] Because collagenase degrades collagen, long-term increases in collagenase and other MMPs likely result in the disorganized and clumped collagen seen in photoaged skin.

Collagen

Collagen gives skin its strength and support – it is the scaffolding of the skin. Fibroblasts (the primary type of skin cells in the dermis) synthesize collagen in a process that requires the presence of ascorbic acid (vitamin C). The addition of vitamin C induces fibroblasts to produce more collagen. Thus, fibroblasts can be spurred by topical skin care products that contain vitamin C to generate new collagen. When UV light hits the skin, it leads to skin aging in several ways but the exposure exerts specific effects on collagen that include: 1) decreased expression of collagen genes, and 2) increased levels of the MMP enzyme collagenase. Retinoids help prevent the loss of collagen by inhibiting the formation of collagenase and blocking the downregulation of collagen gene expression.

Elastin

Elastin confers elasticity (ability to bounce back or rebound) to the skin. After puberty, fibroblasts cannot produce functional elastin. Elastase is the enzyme known to break down elastin. Sunscreens and antioxidants help prevent the loss of elastin, but there are no known ways to increase elastin levels in the skin.

Hyaluronic Acid

HA avidly binds water, affecting skin hydration, volume, and plumpness. It also influences cellular mobilization and communication. HA has become a popular injectable substance (e.g., Belotero, Juvéderm, Restylane, and Voluma) that is used to plump aged skin by increasing the levels of this key dermal component in the skin.[6] In addition, HA is a topical additive to many skin care products because of its humectant properties.

Its ability to penetrate into the skin depends on its size and the formulation of the product.

Glycation

Glycation is caused by the Maillard reaction (see Chapter 2, Basic Cosmetic Chemistry). When glycation occurs, sugar molecules attach to proteins, thus initiating a series of chemical reactions and creating "crosslinked" proteins. These crosslinked proteins, called advanced glycation endproducts (AGEs) emerge in collagen fibers. The formation of the crosslinks that bind collagen fibers to each other may render the skin stiffer. Glycosylated collagen is thought to play a role in the appearance of aged skin.[7] Elastin can also be affected by glycation. Photoaged skin is characterized by the impaired ability to rebound and when seen under a microscope exhibits elastin that is abnormally clumped together. This is known as elastosis. Recent research has found that these clumps are likely caused by glycation, since the adhering elastin is stiff and devoid of its usual springiness. Therefore, glycation most likely plays a role in the damage seen in the collagen and elastin of aged skin.

Mitochondria

Every human cell contains mitochondria inside the cytoplasm, ranging in number based on tissue and cell type. These organelles play a crucial role because they are responsible for the energy production that drives all cellular processes. Diseases of the mitochondria are devastating and dysfunction of the mitochondria is believed to play an important role in aging.[8] The mitochondria produce energy by converting adenosine diphosphate (ADP) to adenosine triphosphate (ATP). This complicated process occurs in the intricate inner membranes of the mitochondria.

During the process of forming ATP, which is called oxidative phosphorylation, the mitochondria use oxygen as a carrier for electrons and the flow of electrons generates energy that is stored in ATP. The electrons are then bound to oxygen and carried off, usually as water. Oxygen is consumed in this process. Energy production in the mitochondria results in an excess number of electrons, many of which are bound to oxygen to form water. The electrons are innocuous when bound to oxygen in even numbers. However, some of the electrons slip out and singly bind oxygen, leading to a superoxide compound also known as a free radical. These free radicals cause damage to the mitochondrial membranes, mitochondrial DNA, and low-density lipoprotein cholesterol, which is a component of cell membranes. Mitochondrial DNA code for proteins present in the membranes of the mitochondria that are necessary for energy production. Mutations of mitochondrial DNA engender disorder in the energy production process and can lead to an increased number of free radicals. The cycle is perpetuated as these free radicals cause more mitochondrial DNA mutations.

Mitochondrial damage must be prevented in order to slow aging but not much is known about how to accomplish this. For the last five to eight years dermatologists who perform copious light and laser procedures have begun to suspect that the wavelengths of light may have effects on the skin that transcend what is presently understood. The currently accepted mechanisms of action of lasers and light-emitting diodes do not adequately explain how skin appearance is ameliorated in these procedures. Scientists have begun to suspect that the light exerts effects on mitochondria.[9] Certain wavelengths may stimulate mitochondria to work more effectively while UV light may deleteriously

affect the mitochondria.[10] The role of mitochondria, lasers, and lights in skin appearance is under active investigation and, ideally, breakthroughs may be seen relatively soon.

Lysosomes

Lysosomes are intracellular organelles that function to degrade or recycle cellular waste products into basic components that can be used as raw materials to form new cellular products. In addition, lysosomes, which are composed of various enzymes, break down toxic waste into less harmful substances. Each enzyme within a lysosome has a specific function. In order for a lysosome to do its job of ridding cells of waste it needs the following: 1) the correct enzymes; 2) the ideal pH (or acidity) for that enzyme to work (different enzymes operate more efficiently under different pH environments); and 3) energy produced by the mitochondria known as ATP. The lysosome membrane contains a pump that requires energy (ATP) to propel hydrogen ions into the lysosome to maintain its acidity.

Dysfunction of the lysosome, which allows cellular waste products to accumulate inside the cell, leads to several disorders, called lysosomal storage diseases (e.g., Tay–Sachs disease and Gaucher's disease). Lysosomes are not able to degrade all cellular waste; what remains from lysosomal digestion is called lipofuscin. The accumulation of lipofuscin is seen in aged cells.[11] Under a microscope and with proper staining, lipofuscin appears fluorescent and is thus easily visualized. Studies have shown that oxidative stress by free radicals leads to an increase in lipofuscin. Accumulation of lipofuscin hampers the ability of lysozymes to work effectively, altering acidity and disrupting the supply of enzymes.[12] In other words, the amassing of lipofuscin cellular waste contributes to cutaneous aging. Treatments to prevent this form of aging would have to achieve one of the following: 1) enhance lysosomal function, 2) increase breakdown of lipofuscin and cellular waste, 3) reduce free radical formation, or 4) enhance lysosomal function.

Medical discoveries often occur first in areas of severe disease because these advances are most needed and may receive the most attention and funding. Gaucher's disease, which is a severe disorder caused by a lack of a lysosomal enzyme, is successfully treated with intravenous infusion of the missing enzyme.[13] Genetic treatments are being developed for Tay–Sachs disease. At this time, there are no published data on skin aging or skin appearance and the role of lipofuscin. Although it is likely that skin with increased lipofuscin appears older, this research has not been conducted. It is not yet known if there are any particular enzyme deficiencies that lead to increased or accelerated skin aging.

Telomere Shortening

Telomeres are repetitive nucleotide sequences that compose the terminal portions of mammalian chromosomes. Their presence at the ends of chromosomes prevents deterioration or fusion with nearby chromosomes. However, the enzyme DNA polymerase cannot replicate the final base pairs of the chromosome curing cellular and chromosomal division. Consequently, these terminal sequences are continuously lost on replication, which results in the shortening of the chromosome. Since telomeres shorten with age, their erosion has become an important measure of cellular aging, a veritable internal clock.[14] Apoptosis, or cell death, is triggered when telomeres become "too short," thus precluding further replication. It is important to note that UV exposure contributes to telomere shortening and signaling through the tumor-suppressor protein p53 after telomere disruption, which is typically observed in skin aging and photodamage.[15] Therefore, telomeres are thought to play a role in extrinsic as well as intrinsic aging.[16]

Telomeres are also thought to play a role in cancer. A recent paper suggests that the photoaging and melanogenesis provoked by UV exposure is linked to telomere-based DNA damage signaling that may actually represent a cancer-avoidance protective response.[17] The enzyme telomerase, which stabilizes or lengthens telomeres, is expressed in approximately 90 percent of all tumors but is absent in many tissues.[14] The epidermis is one of the few regenerative tissues to express telomerase.[18] Telomerase is believed to act against excessive telomere loss in human epidermis throughout the lifelong regeneration process.[19] There are several products that claim to help lengthen or preserve telomeres, but such claims are not well substantiated in the author's opinion. The exact role and importance of telomere length in skin aging is not known.

Sirtuins

Sirtuins (SIRTs) are a family of NAD+ dependent protein deacetylases that regulate the biologic functions of proteins. There are seven known types of SIRTs found in humans, with SIRT1, the most extensively studied, known to guard against cellular oxidative stress and DNA damage. SIRTs are involved in the cutaneous response to UV and are believed to play a role in aging.[20] Interest in SIRTs first emerged when researchers noticed that calorie-restricted rodents lived longer than animals whose calories were not restricted.[21] SIRTs were found to have been upregulated in these calorie-restricted rodents, and that certain types of mice that overexpressed SIRT6 had significantly extended life spans.[21,22] Another study showed that brain-specific overexpression of SIRT1 was also shown to extend the life span.[23] In 2003, investigators learned that small molecules could be used to activate SIRT expression.[24] This generated a search for molecules that would influence SIRTs expression. Suddenly, cosmetic companies began launching products that "stimulate sirtuins expression." Unfortunately, not enough is yet known about SIRTs and their influence on the aging process to warrant such inflated skin care product claims. However, it will be interesting to watch as SIRTs research develops.

Stem Cells

Stem cells have the potential to transform into other types of cells. They are distinguished from other cell types by two important characteristics. First, they are unspecialized cells capable of dividing and forming new "daughter" cells. Second, under certain physiologic or experimental conditions, stem cells can be induced to become specific types of cells with special functions. Stem cells certainly play an important role in medicine and have been used to repair brain, heart, and pancreatic cells among other uses. However, stem cells must be cultured in particular conditions and would not survive in a skin care product on a shelf. Stem cells are being used in chronic wounds, but they are grown in controlled laboratory conditions and do not sit on a shelf in uncontrolled conditions.[25] In addition, the stem cells in skin care products are derived from apples and other nonmammalian sources. There is no reason to believe that these formulations will be efficacious in human skin.

Senescent Cells

Aged cells that lose their ability to divide and respond to environmental changes are known as senescent cells. Cellular senescence is important because it is the way the body naturally rids itself of dysfunctional or damaged cells—they stop functioning and become senescent. Cancer is a disease that occurs when cells lose the ability to become senescent and continue dividing and reproducing even though they are damaged. The accumulation of senescent cells is characteristic of aged skin, and it is believed that the presence of senescent cells leads to cutaneous aging.[26] Inflammation has been believed for several years to play a role in aging, but the mechanism of action has not been elucidated. New research demonstrates how inflammation contributes to an increase in senescent cells, and this may provide a clue as to how inflammation promotes aging.[27] It is likely that the accumulation of these nonfunctioning senescent cells can damage surrounding "healthy" cells. Senescent cells likely gather around fibroblasts and other skin cells rendering them stiffer and unable to function properly. It is possible that senescent cells may secrete proteins and other substances that are deleterious to surrounding cells.

DNA Damage

It is well known that UV radiation leads to DNA damage by formation of thymine dimers. Thymine dimers develop when nucleic acid base pairs bind together causing a disruption of the DNA. Damage to DNA is known to lead to skin cancer but likely plays a role in skin aging. The exact role of DNA damage in skin aging is not known because the genes that cause skin aging have not been identified.

■ PREVENTION OF AGING

Sunscreen prevents aging by minimizing UV damage and blocking or decreasing the formation of free radicals and inflammation. HA may protect collagen from degradation through the activity of interleukin (IL)-1.[28] Antioxidants, such as tocopherol (vitamin E) and ascorbic acid, protect collagen and elastin from glycation and damage by free radicals, which are known to promote aging.[29] Retinoids decrease the breakdown of collagen by lowering MMP levels and increasing collagen synthesis.

Antioxidants

The free radical theory of aging, proposed by Harman in 1956, is one of the most widely accepted theories to explain the cause of aging.[30,31] Free radicals are compounds formed when oxygen molecules combine with other molecules yielding an odd number of electrons. An oxygen molecule with paired electrons is stable; however, oxygen with an unpaired electron is "reactive" because it seeks and seizes electrons from vital components leaving them damaged.[32] DNA, cytoskeletal elements, cellular proteins, and cellular membranes may all be adversely affected by activated oxygen species (see Chapter 2, Basic Cosmetic Chemistry).[33,34]

Antioxidants give oxygen the missing electron it craves and thus neutralize free radicals, rendering them harmless. By neutralizing free radicals, antioxidants are able to mitigate cutaneous damage as well as the effects of aging, "preventing aging" in a sense (see Chapter 46, Antioxidants, for a lengthier discussion).

Free radicals may also increase glycation by more rapidly converting AGE precursors into pernicious AGEs. Although antioxidants are beneficial for many reasons, they do not seem to aid in abrogating the glycation process. This is due to the fact that once the Schiff base is formed, it is unstable. The use of antioxidants may block one pathway, but the Schiff base can move down another pathway that still results in the development of harmful free radicals (see Chapter 2, Basic Cosmetic Chemistry, for details on the Schiff base).

Peptides

Peptides are short chains of amino acids, which are the building blocks of proteins. In typical cellular settings, peptides communicate between DNA and the cellular network. It is thought, then, that peptides can be used to direct cells to maintain youthful behavior, yielding a stable, non-aging manifestation. However, while peptides play several important roles in skin, one of the functions of the skin is to prevent penetration of peptides and proteins. Consequently, most topically applied peptides fail to penetrate into the skin. Some products appear to exert antiaging activity, but most evidence of effectiveness comes from *in vitro* studies, however, or small *in vivo* investigations.

The four main types of peptides used in topical or cosmeceutical products include signal peptides, enzyme-inhibitor peptides, neurotransmitter-inhibitor peptides (or neuropeptides), and carrier peptides.[35] Insulin is an example of a peptide that has useful activity (regulating blood sugar), but it must be injected to penetrate the skin barrier, as topical vehicles such as creams or patches, have failed to achieve absorption. In addition to limited skin penetration, peptides are difficult to formulate in skin care products because they are reactive and tend to interfere with other product ingredients, thus reducing their shelf life. For these reasons, topical peptide-containing creams will likely be shown to have limited utility in treating skin aging until the penetration technology is improved. Popular peptide ingredients seen in antiaging skin care include palmitoyl pentapeptide (Matrixyl) and acetyl hexapeptide-3 (Argireline). A full discussion of peptides is beyond the scope of this text.

Retinoids

In the 1970s, female patients that were being treated with tretinoin for acne noticed that their wrinkles improved.[36] This observation was followed by a clinical trial that showed that patients treated with tretinoin displayed improvement of photodamaged skin.[37] A plethora of clinical trials have confirmed such early observations and now it is well known that retinoids are the most efficacious ingredients to treat photodamaged skin.[38] For this reason, an entire chapter is dedicated to the use of retinoids in antiaging skin care products [see Chapter 83, Retinoids (Retinol)]. The acne section also contains a chapter on the use of retinoids in acne (see Chapter 79, Retinol, Retinyl Esters, and Retinoic Acid).

CONCLUSION

In summary, skin aging is a complex process. Although many of the mechanisms such as the production of MMPs have been deciphered, much remains to be uncovered regarding the role of genes, telomeres, and organelles, such as mitochondria, in the aging process. Although many companies tout products that claim to affect "genes associated with skin aging," these statements are greatly inflated. The genes that are being referred to in these boasts are usually the collagen and HA genes. There are several processes beyond collagen and HA gene biochemistry that lead to cutaneous aging that have not been characterized or are poorly understood. However, we will likely learn much more about the skin aging process in the near future. In the meantime, a daily regimen consisting of sunscreen, antioxidants, and retinoids at night is scientifically justified.

REFERENCES

1. Baumann L, Saghari S. Photoaging. In: Baumann L, Saghari S, Weisberg E, eds. *Cosmetic Dermatology: Principles and Practice*. 2nd ed. New York: McGraw-Hill, 2009:34–35.
2. Uitto J. Understanding premature skin aging. *N Engl J Med*. 1997;337:1463.
3. Farage MA, Miller KW, Elsner P, et al. Intrinsic and extrinsic factors in skin ageing: A review. *Int J Cosmet Sci*. 2008;30:87.
4. Fisher GJ, Datta SC, Talwar HS, et al. Molecular basis of sun-induced premature skin ageing and retinoid antagonism. *Nature*. 1996;379:335.
5. Fisher GJ, Wang ZQ, Datta SC, et al. Pathophysiology of premature skin aging induced by ultraviolet light. *N Engl J Med*. 1997;337:1419.
6. Baumann L, Blyumin M, Saghari S. Dermal fillers. In: Baumann L, Saghari S, Weisberg E, eds. *Cosmetic Dermatology: Principles and Practice*. 2nd ed. New York: McGraw-Hill, 2009:195–200.
7. Pageon H, Bakala H, Monnier VM, et al. Collagen glycation triggers the formation of aged skin in vitro. *Eur J Dermatol*. 2007;17:12.
8. Beal MF. Mitochondria take center stage in aging and neurodegeneration. *Ann Neurol*. 2005;58:495.
9. Karu TI, Pyatibrat LV, Kolyakov SF, et al. Absorption measurements of cell monolayers relevant to mechanisms of laser phototherapy: Reduction or oxidation of cytochrome c oxidase under laser radiation at 632.8 nm. *Photomed Laser Surg*. 2008;26:593.
10. Krutmann J, Schroeder P. Role of mitochondria in photoaging of human skin: The defective powerhouse model. *J Investig Dermatol Symp Proc*. 2009;14:44.
11. Jung T, Bader N, Grune T. Lipofuscin: Formation, distribution, and metabolic consequences. *Ann N Y Acad Sci*. 2007;1119:97.
12. Terman A, Kurz T, Navratil M, et al. Mitochondrial turnover and aging of long-lived postmitotic cells: The mitochondrial-lysosomal axis theory of aging. *Antioxid Redox Signal*. 2010;12:503.
13. Barton NW, Brady RO, Dambrosia JM, et al. Replacement therapy for inherited enzyme deficiency – Macrophage-targeted glucocerebrosidase for Gaucher's disease. *N Engl J Med*. 1991;324:1464.
14. Boukamp P. Ageing mechanisms: The role of telomere loss. *Clin Exp Dermatol*. 2001;26:562.
15. Kosmadaki MG, Gilchrest BA. The role of telomeres in skin aging/photoaging. *Micron*. 2004;35:155.
16. Saghari S, Baumann L. Wrinkled skin. In: Baumann L, Saghari S, Weisberg E, eds. *Cosmetic Dermatology: Principles and Practice*, 2nd ed. New York: McGraw-Hill, 2009:145–147.
17. Gilchrest BA, Eller MS, Yaar M. Telomere-mediated effects on melanogenesis and skin aging. *J Investig Dermatol Symp Proc*. 2009;14:25.
18. Boukamp P. Skin aging: A role for telomerase and telomere dynamics? *Curr Mol Med*. 2005;5:171.
19. Krunic D, Moshir S, Greulich-Bode KM, et al. Tissue context-activated telomerase in human epidermis correlates with little age-dependent telomere loss. *Biochim Biophys Acta*. 2009;1792:297.
20. Benavente CA, Schnell SA, Jacobson EL. Effects of niacin restriction on sirtuin and PARP responses to photodamage in human skin. *PLoS One*. 2012;7:e42276.
21. Guarente L. Calorie restriction and sirtuins revisited. *Genes Dev*. 2013;27:2072.
22. Kanfi Y, Naiman S, Amir G, et al. The sirtuin SIRT6 regulates lifespan in male mice. *Nature*. 2012;483:218.
23. Satoh A, Brace CS, Ben-Josef G, et al. SIRT1 promotes the central adaptive response to diet restriction through activation of the dorsomedial and lateral nuclei of the hypothalamus. *J Neurosci*. 2010;30:10220.
24. Howitz KT, Bitterman KJ, Cohen HY, et al. Small molecule activators of sirtuins extend Saccharomyces cerevisiae lifespan. *Nature*. 2003;425:191.

25. Dabiri G, Heiner D, Falanga V. The emerging use of bone marrow-derived mesenchymal stem cells in the treatment of human chronic wounds. *Expert Opin Emerg Drugs*. 2013;18:405.

26. Dimri GP, Lee X, Basile G, et al. A biomarker that identifies senescent human cells in culture and in aging skin in vivo. *Proc Natl Acad Sci U S A*. 1995;92:9363.

27. Yang HH, Kim C, Jung B, et al. Involvement of IGF binding protein 5 in prostaglandin E(2)-induced cellular senescence in human fibroblasts. *Biogerontology*. 2011;12:239.

28. Nawrat P, Surazyński A, Karna E, et al. The effect of hyaluronic acid on interleukin-1-induced deregulation of collagen metabolism in cultured human skin fibroblasts. *Pharmacol Res*. 2005;51:473.

29. Pillai S, Oresajo C, Hayward J. Ultraviolet radiation and skin aging: Roles of reactive oxygen species, inflammation and protease activation, and strategies for prevention of inflammation-induced matrix degradation – A review. *Int J Cosmet Sci*. 2005;27:17.

30. Harman D. Aging: A theory based on free radical and radiation chemistry. *J Gerontol*. 1956;11:298.

31. Pelle E, Maes D, Padulo GA, et al. An in vitro model to test relative antioxidant potential: Ultraviolet-induced lipid peroxidation in liposomes. *Arch Biochem Biophys*. 1990;283:234.

32. Werninghaus K. The role of antioxidants in reducing photodamage. In: Gilchrest B ed. *Photodamage*. London: Blackwell Science Inc., 1995:249.

33. Greenstock CL. *Free Radicals, Aging, and Degenerative Diseases*. New York: Alan R. Liss, Inc., 1986.

34. Rikans LE, Hornbrook KR. Lipid peroxidation, antioxidant protection and aging. *Biochim Biophys Acta*. 1997;1362:116.

35. Gorouhi F, Maibach HI. Role of topical peptides in preventing or treating aged skin. *Int J Cosmet Sci*. 2009;31:327.

36. Kligman L, Kligman AM. Photoaging – Retinoids, alpha hydroxy acids, and antioxidants, In: Gabard B, Elsner P, Surber C, Treffel P, eds. *Dermatopharmacology of Topical Preparations*. New York: Springer, 2000:383.

37. Kligman AM, Grove GL, Hirose R, et al. Topical tretinoin for photoaged skin. *J Am Acad Dermatol*. 1986;15:836.

38. Baumann L, Saghari S. Retinoids. In: Baumann L, Saghari S, Weisberg E, eds. *Cosmetic Dermatology: Principles and Practice*. 2nd ed. New York: McGraw-Hill, 2009:256–262.

CHAPTER 82

Hydroxy Acids

Activities:

Anti-inflammatory, exfoliating, antiacne, depigmenting, moisturizing

Important Chemical Components:

Mostly carbon, hydrogen, and oxygen
Molecular formulas:
Citric acid: $C_6H_8O_7$
Gluconolactone $C_6H_{10}O_6$
Glycolic acid: $C_2H_4O_3$
Lactic acid: $C_3H_6O_3$
Malic acid: $C_4H_6O_5$
Mandelic acid: $C_8H_8O_3$
Phytic acid: $C_6H_{18}O_{24}P_6$
Salicylic acid: $C_7H_6O_3$
Tartaric acid: $C_4H_6O_6$

Origin Classification:

Acids are all found in natural sources, but are synthesized in the laboratory for use in chemical peels and other products.

Personal Care Category:

Antiaging, exfoliant, brightening, antiacne, moisturizer

Recommended for the following Baumann Skin Types:

DRNW, DRPW, DSNW, DSPW, ORNW, ORPW, OSNW, and OSPW. Hydroxy acids are used in all Baumann Skin Types but the choice of hydroxy acid depends on the individual skin type. All of the acids discussed in this chapter are useful in wrinkle-prone skin types. Acids used for acne indications are discussed in the acne section of this text.

SOURCE

Found in plants but also manufactured in the laboratory, α-hydroxy acids (AHAs), polyhydroxy acids (PHAs), and β-hydroxy acid (BHA) are naturally-occurring organic acids that induce exfoliation and accelerate the cell cycle. The plant source depends on the type of hydroxy acid. There are several types of AHAs: citric acid from citrus fruits; glycolic acid from sugar cane, grapes, sugar beets, and Virginia creeper leaves; malic acid from fruits such as cherries and apples; mandelic acid from bitter almond; lactic acid from dairy as well as fermented vegetables and fruit; phytic acid from rice; and tartaric acid from grapes.[1]

PHAs, also known as polyhydroxy bionic acids (PHBAs), include gluconolactone and lactobionic acid.[2] They were developed to deliver the antiaging efficacy of AHAs without the irritation or increased vulnerability to ultraviolet (UV) radiation due to their antioxidant effects (Table 82-1).

TABLE 82-1
Pros and Cons of Hydroxy Acids

Pros	Cons
Many studies demonstrating efficacy	May cause stinging
Low cost	Increased sun sensitivity (AHAs)
SA exhibits anti-inflammatory and antiacne activity	May interact with other ingredients and products
PHAs have antioxidant capability	Knowledge of chemistry is necessary for proper use
Humectant	

BHA, also known as salicylic acid (SA), is found in willow bark, almonds, water chestnuts, peanuts, and some fruits and vegetables. There is only one type of BHA, as compared to the several types of AHA and PHA. BHA can also be produced in the laboratory from phenylalanine or by hydrolysis of aspirin (acetylsalicylic acid) or oil of wintergreen (methyl salicylate).

HISTORY

Cleopatra was said to have routinely bathed in sour milk.[3] If this is true, it is the first known use of a hydroxy acid (lactic acid) to improve the skin's appearance. Fermented grape skins, rife with tartartic acid, were collected from the bottoms of wine barrels by women in ancient Rome and used topically to enhance beauty.[3] More recently, books (and movies) such as *Gone with the Wind* have referred to the use of buttermilk to remove "sun spots." AHAs, especially lactic acid, were first used in dermatology to treat dry skin, psoriasis, and other conditions. Lactic and glycolic acids have been used therapeutically since the 1970s.[4] In the 1990s, Van Scott and his group noticed that glycolic acid improved photodamaged skin. In 1992, Van Scott and Yu filed a patent on the use of glycolic acid for treating wrinkles and subsequently formed the company NeoStrata.[5] AHAs became one of the most popular antiaging skin ingredients and enjoyed widespread acceptance until the United States Food and Drug Administration (FDA) began questioning their safety with concomitant sun exposure. The FDA ultimately mandated that AHA product labels contain a sun safety label. This FDA scrutiny, along with the desire to develop a less irritating hydroxy acid, provided the impetus for Drs. Van Scott and Yu to later develop PHAs. The most popular PHA marketed today is gluconolactone.[6]

The Greek physician Hippocrates described using willow bark in childbirth for pain in the late 4th century BCE.[7,8] It was not until the 19th century that SA was isolated from the bark of the willow tree by the German chemist Johann Andreas Buchner in 1828.[9] The active extract was called salicin, after the Latin name for the white willow (*Salix alba*). (For a more detailed history on the use of salicylic acid in medicine, see Chapter 78, Salicylic Acid.) In the late 1990s, people began to incorrectly refer to SA as a BHA, most likely to associate it with the popular AHAs that were penetrating the antiaging skin care market at the

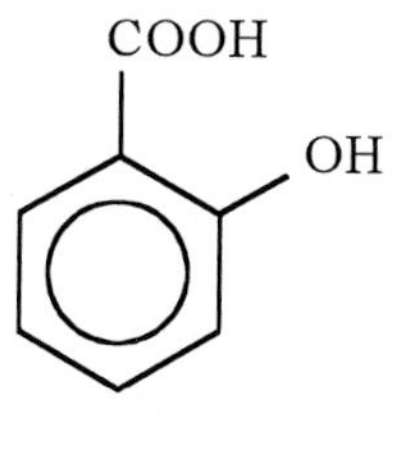

COOH

OH

Salicylic Acid

▲ **FIGURE 82-1** Salicylic Acid. Chemical structure of salicylic acid, with its hydroxy group in the β position.

time. BHA products are not required to contain the "sun safety" label that AHAs are directed to display.

CHEMISTRY

All AHAs have a terminal carboxyl group with one or two hydroxyl groups on the second or α-carbon and a variable length carbon chain. The two shortest carbon chain acids, glycolic (2-hydroxyethanoic) and lactic (2-hydroxypropanoic), are the most commonly used in dermatology.[10]

SA is improperly called a BHA because the aromatic carboxylic acid has a hydroxyl group in the β position (Figure 82-1). This designation is a misnomer insofar as the carbons of aromatic compounds are traditionally given Arabic numerals (1, 2, etc.) rather than the Greek letter designations typical for the nonaromatic structures. However, the term BHA is commonly used.

PHAs, such as lactobionic acid, are carboxylic acids with two or more hydroxyl groups attached to carbon atoms or an alicyclic chain. It is essential that at least one hydroxyl group be attached to the α position. Attaching a sugar molecule to the PHA structure yields a polysaccharide known as bionic acid.

Hydroxy acid solutions contain free acid forms and salt forms that exist in equilibrium based on the pH of the solution. The most important aspect of hydroxy acid strength is the amount of available free acid. The amount of free acid itself is affected by the following: the concentration of hydroxy acid, the pK_a of the hydroxy acid, and the pH of the solution (which is also influenced by the type of vehicle used), and whether or not the peel is buffered. For a detailed discussion of pH and pK_a, see Chapter 2, Basic Cosmetic Chemistry. It is difficult to know the strength of a hydroxy acid-containing product by reading the label because these important details are not listed. The exfoliative, toxic, and abrasive action as well as absorption into the skin of hydroxy acid products increase with higher concentration and lower pH.[1,11]

ORAL USES

Although hydroxy acids are available in food, their oral use has no known role in the treatment of skin conditions at this time.

TOPICAL USES

Multiple studies have demonstrated success using AHA and BHA products in the treatment of photoaging by ameliorating fine lines, ephelides (freckles), lentigines, mottled pigmentation, and surface roughness. Actinic and seborrheic keratoses have also been effectively treated with AHAs and BHA.[12] Topical preparations that contain hydroxy acids exert profound

influence on epidermal keratinization by speeding the cell cycle and decreasing corneocyte cohesiveness, leading to increased desquamation.[13–15] The topical application of AHAs and BHA in high concentrations results in the detachment of keratinocytes (skin cells) and epidermolysis, which can cause erosions and blisters. Application at lower concentrations attenuates intercorneocyte cohesion directly above the granular layer, advancing desquamation and thinning of the stratum corneum (SC) but not the epidermis.[15] Two major effects emerge: acceleration of the cell cycle (which is slowed in aged skin) and increased desquamation, which yields improved skin tone and light reflection (radiance) as well as a smoother skin surface. AHAs confer a moisturizing effect and are beneficial in dry skin because they function as humectants, assisting the skin in holding onto water. They also enhance desquamation thereby normalizing the SC by eliminating the clinging keratinocytes that leave the skin looking rough and scaled. Once desquamation is enhanced, the skin is more flexible and better able to reflect light. Phytic acid was among several bioactive constituents in rice bran incorporated into topical formulations containing niosomes recently found to be effective in imparting antiaging benefits in 30 human volunteers.[16] In addition to photodamage, hydroxy acids have been used to treat a wide range of cutaneous conditions, including actinic keratosis, melasma, ichthyosis, psoriasis, warts, hyperpigmentation, acne, and rosacea.

Glycolic Acid

In 1996, Ditre demonstrated that topically applying AHAs generated significant changes histologically, with a 25 percent increase in skin thickness, increased acid mucopolysaccharides in the dermis, enhanced elastic fiber quality, and augmented collagen density.[17] Two years later, Kim et al. showed *in vitro* that glycolic acid treatments increased fibroblast proliferation and collagen synthesis.[18] A significant decline in wrinkle score and an increase in the amount of collagen synthesized in mice treated with glycolic acid was subsequently reported by Moon et al.[19] In 2001, Bernstein et al. found that topically applied glycolic acid enhanced collagen gene expression in skin biopsy specimens, and increased epidermal and dermal hyaluronic acid immunohistochemical staining between glycolic acid-treated and vehicle-treated skin.[20] Okano et al. further explored these findings two years later, and demonstrated that glycolic acid placed in cell cultures directly accelerated collagen production by fibroblasts, and increased interleukin-1α release from keratinocytes thereby affecting matrix degradation.[21]

Lactic Acid

Antiaging benefits similar to those imparted by glycolic acid have also been associated with lactic acid, which has been hypothesized to be part of the natural moisturizing factor of the skin that plays a role in hydration (see Chapter 7, Moisturizing Agents).[22] Several studies in the 1980s on the activity of buffered 12 percent ammonium lactate lotion documented its moisturizing ability.[23] One study demonstrated an increase in skin firmness and thickness as well as improvement in skin texture and moisturization using 5 and 12 percent lactic acid. These effects were seen only in the epidermis, with no dermal changes in firmness or thickness noted.[24] In 2006, Yamamoto et al. found that longer treatment intervals, once daily for six weeks, with glycolic and lactic acids led to improvements in epidermal as well as dermal constituents, suggesting the suitability of the primary AHAs in ameliorating photodamaged skin.[4]

Rendl et al. investigated the effects of lactic acid-containing creams on the secretion of cytokines by keratinocytes in human reconstructed epidermis, finding that topically applied lactic acid modulated the secretion of vascular endothelial growth factor (VEGF) by keratinocytes.[25] Interestingly, lactic acid is one of the few ingredients available in the United States in the same strength in prescription and over-the-counter (OTC) form. LacHydrin™ is approved by the FDA as a drug for use in dry skin, but not for photoaged skin. OTC products that contain lactic acid to treat photoaged skin are readily available, however.

BHA

In 1992, Swinehart demonstrated that 50 percent SA was effective in treating patients with actinically-induced pigmentary changes on the hands and forearms.[26] These effects are likely due to increased exfoliation and a quickened cell cycle, similar to the effects observed with AHAs. However, unlike AHAs, BHA alters the arachidonic acid cascade and, therefore, exhibits anti-inflammatory capabilities. For this reason, SA is often used in the treatment of acne (see Chapter 78, Salicylic Acid). Notably, BHA has a tendency to dry the skin and, therefore, is not the best choice for individuals with dry skin types.

Polyhydroxy Acids

PHAs, found naturally in humans and other natural sources, are characterized as milder and less irritating than AHAs, but are related to AHAs insofar as they have a hydroxyl group on the α-carbon and share some biochemical properties.[27] The lactonic structure of gluconolactone, one of the most popular PHAs, allows it to conceal its acidic nature, and renders it suitable for sensitive skin.[28] Some PHAs exhibit antioxidant activity due to their ability to chelate metal. Protective antioxidant constituents of PHAs likely account for the fact that these compounds do not increase the number of sunburn cells after UV exposure. One of the most popular PHAs in skin care products is gluconolactone. In 2004, Bernstein et al. exposed fibroblast cultures culled from the skin of transgenic mice to UVB and demonstrated that glycolic acid-treated skin evinced a significant increase in sunburn cells, whereas gluconolactone-treated skin did not.[27] The investigators attributed the protective mechanism of gluconolactone to its ability to function as a metal-chelating agent and its potency in scavenging free radicals.

Uneven Skin Tone and Dyspigmentation

Researchers have not yet completely elucidated how hydroxy acids improve unwanted pigmentation engendered by sun exposure but it appears that these compounds exert separate effects on the keratinocytes and the melanocytes. In the epidermis, the principal effect is diminished superficial keratinocyte (corneocyte) cohesion leading to desquamation of the pigmented keratinocytes with the intention that the newly formed keratinocytes will contain less pigment.[29] It also helps to increase the keratinocyte turnover rate (accelerating and shortening the cell cycle). By speeding up the keratinocyte transition from birth to desquamation known as the cell cycle, this decreases the amount of time that the melanocyte has to produce melanin (pigment) and transfer it to the keratinocytes (see Chapter 32, Overview of the Pigmentation Process).

In addition, hydroxy acids may directly inhibit the formation of melanin by blocking tyrosinase. Support for this was seen in a study that showed that in melanoma cells, AHAs directly inhibited tyrosinase activity leading to decreased melanin formation.[30] A new superficial chemical peel (Theraderm®) that combines AHAs, vitamin C and oxygen was shown by Kim in 2013 to be safe and effective for the treatment of melasma in 25 Korean patients (Fitzpatrick skin types IV and V), with significant improvement of hyperpigmentation observed.[31]

Comparison Studies

In 2008, Oresajo et al. compared the efficacy and clinical tolerance of a glycolic acid peel (20–50 percent) to a 5 to 10 percent capryloyl salicylic acid, a then-new SA-derived peel, in a split-face study in 50 women between 35 and 60 years old with hyperpigmented skin as well as fine lines and wrinkles. Forty-four participants completed the study, with 41 percent of the capryloyl salicylic acid group and 30 percent of the glycolic group experiencing significant improvement in fine lines and wrinkles compared to baseline. Significant reduction in hyperpigmentation compared to baseline was observed in 46 percent of the subjects treated with capryloyl salicylic acid and 34 percent of those treated with glycolic acid. There were no statistically significant differences between the groups, though the investigators cited the apparent superiority of the new product, which, in five to 10 percent concentrations, they found to be generally safe and as effective as 20 to 50 percent glycolic acid in treating signs of photoaging.[32]

The next year, Kornhauser et al. assessed whether topically applied hydroxy acids, specifically glycolic and salicylic, alter the short-term effects of solar simulated radiation in the skin of 14 human subjects. Participants were treated in three of four areas on the mid-back daily Monday through Friday for 3.5 weeks with 10 percent glycolic acid, 2 percent SA, or vehicle, with the fourth area receiving no treatment. Each site was exposed to solar simulated radiation after the final treatment and shave biopsies on each site were collected. The researchers found that sensitivity to solar simulated radiation, as measured by increased erythema, DNA damage, and sunburn cell formation, was amplified by glycolic acid and unaffected by SA.[33]

In 2010, Abdel-Daim et al. evaluated the photo-chemopreventive effect of 35 percent glycolic acid dissolved in distilled water, 30 percent SA in ethanol, and 10 or 35 percent trichloroacetic acid in distilled water on the UV-exposed skin of hairless mice. Tumor formation in the treated area, and beyond, was reduced by all of the peeling agents, with retention of p53-positive abnormal cells and mRNA expression of cyclooxygenase-2 diminished in treated skin. Serum prostaglandin E_2 was also lowered. The investigators concluded that use of these agents could confer a chemopreventive effect by eliminating photodamaged cells.[34]

<h2>■ SAFETY ISSUES</h2>

α-Hydroxy Acids

AHAs increase desquamation, which may leave the epidermis more vulnerable to UV radiation by thinning the SC. Lai et al. demonstrated that combining glycolic acid with UVB exposure inhibited cell proliferation and induced apoptosis (cell death). The mechanisms of apoptosis induced by co-treatment of glycolic acid and UVB are likely related to cell cycle arrest.[35] Another study showed that use of AHA on UV-exposed skin led to an increase in sunburn cells and a lower minimal erythema dose (MED) upon UVB exposure.[36] This sensitivity to UV resolved after one week of stopping the glycolic acid products. Although one study revealed that glycolic acid imparted a photoprotective effect,[37] all subsequent studies have indicated increased photosensitivity following the application of AHAs.[36,38,39] Concern about the safety of AHA use in cosmetic products led to a safety evaluation of AHAs by the Cosmetic Ingredient Review (CIR). The FDA committee reviewed the data and issued a guidance (an interim step prior to a regulation) calling for labels of AHA-containing cosmetic products (see FDA Labeling Guidelines). Although this FDA guidance led consumers to wonder if AHAs "thin the skin," the reverse is actually true. Guinea pigs treated with glycolic acid had approximately a twofold *increase* in epidermal thickness and almost double the number of nucleated cell layers as compared with the control group.[40] In addition, AHAs have been shown to counteract the epidermal thinning that occurs with prolonged topical steroid use.[41] These studies illustrate that although the SC is thinned by AHAs, the overall epidermis is thicker. OTC products are limited to a maximum 10 percent AHA concentration by the FDA.[42]

In 2011, Okuda et al. evaluated *in vitro* the potential skin penetration of lactic and malic acids in rinse-off personal care products, and compared them to rinse-off and leave-on exposures to 10 percent glycolic acid, finding that there is nominal penetration of AHAs. They concluded that UV-induced skin effects of rinse-off shampoos and conditioners that contain AHAs are negligible.[11]

BHA

When ingested, SA exerts a possible ototoxic effect.[43] It can induce transient hearing loss in zinc-deficient individuals. For this reason, high percentages of SA (20–30 percent) should not be applied to the entire body in one session. Instead, different segments of the body should be treated at different times. This is more applicable to the use of in-office peels and not to the OTC preparations that usually contain only 0.5 to 3 percent SA.

There are no studies specifically addressing the safety of topical SA in pregnancy and most dermatologists advise against using it on large areas of the body or in high percentages when pregnant. This caution is due to the risks known to be associated with oral salicylates such as aspirin. Oral SA has not been associated with an increase in malformations if used during the first trimester, but use in late pregnancy has been linked to bleeding, especially intracranial bleeding.[44] The risks of aspirin use late in pregnancy are probably not relevant when considering topical exposure to SA because of the low systemic levels of SA when used topically. Topical SA is common in many OTC dermatologic agents, and the lack of adverse reports suggests a low teratogenic potential.[45] Nevertheless, caution during pregnancy is recommended.

SA overdose can lead to salicylate intoxication, the clinical presentation of which is typically in a state of metabolic acidosis accompanied by compensatory respiratory alkalosis.[46] A 16 percent morbidity rate and a 1 percent mortality rate have been observed in patients presenting with an acute overdose.[46] Topical products should be used sparingly if used simultaneously with oral aspirin to avoid increased levels of salicylates in the body.

Polyhydroxy Acids

PHAs such as gluconolactone and glucoheptonolactone do not cause sunburn cell formation and, in fact, may provide some protection from UV radiation.[27,47]

FDA Labeling Guidelines

The purpose of the FDA labeling "guidance document" is to serve as a nonbinding informational resource to help manufacturers to ensure that their labeling for cosmetic products containing AHAs as ingredients is not false or misleading and to educate consumers about the potential for increased skin sensitivity to the sun from using topically applied AHA-containing cosmetics.[48] The FDA recommends that the following "Sunburn Alert" labeling statement appear prominently on cosmetic products containing AHAs:

> Sunburn Alert: This product contains an alpha hydroxy acid (AHA) that may increase your skin's sensitivity to the sun and particularly the possibility of sunburn. Use a sunscreen, wear protective clothing, and limit sun exposure while using this product and for a week afterwards.[48]

In addition, the FDA provided guidance to manufacturers with Use Conditions for the Sunburn Alert.[48] The alert should be used in the following situations:

1. *"The product contains an AHA as an ingredient (other than as an incidental ingredient as defined in 21 CFR 701.3(l)).*

   FDA recommends 'Sunburn Alert' labeling for cosmetic products containing an AHA as an ingredient. FDA does not recommend 'Sunburn Alert' labeling for cosmetic products containing an AHA only as an incidental ingredient, as defined in 21 CFR 701.3(l).

2. *The product is intended for topical application to the skin or mucous membrane that are exposed to the sun or for application to areas of the body that may result in unintentional application to the skin or mucous membrane that are exposed to the sun. The product may be a "leave on" product that is intended to remain on the skin or mucous membrane or it may be a "discontinuous use" product that is intended to be left on the skin for a short period of time (less than an hour) followed by thorough rinsing.*

   FDA recommends "Sunburn Alert" labeling for cosmetic products that are intended for topical application to the skin or mucous membrane that are exposed to the sun. FDA also recommends "Sunburn Alert" labeling for cosmetic products that are intended for application to areas of the body that may result in unintentional topical application to the skin or mucous membrane that are exposed to the sun. This guidance does not apply to cosmetic products that contain an AHA as an ingredient and that are intended for application to non-sun exposed areas of the body.

3. *The product contains an AHA as an ingredient and does not also contain a sunscreen for sun protection.*

   This guidance does not apply to drug-cosmetic products that contain an AHA as an ingredient and also are labeled to contain a sunscreen for sun protection. FDA intends to address labeling for such products in a future document."[48]

In summary, although BHA, PHAs, exfoliating scrubs, rotating facial brushes, microdermabrasion and other agents that increase desquamation may also thin the SC, only AHAs are required to display this "sunburn alert" on the label. However, it is prudent to recommend to patients and clients to use a daily sunscreen and an antioxidant when using these agents. PHAs often have antioxidant properties that give them a benefit over other desquamating ingredients.[49]

ENVIRONMENTAL IMPACT

Hydroxy acids have been synthesized in the laboratory for the last century. While numerous plants contain these organic acids, few if any are targeted specifically on a large-scale industrial basis; therefore, the likely environmental impact is minimal.

FORMULATION CONSIDERATIONS

Hydroxy acid formulations are acidic and have varying acidity constants (pK_a); therefore, the pH of the formulation, formulation type, combination of ingredients, and order of product application are especially important. For example, some ingredients perform poorly in an acidic environment and, therefore, should not be used just after or at the same time as another hydroxy acid-containing product.

In order to use hydroxy acids properly, one must understand how the pK_a and pH affect the amount of the acid form and the salt form of the hydroxy acid available in the product. The acid form is the "active form" in the product because it causes exfoliation, while the salt form often causes irritation. It is necessary to have the proper balance of the salt and acid forms to produce an efficacious preparation with minimal irritation (see Chapter 2, Basic Cosmetic Chemistry). The pK_a is the pH at which the free acid level is the same as the level of the salt form of the acid. When the pH is less than the pK_a, the free acid form predominates; when the pH is greater than the pK_a, the salt form predominates. The pK_a for AHAs is 3.83; for SA, 2.97.[12,43] Because the pK_a of BHA differs from that of the AHA family, it is difficult to formulate a product combining BHA and an AHA that reaches an optimal pH. For example, in a combination AHA/BHA product with a pH of 3.5, the AHA *acid* form would predominate while the BHA *salt* form would predominate. This would render the effects of BHA suboptimal. The pK_a for PHAs varies depending on the type of hydroxy acid in the preparation.

Some hydroxy acid formulations are "buffered" to increase their tolerability to the skin. Buffering results when a base, such as sodium bicarbonate or sodium hydroxide, is added to the solution. This raises the level of the salt form, which yields less free acid and a higher pH. Buffered solutions resist pH changes when a salt or an acid is added to the preparation. Fewer side effects are associated with these solutions due to the lower pH and reduced free acid, but there may also be a decrease in efficacy.

USAGE CONSIDERATIONS

Knowing the pK_a and pH of hydroxy acid formulations is critical when designing a skin care regimen for a patient. In addition, their Baumann Skin Type (see Chapter 1, The Importance of Skin Type: The Baumann Skin Type System) should be taken into consideration. S_3 stinging types often cannot consider a hydroxy acid product with a substantial level of free acid because they would not be able to tolerate the resultant stinging.[50] The "lactic acid stinging test" was previously used to identify such stinging skin types.[51] In a study with 30 young adult student volunteers, Frosch and Kligman applied 5 percent lactic acid to the nasolabial fold and cheek in each subject.[52] Approximately 20 percent of the participants reported experiencing an unpleasant sensation. However, not all S_3 stinging

skin types test positive to the lactic acid stinging test, implying that the response is due to more than just the low pH. A fuller explanation is thus far elusive. At this time, it is correct to say that individuals whose Baumann Skin Type tests indicate they have an S_3 skin type are more likely to sting from hydroxy acids than those revealed to have a resistant type skin.

Although hydroxy acids tend to thin the SC, it appears that they do not impair the barrier or facilitate the penetration of other ingredients, unless the ingredient penetration is affected by pH changes. In 1999, Hood et al. evaluated the barrier integrity of hairless guinea pigs after treatment with 5 and 10 percent glycolic acid at a pH of 3.[40] They found no increase in skin penetration of exogenously applied hydroquinone, musk xylol, and 3H water when compared to controls. In fact, evidence suggests that hydroxy acids, particularly PHAs, can improve the skin barrier function.[15]

The pH and effects on the skin barrier may increase or decrease absorption of other ingredients and should be considered when designing a skin care regimen. In addition, the low pH of the hydroxy acid may influence the efficacy of other skin care ingredients in the formulation or skin care regimen. The antioxidant properties of PHAs may help prevent oxidation of labile ingredients. For example, gluconolactone may prevent the oxidation of hydroquinone and other rapidly oxidized ingredients.[49]

SIGNIFICANT BACKGROUND

Topical preparations that contain AHAs have long been known to exert significant influence on epidermal keratinization and have been used since the 1970s to treat dry skin conditions.[13] The cosmetic effects of hydroxy acids include normalization of SC exfoliation resulting in increased plasticization and decreased formation of dry scales on the skin surface. Hydroxy acids function by degrading desmosomes and allowing desquamation to proceed. They also modify corneocyte cohesiveness at the basement levels of the SC, where they affect its pH, and enhance desquamation.[14,15] An SC that has been thinned in this fashion is left more pliable and compact, giving the skin a more youthful appearance. This increased flexibility rendered by the use of AHAs has been shown to persist even in low-humidity situations.[53] A thinner, more compact SC is also desirable because it better reflects light, making the skin appear more luminous.[15]

AHAs and PHAs possess strong humectant properties and are frequently added to moisturizers. Humectants draw water into the skin, provoking a slight swelling of the SC that gives the perception of smoother skin with fewer wrinkles. SA is lipophilic and breaks down occlusive lipids on the skin surface and can lead to dryness. Therefore, SA is an appropriate treatment option for individuals with oily skin whereas AHAs and PHAs are suitable for dry skin.

CONCLUSION

Hydroxy acids join sunscreens, retinoids, and ascorbic acid as the most effective antiaging agents. To increase safety and efficacy, hydroxy acids should always be used in conjunction with sunscreens. Long-term use of hydroxy acids has been proven to enhance skin appearance by improving fine lines, increasing skin radiance, evening skin tone, and augmenting epidermal thickness. Use of hydroxy acids thins the SC and may not be tolerated by individuals with S_3 type sensitive skin.

REFERENCES

1. Babilas P, Knie U, Abels C. Cosmetic and dermatologic use of alpha hydroxyl acids. *J Dtsch Dermatol Ges.* 2012;10:488.
2. Green BA, Briden E. PHAs and bionic acids: Next generation of hydroxy acids. In: Draelos ZD, ed. *Cosmeceuticals.* 2nd ed. Amsterdam: Elsevier Inc; 2009:209–215.
3. Clark E, Scerri L. Superficial and medium-depth chemical peels. *Clin Dermatol.* 2008;26:209.
4. Yamamoto Y, Uede K, Yonei N, et al. Effects of alpha-hydroxy acids on the human skin of Japanese subjects: The rationale for chemical peeling. *J Dermatol.* 2006;33:16.
5. U.S. Patent number 5385938.
6. Kornhauser A, Coelho SG, Hearing VJ. Applications of hydroxy acids: Classification, mechanisms, and photoactivity. *Clin Cosmet Investig Dermatol.* 2010;3:135.
7. Klessig DF, Malamy J. The salicylic acid signal in plants. *Plant Mol Biol.* 1994;26:1439.
8. Raskin I. Role of salicylic acid in plants. *Annu Rev Plant Physiol Plant Mol Biol.* 1992;43:439.
9. Fischer J, Ganellin CR, Ganesan A, et al. Acetylsalicylic acid (aspirin). In: Fischer J, Ganellin CR, eds. *Analogue-based Drug Discovery II.* Weinheim: Wiley; 2010:33.
10. Baumann L, Allemann IB. Depigmenting agents. In: Baumann L, Saghari S, Weisberg E, eds. *Cosmetic Dermatology: Principles and Practice.* 2nd ed. New York: McGraw-Hill; 2009:287.
11. Okuda M, Donahue DA, Kaufman LE, et al. Negligible penetration of incidental amounts of alpha-hydroxy acid from rinse-off personal care products in human skin using an in vitro static diffusion cell model. *Toxicol In Vitro.* 2011;25:2041.
12. Baumann L, Saghari S. Chemical peels. In: Baumann L, Saghari S, Weisberg E, eds. *Cosmetic Dermatology: Principles and Practice.* 2nd ed. New York: McGraw-Hill; 2009:148–162.
13. Van Scott EJ, Yu RJ. Control of keratinization with alpha-hydroxy acids and related compounds. I. Topical treatment of ichthyotic disorders. *Arch Dermatol.* 1974;110:586.
14. Van Scott EJ, Yu RJ. Hyperkeratinization, corneocyte cohesion, and alpha hydroxy acids. *J Am Acad Dermatol.* 1984;11:867.
15. Berardesca E, Distante F, Vignoli GP, et al. Alpha hydroxyacids modulate stratum corneum barrier function. *Br J Dermatol.* 1997;137:934.
16. Manosroi A, Chutoprapat R, Abe M, et al. Anti-aging efficacy of topical formulations containing niosomes entrapped with rice bran bioactive compounds. *Pharm Biol.* 2012;50:208.
17. Ditre CM, Griffin TD, Murphy GF, et al. Effects of alpha-hydroxy acids on photoaged skin: A pilot clinical, histologic, and ultrastructural study. *J Am Acad Dermatol.* 1996;34:187.
18. Kim SJ, Park JH, Kim DH, et al. Increased in vivo collagen synthesis and in vitro cell proliferative effect of glycolic acid. *Dermatol Surg.* 1998;24:1054.
19. Moon SE, Park SB, Ahn HT, et al. The effect of glycolic acid on photoaged albino hairless mouse skin. *Dermatol Surg.* 1999;25:179.
20. Bernstein EF, Lee J, Brown DB, et al. Glycolic acid treatment increases type I collagen mRNA and hyaluronic acid content of human skin. *Dermatol Surg.* 2001;27:429.
21. Okano Y, Abe Y, Masaki H, et al. Biological effects of glycolic acid on dermal matrix metabolism mediated by dermal fibroblasts and epidermal keratinocytes. *Exp Dermatol.* 2003;12(Suppl 2):57.
22. Middleton J. Sodium lactate as a moisturizer. *Cosmet Toiletries.* 1978;93:85.
23. Wehr R, Krochmal L, Bagatell F, et al. A controlled two-center study of lactate 12 percent lotion and a petrolatum-based creme in patients with xerosis. *Cutis.* 1986;37:205.
24. Smith WP. Epidermal and dermal effects of topical lactic acid. *J Am Acad Dermatol.* 1996;35:388.
25. Rendl M, Mayer C, Weninger W, et al. Topically applied lactic acid increases spontaneous secretion of vascular endothelial growth factor by human reconstructed epidermis. *Br J Dermatol.* 2001;145:3.
26. Swinehart JM. Salicylic acid ointment peeling of the hands and forearms. Effective nonsurgical removal of pigmented lesions and actinic damage. *J Dermatol Surg Oncol.* 1992;18:495.
27. Bernstein EF, Brown DB, Schwartz MD, et al. The polyhydroxy acid gluconolactone protects against ultraviolet radiation in an in vitro model of cutaneous photoaging. *Dermatol Surg.* 2004;30:189.
28. Rona C, Vailati F, Berardesca E. The cosmetic treatment of wrinkles. *J Cosmet Dermatol.* 2004 Jan;3(1):26–34.
29. Slavin JW. Considerations in alpha hydroxy acid peels. *Clin Plast Surg.* 1998;25:45.
30. Usuki A, Ohashi A, Sato H, et al. The inhibitory effect of glycolic acid and lactic acid on melanin synthesis in melanoma cells. *Exp Dermatol.* 2003;12(Suppl 2):43.
31. Kim WS. Efficacy and safety of a new superficial chemical peel using alpha-hydroxy acid, vitamin C and oxygen for melasma. *J Cosmet Laser Ther.* 2013;15:21.
32. Oresajo C, Yatskayer M, Hansenne I. Clinical tolerance and efficacy of capryloyl salicylic acid peel compared to a glycolic acid peel in subjects with fine lines/wrinkles and hyperpigmented skin. *J Cosmet Dermatol.* 2008;7:259.
33. Kornhauser A, Wei RR, Yamaguchi Y, et al. The effects of topically applied glycolic acid and salicylic acid on ultraviolet radiation-induced erythema, DNA damage and sunburn cell formation in human skin. *J Dermatol Sci.* 2009;55:10.
34. Abdel-Daim M, Funasaka Y, Kamo T, et al. Effect of chemical peeling on photocarcinogenesis. *J Dermatol.* 2010;37:864.
35. Lai WW, Hsiao YP, Chung JG, et al. Synergistic phototoxic effects of glycolic acid in a human keratinocyte cell line (HaCaT). *J Dermatol Sci.* 2011;64:191.
36. Kaidbey K, Sutherland B, Bennett P, et al. Topical glycolic acid enhances photodamage by ultraviolet light. *Photodermatol Photoimmunol Photomed.* 2003;19:21.
37. Perricone NV, Dinardo JC. Photoprotective and antiinflammatory effects of topical glycolic acid. *Dermatol Surg.* 1996;22:435.
38. Tsai TF, Bowman PH, Jee SH, et al. Effects of glycolic acid on light-induced pigmentation in Asian and caucasian subjects. *J Am Acad Dermatol.* 2000;43:238.
39. Draelos ZD. Therapeutic moisturizers. *Dermatol Clin.* 2000;18:597.
40. Hood HL, Kraeling ME, Robl MG, et al. The effects of an alpha hydroxy acid (glycolic acid) on hairless guinea pig skin permeability. *Food Chem Toxicol.* 1999;37:1105.
41. Lavker RM, Kaidbey K, Leyden JJ. Effects of topical ammonium lactate on cutaneous atrophy from a potent topical corticosteroid. *J Am Acad Dermatol.* 1992;26:535.
42. Thomas JR, Dixon TK, Bhattacharyya TK. Effects of topical on the aging skin process. *Facial Plast Surg Clin North Am.* 2013;21:55.
43. Clark CP 3rd. Alpha hydroxy acids in skin care. *Clin Plast Surg.* 1996;23:49.
44. Draelos Z. Hydroxy acids for the treatment of aging skin. *J Geriatric Dermatol.* 1997;5:236.
45. Zhai H, Hannon W, Hahn GS, et al. Strontium nitrate suppresses chemically-induced sensory irritation in humans. *Contact Dermatitis.* 2000;42:98.
46. Kreplick LW. Salicylate toxicity in emergency medicine. *eMedicine Journal.* 2001;2(6), June 7. http://www.emedicine.com. Accessed February 18, 2014.
47. Green BA, Wildnauer RH, Edison BL. Polyhydroxy acids (PHAs) provide conditioning effects to skin without increasing sensitivity to UV light. American Academy of Dermatology poster exhibit, New Orleans, LA, February 22–27, 2002. http://www.neostratapro.com/images/neostratapro/en_us/local/landing/2002_phas_uv_light.pdf. Accessed January 14, 2014.
48. U.S. Food and Drug Administration Guidance for Industry: Labeling for Topically Applied Cosmetics Containing Alpha Hydroxy Acids as Ingredients, January 10, 2005. http://www.fda.gov/Cosmetics/GuidanceComplianceRegulatoryInformation/GuidanceDocuments/ucm090816.htm. Accessed January 15, 2014.
49. Green B. After 30 years... the future of hydroxyacids. *J Cosmet Dermatol.* 2005;4:44.
50. Baumann L. Sensitive skin. In: Baumann L, Saghari S, Weisberg E, eds. *Cosmetic Dermatology: Principles and Practice.* 2nd ed. New York: McGraw-Hill; 2009:95–96.
51. Baumann L, Castanedo-Tardan MP. Bioengineering of the skin. In: Baumann L, Saghari S, Weisberg E, eds. *Cosmetic Dermatology: Principles and Practice.* 2nd ed. New York: McGraw-Hill; 2009: 335–96.
52. Frosch PJ, Kligman AM. A method for appraising the stinging capacity of topically applied substances. *J Soc Cosmet Chem.* 1977;28:197.
53. Takahashi M, Machida Y. The influence of hydroxyacids on the rheological properties of the stratum corneum. *J Soc Cosmet Chem.* 1985;36:177.

CHAPTER 83

Retinoids (Retinol)

Activities:

Antiaging, antiacne, depigmenting

Important Chemical Components:

Natural retinoids: The major naturally-occurring retinoids are tretinoin (all-*trans* retinoic acid, also known simply as retinoic acid), the stereoisomers of tretinoin [isotretinoin (13-*cis*-retinoic acid) and alitretinoin (9-*cis*-retinoic acid)], retinol, retinaldehyde, and retinol esters (retinyl acetate, retinyl palmitate, retinyl propionate).
Synthetic retinoids: The retinoids that have been designed in the laboratory to increase stability are tazarotene (molecular formula: $C_{21}H_{21}NO_2S$), adapalene (molecular formula: $C_{28}H_{28}O_3$), and retinyl retinoate (an ester of retinoic acid and all-*trans* retinol).

Origin Classification:

Retinoids are natural and synthetic derivatives of vitamin A (also known as all-*trans* retinol). As ingredients in skin therapy, these products are laboratory made.

Personal Care Category:

Antiaging, antiacne

Recommended for the following Baumann Skin Types:

DRNW, DRPT, DRPW, DSNW, DSPT, DSPW, ORNW, ORPW, ORPT, OSPW, OSNW, and OSPT

SOURCE

Vitamin A is found naturally in the skin and other parts of the body and is obtained through the diet from carotenoid-containing foods, such as sweet potatoes, carrots, dark green leafy vegetables, tomatoes, squash, apricots, cantaloupe, red pepper, and tropical fruits (e.g., mangoes and papayas).[1,2] Like β-carotene, lutein, lycopene, and other carotenoids, retinoids are derived from vitamin A (all-*trans* retinol). The retinoid family includes natural (e.g., tretinoin, isotretinoin, alitretinoin, retinol, and retinaldehyde) and synthetic (e.g., tazarotene, adapalene, and retinyl retinoate) forms. Retinol and retinyl esters represent 99 percent of cutaneous retinoids naturally present in the skin.[3] The retinoids used in prescription products and over-the-counter (OTC) skin care formulations are synthesized in laboratories.

Retinoids have demonstrated salutary benefits in the treatment of various cutaneous conditions, including acne, psoriasis, ichthyosis, and photoaging. In fact, retinoid efficacy has been reported in more than 125 distinct dermatologic disorders.[4] Two prescription retinoids, tretinoin (retinoic acid) and tazarotene, have been approved by the United States Food and Drug Administration (FDA) for use in the treatment of photoaging,

TABLE 83-1
Pros and Cons of Retinoids

Pros	Cons
Variety of products	Unstable
Excellent research on efficacy, with significant evidence from randomized controlled trials	Difficult to formulate
Irritation lessens with time	Many products do not work because of packaging and stability issues
Treats acne and skin pigmentation as well as wrinkles	Causes irritation especially in S_2 rosacea types
Protects skin from sun damage	Prevalent myth, actually based on *in vitro* and animal studies,[3] that retinoids make skin more photosensitive
	Should be used at night only

although isotretinoin (the 13-*cis* isomer of tretinoin), and several synthetic retinoids are deployed for therapeutic applications (Table 83-1).[3] In addition, retinol, though it has not been approved by the FDA to treat photoaging or included among the FDA monograph ingredients for that purpose, is known to impart antiaging activity. The retinoids used in effective skin care products include retinoic acid (tretinoin), retinol, retinaldehyde, adapalene, or tazarotene. Retinyl esters such as retinyl palmitate (RP) are used in several OTC formulations, but the efficacy is questionable because penetration rates are minimal.

HISTORY

Vitamin A was recognized in 1928 by Green and Mellanby as having anti-infective properties.[3,5] The structure of retinol was ascertained just three years later by Karrer et al.[6] In 1937, Karrer was a corecipient of the Nobel Prize in Chemistry for this and related work. In 1943, the first study to document the use of vitamin A for the treatment of acne was published.[7] Tretinoin was first used in dermatologic therapy in 1959 by Stüttgen.[7–9] In 1969, Kligman et al. reported that topically applied tretinoin was efficacious in the treatment of acne vulgaris.[8,10]

The apparent ameliorative effects of retinoids on aged skin were recognized serendipitously by Kligman et al. in the mid-1980s in examinations of female acne patients who reported that their skin felt smoother and less wrinkled after treatment.[11] A small subsequent clinical trial revealed that daily topical application of 0.05 percent tretinoin to the forearm and face diminished ultraviolet (UV)-induced epidermal atrophy, dysplasia, keratosis, and dyspigmentation compared to vehicle control.[12] These observations have since been duplicated in numerous studies.

A metabolic precursor to tretinoin, retinol is often incorporated in OTC "antiwrinkle" creams. There is currently no FDA-approved monograph for the use of retinol in cosmetics and personal care products; however, one may be developed in the future.

CHEMISTRY

Vitamin A is found in various forms, with multiple precursors to retinoic acid.

Retinoids

Over the last several decades, myriad synthetic retinoids have been developed, with the vitamin A or "retinoid" family now including retinyl esters (such as RP), retinol, tretinoin (retinoic acid), adapalene, tazarotene, and oral isotretinoin (Accutane) in addition to four carotenoids such as β-carotene.

Retinoids regulate growth and differentiation in epithelial cells and suppress tumor promotion during experimental carcinogenesis, thus hampering malignant cell growth, quelling inflammation, and supporting the immune system.[13] This is accomplished at the molecular level through the regulation of gene transcription and influencing cellular differentiation as well as proliferation. Retinoids act directly by initiating transcription from genes with promoter regions containing retinoid response elements or indirectly by precluding the transcription of particular genes.[14]

The use of topical retinoids has been shown clinically and histologically to be effective in reversing some of the physical alterations and cutaneous manifestations induced in humans by excessive sun exposure. Irritant reactions, such as xerosis, erythema, and scaling, tend to be the worst of any adverse responses to retinoid compounds (i.e., tretinoin, isotretinoin, retinaldehyde, and tazarotene).[8] This irritation is dose related and resolves with continued use (tachyphylaxis).

Retinaldehyde, retinol, and retinyl esters, all natural retinoic acid precursors, are the retinoids used in cosmeceuticals.[3,15] Retinol is the most efficacious and the most irritating of the forms of retinol available without a prescription. Though less irritating, retinyl esters and retinaldehyde typically have less clinical efficacy, due to decreased penetration. Retinaldehyde, which exhibits slightly more efficacy than retinyl esters, is generally well tolerated, and appears to renew epidermal cells, blunt the effects of photoaging, and limit oxidative stress and bacterial flora on the skin.[3]

Lipophilic retinoids such as retinol, tretinoin, adapalene, and tazarotene easily penetrate the epidermis.[3] Some protocols have suggested short contact time such as 15 minutes with retinoid products to decrease the amount of absorption. This ease of penetration of retinoids is unique among antiaging products; most products cannot penetrate into the skin, greatly reducing their efficacy. (Retinoid esters such as RP are an exception, and do not penetrate well due to their chemical structure.) All retinoids, by definition, bind the retinoic acid receptor and therefore should improve photoaged skin; however, only tretinoin (Renova) and tazarotene (Avage) are approved by the FDA to treat photoaged skin.

Retinoid Receptors

Although retinoids have been extensively studied for several years, much remains to be elucidated regarding the mechanisms of action of these compounds. In the 1970s, retinoid-binding proteins were discovered and, in 1987, retinoic acid receptors were identified, leading to the insight that tretinoin functions as a hormone.[16–18] The biologic effects of retinoic acid are mediated by binding proteins such as cellular retinoic acid-binding proteins (CRAB) I and II; cellular retinol-binding protein (CRBP); and the nuclear receptors retinoic acid receptors (RARs) and retinoid X receptors (RXRs), both sets of which consist of α, β, and γ isotypes.[11,19,20] RARs heterodimerize with RXRs in order to interact with their retinoic acid response elements (RAREs), with RXR-α and RAR-γ heterodimers serving as the primary cutaneous retinoid receptors in humans.[20] (See Chapter 79, Retinol, Retinyl Esters, and Retinoic Acid, for more information on retinoid receptors.)

Adapalene and tazarotene bear no structural resemblance to natural retinoids but are categorized as retinoids because they activate retinoic acid receptors and share several functional traits.[20] Adapalene is marketed as Differin and EpiDuo. Tazarotene, marketed as Tazorac and Avage, is selective for RAR-β and RAR-γ and is FDA approved to treat psoriasis, acne, and photoaging.[21,22]

ORAL USES

Isotretinoin (Accutane) is used orally to treat acne. Oral retinoids are rarely used for photoaging because of the risk of teratogenicity. One study showed that a dose of 10 to 20 mg three times a week for two months led to improvement of skin aging signs such as wrinkles.[23] A discussion of oral retinoid compounds is beyond the scope of this text.

TOPICAL USES

In the author's opinion, retinoids are the most important ingredients to treat and prevent skin aging. Their use is backed up by multiple studies. Retinoids elicit their effects at the molecular level by regulating gene transcription and affecting activities such as cellular differentiation and proliferation. All-*trans* retinoic acid (tretinoin) has been shown in various studies to decrease wrinkles and is the most frequently studied retinoid for photoaging treatment.[12,20] Much work has been performed to characterize this mechanism.[24–27] In general, retinoids treat and prevent photoaging by inhibiting the breakdown and loss of collagen and stimulating skin cells (fibroblasts) to increase collagen synthesis.[27–30]

The use of retinoids to prevent or treat the cutaneous signs of photoaging has been investigated in several studies. The first clinical trials demonstrating clinical improvement of photoaged skin using tretinoin were published in 1986 and 1988.[12,31] The findings by Kligman et al. and Weiss et al. have since been duplicated numerous times. In one randomized, single-center study performed by Griffiths et al. in 1995, 100 subjects were divided into two tretinoin treatment groups (0.1 and 0.025 percent) and a vehicle cream group.[32] Statistically significant improvements were seen in both tretinoin groups compared with vehicle.

A cascade of histologic changes have been associated with retinoid use, including the abrogation of cellular atypia, increased compacting of the stratum corneum (SC), diminished clumping of melanin in basal cells, and polarity correction of keratinocytes, with more orderly differentiation as cells move upward. The ultrastructural changes induced by retinoid use include hyperproliferation of keratinocytes (e.g., larger nuclei, increased ribosomes, etc.) and melanosome size reduction. The topical application of tretinoin 0.1 percent to photodamaged skin has been shown to prevent the breakdown of collagen and promote collagen synthesis, partially restoring collagen type I levels and increasing anchoring fibrils (collagen type VII).[33]

Although tretinoin and tazarotene are FDA approved to treat photoaged skin, which means that the efficacy of these retinoids is proven, retinol has not undergone the FDA approval process. Retinol is considered a cosmetic ingredient. Nevertheless, a number of studies have demonstrated its efficacy in treating aged skin but no company has made the large monetary investment and time commitment required to seek FDA approval. In spite of the lack of FDA approval to treat photoaged skin, several studies support the use of retinol to treat aged skin. Many of these were performed by the same team responsible for the original work on the FDA-approved forms of retinoic acid: John Voorhees, Chair of Dermatology at the University of Michigan, and Sewon Kang, Chair of Dermatology at Johns Hopkins School of Medicine. These studies are published in reputable peer-reviewed journals such as the *Journal of Investigative Dermatology*.[34-38] For this reason, the author believes that using OTC retinol can achieve the same results as using a prescription retinoid.

Retinol has been shown to penetrate skin better than retinoic acid.[37] One study demonstrated that retinol improves the appearance of wrinkles in sun-protected areas.[39] Biopsies of treated skin show that retinol does induce cellular and molecular changes similar to those observed with the application of 0.025 percent retinoic acid.[37] A separate study showed that 1.6 percent retinol induced significant epidermal thickening and other skin changes similar to those produced by retinoic acid but without measurable irritation.[38] An elegant and frequently quoted randomized, double-blind, vehicle-controlled, left and right arm comparison study by Kafi et al. in 2007 showed that skin treated with 0.4 percent retinol showed increased glycosaminoglycans and collagen in biopsies as compared to those treated with vehicle.[39] Visual scales also showed improvement of skin wrinkling in the retinol-treated group. Another study by Tucker-Samaras et el. showed that 0.1 percent stabilized retinol improved photoaged skin as compared to vehicle.[40]

Retinol and RP are the two most frequently used retinoids in OTC products. They are typically listed as excipient or "inactive" ingredients based on their status as "cosmetic" ingredients according to the FDA. Retinol is now well known for its photoinstability, but using it at night, along with the addition of an antioxidant to the regimen or formulation, circumvents this problem. Significantly, retinol is now recognized for exerting similar effects on the retinoic acid receptor as tretinoin.

Retinyl Palmitate

RP, a storage and ester form of retinol and the main type of vitamin A present naturally in the skin,[41] has steadily gained popularity over the last two decades and is incorporated into more than 600 skin care products, including cosmetics, sunscreens, as well as FDA-approved OTC and prescription drugs.[42] However, Xia et al., who had earlier demonstrated that irradiation of RP with UVA yields photodecomposition products, synthesis of reactive oxygen species, and lipid peroxidation induction, obtained similar findings identifying RP as a photosensitizer after irradiation with UVB.[43] Four years later, the Environmental Working Group (EWG) issued a consumer warning about the potential photocarcinogenicity of RP-containing sunscreens. The EWG's methodology and conclusions, which the organization stood by, were roundly criticized in a debate that wound up in the pages of the *Journal of the American Academy of Dermatology*.[44] While current evidence is inconclusive, the weight of extant evidence and clinical experience suggests that RP does not easily penetrate into the skin. Retinol rather than RP, even though it is easier to formulate,[22] is thus the recommended choice.

Retinyl Retinoate

In 2011, Kim et al. conducted a 12-week, randomized, double-blind, controlled trial to investigate the efficacy of retinyl retinoate, a new synthetic hybrid of retinoic acid and retinol, in treating the periorbital wrinkles of 11 Korean women over the age of 30. The researchers observed a statistically significant reduction in facial wrinkles in all 11 participants. Compared to 0.075 percent retinol cream, 0.06 percent retinyl retinoate treatment over three months resulted in diminished wrinkle depth and size. In addition, the test cream outperformed retinol by 22 percent in terms of visual wrinkle improvement and the maximum roughness improvement rate. The authors concluded that retinyl retinoate reduced facial wrinkles while exhibiting greater photostability and provoking less irritation than earlier generations of retinoids.[45]

A year earlier, several of the same team performed two similar clinical studies, with a total of 46 Korean women with periorbital wrinkles. Twenty-four subjects applied 0.06 percent retinyl retinoate to one side of the face twice daily and a placebo ointment to the other side for 12 weeks in the first study. Twenty-two patients in the second study, conducted over eight weeks, applied 0.06 percent retinyl retinoate twice daily to one side of the face and 0.075 percent retinol to the other side. Assessments by investigators and subjects indicated greater improvements in wrinkles on skin treated with retinyl retinoate compared to placebo or retinol, with no reported side effects. In addition, average roughness was significantly diminished by retinyl retinoate based on skin replica analysis. The investigators concluded that twice-daily application of retinyl retinoate was significantly more effective in treating periorbital wrinkles than placebo or retinol.[46]

SAFETY ISSUES

Erythema, skin irritation, and desquamation are the most common adverse side effects of topical retinoids. The type and dose of retinoid influences such reactions, which typically occur within two to four days of beginning topical treatment.[47] When retinoid products were first commercialized, many believed that the redness and inflammation were a prerequisite for improvement of aged skin. It has now been established that benefits can be derived from using retinoids without incurring irritation. Indeed, the attenuating effects on photoaging can be separated from the irritation reliably produced by retinoids. Griffiths et al. showed this in 1995 in their double-blind, vehicle-controlled experiment with two different strengths of tretinoin (0.1 and 0.025 percent) used to treat photoaging. Although the formulations were equally efficacious, the degree of irritation varied substantially between the two treatment groups, with the 0.1 percent tretinoin-treated group displaying almost a threefold greater incidence of irritation than those treated with the 0.025 percent preparation.[32] New ingredients are being investigated to block the irritation of retinoids without affecting the efficacy.

Erythema, flushing, and facial stinging – common side effects of topical retinoids – can be reduced by applying the retinoid on top of a moisturizer to limit penetration and by decreasing the amount and frequency of application until the retinoid can be tolerated as tachyphylaxis occurs. Care should be taken when designing the skin care regimen to include anti-inflammatory ingredients and reduce ingredients that increase skin penetration when retinoid treatments are being initiated.

It is well established that teratogenicity is a significant risk associated with the use of oral retinoids. Long debated is the advisability of topical retinoid use by women of childbearing age due to the potential risk of systemic absorption. As a general rule, great care should be taken when prescribing retinoids (even OTC retinol) to women of childbearing age, although no studies have convincingly demonstrated harm from use during pregnancy. A 1993 study by Jick et al. demonstrated no significant rise in the fetal malformation rate in 215 women treated with topical tretinoin during the first trimester of pregnancy, as compared with 430 age-matched nonexposed women.[48]

The topical application of tretinoin has been thought by many to augment photosensitivity because its daily use engenders thinning of the SC, rendering it more compact. Such concern arose partly as a result of admonitions to early tretinoin users to apply the product only at night. This warning was based solely on the poor stability of tretinoin upon UV light exposure. Retinoids are now known not to have photosensitizing or phototoxic properties, and may actually protect the skin from the deleterious sequelae of UV exposure.[27]

ENVIRONMENTAL IMPACT

There is no environmental impact of commercial topical retinoid formulation manufacture known by the author.

FORMULATION CONSIDERATIONS

It is important to understand that not all retinol-containing products are equal. Retinol is very unstable and loses biologic activity on exposure to UV light, air, heat, water, and lipid peroxidation.[46] When it is formulated and packaged retinol must remain in an airless system with no exposure to light. Proper packaging of retinol is in an aluminum tube with a small mouth or an airless pump. Retinol must be manufactured, formulated, and packaged properly to avoid oxidation and loss of potency. Also, the amount of retinol in the product must be high enough to be effective. New stabilized forms of retinol have been shown to exhibit greatly increased efficacy in aging skin.[49] Nanoparticles have displayed potential in enhancing the efficacy, stability, and tolerability of retinoid agents, particularly those more prone to elicit irritant reactions such as tretinoin and tazarotene.[50]

In 2011, Ourique et al. showed that nanoencapsulation of tretinoin with lipid-core polymeric nanocapsules yielded improved photostability, with hydrogels containing nanoencapsulated tretinoin manifesting a half-life seven times longer than the nonencapsulated tretinoin after eight hours of UVA irradiation. Their experiments also revealed that nanoencapsulation led to extended retention of the drug on the skin surface and decreased skin permeation.[51]

USAGE CONSIDERATIONS

The side effects commonly seen in patients on retinoid therapy can usually be alleviated by directing the patient to apply small amounts of the retinoid at less frequent intervals. The lowest available dose should be started initially. For individuals with sensitive skin, topical retinol can be used every third night for the first two weeks. If no redness or irritation results, the retinoid can be increased to every other night for two weeks. Eventually most patients can tolerate nightly use. Once the patient is consistently applying the retinol nightly, the strength of the retinol can be increased. Once the maximal retinol strength is reached, the patient can be seamlessly switched to a prescription retinoid if desired.

A 1997 study by Olsen et al. suggested that after a 48-week regimen of once-daily 0.05 percent tretinoin emollient cream, the benefits of tretinoin could be sustained by *at least* three applications each week for an additional 24 weeks. The investigators found that once-weekly treatment was insufficient for maintaining the previously seen clinical improvement. In addition, they noted that discontinuation of therapy for 24 weeks led to the abrogation of the earlier benefits derived from the tretinoin regimen.[52]

SIGNIFICANT BACKGROUND

Although tretinoin has long been approved for the *treatment* of photoaging, evidence suggests that it also plays a role in the *prevention* of cutaneous aging. The inhibitory effects of retinoids on harmful matrix metalloproteinases (MMPs) are thought to be responsible for this potential benefit. UVB exposure dramatically upregulates MMP synthesis. Activation of the genes of these collagen-degrading enzymes leads to the production of collagenase, gelatinase, and stromelysin, all of which have been shown to fully degrade cutaneous collagen.[53] Fisher et al. showed in 1996 that topical tretinoin application suppresses the induction of all three of these detrimental MMPs.[27]

In addition to elevating MMP levels, UV exposure has also been demonstrated to reduce collagen production. In 2000, Fisher et al. showed that expression of collagen types I and III was markedly diminished within 24 hours after one UV exposure. They found that pretreating the skin with tretinoin mitigated such a decline in procollagen production.[54] Consequently, the consistent pretreatment of skin with topical retinoids is thought to likely contribute to the prevention as well as treatment of photodamage.[55]

Significantly, the use of topical retinoids (especially tretinoin, isotretinoin, and tazarotene) is the only therapeutic option established through randomized clinical trials to improve the clinical appearance of photoaged skin. In addition, to elaborate on the above, topically applied retinoids show indications of being able to prevent photoaging and possibly altering the course, and blunting the effects, of intrinsically aging skin.[56] It is important to note that, to date, the cogent evidence in support of topical retinoids for photoaging correlates to mild-to-moderate photodamage.[20]

Stabilized, Low-irritancy Retinol

Tucker-Samaras et al. conducted an eight-week, double-blind, split-face, randomized clinical study in 2009 to evaluate the effects of once-daily application of stabilized 0.1 percent retinol-containing moisturizer in 36 subjects with moderate facial photodamage. The vehicle was used in 28 control subjects. With some improvement evident and significant at week 4, after eight weeks, the retinol moisturizers were found to be significantly more efficacious than the vehicle in reducing overall signs of photodamage, specifically improving elasticity and firmness and diminishing lines and wrinkles. The investigators concluded that a stabilized retinol formulation was safe and effective in enhancing the appearance of photoaged facial skin.[40]

Also that year, Kikuchi et al. conducted a randomized, blinded, vehicle-controlled study to assess the efficacy of once-nightly applied 0.075 percent retinol cream in treating mild photoaging in 57 middle-aged Japanese females. Fifty-four of 57 participants completed the 26-week study, with three withdrawing due to irritation. Signs of photoaging (fine and deep wrinkling) were significantly reduced on the retinol-treated side of the face versus control [27 on retinol (50 percent) vs. 13 (24 percent) for fine wrinkling and, for deep wrinkling, 15 (28 percent) vs. 1 (2 percent)].

The investigators also led a 13-week study using a 0.04 percent retinol cream, with less salient improvements in fine wrinkling revealed but minimal irritation elicited. They concluded that retinol creams, particularly the 0.04 percent formulation, are appropriate for daily use, even by those with sensitive skin, because of low irritancy.[57]

Retinoids in Combination

In a 2010 literature review of combination treatments for photoaging, Tierney and Hanke identified 10 studies documenting histologic evidence that several combination approaches, including the use of topical retinoids, yielded cutaneous repair of photodamaged skin.[58] Retinoids should be combined with daily sunscreen, antioxidants, and other treatment solutions depending on the patient's skin type.

◼ CONCLUSION

Retinoid therapy is appropriate for all patients that are wrinkle-prone types within the BSTS. OTC retinol appears to be just as effective as prescription retinoids in conferring improvement to photoaged skin, but with less irritation. The author recommends combining retinol with an antioxidant and a daily sunscreen for optimal benefit. Patients should be carefully instructed on the use of retinoids and taught to slowly increase the frequency, amount used, and strength to avoid excessive irritation. They should be educated that retinoids do not increase sun sensitivity and can help protect them from the ravages of UV exposure. Care should be taken to recommend a retinol that has a stable formulation and proper packaging. The product should be discarded after six months because retinol loses its activity, especially after being opened. RP is less effective than other retinoids and its safety is a controversial issue; for this reason the author recommends avoiding retinyl palmitate and other retinyl esters.

REFERENCES

1. Schweiggert RM, Kopec RE, Villalobos-Gutierrez MG, et al. Carotenoids are more bioavailable from papaya than from tomato and carrot in humans: A randomised cross-over study. *Br J Nutr.* 2014;111:490.
2. Khan NC, West CE, de Pee S, et al. The contribution of plant foods to the vitamin A supply of lactating women in Vietnam: A randomized controlled trial. *Am J Clin Nutr.* 2007;85:1112.
3. Sorg O, Antille C, Kaya G, et al. Retinoids in cosmeceuticals. *Dermatol Ther.* 2006;19:289.
4. Kligman AM. The growing importance of topical retinoids in clinical dermatology: A retrospective and prospective analysis. *J Am Acad Dermatol.* 1998;39:S2.
5. Green HN, Mellanby E. Vitamin A as anti-infective agent. *Br Med J.* 1928;II:691.
6. Karrer P, Morf R, Schopp K. Zur kenntnis des vitamin-a aus fischtranin. *Helv Chim Acta.* 1931;14:1036.
7. Darlenski R, Surber C, Fluhr JW. Topical retinoids in the management of photodamaged skin: From theory to evidence-based practical approach. *Br J Dermatol.* 2010;163:1157.
8. Stratigos AJ, Katsambas AD. The role of topical retinoids in the treatment of photoaging. *Drugs.* 2005;65:1061.
9. Torras H. Retinoids in aging. *Clin Dermatol.* 1996;14:207.
10. Kligman AM, Fulton JE Jr, Plewig G. Topical vitamin A acid in acne vulgaris. *Arch Dermatol.* 1969;99:469.
11. Kligman L, Kligman AM. Photoaging - Retinoids, alpha hydroxy acids, and antioxidants. In: Gabard B, Elsner P, Surber C, Treffel P, eds. *Dermatopharmacology of Topical Preparations.* New York: Springer; 2000:383.
12. Kligman AM, Grove GL, Hirose R, et al. Topical tretinoin for photoaged skin. *J Am Acad Dermatol.* 1986;15:836.
13. Keller KL, Fenske NA. Uses of vitamins A, C, and E and related compounds in dermatology: A review. *J Am Acad Dermatol.* 1998;39:611.
14. Chandraratna RA. Tazarotene – first of a new generation of receptor-selective retinoids. *Br J Dermatol.* 1996;135(Suppl 49):18.
15. Serri R, Iorizzo M. Cosmeceuticals: Focus on topical retinoids in photoaging. *Clin Dermatol.* 2008;26:633.
16. Chytil F, Ong D. Cellular retinoid-binding proteins. In: Sporn MB, Roberts A, Goodman D, eds. *The Retinoids.* Vol. 2. Orlando: Academic Press; 1984:89–123.
17. Giguere V, Ong ES, Segui P, et al. Identification of a receptor for the morphogen retinoic acid. *Nature.* 1987;330:624.
18. Petkovich M, Brand NJ, Krust A, et al. A human retinoic acid receptor which belongs to the family of nuclear receptors. *Nature.* 1987;330:444.
19. Pfahl M. The molecular mechanism of retinoid action. Retinoids today and tomorrow. *Retinoids Dermatol.* 1996;44:2.
20. Antoniou C, Kosmadaki MG, Stratigos AJ, et al. Photoaging: Prevention and topical treatments. *Am J Clin Dermatol.* 2010;11:95.
21. Ogden S, Samuel M, Griffiths CE. A review of tazarotene in the treatment of photodamaged skin. *Clin Interv Aging.* 2008;3:71.
22. Stefanaki C, Stratigos A, Katsambas A. Topical retinoids in the treatment of photoaging. *J Cosmet Dermatol.* 2005;4:130.
23. Hernandez-Perez E, Khawaja HA, Alvarez TY. Oral isotretinoin as part of the treatment of cutaneous aging. *Dermatol Surg.* 2000;26:649.
24. Lever L, Kumar P, Marks R. Topical retinoic acid for treatment of solar damage. *Br J Dermatol.* 1990;122:91.
25. Leyden JJ, Grove GL, Grove MJ, et al. Treatment of photodamaged facial skin with topical tretinoin. *J Am Acad Dermatol.* 1989;21:638.
26. Weinstein GD, Nigra TP, Pochi PE, et al. Topical tretinoin for treatment of photodamaged skin. A multicenter study. *Arch Dermatol.* 1991;127:659.
27. Fisher GJ, Datta SC, Talwar HS, et al. Molecular basis of sun-induced premature skin ageing and retinoid antagonism. *Nature.* 1996;379:335.
28. Chaqour B, Bellon G, Seite S, et al. All-trans-retinoic acid enhances collagen gene expression in irradiated and non-irradiated hairless mouse skin. *J Photochem Photobiol B.* 1997;37:52.
29. Griffiths CE, Russman AN, Majmudar G, et al. Restoration of collagen formation in photodamaged human skin by tretinoin (retinoic acid). *N Engl J Med.* 1993;329:530.
30. Schwartz E, Cruickshank FA, Mezick JA, et al. Topical all-trans retinoic acid stimulates collagen synthesis in vivo. *J Invest Dermatol.* 1991;96:975.
31. Weiss JS, Ellis CN, Headington JT, et al. Topical tretinoin improves photoaged skin: A double-blind vehicle-controlled study. *JAMA.* 1988;259:527.
32. Griffiths CE, Kang S, Ellis CN, et al. Two concentrations of topical tretinoin (retinoic acid) cause similar improvement of photoaging but different degrees of irritation. A double-blind, vehicle-controlled comparison of 0.1% and 0.025% tretinoin creams. *Arch Dermatol.* 1995;131:1037.
33. Woodley DT, Zelickson AS, Briggaman RA, et al. Treatment of photoaged skin with topical tretinoin increases epidermal-dermal anchoring fibrils. A preliminary report. *JAMA.* 1990;263:3057.
34. Fisher GJ, Reddy AP, Datta SC, et al. All-trans retinoic acid induces cellular retinol-binding protein in human skin in vivo. *J Invest Dermatol.* 1995;105:80.
35. Duell EA, Kang S, Voorhees JJ. Retinoic acid isomers applied to human skin in vivo each induce a 4-hydroxylase that inactivates only trans retinoic acid. *J Invest Dermatol.* 1996;106:316.
36. Duell EA, Derguini F, Kang S, et al. Extraction of human epidermis treated with retinol yields retro-retinoids in addition to free retinol and retinyl esters. *J Invest Dermatol.* 1996;107:178.
37. Duell EA, Kang S, Voorhees JJ. Unoccluded retinol penetrates human skin in vivo more effectively than unoccluded retinyl palmitate or retinoic acid. *J Invest Dermatol.* 1997;109:301.
38. Kang S, Duell EA, Fisher GJ, et al. Application of retinol to human skin in vivo induces epidermal hyperplasia and cellular retinoid binding proteins characteristic of retinoic acid but without measurable retinoic acid levels or irritation. *J Invest Dermatol.* 1995;105:549.
39. Kafi R, Kwak HS, Schumacher WE, et al. Improvement of naturally aged skin with vitamin A (retinol). *Arch Dermatol.* 2007;143:606.

40. Tucker-Samaras S, Zedayko T, Cole C, et al. A stabilized 0.1% retinol facial moisturizer improves the appearance of photodamaged skin in an eight-week, double-blind, vehicle-controlled study. *J Drugs Dermatol.* 2009;8:932.

41. Yan J, Xia Q, Cherng SH, et al. Photo-induced DNA damage and photocytotoxicity of retinyl palmitate and its photodecomposition products. *Toxicol Ind Health.* 2005;21:167.

42. Burnett ME, Wang SQ. Current sunscreen controversies: A critical review. *Photodermatol Photoimmunol Photomed.* 2011;27:58.

43. Xia Q, Yin JJ, Wamer WG, et al. Photoirradiation of retinyl palmitate in ethanol with ultraviolet light – Formation of photodecomposition products, reactive oxygen species, and lipid peroxides. *Int J Environ Res Public Health.* 2006;3:185.

44. Wang SQ, Dusza SW, Lim HW. Safety of retinyl palmitate in sunscreens: A critical analysis. *J Am Acad Dermatol.* 2010;63:903.

45. Kim H, Koh J, Baek J, et al. Retinyl retinoate, a novel hybrid vitamin derivative, improves photoaged skin: A double-blind, randomized-controlled trial. *Skin Res Technol.* 2011;17:380.

46. Kim H, Kim N, Jung S, et al. Improvement in skin wrinkles from the use of photostable retinyl retinoate: A randomized controlled trial. *Br J Dermatol.* 2010;162:497.

47. Baumann L, Saghari S. Retinoids. In: Baumann L, Saghari S, Weisberg E, eds. *Cosmetic Dermatology: Principles and Practice.* 2nd ed. New York: McGraw-Hill; 2009:256–262.

48. Jick SS, Terris BZ, Jick H. First trimester topical tretinoin and congenital disorders. *Lancet.* 1993;341:1181.

49. Kligman LH, Gans EH. Re-emergence of topical retinol in dermatology. *J Dermatol Treat.* 2000;11:47.

50. Mukherjee S, Date A, Patravale V, et al. Retinoids in the treatment of skin aging: An overview of clinical efficacy and safety. *Clin Interv Aging.* 2006;1:327.

51. Ourique AF, Melero A, de Bona da Silva C, et al. Improved photostability and reduced skin permeation of tretinoin: Development of a semisolid nanomedicine. *Eur J Pharm Biopharm.* 2011;79:95.

52. Olsen EA, Katz HI, Levine N, et al. Sustained improvement in photodamaged skin with reduced tretinoin emollient cream treatment regimen: Effect of once-weekly and three-times-weekly applications. *J Am Acad Dermatol.* 1997;37:227.

53. Fisher GJ, Wang ZQ, Datta SC, et al. Pathophysiology of premature skin aging induced by ultraviolet light. *N Engl J Med.* 1997;337:1419.

54. Fisher GJ, Datta S, Wang Z, et al. c-Jun-dependent inhibition of cutaneous procollagen transcription following ultraviolet irradiation is reversed by all-trans retinoic acid. *J Clin Invest.* 2000;106:663.

55. Fisher GJ, Talwar HS, Lin J, et al. Molecular mechanisms of photoaging in human skin in vivo and their prevention by all-trans retinoic acid. *Photochem Photobiol.* 1999;69:154.

56. Singh M, Griffiths CE. The use of retinoids in the treatment of photoaging. *Dermatol Ther.* 2006;19:297.

57. Kikuchi K, Suetake T, Kumasaka N, et al. Improvement of photoaged facial skin in middle-aged Japanese females by topical retinol (vitamin A alcohol): A vehicle-controlled, double-blind study. *J Dermatolog Treat.* 2009;20:276.

58. Tierney EP, Hanke CW. Recent advances in combination treatments for photoaging: Review of the literature. *Dermatol Surg.* 2010;36:829.

Index

335